CONTENTS

KU-360-344

ACKNOWLEDGEMENTS		IV
ABOUT THE AUTHORS		VI
FOREWORD		VIII
INTRODUCTION – HOW TO USE THIS TEXTBOOK		IX
ARE YOU READY FOR WORK?		X
GENERIC:		
ANATOMY AND PHYSIOLOGY		1
LEGISLATION		91
201	**WORKING IN BEAUTY-RELATED INDUSTRIES**	114
202	**FOLLOW HEALTH AND SAFETY PRACTICE IN THE SALON**	141
203	**CLIENT CARE AND COMMUNICATION IN BEAUTY-RELATED INDUSTRIES**	165
205/213	**PROMOTE PRODUCTS AND SERVICES/ DISPLAY STOCK**	189
216	**SALON RECEPTION DUTIES**	237
SKIN CARE:		
204/224	**PROVIDE FACIAL SKIN CARE/FACIAL CARE FOR MEN**	261
HAIR REMOVAL:		
206/219	**REMOVE HAIR USING WAXING/ THREADING TECHNIQUES**	325
NAIL SERVICES:		
207/208	**PROVIDE MANICURE/PEDICURE TREATMENTS**	384
214	**PROVIDE AND MAINTAIN NAIL ENHANCEMENT**	439
215	**PROVIDE NAIL ART**	472
MAKE-UP:		
209/211/220	**MAKE-UP APPLICATION/INSTRUCTION**	496
212	**CREATE AN IMAGE BASED ON A THEME WITHIN THE HAIR AND BEAUTY SECTOR**	542
LASH AND BROW:		
210/218/225	**PROVIDE EYELASH AND EYEBROW SHAPING/ EYELASH PERMING/COLOURING TREATMENTS**	560
TEST YOUR KNOWLEDGE ANSWERS		601
INDEX		602

ACKNOWLEDGEMENTS

Thanks to all those who have given me time, advice and support during the writing of this book. Thanks in particular to my family: Howard, Connor, Alex and Hazel for their love and understanding. Lastly to my wonderful team at Hebe, in particular Hannah, Julie and Kathy.

Helen

I would like to say personal, heartfelt thanks to my mum for her constant support throughout my training and career. My son, Daniel, and partner, Ben, have kept me going during drafts and more drafts! My friend and colleague, Nicki, has provided unrivalled enthusiasm and help when piecing together parts of the book and contributing greatly to the photoshoot. Additionally, other work colleagues contributed hugely to the photoshoots that took place at Andover College – a big thank you to Emma, Carla and Amanda. Finally, a huge thank you to my mentor, Judith Ifold, who taught me during my formative years and inspired me to work in the industry as well as mentoring me when I first started teaching.

Kelly

City & Guilds would like to sincerely thank the following:

For invaluable beauty therapy expertise
Anita Crosland, Dee Gerrard, Marie Roberts, Marisol Martinez-Lees and Sarah Farrell.

For invaluable hairdressing expertise
Keryl Titmus, Diane Mitchell, Jacky Jones, Gail Brown and Elizabeth McNamara.

For their help with the cover photoshoot
Andrew Buckle (photography), Kate MacLellan (hairdressing), Kym Menzies-Foster (make-up), Models1 (model supply).

For their help with taking pictures
Kelly Rawlings at Andover College.

For contributing their photographs
Saks, Professional Beauty, Dove Spa, Jessica Nails, Sally Cosmetics, HIVE, Ellisons, Beauty Express, IPL, Ultrasonic, Krolan, Disney, Universal, Nail Delights, Decleor.

Picture credits
Every effort has been made to acknowledge all copyright holders as below and the publishers will, if notified, correct any errors in future editions.

Alamy: p94, p194, p219, p505, p533, p553; **Andover College:** p99, p100, p104, p106, p109, p111, p117, p118, p131, p133, p134, p146, p147, p162, p163, p170, p172, p173, p185, p224, p226, p227, p230, p231, p277, p279, p282, p283, p288, p289, p290, p291, p295, p296, p297, p298, p299, p300, p301, p302, p314, p327, p334, p351, p442,

I have worked in the beauty therapy industry since I left college – 28 years ago! During this time I have worked for several salons and have been a Qualification Consultant for City & Guilds for over 10 years. In the past I have also been an international examiner for CIBTAC – The Confederation of International Beauty Therapy and Cosmetology. For the last 8 years I have owned my own beauty and holistic therapies salon – somehow I still find the time to manage it too! I believe this helps me to continuously develop new skills and keep abreast of industry changes. I am passionate about adding new therapies to my skills each year. I also teach in higher education on a foundation degree in complementary therapies.

Reading the above makes me feel proud and amazed that I have achieved so much – it shows what a great industry beauty therapy is. If you are prepared to work hard in this industry there are opportunities to have a really fun and varied career.

Helen Beckmann

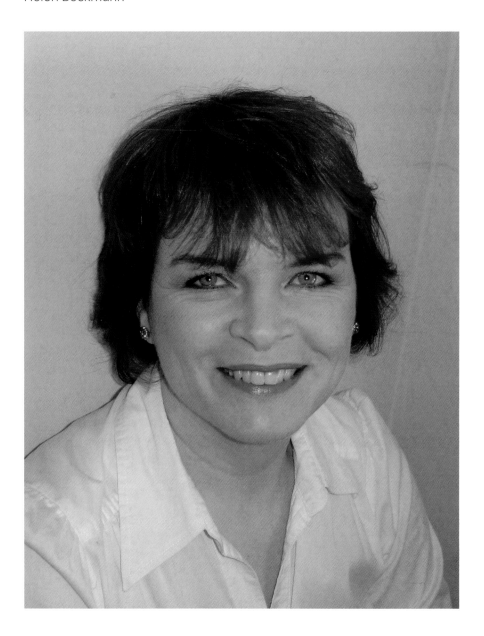

From an early age my interests and passion often included anything that involved styling. When I went to college there was only ever one choice of course to do. Three years later I had various hairdressing and beauty therapy qualifications, and soon decided I wanted my own business. I eventually moved into my own salon with three treatment rooms focusing largely on beauty treatments. I had a great 5 years in my salon, but then decided that I wanted to train young, aspiring therapists and applied for a job at a local college while working towards my teachers' qualification.

I have loved being able to combine teaching with beauty therapy. I have had the pleasure of watching my students progress into budding therapists, looking to make inroads into the industry. It is opening up these opportunities and showcasing the wonders of beauty therapy to others which led me to this book. I hope by reading this textbook and using it to develop your skills that you, like me, will discover a passion for the industry. Enjoy it and be creative!

Kelly Rawlings

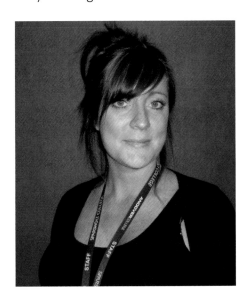

I have had a really varied career spanning 30 years of working in this fabulous industry, ranging from working in spas, health farms and salons to teaching for 15 years in the education market. During my time in education I have worked as a Qualification Consultant, Chief Examiner and Consultant for City & Guilds, as well as being a published author. I have had the pleasure of working with exceptional people and have been surprised by the opportunities that opened up to me after I gained my own beauty therapy qualifications.

This City & Guilds textbook brings beauty therapy alive, with visual step-by-steps, handy hints and industry tips, as well as valuable information based on the theory part of the qualification. Helen and Kelly are inspirational tutors and experts in their own right, which makes them ideal authors of this textbook.

The beauty industry is a diverse and exciting one, and whichever pathway you choose the work will be inspirational, challenging and exciting. What a wonderful industry to work in! I want to take this opportunity to wish all who are studying the City & Guilds Level 2 Beauty Therapy qualification the best of luck throughout their career.

Anita Crosland
Beauty Therapy Portfolio Manager, City & Guilds

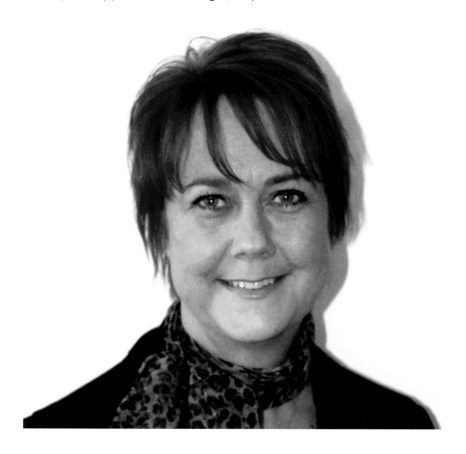

INTRODUCTION – HOW TO USE THIS TEXTBOOK

You will find that your City & Guilds VRQ Level 2 Beauty Therapy textbook is laid out in the same way as your City & Guilds VRQ Level 2 Beauty Therapy logbook to aid your navigation and understanding of both.

Each chapter in your textbook covers everything you will need to understand in order to complete your written or online tests and practical assessments.

The chapters in your logbook and in this textbook are divided into colour-coded sections as follows: 'generic', 'skin care', 'hair removal', 'nail services', 'make-up', 'lash and brow' and 'hair services'.

Throughout this textbook you will see the following features:

HANDY HINTS

Toner is also available as a spray which is ideal for male clients as it eliminates the risk of getting cotton wool caught in facial hair. It is also more cost-effective to use toner in a spray format.

Handy hints are particularly useful tips that can assist you in your revision or help you remember something important.

Strip lashes

Very dramatic artificial lashes that are applied to the length of the eye.

Words in bold in the text are explained in the margin to aid your understanding.

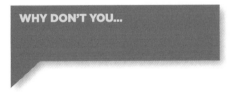

WHY DON'T YOU...

Why don't you – These hints suggest activities for you to try to help you practise and learn.

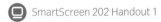

ACTIVITY

Activities – The activities help to test your understanding and learn from your colleagues' experiences.

⊙ SmartScreen 202 Handout 1

SmartScreen – These icons refer to the City & Guilds SmartScreen resources and activities. Ask your tutor for your log-in details.

At the end of each chapter are some 'Test your knowledge' questions. These are multiple choice questions, designed to prepare you for your written or online tests and to identify any areas where you might need further training or revision.

ARE YOU READY FOR WORK?

Sara Wilce has been a therapist for a number of years and has had an amazing career. Read her story below and learn from her career advice!

SARA WILCE

I have been a therapist for a number of years and have been fortunate enough to have had an amazing career. Gone are the days when the only options open to therapists were a job in the local salon, a beauty counter in a department store or as a TV make-up artist. Today the sky really is the limit!

There are opportunities to be found in salons, spas, on cruise liners, private jets, private yachts, health farms, holiday centres, television, with photographic or theatre and film make-up…the list is endless. A Government recognised qualification, such as a VRQ, can take you all over the world – I have worked in England, Hong Kong, South Africa, Morocco, Majorca, and even on Richard Branson's island, Necker, in the British Virgin Islands! I have owned my own salon, been a college lecturer, managed the in-flight beauty therapy service for a large airline and set up and run spas. I have also helped to develop a skin care range!

My current position finds me working for ARK Age Aware skin care in Putney, South West London – a fast-growing company that has three salons and, uniquely, their own product range based on skin age rather than skin type. My role has been to plan and set up a training academy for them to make sure all the therapists are highly skilled at what they do, to deliver training to those salons that take on our product range and to offer a range of courses to anyone who wants to learn to be a therapist or just develop their skills. I also deal with all the recruitment for the salons.

Having worked and recruited for what is probably the biggest employer of beauty therapists in this country, I think I know what I am talking about when it comes to the dos and don'ts of applying for a job, something you will probably all need to do at some time in your career! So …………

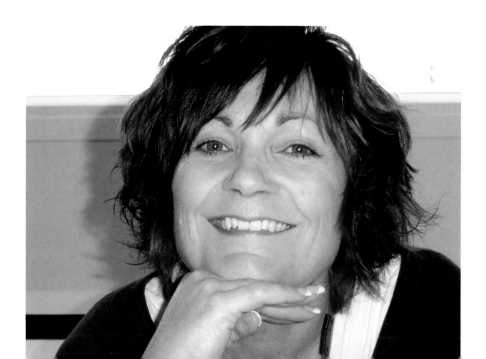

JOB ADVERTISEMENT – WHAT TO LOOK FOR

When you are replying to an advertisement, read it through carefully first. What is the employer looking for? What will they need you to do? What qualifications do they want? Make sure that the experience you have on your CV matches some of the key words/sentences in the advert. Below is an example with the key terms in bold.

Here at Ark Health and Beauty we are renowned for our unique approach to skin care and our philosophy of **encouraging our clients' own natural health and beauty**. As a company we are committed to maintaining professional treatment standards and ensuring the **highest level of customer service**.

We are at the beginning of a strong period of growth and are therefore looking for **experienced beauty therapists** for three sites in Fulham, Putney and Wimbledon. You will need a **passion** for your trade and should possess the desire to build a business based on honesty, high-quality products and exceptional customer service, all within a unique **team environment**.

You must possess VRQ Level 3 or equivalent beauty therapy qualifications.

You also need to be **articulate, well-presented and really want to make a difference**.

This advert is telling you that we believe in natural products, we expect outstanding customer service, we are looking for therapists (not apprentices or students on work experience), we want people who are passionate about beauty and we want people who can work as a team. Now all you have to do is make sure your CV shows that you are that person!

HOW TO WRITE A CV

BASIC RULES

- Spelling: check the spelling, then check again, then check once more, then use your spell check and lastly get someone else to check! I will often discard CVs that contain bad spelling errors – if you cannot be bothered to make sure your spelling and punctuation are correct then you might not be bothered to make sure my customers are happy!

- Use straightforward language – no lengthy paragraphs or long, complicated words. But make sure what you are saying makes sense! And write it yourself – get help if you need it but make sure that the language you use is how you would speak; an interviewer will soon work out that you do not understand what you have said!

- Do not lie; you will gain nothing and will get found out! Highlight your strengths and do not be afraid to mention weaknesses, but show that you are willing to work at improving/developing them.

- Email address: keep the fun, funky addresses for your personal emails; make sure you have a plain, more serious one for job applications. You will not come across as professional if the email address the employer sees is something like 'prettyfluffyprincess@…'!

- Make sure your CV is no more than two pages long and put the most important information about you first – interviewers get a lot of CVs and they need to see at a glance that you have the basic skills that they are looking for, not what hobbies you have.

- Try to keep it as concise as possible but include all the relevant information. Think to yourself – what do they need to know about me and my experience in order for them to think I am able to do this job?

LAYOUT

There are many ways to set out your CV. I think this is a good one:

Name

Address and contact numbers plus email address

Personal profile

Tell them a bit about yourself, what your strengths are, eg 'An enthusiastic beauty therapist with good communication and organisational skills'.

Tell them what you think your experience will enable you to do.

Talk about ways of working, eg 'I am able to work effectively and unsupervised both as an individual and as part of a team'.

Professional qualifications

List your main qualifications, eg VRQ Level 2.

List any extra training you have done, eg Caflon Professional Ear Piercing, Introductory Skin by Sterex Course.

List membership of any professional organisations, eg BABTAC/FHT.

Relevant work experience and work history

Give the company name and the dates you were there.

Give the title of the role.

List your key responsibilities or achievements.

For example:

Ark Age Aware Skincare
April 2012
Beauty Therapist

Key accountabilities:
- Deliver an exceptionally high-class customer service experience, treating clients using the ARK service and treatment techniques, providing beauty treatments to the highest standard.
- Work as part of a team to establish a professional and profit-making salon business.
- Involved in 'launch events' for new products.
- Consistently meet set retail targets.
- Take accurate appointment details using a computerised system.

Other qualifications

List GCSEs and grades.

Include anything that highlights your strengths as a person, such as first-aid certificates, Duke of Edinburgh award (proves you can work as part of a team), key skills qualifications.

Personal details

Date of birth, full driving licence held? Smoker or non-smoker?

This information is not essential (unless you are applying for a sales position, when you will need a driving licence!) and no employer can make you give it. However, it does help a potential employer to build up a picture of you.

You do not need to add references at this stage, just say that they can be arranged if required. You also do not need to go into your hobbies unless you do something that directly relates to your role as a therapist, ie 'I like doing make-up for my friends'.

HOW TO WRITE A COVERING LETTER

In order to give yourself another chance to tell the employer about your strengths and how they match what the employer is looking for, always write a covering letter to go with every application and change it slightly with every application – make a direct link to the advert.

It should state which job role you are applying for and highlight some of the things you have done or achieved that again match the job profile in the advertisement, but keep it short and concise!

Your address

Date

Address of company

Dear ....

APPLICATION FOR POST OF ....

In response to the post advertised on .... please find enclosed/attached a copy of my CV.

Say what you have been doing: 'I have been training/working as a therapist for the past .... I am now looking for a new and exciting challenge where I can use my experience.'

Tell them what you can offer – make sure this picks up on some of the key words in the advert: 'I feel that I could be the right person to ....'

Tell them how much you would like to work for their company.

Give them some contact information in case they want to get in touch and sign off appropriately.

HOW TO PRESENT YOURSELF AT INTERVIEW

The above advertisement example also tells you that how you present yourself will be important! To make sure you make the best of impressions, follow the rules below:

1 **Dress to impress!** That means SMART; jeans and leggings are a definite NO!
   - Make sure that what you wear is clean, tidy, ironed and suitable – no really short skirts or low-cut tops!

- If long, make sure your hair is tied back and secured neatly away from your face – employers will want to see that you understand that this is how you will need to look and that you can achieve that look. Make sure it is clean and well-brushed.
- Wear a light day make-up and make sure nails are short, clean, well-manicured and free of nail varnish or coloured gels.
- Look as if you care and have really made an effort – you are representing the beauty industry so look the part!

If you look good, then employers will feel confident that you will represent their salon well and will also make the clients look good!

2 **Research!** Show you have researched the company – look it up on the Internet and try and remember some key facts about them.
- Try and visit the salon and get an idea about what treatments it offers – ask for a price list.
- Find out what products the salons use and see if you can find out a bit about them.

All these things will show the employer that you are really interested in working for the them.

3 **Listen!** Make sure you listen carefully to the questions you are being asked so that you can be sure you are giving the appropriate answer. If you are not sure what the interviewer means, ask them to explain. Never worry about taking your time to answer, interviewers like to see people thinking!

4 **Speak clearly!** Do not talk too fast, do not mumble, do not use slang words and most importantly – DO NOT SWEAR!

INTERVIEW QUESTIONS – TIPS FOR HOW TO ANSWER AND QUESTIONS TO ASK – OR NOT ASK!

Remember, interviews are for the employer to find out about you, the person you are and what you can do. They want to know that you can 'do the job' but that you will also fit in well with the rest of the team. Most importantly, they are not there to 'trip you up'; there is often no right or wrong answer to a question, it will just be your thoughts or ideas they are looking for.

GENERAL, WARMING-UP QUESTIONS

All employers recognise how nerve wracking an interview can be and will do their best to get you to relax and put you at ease. They will do this by asking general questions, such as:
- Why did you choose to become a beauty therapist?
- What is your favourite treatment?
- Where do you want to be in 5 years' time?
- What are your goals?

COMPANY-SPECIFIC QUESTIONS

They will then want to see how much research you have done into the company; they want to see how much you want the role, how important it is to you, how much effort you are prepared to make to get it. They will ask questions, such as:

- Why are you interested in this role?
- What do you know about ARK?
- Do you have any experience of working to targets? (Retail is very important in salons; today it is a crucial part of their income.)

COMPETENCY QUESTIONS

Employers will often use this type of question when they want to know about your past experience and how you deal with certain situations that you might come across in the role. Typical questions are:

Can you tell me about a time when you feel you have received poor customer service? What was it that made it poor? How did it make you feel?

Can you tell me about a time when you have gone 'above and beyond' for a customer?

Can you tell me about a time when you have had to deal with a difficult situation involving a customer?

For each question like this, answer as if you are telling a story, although try to keep it short! Tell the interviewer what happened and what you did/how you felt.

Interviews are also about you finding out if the company/job role is the right one for you, so do not be afraid to ask questions. However, bear in mind the following rules:

Do ask about:

- the salon – how many people work there, what treatments they offer (if you have not been able to find out)
- the working hours – you need to make sure these will be suitable for you. Take any travelling time into account
- the uniform – find out whether there is a set uniform and whether that is provided.

Do not ask about:

- money – that can come later if the employer invites you back for a second interview or trade test
- holidays – you want to be seen to be keen to work!
- whether you get paid for being sick – this will look as if you are already planning how you can get time off!

It might sound really daunting, but a little pre-preparation will give you the best chance of success and set you off on your chosen path. Good luck with it, and I really hope that you reach you goals. Remember – go to bed with a dream and wake up with a purpose!

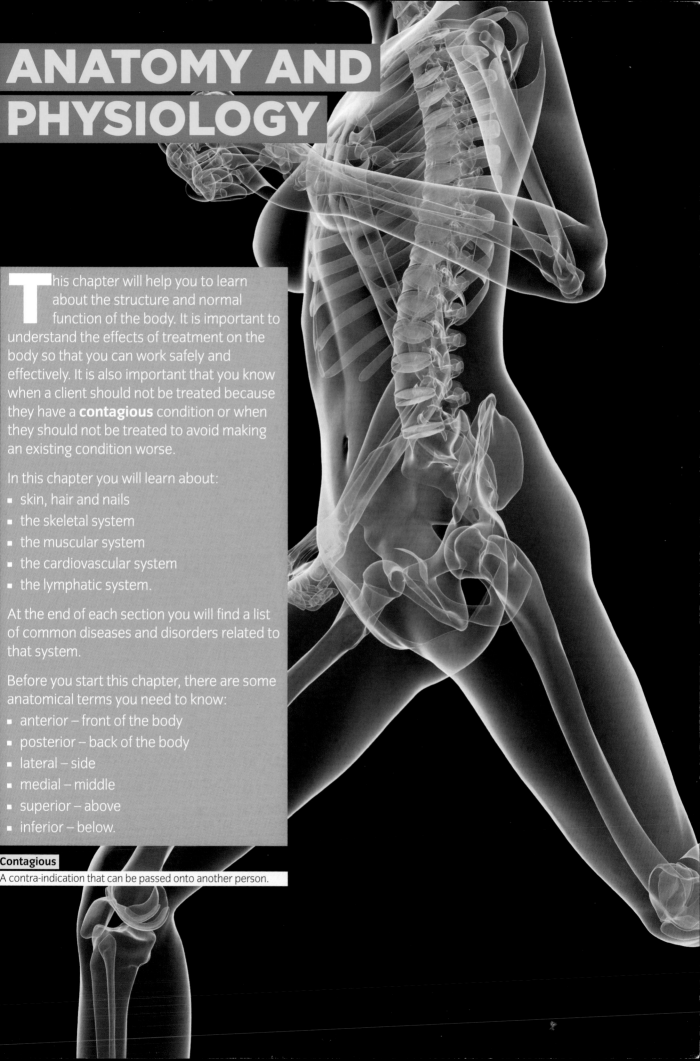

ANATOMY AND PHYSIOLOGY

This chapter will help you to learn about the structure and normal function of the body. It is important to understand the effects of treatment on the body so that you can work safely and effectively. It is also important that you know when a client should not be treated because they have a **contagious** condition or when they should not be treated to avoid making an existing condition worse.

In this chapter you will learn about:

- skin, hair and nails
- the skeletal system
- the muscular system
- the cardiovascular system
- the lymphatic system.

At the end of each section you will find a list of common diseases and disorders related to that system.

Before you start this chapter, there are some anatomical terms you need to know:

- anterior – front of the body
- posterior – back of the body
- lateral – side
- medial – middle
- superior – above
- inferior – below.

Contagious
A contra-indication that can be passed onto another person.

SKIN

The skin is the body's largest organ. The skin's condition is subject to constant change and can therefore reflect the general health of an individual.

In this part of the chapter you will learn about:

- the normal structure of the skin
- the functions of the skin
- the **characteristics** of the skin
- skin tones, types and conditions
- common skin diseases and disorders.

Characteristics
Qualities or features of a product, service or treatment.

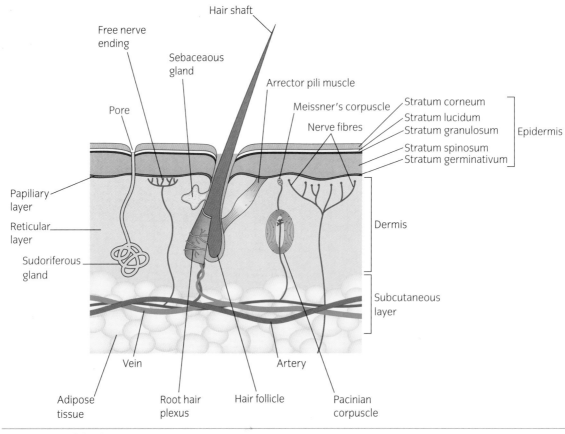

Cross-section of the skin

NORMAL STRUCTURE OF THE SKIN

The skin has three distinct layers:

- epidermis
- dermis
- hypodermis or subcutaneous.

The surface of the skin is covered by an acid mantle, which is a water in oil **emulsion** formed from a mixture of sweat and sebum. It makes the skin's surface slightly acidic. It is also covered with mineral and organic **substances**, such as **urea**, lactic acid and **amino acids**.

Emulsion
A creamy liquid.

Substance
A chemical.

Urea
A chemical found in urine.

Amino acids
The building blocks of protein. When you break protein down you are left with amino acids.

> **INDUSTRY TIP**
>
> The skin, hair and nails are part of the integumentary system.

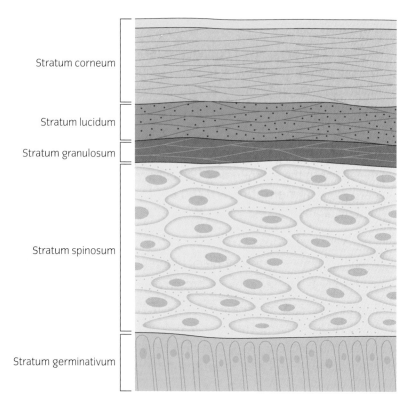

Stratum corneum

Stratum lucidum

Stratum granulosum

Stratum spinosum

Stratum germinativum

EPIDERMIS

The epidermis has five layers which are formed of sheets of **cells**. These five layers are called:

1 stratum corneum (horny layer)

2 stratum lucidum (clear layer)

3 stratum granulosum (granular layer)

4 stratum spinosum (prickle cell layer)

5 stratum germinativum (basal layer).

The skin cells in the epidermis move upwards from the stratum germinativum (where they are produced) to the stratum corneum (where they die). This process takes on average between 24 and 42 days. As we get older this process takes longer.

The average thickness of the epidermis is 0.12 mm. It is thickest on the soles of the feet (1.5 mm) and thinnest on the eyelids (0.05 mm).

There are several different types of cells in the epidermis.

Cells
The building blocks of the human body. Cells are **microscopic** and have a slightly different structure and shape depending on their location and activity in the body. Our body is always renewing cells to replace worn out cells.

Microscopic
Something that can only be seen by looking through a microscope.

Cell name	Function
Keratinocytes 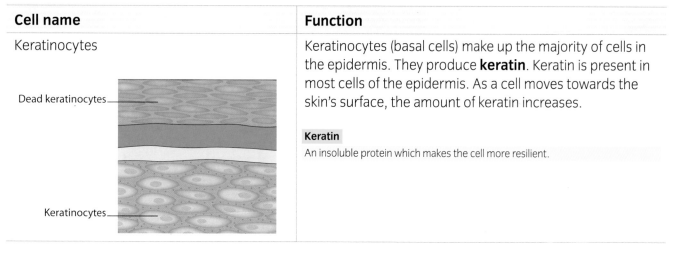	Keratinocytes (basal cells) make up the majority of cells in the epidermis. They produce **keratin**. Keratin is present in most cells of the epidermis. As a cell moves towards the skin's surface, the amount of keratin increases. **Keratin** An insoluble protein which makes the cell more resilient.

Cell name	Function
Melanocytes 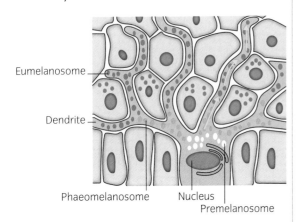 Eumelanosome Dendrite Phaeomelanosome — Nucleus — Premelanosome	Melanocytes are cells of connective tissue. They produce the pigment **melanin** which gives colour to the skin and hair. Tyrosine (an amino acid) causes a series of chemical reactions in the melanocytes to produce melanin. Melanin granules are formed in the melanocytes which pass along finger-like **projections** called dendrites that inject melanin into the surrounding skin cells. When dendrites are damaged **pigmentation** is distributed unevenly causing patchy pigmentation. There are two types of melanin: ▪ eumelanin – a brown or black pigment ▪ pheomelanin – a yellow or brown pigment.
Langerhans cells 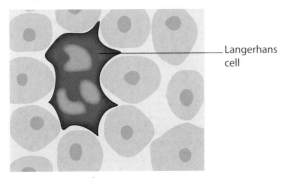 Langerhans cell **Macrophage** Small white cells of the immune system which move through tissues and remove cell debris and pathogens.	Langerhans cells are specialised white blood cells which circulate in the skin. They move around by squeezing through the connective tissue. They are a type of **macrophage** and alert the **immune system**'s **pathogens** in the skin. They also affect the skin's reaction to infection and **inflammation**. **Immune system** The system which protects the body from micro-organisms. **Pathogen** A collective term used to describe a type of microbe. It includes viruses, bacteria, fungi and parasites. A pathogen has the potential to cause harm. **Inflammation** Swelling and tenderness.

Melanin
Substance that determines the skin's natural colour. For example, someone who is fair-skinned will have a lot less melanin in their skin than someone who is dark-skinned.

Projection
A part that sticks out.

Pigmentation
The colouration of tissues by pigment. This is what gives skin and hair its colour.

Soluble
Able to dissolve.

Lipids
A group of organic molecules that don't like water. They include fats, oils, waxes and fat soluble vitamins.

Ceramides
Natural lipids (fats) that help the skin stay hydrated.

Stratum corneum (horny layer)

This is the uppermost layer of the epidermis. Its surface is in direct contact with the environment. The dead cells are hard and flat. They do not have a nucleus. Dead skin cells shed continually. About 90 per cent of household dust is made up of dead skin cells. The thickness of the stratum corneum varies with age – it gets thicker as we grow older. This thickening makes the signs of ageing more obvious.

One function of the stratum corneum is to stop the skin dehydrating. This is achieved by the natural moisturising factor (NMF), which is a collection of water **soluble** substances that absorb water from the air and combine it with their own water content. This allows the stratum corneum to remain hydrated despite exposure to the environment.

Lipids (eg **ceramides**, cholesterol and fatty acids (sebum)) also help to control water loss and prevent the entry of water soluble agents and harmful bacteria by providing a waterproof layer on the skin's surface. Lipids also keep the skin supple, preventing it from cracking and breaking which would allow pathogens to enter the skin and could cause an infection.

Stratum lucidum (clear layer)

This layer has flat transparent cells, hence the name clear layer. There is no melanin present. The stratum lucidum forms a waterproof barrier.

Stratum granulosum (granular layer)

The cells take on a distinctive flattened shape and a granular appearance as a result of **keratinisation**. As the cells lose their **nuclei** the cell functions begin to decrease dramatically.

Stratum spinosum (prickle cell layer)

This layer includes Langerhans cells which help to support our immune system. Keratin production begins in this layer and is injected into the cells. The stratum spinosum is several layers deep. The cells have connection threads called fibrils which give the cells a prickly appearance.

Stratum germinativum (basal layer)

This is the deepest layer of the epidermis. Skin cells are produced here by a process called **cell mitosis**, which produces new **epithelium** cells. One cell remains in the stratum germinativum and continues to reproduce while the other migrates through the layers to the stratum corneum.

The stratum germinativium also contains keratinocytes and melanocytes. The melanocytes help to protect the skin against harmful UV rays. Eighty per cent of the moisture required for maintaining healthy skin is found in this layer.

DERMIS

The dermis is the layer of skin that lies below the epidermis. It is a 3–5 mm thick layer of extra-cellular tissue. The dermis has a high water content. It contains most of the living structures of the skin including blood vessels, sweat glands and sebaceous glands.

The main functions of the dermis are:
- to provide strength and flexibility
- to provide a system of capillaries to nourish the cells of the lower layers of the epidermis and to remove waste products
- to control temperature and blood pressure.

The dermis has two layers:
1 papillary layer
2 reticular layer.

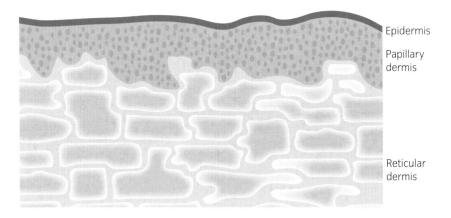

Epidermis

Papillary dermis

Reticular dermis

Papillary layer

The papillary layer is made up of loose connective tissue. The surface of the papillary layer is covered with tiny, irregularly shaped projections called dermal papillae. These fit into the underside of the epidermis

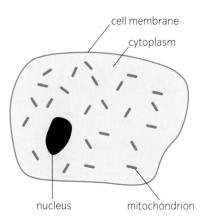

cell membrane

cytoplasm

nucleus

mitochondrion

Granular
Microscopic particles.

Keratinisation
The process by which living cells change into hard, flat, dead cells. It is caused by the production of a protein called keratin and the **degeneration** of the nucleus.

Degeneration
Fallen below normal amounts.

Nucleus
Singular of nuclei. The part of the cell that contains the **genetic** structure. The nucleus is the control centre of the cell.

Genetic
Relating to genes.

Cell mitosis
A method of cellular division that produces two daughter cells each with exactly the same genetic make-up as the parent cell.

Epithelium
Type of tissue found covering the body, lining cavities, hollow organs and tubes.

forming a secure bond (eg like Velcro). They contain intricate networks of blood and lymphatic capillaries and nerve endings. These networks nourish the lower layers of the epidermis and hair follicles, carry oxygen to the tissues and remove waste from the tissues.

Reticular layer
This is made up of thick tough **fibrous** connective tissue which helps to hold and support the dermis. It connects the dermis to the hypodermis.

CELLS OF THE DERMIS
The main cells of the dermis are fibroblasts, mast cells and phagocytic cells.

Fibroblasts/fibre cells
Fibroblasts are important for tissue repair following tissue damage. Fibroblasts produce two important proteins – collagen and elastin. The production of collagen and elastin slows down as we age causing wrinkles and a loss of skin tone.

Collagen
Collagen fibres provide strength and elasticity. These wavy white fibres form a network and hold bodily tissues, such as skin, bone and muscles together. The wave allows the fibres' length to be **extended**, and the fibres to run in a specific direction, following the contours of the body. Collagen makes up 75 per cent of the skin's weight.

Elastin
Elastin holds collagen in place and forms an organised network of elastic fibre cells in the dermis. Elastin is a very stretchy yellow fibre. Just like an elastic band, elastin can stretch and return back to its original shape. However, if the skin is overstretched the elastin fibres will break, causing stretch marks. Elastin accounts for 5 per cent of the body's weight.

Fibrous
Containing fibres.

Extend
Reaches down or into.

> **INDUSTRY TIP**
> Skin is looser around the joints to allow movement without damaging the skin.

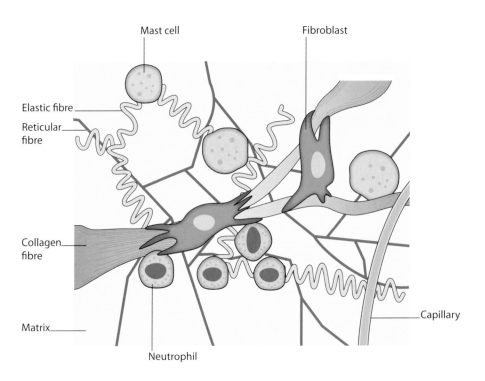

Mast cell · Fibroblast · Elastic fibre · Reticular fibre · Collagen fibre · Matrix · Neutrophil · Capillary

Mast cells

Mast cells release **histamine** in response to damage to local tissues caused by **micro-organisms**. Histamine causes the blood vessels to leak so that the immune system has better access to the damaged tissues and can fight the micro-organisms. White blood cells are also attracted to histamine, drawing them to the damaged tissue.

Phagocytic cells

Phagocytic cells are white blood cells which move through the skin's tissues destroying pathogens and other cell debris.

Hyaluronic acid

Hyaluronic acid is a naturally occurring substance found in the **extra-cellular matrix** of the dermis. It helps to keep the skin hydrated. It is able to attract and hold water up to 1000 times its weight. It plays a **crucial** role in skin repair by supporting the formation of collagen and elastin. As we age the skin produces less hyaluronic acid and contributes to the appearance of ageing.

Sensory nerve endings

The skin is packed with sensory nerve endings which relay information about **tactile** sensation to the brain. Different nerve receptors respond to different sensations.

Nerve receptor	Sensation
Meissner's corpuscles	Movement and light touch
Ruffini corpuscles	Skin stretching and temperature
Pacinian corpuscles	Pressure and vibration
Krause corpuscles	Cold
Free nerve endings	Pain, touch and temperature

Histamine

A substance produced in the body in response to an allergic reaction.

Micro-organism

A very small living thing that can only be seen through a microscope.

INDUSTRY TIP

The direction of collagen fibres can be determined by pinching the skin and seeing which way it folds most easily into wrinkles.

Extra-cellular matrix

A substance outside the cells that contains non-living tissue (eg fibres) which supports the surrounding cells.

Crucial

Really needed, vital.

INDUSTRY TIP

Hyaluronic acid is found as an ingredient in skin care products to help maintain skin **hydration**.

Hydration

Combining with water.

Tactile

To touch and feel.

INDUSTRY TIP

The most sensitive skin is on your lips.

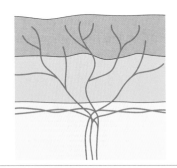

Free nerve endings

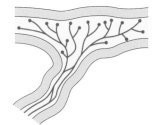

Ruffini corpuscle

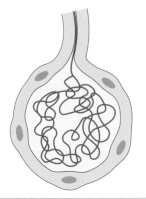

Krause corpuscle

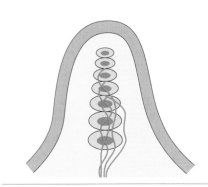

Meissner's corpuscle

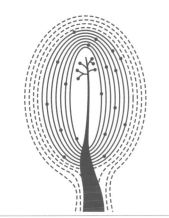

Pacinian corpuscle

Vasodilation

When the muscles relax in the wall of the blood vessels, the blood vessels dilate and allow blood to flow more freely.

Vasoconstriction

When the muscles contract in the wall of the blood vessels, the blood vessels constrict (shrink in size) and restrict blood flow.

Nutrients

Substances that help us grow.

> **HANDY HINTS**
>
> See the section on the lymphatic system on pages 82–88 for more detail.

Regulate

Controlling or maintaining.

Eliminate

Getting rid of something

Excrete

To eliminate waste, eg sweat, from the skin.

Secrete

To release a substance from a cell or gland.

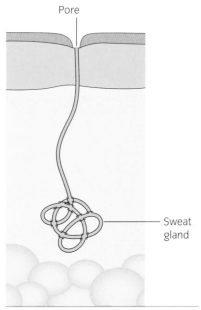

Cross-section of a sweat gland

Emollient

Something that has a softening effect.

Comedones

Blackheads.

Papule

A small raised solid area of infected unbroken skin that often develops into a pustule.

Pustule

A small collection of pus that is visible through a raised portion of the epidermis.

Blood vessels

The dermis contains a rich, delicate network of blood vessels. The small blood vessels in the outer areas of the skin are known as the micro-circulation and are prone to **vasodilation** and **vasoconstriction**. The circulation of blood brings oxygen and **nutrients** to the dermis, the hair follicle and the epidermis and removes the waste products made during cellular activity.

Lymphatic vessels

A network of lymphatic capillaries nourish the cells in the dermis. These vessels allow lymphatic fluid to leave and move around the network of cells as tissue fluid. Tissue fluid moves back into the lymphatic vessels to take with it waste from the extra-cellular tissues.

Sweat glands

The two main purposes of sweat glands are:

1 to help **regulate** the temperature of the body

2 to help **eliminate** waste.

Sweat cools down the body by removing heat from the skin's surface. It helps to maintain hydration of the skin's surface. Sweat is **excreted** as a clear watery fluid. It takes away waste substances, eg water, sodium and potassium chloride (salts), ammonia and urea. There are two types of sweat glands:

1 apocrine glands

2 eccrine glands.

Apocrine glands

Apocrine glands are found under the arms and around the groin. Most apocrine glands open into hair follicles.

Eccrine glands

Eccrine glands are found all over the body. Eccrine sweat is formed when sodium is **secreted** into the base of a sweat gland. The sodium attracts water from the surrounding tissues and is excreted onto the surface of the skin. Sweat from eccrine glands also contains urea.

Sebaceous glands

Sebaceous glands can be found all over the skin, except on the palms of the hands and soles of the feet. Most sebaceous glands open into hair follicles where they secrete sebum but some open directly onto the skin. Sebaceous glands produce sebum (a lipid). Sebum is the skin's natural **emollient** and prevents the skin from drying out. It forms a barrier to keep moisture in. Sebum helps to prevent the growth of bacteria as long as the sebum does not become excessive. Too much sebum will cause the skin to become oily and look shiny particularly around the nose, chin and forehead. Very oily skin attracts surface dirt and the pores might become blocked causing **comedones**, **papules** and **pustules**.

Arrector pili muscle

These are tiny muscle fibres that are attached to the hair follicle. When they contract they pull the hair up and away from the skin. These muscles cause goosebumps when we are cold or frightened. The raised hairs trap air and help to keep the skin warm.

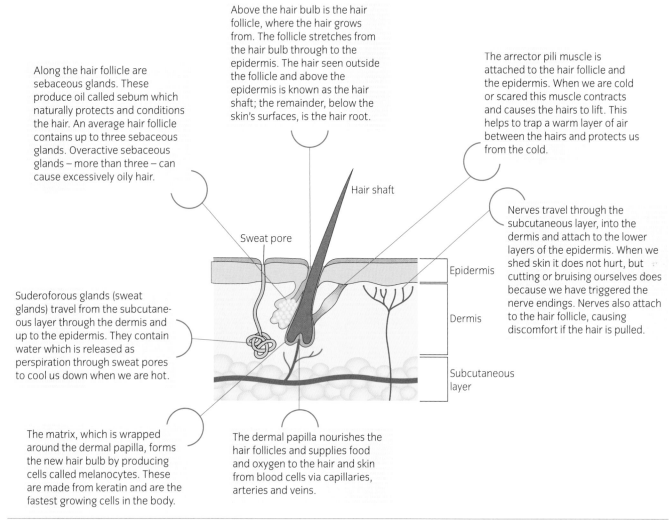

Along the hair follicle are sebaceous glands. These produce oil called sebum which naturally protects and conditions the hair. An average hair follicle contains up to three sebaceous glands. Overactive sebaceous glands – more than three – can cause excessively oily hair.

Above the hair bulb is the hair follicle, where the hair grows from. The follicle stretches from the hair bulb through to the epidermis. The hair seen outside the follicle and above the epidermis is known as the hair shaft; the remainder, below the skin's surfaces, is the hair root.

The arrector pili muscle is attached to the hair follicle and the epidermis. When we are cold or scared this muscle contracts and causes the hairs to lift. This helps to trap a warm layer of air between the hairs and protects us from the cold.

Nerves travel through the subcutaneous layer, into the dermis and attach to the lower layers of the epidermis. When we shed skin it does not hurt, but cutting or bruising ourselves does because we have triggered the nerve endings. Nerves also attach to the hair follicle, causing discomfort if the hair is pulled.

Suderoforous glands (sweat glands) travel from the subcutaneous layer through the dermis and up to the epidermis. They contain water which is released as perspiration through sweat pores to cool us down when we are hot.

The matrix, which is wrapped around the dermal papilla, forms the new hair bulb by producing cells called melanocytes. These are made from keratin and are the fastest growing cells in the body.

The dermal papilla nourishes the hair follicles and supplies food and oxygen to the hair and skin from blood cells via capillaries, arteries and veins.

Hair shaft

Sweat pore

Epidermis

Dermis

Subcutaneous layer

The sebaceous gland

HYPODERMIS (SUBCUTANEOUS LAYER)

The subcutaneous layer is a layer of fat cells located beneath the dermis. It provides some cushioning from external pressure and some thermal **insulation**. It varies in thickness depending on a person's gender and the area of the body.

Insulation
Reduces heat loss.

FUNCTIONS OF THE SKIN

The skin has seven functions:

1 sensation
2 temperature regulation
3 absorption
4 protection
5 excretion
6 secretion
7 production of vitamin D.

SENSATION

The skin contains approximately 5 million tiny sensory cells which enable us to respond to sensations that are applied to the surface of the skin, eg touch, pressure and vibration. These cells respond to environmental changes and send information to the brain where the sensation is perceived. Sensory nerve endings are mainly located in the dermis but some free nerves end in the epidermis.

TEMPERATURE REGULATION

The body needs to be maintained at a constant temperature of about 36.8°C to help it to function properly. The skin responds to an increase in temperature by dilating the blood vessels in the dermis (vasodilation) to radiate heat away from the skin where it is **exposed**. The skin also begins to sweat. As sweat **evaporates** it helps to cool the body. At room temperature water evaporation from the skin's surface can account for up to 15 per cent of heat loss.

Exposed

Open to the elements.

Evaporate

To disappear or vanish.

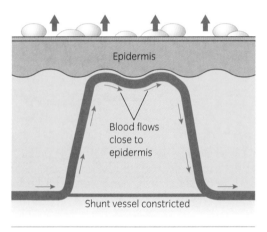

Vasodilation

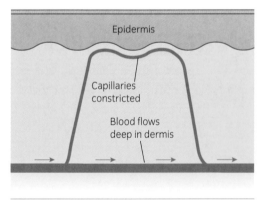

Vasoconstriction

Essential

Extremely important.

Limited

Restricted in size or amount.

If the body gets too cold the blood vessels constrict (vasoconstriction) to keep heat nearer to the **essential** organs of the body. Shivering makes the muscles contract and produces additional heat. Heat loss is affected by the environment and the amount and type of clothing worn.

ABSORPTION

The skin is not totally waterproof. It allows certain substances through, eg hormones, in a **limited** capacity. Substances that can enter the skin do so:

- between the cells of the epidermis
- through sweat glands
- through hair shafts.

PROTECTION

The skin forms a water resistant seal over the body. It is very hard-wearing and acts as a defence against chemicals, micro-organisms, dehydration and damage. Sebum, water and other substances are secreted onto the skin to keep it waterproof, supple and flexible. The surface of skin is slightly acidic (pH4.5–5.5), which prevents harmful bacteria growing. Melanin acts as a chemical **filter** absorbing and reflecting UV **radiation**.

The subcutaneous layer cushions the **underlying** bone structure and organs to help prevent damage from external forces and pressure. The hypodermis and dermis act together to protect the body against temperature changes.

EXCRETION

The skin is a minor excretory organ. It excretes sweat which contains water, sodium and potassium chloride (salts), urea and uric acids and an **aromatic** substance that gives the skin its personal odour. If we do not wash our skin and clothes regularly we will start to smell because bacteria break down the sweat and cause unpleasant odours.

SECRETION

Sebum is secreted into the hair follicles and onto the skin. Sebum is an oily substance that keeps the hair and skin soft, supple and flexible. It can also give the skin and hair a shiny appearance. Sebum contains **antibacterial** substances to prevent the growth of harmful micro-organisms on the skin's surface.

PRODUCTION OF VITAMIN D

Vitamin D is produced in the skin as a response to exposure to UVB radiation. **Cholecalciferol** is produced when the sun **penetrates** the skin. Cholecalciferol is taken to the liver where it is made into calcidol and stored as vitamin D.

If you block UVB you block the production of vitamin D. Dark skin needs more exposure to UVB to produce the same amount of vitamin D as light skin as melanin restricts the absorption of UVB.

SKIN REPAIR AND SCAR TISSUE

Although the body is able to repair tissue damage there is always some scar tissue.

When the skin is broken, blood cells move into the wound and the blood clotting process starts. A protein in the blood plasma called fibrinogen is released and this starts to form a mesh over the surface. This mesh prevents further blood leaking out. The mesh dries out to form a scab.

Filter
Method of allowing some but not all substances through.

Radiation
A process in which particles or waves travel through space, eg the heat from an infra red lamp.

Underlying
Found under something.

Aromatic
Fragrant smell or perfume.

Antibacterial
A substance that prevents the growth of bacteria.

Cholecalciferol
A form of vitamin D.

Penetrate
When something, eg a substance, enters into another thing.

 SmartScreen 210 Worksheet 6

INDUSTRY TIP

We all need to go outside into the sunlight for 20 minutes each day to make sure we produce enough vitamin D. This does not mean sunbathing but general exposure.

INDUSTRY TIP

The skin repairs and renews itself three times faster at night so it is important to get a good night's sleep. Specialised products to help repair the skin should be used at night.

Histamine is released to make the blood vessels dilate. Vasodilation allows blood cells to leak out from the blood vessels to help in the healing process. The cells can also attack unwanted micro-organisms that might have entered through the open wound. The increased circulation gives the area an inflamed red appearance.

Fibroblast cells begin to produce new collagen cells and a protein called actin. Actin helps to slowly draw the edges of the wound together as it is able to contract. It takes the epidermis about 48 hours to heal but the deeper tissues take much longer and the area might look red for 2–4 weeks. Some very deep damage might take even longer to fully repair. Working over scar tissue is **contra-indicated** as the healing process could be on-going even though the epidermis has healed.

Contra-indicated

A reason why a treatment cannot be carried out. This might be that the treatment should be adapted or restricted, or it might be an absolute contra-indication in that the treatment cannot be carried out at all (prevented).

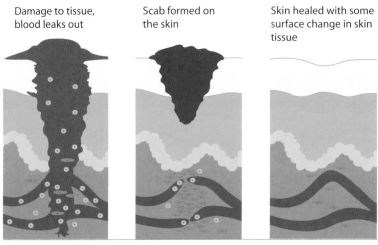

Damage to tissue, blood leaks out

Scab formed on the skin

Skin healed with some surface change in skin tissue

The process of skin healing

SKIN CHARACTERISTICS

Both internal and external factors affect the health and appearance of the skin.

INTERNAL FACTORS

Factor	Result
Family history	If your parents have good skin and have aged slowly it is likely that you will too.
Sleep patterns	A lack of sleep affects the skin's ability to renew itself **efficiently**.
Stress	This inhibits the body's ability to function at its best and negatively affects most of the systems of the body.
Hormones	Hormonal changes can bring a variety of changes to the function and appearance of the skin. Excessively oily skin can be caused by the androgen hormone during puberty. The menopause causes the hormone oestrogen to decline. Oestrogen has an important role in the cellular activity of the skin and skin hydration. Thyroid problems can cause the skin to become dry.

Efficient

Performing in the best possible way without wasting time.

EXTERNAL FACTORS

Factor	Result
Smoking	When a smoker inhales they purse their lips and often squint against the smoke. These frequent actions cause fine lines to develop around the lips and eyes. Smoking uses up vitamin C which is important as it preserves collagen in the skin and is essential for healthy blood vessels to transport nutrients around the body. Smoking also affects the amount of oxygen the skin receives giving it a sallow grey appearance.
Skin care	Incorrectly using products or using products that are abrasive or harsh will increase rather than reduce the appearance of ageing.
Diet	A balanced diet is essential to the health and appearance of the skin. Skin needs to be provided with all the essential nutrients to repair itself and to function properly. Vitamins B, C and E and the minerals zinc and selenium are very important for healthy skin.
Overexposure to UV rays	Too much sun on one day or over the years causes collagen and the skin's natural moisture factor to change. The stratum corneum thickens making lines and wrinkles more noticeable.
Stress	Stress causes the skin to lose its healthy glow as it affects the immune system and the circulation.
Unhealthy lifestyle	A lack of physical activity and a poor diet means **enzymes** become slow and sluggish and allow toxins to accumulate in the tissues.
Environmental factors	Air conditioning and central heating cause the skin to lose moisture as they tend to create a dry **atmosphere**. The chemicals in air pollution, especially carbon dioxide, disrupt the skin's normal functions.

INDUSTRY TIP

A balanced diet should have:

- protein: 15 per cent
- carbohydrates: 55 per cent
- good fats: 30 per cent (remember, not all fats are bad!)
- vitamins and minerals.

Enzymes

The proteins that speed up chemical reactions.

Atmosphere

In the air.

INDUSTRY TIP

Alcohol deprives the body of its vitamin reserves, including vitamins B and C, causing dehydration.

INDUSTRY TIP

A vitamin A **deficiency** can cause **hyper-keratinisation**. A vitamin B deficiency can cause cracks at the corner of the mouth. A vitamin C deficiency can cause wounds to heal slowly and premature ageing. A severe vitamin C deficiency causes scurvy.

Hyper-keratinisation

The excessive production of keratin in the epidermis causing an abnormal thickening of skin in the palms of the hands and soles of the feet.

Deficiency

Something lacking.

Prone

Likely to suffer from.

Counteract

To oppose.

EFFECTS OF AGEING ON THE SKIN

Ageing is dependent on lots of factors. Some ethnic groups have a slower ageing process than others. The suppleness and large amounts of collagen in Afro-Caribbean skin allows it to prevent some of the effects of ageing. Caucasian (white) skin tends to be thinner, more **prone** to damage and less able to **counteract** the damaging effects of the sun and environmental exposure.

Age	Skin's appearance
Mid twenties	The skin's ability to renew itself and repair damaged cells starts to decrease. Each cell division passes genetic information and as we grow older tiny pieces of genetic information are lost. This means that the next generation of cells produced do not carry the same information as the previous one.
Mid thirties	The skin **contours** become less defined and the skin starts to sag. As the skin ages the structure of new collagen is more uneven. Elastin fibres show signs of cross linking and hardening. The fat cells that plump out the skin begin to reduce causing the skin to sag, thin and become crepe-like. The skin retains less moisture which causes it to lose its plump appearance. The blood vessels of the dermis become more fragile and are more easily damaged. The production of sebum from the sebaceous glands declines causing a reduction in the surface lipids and the skin becomes visibly drier. **Contours** Outline shape of the skin.
Forties	The ageing becomes more obvious with lines deepening, particularly along the expression lines, which are creases in the skin caused by muscle movement.
Fifties	The skin is more wrinkled and elasticity loss is more noticeable, especially around the facial contours. Older skin often has a sallow or yellow tone caused by changes in the skin's brown pigment. Melanin is no longer spread evenly throughout the skin and becomes patchy leaving the skin with uneven pigmentation, age spots and **lentigines**. **Lentigines** Also called liver spots or age spots. An area of hyper-pigmentation.

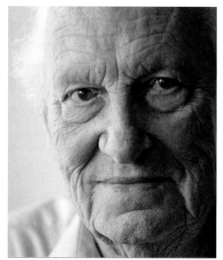

Elderly skin

WRINKLES

Whenever we smile, laugh or frown, natural expression lines appear on our face. Fine or deep lines are created in the skin's structure as a result of muscular movement. Wrinkles are a depression in the skin's surface. A wrinkle occurs as result of:

- the skin becoming thinner
- changes in the muscle density
- changes in the structure and position of elastin and collagen
- dehydration
- a decline in hyaluronic acid.

HANDY HINTS

See Diseases and disorders of the skin on page 18 for more information about lentigines.

 SmartScreen 204 Worksheet 11

INDUSTRY TIP

It is no coincidence that 'tanning' – the term used to describe the skin's change of colour through exposure to UV rays – also means 'to turn animal skin into leather by drying it out in sunlight'.

INDUSTRY TIP

The hormone oestrogen has water attracting properties and influences the amount of moisture held in the skin. When oestrogen levels drop following the menopause the skin's ability to hold moisture is affected.

SKIN TONES

All skin has the same number of **melanocytes** but they have a slightly different structure and are more active in darker skin. Melanin, which gives skin its colour, is produced in a specialised area of the melanocytes called melanosomes. Darker skin has a greater quantity of melanin in the melanosomes. The depth of colour depends on how the melanosomes are spread out in the epidermis. The size and quantity of sebaceous glands also differs between ethnic groups.

Melanocytes

The cells that produce melanin. Melanocytes contain melanosomes.

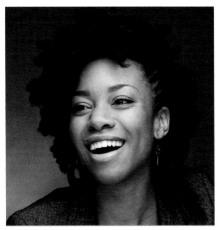

Afro-Caribbean skin

AFRO-CARIBBEAN SKIN

Afro-Caribbean skin has larger sebaceous glands (approximately 10 per cent larger) than Caucasian skin. The sebaceous glands often open directly onto the skin's surface rather than into the hair follicle. Also, the sebum is richer in amino acids. This does not necessarily mean that the skin will be oily or shiny in appearance.

Afro-Caribbean skin can be sensitive to sun damage but it is harder to detect. The melanocytes in darker skin have longer and thicker dendrites and spread out melanin differently.

Afro-Caribbean skin is prone to hyper-pigmentation, which are patches of increased skin pigment, following skin damage. Ageing tends to be slower due to the extra protection given by increased melanin in the skin. Afro-Caribbean skin is prone to **keloid scar** tissue.

Keloid scarring

When the skin produces too much collagen following an injury and continues to produce it so that the resulting scar is bigger than the original wound.

CAUCASIAN (WHITE) SKIN

The melanosomes are smaller and rounder than in Afro-Caribbean skin. The cells are spread out in groups called clusters. The spaces between the cells give the skin a lighter appearance. Sensitivity to UVB is more visible on the skin's surface as pale skin is more translucent. Caucasian skin is more likely to be damaged by the sun than other skin types as there is not the same level of melanin protection against UVB. Not all Caucasian skin is sensitive and some pale skin can produce a golden tan on exposure to UVB. Sebum is secreted into the hair follicles rather than directly onto the skin.

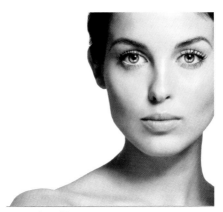

Caucasian skin

ASIAN SKIN

Asian skin takes its orange or red tone from a higher level of caretone, which is a strongly-coloured red–orange pigment. Asian skin has the widest range of pigment colouring but is prone to uneven pigmentation patches. Light Asian skin tends to age far more slowly than dark Asian skin. Asian skin is typically smooth and sebaceous pores are less visible. Sweat glands are larger and found in larger numbers than in Caucasian skin, which gives the skin a sheen.

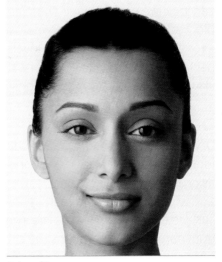

Asian skin

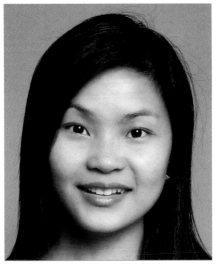

Oriental skin

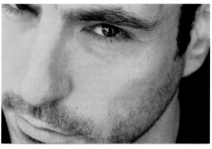

Male skin is more coarse than female skin

Testosterone/androgen

Hormones that stimulate male characteristics.

Imperfections

Flaws in the skin, such as moles or skin tags.

Abnormalities

Something that is not normal.

Exfoliated

Peeling off or removing dead skin cells.

Acidity

The amount of acid in the skin that affects how oily or dry the skin is.

Lubricate

To apply a substance that reduces friction and allows smooth movement.

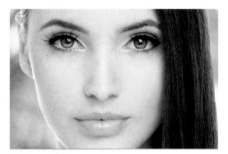

Balanced skin

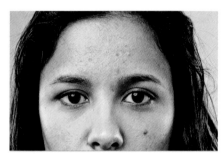

Oily skin

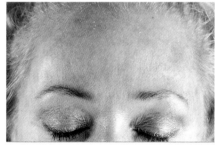

Dry skin

MALE SKIN

The male hormone **testosterone** stimulates fibroblasts to produce collagen at puberty, which means that male skin has a thicker dermis. On average male skin has 32 per cent more collagen than female skin. One of the benefits of this additional collagen is that male skin tends to age slower. Men have a higher **androgen** level making the skin secrete more sebum. This makes the skin more oily and the pores more obvious. This combination gives male skin a coarser texture.

SKIN TYPES

There are four main skin groups:

1 balanced (normal)

2 oily

3 dry

4 combination (a mixture of oily and dry).

Skin can also be described by its condition which might be:

- mature
- dehydrated
- sensitive.

Any skin type can have one or more of these conditions.

BALANCED (NORMAL) SKIN

It is very unlikely that you will see truly balanced skin in an adult. Balanced skin is perfect. It is free from blemishes or **imperfections**. It is neither dry nor oily as secretion levels are balanced. Pigmentation is evenly spread out and there are no **abnormalities**. The skin is bright and looks healthy.

OILY SKIN

Oily skin suffers from over-secretion of sebum. The skin looks shiny and sallow from the residue of surface oil. The skin cells do not easily **exfoliate** naturally as they stick to the oily surface. Very oily patches give skin a rough texture. Pores are relaxed and are more visible on the skin's surface due to the over-activity of the sebaceous glands. The skin can look like orange peel. There are usually comedones present and blocked pores. Oily skin can feel tacky and is cool to the touch. The excess oil lowers the **acidity** levels of the skin making it easier for bacteria to multiply so it is prone to blemishes, papules and pustules. A skin with excessive oily secretions is called seborrhoeic.

DRY SKIN

Dry skin lacks the natural lipids (including sebum) that are responsible for keeping the skin lubricated and hydrated. The surface cells look more flaky and are visible to the eye. Dry skin has a crepe-like appearance. The skin will look matte and feel slightly warm to the touch. The lack of surface **lubrication** leaves the skin feeling tight. The skin is often more transparent and this means the circulation is more visible giving the skin a rosy appearance.

COMBINATION SKIN

Typically the person will have an oily T-zone on the forehead, nose and chin where the sebaceous glands are more concentrated. The cheeks and neck are commonly dry. Around 75 per cent of skin is combination skin.

SKIN CONDITIONS

All skin can also be sensitive or dehydrated.

SENSITIVE SKIN

Sensitive skin can be **allergic** or **reactive**. At some point most of us will experience sensitive skin. An allergic skin is sensitive to one or more products or chemicals. A reactive skin responds to touch and **stimulation** quickly and produces a more defined **erythema**. Sensitive skin might be more highly coloured and easily become red, blotchy and irritated.

DEHYDRATED SKIN

Dehydrated skin lacks the moisture it needs to keep it hydrated and the skin's cells plump. To check if skin is dehydrated gently lift the skin with the thumb and index finger – if very fine lines can be seen the skin is dehydrated. The skin often feels tight and looks extremely dry. Causes include:

- central heating
- air conditioning
- drinks containing caffeine and/or alcohol
- smoking
- **insufficient** water intake
- using products that are too harsh and strip the skin of its natural oils and moisture
- illness
- some medication
- excessive exposure to the elements (wind or sun) or temperature (too hot or too cold).

There might not be any obvious signs of dehydration until a product has soaked into the skin. Oily skin is just as likely to be dehydrated as dry skin.

DISEASES AND DISORDERS OF THE SKIN

It is important that you can recognise common skin diseases and disorders. You need to know whether or not they are contagious and whether treatments can be given (or given once you have **modified** them).

You should never feel under pressure to treat anyone you feel is unwell or treat any area that has signs of a contagious infection. Remember, if you catch something you will risk passing the disease on. You will be unable to work while you are ill or you might have your work activities **restricted**.

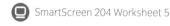 SmartScreen 204 Worksheet 5

Allergic reaction
When someone has a reaction to a product, eg redness, swelling or itchiness.

Reactive
When skin quickly responds to touch and stimulation, producing redness.

Stimulating
Energising or encouraging.

Erythema
Redness of the skin due to increased blood supply to the affected area.

Insufficient
Not having enough.

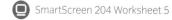 SmartScreen 204 Worksheet 5

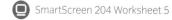 SmartScreen 209 Worksheet 4

Modified
Changing or adapting.

Restricted
To make something limited.

PIGMENTATION DISORDERS

Several common disorders can affect the pigment of the skin. Skin pigment can be lost – hypo-pigmentation – or increased – hyper-pigmentation. In many cases the changes cannot be reversed. Avoiding sun exposure will help improve hyper-pigmentation. It takes a very long time for pigmentation to even out and, as most clients will not keep affected areas out of the sun completely, their skin will not have a chance to recover.

Disorder	Description and cause	Contra-indications and general precautions	Advice for client
Nevi (birthmark)/mole	A raised, pigmented skin growth caused by a cluster of melanocytes between the epidermis and dermis or in the dermis. A mole can vary in size from a pinhead to several centimetres, and in colour from tan to bluish black. Some raised moles have hairs growing from them.	Not contra-indicated. Keep a note on the client's record and be aware of any sudden changes in colour or size or if the mole begins to weep or bleed. Avoid excessive stimulation over and around the mole.	Use sunblock over the mole.
Ephilides (freckles)	Melanin is spread out in clusters of pigment. These small areas of pigmentation become more prominent after exposure to UV radiation.	Not contra-indicated.	Use sunblock or a high **SPF** sunscreen to **minimise** any further changes in pigmentation. Give advice on camouflage make-up if appropriate. **SPF** This stands for sun protection factor and the number following it, eg 30, indicates the amount of protection that the sunscreen will provide when the skin is exposed to UV light. **Minimise** To reduce the impact of.
Lentigines (liver spots)	Also called age spots. Areas of darkened pigmentation about 1 cm in size caused by an abnormality in the production of melanin. Skin is often slightly raised. Changes in the skin can be felt by touching the surface of the lentigines. Commonly found on the back of the hands, face and upper chest of mature clients.	Not contra-indicated.	Use sunblock or a high SPF sunscreen to minimise further pigmentation changes. Give advice on camouflage make-up if appropriate.

Disorder	Description and cause	Contra-indications and general precautions	Advice for client
Chloasma	A cluster of pigmentation in the skin. Commonly found on the upper cheeks, nose and forehead. Caused by hormonal stimulation (eg pregnancy or taking the contraceptive pill). Sometimes disappears once hormones settle down but might be permanent. Perfume can react to skin and sunlight and cause hyper-pigmentation.	Not contra-indicated.	Use sunblock or a high SPF sunscreen to minimise further pigmentation changes. Spray perfume on clothing rather than the skin. Give advice on camouflage make-up if appropriate.
Vitiligo	A lack of skin pigmentation. Where melanocytes have been destroyed white patches of skin can be seen. Thought to be an autoimmune disorder (when the body attacks its own tissues) or one triggered by stress or severe sunburn. Hair growing in the area will also be white. The skin around the edge of the area might look darker due to the contrast with the surrounding darker skin.	Be cautious. Treatment should not be carried out, depending on the severity of the vitiligo. However, most treatments would not be contra-indicated.	Use a total sunblock in the areas affected as there is no melanin to absorb UV radiation and the skin will burn easily. Give advice on camouflage make-up if appropriate.
Albinism	The total destruction of melanocytes means there is no pigmentation. Hair and skin will be white; eye colour might vary but is often pale blue.	Contra-indicated, depending on treatment. Tanning treatments would be unsuitable. The skin is often very sensitive so carry out a sensitivity test.	Avoid unnecessary exposure to the sun.

CIRULATION DISORDERS

There is a wide range of disorders that affect the skin's circulation. Some of these changes are permanent while others come and go. Some conditions are **hereditary** or are present at birth, eg birthmarks. Others develop over time and are the result of ageing.

Hereditary
Passed on in the genes (instructions) in our cells.

Disorder	Description and cause	Contra-indications and general precautions	Advice for client
Telangiectasias (dilated capillaries)	Permanently dilated capillaries visible through the skin. Repeated changes in temperature both internal (eg hot flushes) and external (eg air conditioning, central heating and extremes of weather) **aggravate** the condition. Also aggravated by lack of skin care, eating hot spicy food and alcohol. **Aggravate** Make worse.	Not contra-indicated but take care with some treatments, eg steaming and skin warming. Avoid extremes of temperature.	Can be treated using advanced electrolysis techniques. Keep skin protected with a good moisturiser. Give advice on camouflage make-up if appropriate.
Rosacea	A chronic long-term skin disorder causing redness and swelling, mainly of the face. It can be caused by congestion and enlargement of the superficial blood capillaries. It usually affects the nose, cheeks and centre of the forehead (butterfly pattern). The skin's surface becomes thickened and is superficially dry and flaky in texture. Pustules and papules might be present in more severe cases and are thought to be caused by an immune system response. It can be hereditary.	Not contra-indicated. Not contagious. Treatment will depend on how severe the condition is. Treat the skin with care and avoid extremes of temperature and **over-stimulation**. **Over-stimulation** Energising and encouraging more than is necessary.	Avoid stress, smoking, spicy foods and alcohol. Use a gentle anti-inflammatory skin care range, with a protective moisturiser and high SPF. Give advice on camouflage make-up and make-up colours to avoid if appropriate.

Disorder	Description and cause	Contra-indications and general precautions	Advice for client
Vascular **nevi**	Caused by an abnormality of the capillary blood vessels. These cluster together to form a very red raised area of skin. There are different types and most are **congenital**.	Not contra-indicated. Avoid excessive stimulation over and around the nevi.	Use sunblock over the area. Give advice on camouflage make-up if appropriate.
Allergies	When an allergic reaction occurs the immune system produces antibodies in response to **allergens** that most other people would not find harmful. Common allergic conditions include hay fever, allergic asthma, urticaria, dermatitis and eczema. **Anaphylactic shock** is a dangerous allergic reaction.	Contra-indicated depending on the allergy. Include allergies on the client's record card.	Check product labels and make sure you avoid ingredients that you know the client's skin is reactive to.
Urticaria (hives)	Also called nettle rash. An allergic reaction characterised by red blotchy skin, **wheals** and severe itching. The skin will feel very warm.	Contra-indicated. If the client is already suffering with an allergic reaction allow the body to heal before treatment. If this occurs as an allergic contra-action to a product used during a treatment, remove all traces of the product from the skin and wash the area with lukewarm water. Do not continue with any further treatment.	Check product labels and make sure you avoid ingredients you know your client's skin is reactive to. Avoid excessive heat if there is a history of urticaria.

Nevi
Lesions of the skin (eg birthmarks).

Congenital disorder
A disorder with which a person is born.

Allergen
Any foreign substance which can trigger an inflammatory response in the body.

Anaphylactic shock
A rare but severe acute allergic reaction that affects the whole body. Symptoms can start within minutes of the client coming into contact with something they are allergic to. Symptoms include swelling and irritation in the area of contact, sickness, rashes, wheezing, a drop in blood pressure and a rapid pulse. If you think a client is going into anaphylactic shock you should call for an ambulance *immediately*.

Wheal
A raised fluid-containing area of flesh-coloured or white skin surrounded by a red area. It can look like a cat scratch.

WHY DON'T YOU...
make a list of all the products in your salon that could potentially cause an allergic reaction.

SEBACEOUS GLAND DISORDERS

Some of the most common skin disorders that a therapist will come in contact with will be linked to the sebaceous glands. These glands are very reactive during hormonal changes particularly during puberty. These conditions are often easily irritated by the use of incorrect products and skin care. It is important to treat the skin gently and not to remove all the natural oils that the skin needs for protection.

Disorder	Description and cause	Contra-indications and general precautions	Advice for client
Milia (whiteheads)	Milia are small cysts. They appear as white pearly lumps on the skin and might include uric acid or sebum. Common around the eye area and on skin which is very dehydrated. Might be caused by inappropriate skin care products.	Not contra-indicated.	Check that skin care products are appropriate for the skin type. Skin must be kept moisturised to prevent dehydration. Avoid mineral-based products around the eye. Advise on facial treatments to stimulate and improve the skin's functions and to keep the skin soft. Milia can be removed using advanced electrolysis or with a microlance which gently lifts the skin so the milia can be easily extracted.
Comedones (blackheads)	A grey spot caused by hardened sebum blocking the hair follicle. The change in colour is caused by the **oxidation** of keratin in the sebum as it comes into contact with the air. Further change in colour is caused by the attraction of surface pollution to the oil.	Not contra-indicated. **Oxidation** Interaction between oxygen molecules and other substances.	Recommend deep cleansing and exfoliating treatments and a suitable home skin care regime.

INDUSTRY TIP

Forty to fifty per cent of adults between the ages of 20 and 40 have persistent oily or acne skin. Acne begins with whiteheads and blackheads and progresses to papules and pustules. Medical treatment might be required if the skin becomes very infected and pustular. Finally, the skin develops cysts and nodules. Medical treatment is essential to prevent scarring.

HANDY HINTS

See Chapter 204/224 for how to remove comedones.

HANDY HINTS

The technique for removing milia using a microlance is taught at Level 3.

Disorder	Description and cause	Contra-indications and general precautions	Advice for client
Sebaceous cyst	Caused by a plug of hardened sebum in the sebaceous gland blocking the follicle and causing it to expand. There are two types of sebaceous **cyst**: ■ epidermal cysts which can appear anywhere on the skin ■ pilar cysts which are commonly found on the scalp.	Not contra-indicated unless the cyst is very large or infected, then the area must be avoided. **Cyst** A small rounded swelling that might contain fluid, semi-solid or solid material. It extends both above and below the surface of the skin.	Recommend that the client seeks medical advice if the cyst is causing irritation or if they are concerned.
Acne vulgaris	A bacterial infection of the sebaceous glands of the face, neck, chest, shoulders, back, thighs and bottom. It can affect one or more areas. Facial acne normally starts around the nose and spreads out over the face. Usually caused by a hormonal imbalance that can be aggravated by stress and poor diet. It might also be caused by exposure to certain chemicals and the use of certain drugs.	Contra-indicated. Avoid contact with the infected areas to prevent further spread of infection on the client's skin. Only use very limited facial treatment to avoid aggravating the condition.	Seek medical attention early to avoid scarring and to treat any skin infection. Advise on make-up application and the use of matte make-up and oil-free products to protect the skin where appropriate.
Seborrhoea	Excessively oily skin. Skin is very shiny and tacky with a sallow grey tone caused by the oily surface residue. Lots of comedones. Caused by a hormonal imbalance. Can develop into acne vulgaris.	Not contra-indicated. Do not over-stimulate the skin during treatment.	Recommend deep cleansing and exfoliating treatments and a suitable home skin care regime.

SKIN DISORDERS INVOLVING ABNORMAL GROWTH

Therapists commonly see abnormal skin growths, eg thickening of skin on the soles of the feet and abnormal skin tags, which are a nuisance to the client. A therapist is unable to improve these disorders directly.

Disorder	Description and cause	Contra-indications and general precautions	Advice for client
Seborrhoeic **keratosis** (senile warts)	A brown thickening on the surface of the skin. Size ranges from 3 mm to 35 mm. Exact cause is unknown. Not caused by exposure to UV radiation.	Not contra-indicated.	Can be removed by a medical practitioner.
Skin tags	Tiny skin **extensions** of loose fibrous tissue. Many have no known cause. Others might be caused by surface stimulation, eg along the neckline or under a bra strap.	Not contra-indicated. If there are clusters avoid stimulation and exfoliation over the area. **Extension** A part that is continued from another part.	If the client is concerned refer them to an advanced electrolysis practitioner.
Psoriasis	Skin cells are produced very quickly and build up on the skin's surface leaving very itchy scaly patches with a white pearly surface. Skin can crack and bleed. The exact cause is unknown. It is linked to stress and is often hereditary.	Not contra-indicated. Not contagious. Avoid affected areas to prevent skin irritation. Client can be safely treated unless the condition is severe.	Recommend relaxing treatments to help reduce stress. Recommend your client sees their medical practitioner for specialised treatment, eg UV treatment, coal tar treatment or cortisone-based medicine.
Hyper-keratosis	Thickening of the skin caused by an excessive amount of keratin. This thickening is often produced to protect the underlying tissue from rubbing, pressure and irritation. Commonly affects elbows, knees, and the soles and heels of the feet.	Not contra-indicated.	Exfoliation will help improve the skin's texture.

Disorder	Description and cause	Contra-indications and general precautions	Advice for client
Corns and calluses	An area of hard skin produced by the body to provide additional protection from pressure or friction (eg from poorly fitting shoes). Corns are smaller and appear on the top of toes or between toe joints. Some people have a corn on their middle finger caused by holding a pen (writer's lump). Calluses are larger and flatter and occur on the heels and palms.	Not contra-indicated.	Choose shoes carefully. Regular pedicures and manicures will help soften the skin. Use a pen with a soft cushion design. Refer to a **podiatrist**. **Podiatrist** A foot specialist.
Malignant tumours	- A tumour may be benign (non-cancerous) or malignant (cancerous). Caused by cells reproducing in an abnormal way. A tumour might be in or on the body. It might be contained in one area or spread into the surrounding tissues and organs. - Malignant melanoma develops in the pigment cells and is associated with excessive exposure to UV radiation. - Basal cell carcinoma develops in the epidermis.	Contra-indicated. A client should not be treated during cancer treatment. It is not contagious.	A client having cancer treatment should seek medical advice before any treatment takes place.

SKIN DISORDERS INVOLVING ABNORMAL CELLULAR GROWTH

Disorder	Description and cause	Contra-indications and general precautions	Advice for client
Eczema	Areas of extreme dryness. Described as wet eczema when there are **vesicles** present. (There are over 25 varieties of eczema.) The irritated skin is itchy. Can be caused by an internal irritant (eg a food intolerance) or by contact with an external allergen (eg animal hair or a product). Eczema can be inherited and is often linked to asthma.	Only contra-indicated if severe and the skin is open. Avoid direct contact with any area with open skin. Only use gentle products with a natural base. Avoid abrasive products and touching the skin too much. **Vesicle** A small blister filled with liquid.	Seek medical advice as medical products can help to relieve the symptoms.
Dermatitis	Symptoms include: ■ redness ■ scaling/flaking ■ blistering ■ weeping ■ cracking ■ swelling. *Irritant contact dermatitis (ICD)* can happen when there is contact with either a strong **irritant** or a weaker irritant over long periods of time. Irritants in the salon include hand washes, essential oils, dust and wet work (ie constant washing of hands to maintain hygiene). *Allergic contact dermatitis (ACD)* can happen when someone develops an **allergy** to something that comes into contact with their skin. Any contact with the **allergen** will cause an allergic response. Allergens in the salon include glue adhesives, nail enamel and skin care products.	Contra-indication will depend on symptoms and level of severity. Avoid affected areas. Ask your tutor for help if you are not sure. **Irritant** A substance, product or chemical that damages the skin and makes it inflamed. **Allergy** A hyper-sensitive reaction of the immune system. **Allergen** A substance that causes your immune system to react abnormally.	When you are washing hands, make sure you dry them properly. Apply moisturiser regularly. Use special creams when recommended by a medical practitioner.

ACTIVITY

Working with your colleagues, list anything that you know someone is allergic to.

VIRAL INFECTIONS

Viral infections are very contagious and you should not feel under pressure to treat anyone you feel is unwell or treat any area that has signs of a viral infection.

Disorder	Description and cause	Contra-indications and general precautions	Advice for client
Herpes simplex (cold sores)	Starts with itching or irritation in the area where the cold sore is going to occur, develops into a red patch followed by blisters. These turn into a moist crusty patch. Tend to develop when the person is run down, under stress or after overexposure to the sun and wind. The **virus** remains **dormant** after the infection has cleared up.	Contra-indicated. Contagious. Do not treat the area around a cold sore. **Transmitted** by direct or indirect contact with an infected area where blisters are present. If a client requests a facial treatment ask them to return once the cold sore has gone so they can fully enjoy their treatment.	There is no cure but over-the-counter treatments might relieve symptoms. **Virus** A micro-organism that multiplies within a living organism. **Dormant** Not growing or active. **Transmitted** Passing on or spreading.
Human papilloma virus (HPV) (warts and verrucae)	The virus enters the skin through a small cut or scratch. It can lie dormant for many months. Keratin is produced too fast and causes a hard, raised cauliflower looking growth of skin. The tiny black dots are blood capillaries which get caught as the wart grows. About 70 per cent of warts are *common warts*, which occur singularly or in clusters. *Verrucae (plantar warts)* occur on the soles of the feet. The weight of the body makes the wart grow inwards. Particularly contagious in damp warm moist conditions.	Contra-indicated. Damaged warts are contagious as the viral spores are exposed. A verrucae prevents a pedicure. Transmitted through direct and indirect contact.	Most people will develop a wart at some point. Usually the body develops an **immunity** to the virus and the wart disappears within 2 years. **Immunity** Being protected from a disease.

Disorder	Description and cause	Contra-indications and general precautions	Advice for client
Herpes zoster (shingles)	Caused when the chickenpox virus is reactivated after lying dormant in the nervous system. Symptoms include tingling and extreme sensitivity along the nerve pathways followed by pain, itching and blisters. The client might feel run down and the pain might last for many months. Physical symptoms disappear after a week.	Contra-indicated. Although shingles is not contagious you can catch chickenpox from someone who has active shingles.	Seek medical advice.

Bacteria

Tiny single-celled organisms. They come in different shapes. Some are harmful to us and others are important for our health.

BACTERIAL INFECTIONS

Our body is covered with millions of tiny **bacteria**. Bacteria can be good as well as bad. Some bacterial infections are very contagious and you should not feel under pressure to treat any infected area.

Disorder	Description and cause	Contra-indications and general precautions	Advice for client
Furuncles (boils) and carbuncles	An infection of the hair follicle. Starts with an inflamed tender area, which develops into a large painful pustule. Caused by the staphylococcus aureus bacteria and linked with poor hygiene and stress. A carbuncle is a collection of boils with several pustule-like heads. A scar is often left when the area has healed.	Contra-indicated. Contagious. Avoid area to prevent cross-infection.	Leave the area alone. Seek medical advice if appropriate.
Impetigo	Caused by the staphylococci and streptococci bacteria. Commonly found on the face around the nose and mouth but can occur anywhere with broken skin. Raised red areas of skin quickly form small blisters, followed by honey-coloured crusts.	Contra-indicated. Contagious. Transmitted by direct and indirect contact.	Seek medical advice.

INDUSTRY TIP

Clients do not always have to see their doctor for medical advice. Often appropriate advice can be given by a pharmacist.

Disorder	Description and cause	Contra-indications and general precautions	Advice for client
Conjunctivitis	Caused by the staphylococci bacteria or occasionally by a virus. Inflammation of the mucus membrane lining and covering of the eye. Eyes look red and swollen, feel gritty and itchy. There might be some sensitivity to light. The discharge might contain pus, causing the eyelids to stick together in the mornings.	Contra-indicated. Very contagious. Transmitted by direct contact and indirect contact (eg by sharing make-up brushes).	Seek medical advice.
Hordeolum (stye)	A staphylococcal bacterial infection of one or more follicles of the eyelashes. A small red area on the edge of the eyelid causes irritation. It becomes a small red lump which might contain pus.	Contra-indicated. Contagious. Do not treat the area to avoid cross-infection.	Seek medical advice.

FUNGAL DISEASES

You should be able to recognise tinea pedis/athlete's foot. It is one of the most common conditions that clients will present to you.

Disorder	Description and cause	Contra-indications and general precautions	Advice for client
Tinea corporis (ringworm of the body)	Initially appears as a pink circular patch, sometimes scaly, with a defined red outer ring. The skin heals from the centre as the infection spreads outwards.	Contra-indicated. Contagious. Transmitted by direct or indirect contact.	Seek medical advice.
Tinea pedis (athlete's foot)	Symptoms include irritation and sometimes a distinct odour. The **fungus** lives on keratin and likes a moist warm environment. White spongy looking skin might crack, split and peel. Commonly found between the toes but can also affect larger areas of the foot.	Contra-indicated. Contagious. Transmitted by direct or indirect contact. **Fungus** A tiny plant micro-organism.	Seek medical advice. Wash and dry feet well particularly between the toes. Change socks at least once a day. Wear breathable fabrics which keep the feet dry.

Disorder	Description and cause	Contra-indications and general precautions	Advice for client
Tinea capitis (ringworm of the scalp)	As for tinea corporis but hair becomes brittle and breaks away leaving short stubs. Scalp becomes patchy, with white or grey scales.	Contra-indicated. Contagious. Transmitted by direct or indirect contact.	Seek medical advice.
Tinea barbae (ringworm of the beard)	Small pustules at the tip of the hair follicle from which broken hair protrudes.	Contra-indicated. Contagious. Transmitted by direct or indirect contact, eg via dirty towels or contaminated razors.	Seek medical advice.

INFESTATIONS

Infestation

When a living animal enters the body and survives by feeding off blood and living tissue.

Most **infestations** are conditions that you are unlikely to come across in the salon but it is still important that you are familiar with the conditions and are able to recognise them. It is always a possibility that you might be exposed to them.

Disorder	Description and cause	Contra-indications and general precautions	Advice for client
Pediculosis corporis (body lice)	Caused by a tiny blood-sucking insect that lays its eggs on clothing and feeds on the skin. Symptoms include intense itching at the site of infestation, usually in the skin's creases (eg the elbows).	Contra-indicated. Contagious. Transmitted by direct or indirect contact.	Seek medical advice.
Sarcoptes scabiei (scabies)	Also known as itch mites. Small **parasites** burrow into the skin and lay eggs. Causes intense itching which is worse at night. The infestation is visible by inflammation and irritation of the infected area and small grey swellings caused by the burrowing mites. Commonly found between the fingers and on the wrist but can also be found under the arm and around the groin.	Contra-indicated. Highly contagious. Transmitted by direct or indirect contact. **Parasite** An organism that lives on or in another organism (a host) to which it causes harm. Parasites include fungus, bacteria and worms.	Seek medical advice.

HAIR

Protein makes up 70 to 80 per cent of hair in the form of thread-like structures of dead **keratinised** cells. The rest of the hair is made up of water, minerals, lipids and melanin (which give hair its colour). Hair grows from the hair follicle as new cells are produced.

The main function of the hair is protection. Hair covers the head to keep it warm and to protect it from injury and overexposure to the sun. Eyelashes and eyebrows (supercilia) shield the eyes. They prevent objects from entering the eyes and catch perspiration.

Hair also provides a larger surface area for sweat to evaporate from to cool the body. When we are cold the arrector pili muscle, which is attached to the hair follicle, pulls the hair shaft up to trap air against the body. Tiny hairs in the ears and nostrils, called cilia, catch and filter out dust particles to prevent them entering the body.

In this part of the chapter you will learn about:

- the hair follicle
- the structure of the hair shaft
- hair types
- the hair growth cycle
- the basic hair types and where they are found
- hair diseases and disorders.

HAIR FOLLICLE

The hair follicle is a complex structure that produces hair. It extends deep into the dermis.

INNER ROOT SHEATH AND OUTER ROOT SHEATH

The follicle has an inner and an outer root **sheath**.

Inner root sheath

The inner root sheath has three layers:

1 the cuticle, which holds the hair in place

2 the Huxley layer

3 the Henles layer.

Keratinisation

The process by which living cells change into hard, flat, dead cells. It is caused by the production of a protein called keratin and the **degeneration** of the nucleus.

Degeneration

Fallen below normal amounts.

Sheath

A cover around the follicle root.

INDUSTRY TIP

A wood's light (used for skin analysis) can be used to detect ringworm as the fungus glows under the UV light.

Static
Not moving.

Outer root sheath
The outer root sheath is continued from the stratum germinativum and surrounds the inner root sheath. This sheath remains **static** in the skin and does not grow with the hair.

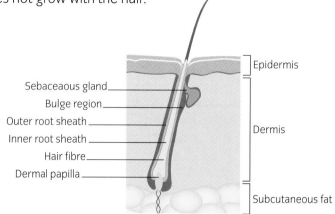

Sebaceaous gland

Bulge region

Outer root sheath

Inner root sheath

Hair fibre

Dermal papilla

Epidermis

Dermis

Subcutaneous fat

The hair follicle

SEBACEOUS GLAND
The sebaceous gland is usually located two-thirds of the way up the hair follicle. It produces sebum which is secreted into the follicle. In larger hair follicles there might be more than one sebaceous gland.

CONNECTIVE SHEATH
This sheath surrounds the follicle and the sebaceous gland. It provides the hair with nerve endings and blood vessels.

DERMAL PAPILLA
At the base of the hair follicle is a mass of loose connective tissue that contains tiny capillaries to nourish the cells of the follicle. Just above the papilla is a group of cells that produce the hair.

ARRECTOR PILI MUSCLE
This is a small muscle that is attached to the hair shaft. It supports the follicle and when we are cold pulls the hair upright causing goose bumps.

STRUCTURE OF THE HAIR SHAFT
The hair shaft is the part of the hair that is visible above the skin. The part embedded in the skin is called the root. The hair shaft is made up of three layers of keratinised cells:

1 the medulla

2 the cortex

3 the cuticle.

MEDULLA
The medulla is the most central layer of the follicle. It is not always found in vellus hair. It is formed of loosely connected, keratinised cells with air spaces in between. It reflects light and makes hair look shiny.

ACTIVITY
See if you can find a hair with a split end and write down how the hair looks. Can you see any definite parts of the hair structure?

CORTEX

The cortex surrounds the medulla and creates the bulk of the hair. It contains melanin and gives hair its colour. It has elongated keratinised cells bound together. These strands are able to stretch and flex and return to their original shape.

CUTICLE

The outermost layer is made up of overlapping scales of keratinised cells that provide a protective coat. If you take a strand of hair and run your fingers towards the root you will feel these scales. The cuticle has no colour and is quite a thin layer.

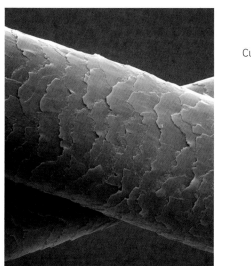
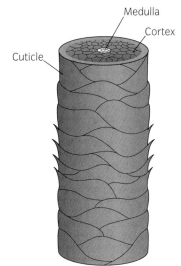

Structure of the hair shaft

HAIR TYPES

HAIR TEXTURE

The texture or thickness of a hair depends on the diameter and shape of the hair follicle and the proportion of the cuticle around the hair. In coarse hair the cuticle makes up around 10 per cent of the volume and the cortex around 90 per cent. In fine hair the cuticle makes up about 40 per cent of the volume and the cortex around 60 per cent.

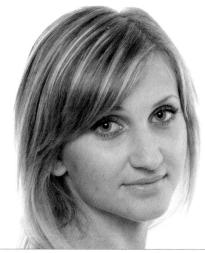

Straight hair

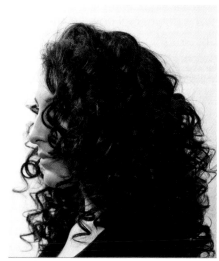

Curly hair

SmartScreen 206 Worksheet 5

HAIR GROWTH CYCLE

The hair follicle has three stages of growth. These stages include periods of activity and rest. They vary from person to person. The growth rate varies in different parts of the body. The hair on the head has a growth cycle of around 2–8 years while the growth rate of eyelashes is about 4 months. The three stages of the hair growth cycle are:

1 **a**nagen

2 **c**atagen

3 **t**elogen.

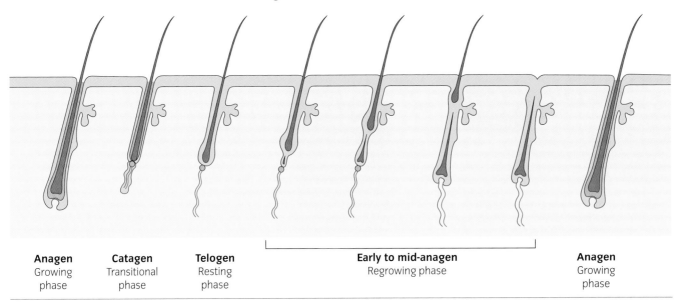

Anagen	Catagen	Telogen	Early to mid-anagen	Anagen
Growing phase	Transitional phase	Resting phase	Regrowing phase	Growing phase

The hair growth cycle

ANAGEN

During anagen the hair is in the active growth stage. The cells in the root sheath divide and grow down deeper into the dermis. At the same time cells move up the follicle to form the inner root sheath and the hair itself. The hair becomes injected with keratin and becomes keratinised. As the hair matures the growth slows down. Around 80 to 90 per cent of the hair on our head is in the anagen phase of growth at any one time.

CATAGEN

When the hair growth is complete the hair goes through a state of change which lasts about 2 weeks. During this time the cell activity slows down until no new cells are produced. There is no melanin pigmentation so the hair produced in these final growth stages has no colour. The bulb of the hair begins to wither and die and forms a club shape at the end. The follicle begins to shorten and shrink and becomes detached from the dermal papilla. A small cord forms between the dermal papilla and the club end of the hair. Around 1 per cent of the hair on the scalp is in the catagen phase of growth.

TELOGEN

In this final stage the hair is dead and is shed from the follicle. The follicle rests until it is stimulated to begin the cycle again. This stage lasts around 3–4 months. Sometimes a new hair begins to grow pushing the old hair out of the skin straight away. Around 13 per cent of head hair is resting in the telogen phase of growth.

WHY DON'T YOU...
run your fingers through your hair and pull at the ends gently. Look at the hair you have in your hand. The telogen hair will have a distinct white ball at the end and you will see the loss of hair colour towards the final hair growth. Now compare this to a hair that has been removed from an eyebrow using tweezers.

INDUSTRY TIP
Remember the word ACT to help you recall the hair growth cycle and its sequence.

ACTIVITY

Examine a hair that has been plucked from an eyebrow and see if you can see what stage of hair growth it is at. Does it have a nice well-formed bulb or a round white club end?

ACTIVITY

Wax an underarm with hot wax. Turn the wax over and look at the hairs. Can you see the different hair growth stages?

ACTIVITY

Discuss with colleagues what impact waxing and threading has on the hair growth cycle.

BASIC HAIR TYPES AND WHERE THEY ARE FOUND

There are three hair types:

1 vellus

2 terminal

3 lanugo.

VELLUS HAIR

This is the soft fine downy hair which is found all over the body with the exception of the soles of the feet and palms of the hands. It usually lacks any pigmentation. This hair has shallow roots.

TERMINAL HAIR

At birth this type of hair is found on the scalp, eyelashes and eyebrows. During puberty it grows under the arms and in the groin areas. During male puberty it grows on the lower legs and chest and as a beard. It has a well-developed root and bulb with a strong blood supply. The follicle extends deep into the dermis during anagen growth.

LANUGO HAIR

The very soft fine hair that covers the baby in the womb and disappears a few months after birth.

WHY DON'T YOU...
draw a table with two columns. Head one 'vellus' and the other 'terminal'. In the relevant column write down the differences between vellus and terminal hair.

ACTIVITY

Ask some of your colleagues with different hair colour, shape and thickness to brush their hair and collect any loose hairs. Compare the hairs. Discuss your findings.

ACTIVITY

Find a vellus hair and a terminal hair and compare the visible appearance and structure.

HAIR DISEASES AND DISORDERS

PARASITIC INFECTIONS OF THE SCALP

Parasitic infections of the scalp are very common. We tend to think of them affecting children but adults can get them just as easily.

Disorder	Description and cause	Contra-indications and general precautions	Advice for client
Pediculosis capitis (head lice)	Caused by a small wingless flat insect which feeds on blood. The eggs (nits) take 7 to 10 days to hatch. It takes 7 to 14 days for the lice to mature and mate. They survive for several weeks. Symptoms include intense itching at the site of infection. Nits look like grey-coloured beads attached to the hair shaft close to the scalp.	Contra-indicated. Contagious. Direct contact is required for the lice to jump from head to head.	Seek medical advice. Treatment must be on-going for a minimum of 14 days. Use a special comb to loosen and remove nits and lice.
Pediculosis pubis (pubic lice)	These tiny insects look like crabs or scabs. The females lay eggs that hatch after 8 days. Pubic lice can be found under the arms, in beards and in eyebrows. Symptoms include intense itching at the site of the infestation.	Contra-indicated. Contagious. Transmitted by direct contact.	Seek medical advice.

BACTERIAL INFECTIONS AFFECTING THE HAIR FOLLICLE

Disorder	Description and cause	Contra-indications and general precautions	Advice for client
Folliculitis	A common result of poor hygiene. Can occur following waxing and shaving. Inflammation of one or more hair follicles. Commonly found around the neck, bikini line, beard and armpits. Pseudo-folliculitis is when hair grows inwards causing further inflammation.	Contra-indicated. There is a risk of cross-infection. Follow very thorough aftercare advice.	Seek medical advice. Follow very thorough home care advice.

COMMON SCALP AND HAIR CONDITIONS

At Level 2 you do not generally deal with the hair during treatments. However, you might come across these common conditions and you will find it useful to have some basic knowledge and understanding about them.

Disorder	Description and cause	Contra-indications and general precautions	Advice for client
Fragilitis crinium (split ends)	Hair end is split. Hair has been exposed to harsh physical treatment (eg excessive heat, brushing, overstretching when wet) or chemical abuse (eg bleaching).	Not contra-indicated.	Protect the hair and minimise exposure to harsh treatment to avoid further damage. Cut off the damaged ends. Make sure hair is trimmed regularly.
Alopecia	Can be patches of hair loss (alopecia areata) or total hair loss (alopecia universalis). Can be caused by stress, shock, illness or medication (chemotherapy).	Not contra-indicated. **INDUSTRY TIP** Androgenic alopecia is male pattern baldness in women. Here the hair growth begins to thin, often starting at the crown, and the hair line recedes. It can be hereditary or caused by hormonal changes. Androgens cause the hair growth to alter and the hair becomes shorter and finer until it stops growing, leaving the scalp hairless or with a fine covering of vellus hair.	Stimulate the blood supply to the area to encourage healthy circulation. Recommend they see a **tricologist** for additional advice and treatment. **Tricologist** A person who specialises in hair and scalp problems.

NAILS

A perfect healthy nail is smooth, unmarked and can be flexed without breaking or splitting. It is usually a delicate pink colour which shows that there is a healthy circulation to the nail bed. The nail is an extension of the stratum lucidum (clear layer). It is made up of dense keratinised cells, water, minerals (including **calcium** and zinc) and a small amount of lipids.

Calcium
A mineral in the body.

In this part of the chapter you will learn about:
- the function of the nails
- the structure of the nail
- the growth cycle of the nail
- nail shapes
- diseases and disorders of the nail.

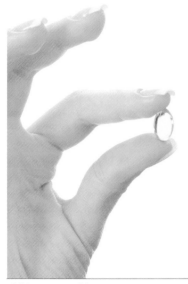

Picking up small items

FUNCTION OF THE NAILS

Nails have three functions:

1 to protect the nail bed and, through the nail plate, to protect the soft sensitive fingers and toes

2 to enhance the fingertips' sensitivity

3 to assist the fingers when picking up objects or scratching.

STRUCTURE OF THE NAIL

The following structures make up the nail:

- matrix
- nail plate
- free edge
- hyponychium
- nail bed
- lunula
- cuticle
- eponychium
- perionychium.

MATRIX

The matrix is the living part of the nail structure and is an extension of the stratum germinativum (granular layer). The matrix is sometimes referred to as the root of the nail. It lies underneath the nail fold or mantle. It is nourished by a large supply of blood vessels. It is here that new cells divide to produce the nail so any injury to this area can cause damage to the nail's structure. The shape of the matrix determines the size and shape of the nail.

NAIL PLATE

Sulphur bonds
One or more sulphur molecules attached together.

The nail plate is the visible part of the nail and is made up of hundreds of layers. These are found in three sections of keratinised cells bound together by **sulphur bonds**, moisture and fat. The middle section makes up 75 per cent of the nail plate. Unlike the skin the nail cells cannot be easily exfoliated. The nail plate is attached to the finger by the nail bed. It is dead and has no nerves or blood supply. The cells of the nail plate are able to absorb moisture and too much moisture can cause the nail to split or peel.

FREE EDGE

This is the part of the nail plate that extends beyond the fingertip. It protects the hyponychium at the edge of the nail bed. This is the part of the nail that can be filed into shape.

HYPONYCHIUM

The hyponychium lies at the edge of the nail bed and just beneath the free edge. It has a seal that protects the nail bed from infection.

ACTIVITY

Gently pull the skin back and look under the free edge of your nail. What can you see?

NAIL BED

The nail bed lies under the nail plate. It has a series of ridges and grooves.

ACTIVITY

Look carefully under the free edge of your nail. Can you see the thickened area and some ripples in the skin's structure? This is the nail bed.

LUNULA

This is the visible part of the matrix. It is the very pale pink area at the base of the nail plate. It is a different colour because the circulation is less efficient and also because the cells are not fully keratinised. Most people only have visible lunula on their thumbs.

CUTICLE

The cuticle is formed from thickened stratum corneum (the horny layer) and is constantly being shed. The cuticle has two parts: the eponychium and the perionychium.

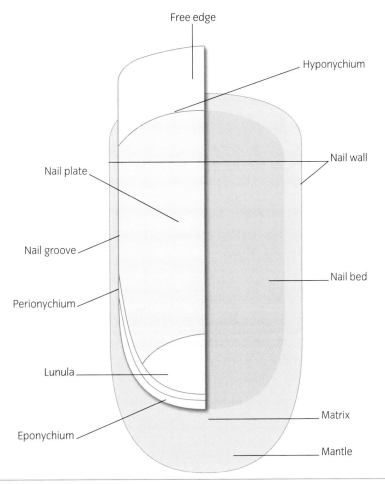

The structure of the nail

Eponychium

The eponychium is the fold of skin which overlaps the lunula at the base of the nail plate. It forms a seal to prevent micro-organisms entering into the surrounding tissues. A healthy eponychium should be soft, supple and secure. This is the part of the nail that is freed from the nail plate during a manicure.

Perionychium

This covers the outer portion and sides of the nail.

GROWTH CYCLE OF THE NAIL

NAIL FORMATION

The nail grows as new cells are produced in the nail matrix pushing the older cells forward.

FACTORS AFFECTING GROWTH AND GROWTH RATES

Fingernails grow at a rate of about 3–5 mm a month. It takes 3–5 months to grow from the matrix to the free edge. Toenails grow at about half this speed. It takes 8–9 months to grow a full new toenail. The growth of the nail is affected by several factors.

Dominant hand

If you are right-handed your dominant hand is your right hand.

SmartScreen 208 Worksheet 6 and Worksheet 7

SmartScreen 207 Worksheet 4

Factor	Effect on nail growth
Activity levels or what you do	The nails on the **dominant hand** grow more quickly because that hand is more active. Similarly thumbnails grow faster than fingernails as thumbs are more active.
	Toenails grow more slowly as although we use our feet all the time we do not flex our toes like we do our fingers.
Circulation	Nails grow faster in the summer when we are warmer and our circulation is improved and slower in the winter when we are cold and the circulation more restricted.
	The circulation has to work harder to reach the feet, which is another reason why toenails grow more slowly than fingernails.
	Buffing nails stimulates the circulation and helps to encourage smooth healthy nail growth.
Age	As we get older cellular activity slows down and the circulation becomes less efficient. Nail growth is slower and the growth is more likely to show flaws or imperfections on the nail plate.
Diet	A poor diet which has insufficient minerals and nutrients will affect the health of the nail.

NAIL SHAPES

The natural nail shape is **determined by** the matrix. The free edge can be manicured into different shapes including squoval, tapered and pointed.

NATURAL NAIL SHAPES

Nail shape	Description	
Fan/tapered	Fan-shaped nails are wider at the free edge than at the base of the nail. The nail plate might be quite short in length. The nail base is usually very curved but the hyponychium might be quite straight.	Fan
Narrow	The nail plate is long and slim with a delicate oblong shape.	Narrow
Square	The nail plate is the same length as its width. The base of the nail and hyponychium tend to be quite straight.	Square
Oval	An oval nail has a delicately curved hyponychium and cuticle giving the nail plate an oval appearance.	Oval
Round	These naturally have a very curved base and hyponychium and a short nail plate.	Round
Ski jump	As the nail grows and extends beyond the free edge the nail plate curves upwards.	Ski jump
Hook	Hook nails are also called claw nails because the nail has an exaggerated curve causing the free edge to fold over the end of the finger.	Hook

Determined by

Decided by.

MANICURED NAIL SHAPES

WHY DON'T YOU...
copy the list of natural nail shapes. Examine your colleagues' hands and write down everyone's natural nail shape. Look at the line of the free edge and the line of the cuticle, not the shape that the nail might have been filed into. Which shape is the most common? Now write down everyone's manicured nail shape. How does this compare?

HANDY HINTS

See Chapter 207/208 for more information about contra-indications to nail services.

Nail shape	Description	
Pointed/ stiletto	A pointed filed shape.	Pointed
Squoval	The nail is cut straight across with gently rounded corners.	Squoval

Nail disorder

Change in the structure of a healthy nail.

NAIL DISEASES AND DISORDERS

The majority of **nail disorders** can be treated. Regular manicures or pedicures will help to improve the circulation, the condition of the nail and surrounding skin, and the appearance of the nail plate. A nail disease is usually more serious and your client might need to see their doctor.

NAIL DISEASES AND DISORDERS THAT CAN RESTRICT TREATMENT

Disorder	Description and cause	Contra-indications and general precautions	Advice for client
Anonychia (an-uh-nik-ee-uh)	The total congenital absence of a nail.	Not contra-indicated. This obviously limits treatment as there is no nail to treat or enamel. The fingers or toes will be more sensitive without the protection of the nail plate.	None.
Beau lines	Distinct horizontal depressions (dips) on all the nails. When seen on all the nails they can mean that there has been a serious acute illness. Can also be caused by medication. Can be seen in **conjunction** with severe dermatitis.	Not contra-indicated. **Conjunction** Linked or combined.	Draw their attention to the damage and see if they are aware of why it has happened.

Disorder	Description and cause	Contra-indications and general precautions	Advice for client
Koilonychia (spoon-shaped nails) (*keel-oh-nik-ee-uh*)	Nail plate grows with a distinct **concave** shape. Often the nail is thin, soft and very flexible. Causes include iron deficiency (**anaemia**), over use of chemicals, heart disease and some endocrine diseases. Can also be an inherited nail shape. **Concave** Dipped or hollowed. **Anaemia** Not having enough iron.	Not contra-indicated. Treat gently.	Use a protective nail treatment base coat or nail conditioner to help strengthen the nails.
Leukonychia (white spots) (*lou-co-nik-ee-uh*)	Caused by the separation of the nail plate layers. A white spot is an sign of trauma, eg knocking a nail. When white spots are seen in a similar line on all nails they can be a result of an illness (high temperature). Not caused by a lack of calcium.	Not contra-indicated.	Let the client know what causes the condition so they can take care to avoid further damage. It might be worth checking with the client how their health was a few months back.
Habit tic	Caused by repeated self-harming trauma or picking of the nail plate, leaving it ridged and uneven.	Not contra-indicated.	Using a dark-coloured nail polish can help to draw attention to the nails so the client becomes more aware of their habit. Buffing will help to smooth the nail.
Longitudinal furrows	Damage to the nail matrix causes deep ridges in the nail plate. This can be caused by a single event or by a **systemic** illness. **Systemic** An illness affecting one of the systems of the body.	Not contra-indicated.	A ridge filler will help to improve the appearance and surface of the nail plate. Regular buffing will help to smooth the nail plate and increase the circulation to encourage healthy nail growth.

Disorder	Description and cause	Contra-indications and general precautions	Advice for client
Onychophagy (nail biting) (*on-i-kof-uh-jee*)	A nervous condition. The free edge of the nail and sometimes the skin around it is bitten off. The flesh at the top of the finger appears to be bulging as there is no nail plate to cover it.	Not contra-indicated. Severely bitten nails might restrict nail services. It might be best not to recommend nail enhancements. It is difficult to attach them securely to the remaining nail plate area.	The nails can be coated with a special bitter tasting nail product to discourage nibbling. Keep the cuticles soft to help prevent nibbling hard skin. File away any free edge to reduce the area that can be bitten.
Onychocyanosis (blue nail) (*on-ee-choc-an-o-sis*)	Nails have a blue **tinge** caused by poor circulation. **Tinge** A trace of colour.	Not contra-indicated *but* it might be a sign of a heart condition. If the client has very blue nails ask them what their circulation is like. Do they get very cold hands?	Massage will benefit the circulation and encourage healthy nail growth.
Splinter haemorrhage	Trauma can cause a small section of the nail plate to lift from the nail bed leading to bleeding under the nail plate. It looks like there is a splinter in the nail plate. This can happen when nails are too long and put pressure on the nail bed at the free edge causing it to lift along the hyponychium.	Not contra-indicated. Take care as the bruise can be caused by damage to the nail plate. Avoid any pressure on the nail plate. Do *not* buff.	Shorten very long nails.

Disorder	Description and cause	Contra-indications and general precautions	Advice for client
Lamella dystrophy	When the nail plate becomes very dry the layers separate. Look for peeling or flaking along the free edge.	Not contra-indicated. Avoid products which might dehydrate the nail plate (eg overuse of nail enamel remover).	Do not file across the nail. Use a conditioning product to nourish and hydrate the nail. Buff the nail gently to remove any loose nail and smooth the nail. This will stimulate the circulation and encourage healthy nail growth.
Pitting	Tiny pits in the nail plate (as if someone has taken a pen and tapped it) are a symptom of psoriasis.	Not contra-indicated. This condition is difficult to improve.	Buffing the nail will help to stimulate the circulation and encourage healthy nail growth.
Onychorrexis (brittle nail syndrome) (*on-i-ko-rek-sis*)	Very common. Brittle nail plates break easily. There are often longitudinal ridges in the nail plate. Can lead to other conditions, eg peeling. Can be a symptom of hypothyroidism (when the thyroid gland does not make enough thyroid hormone) or anaemia.	Not contra-indicated. Avoid harsh chemicals or products that will dry the nail plate further (eg nail enamel remover).	Condition hands and nails to help rehydrate the nail.

SmartScreen 208 Worksheet 2

NAIL DISEASES AND DISORDERS REQUIRING CAUTION

Disorder	Description and cause	Contra-indications and general precautions	Advice for client
Severely bruised nail	A blackened area of tissue under the nail plate. Nail trauma, eg a heavy blow or regular long distance running, damages the blood vessels which causes blood to seep into the surrounding tissues. It will grow out with the nail.	Contra-indicated. Avoid the bruised nail to prevent further damage. The nail plate could be loose if the damage was severe.	Monitor affected toenails for possible lifting as the nail grows out. Avoid any pressure on the nail.
Onychogryphosis (*on-e-koh-gri-foh-sis*)	Crooked, curved, thickened nails. The nail plate becomes enlarged and misshapen. The nail can become claw like or curve forward or sideways. Usually only affects toenails. Usually caused by poor circulation.	Not contra-indicated. The nails might be very difficult to cut.	Refer client to a podiatrist if the nails are difficult to cut.
Onychauxis (hypertrophy) (*on-e-corx-is*)	Causes extreme thickening of the nail plates on one or more toenails.	Not contra-indicated. Caution required. Thickened toenails can be very difficult to cut.	Refer the client to a podiatrist who will have more specialised tools.
Onychoptosis (*on-ee-chop-toe-sis*)	**Shedding** of the nail plate from the finger or toe. **Shedding** When the nail falls off.	Not contra-indicated. Treatment will have to be changed.	**Monitor** pressure on the nail (eg running shoes on toenails) to see if there is a link. **Monitor** Keeping an eye on.

Disorder	Description and cause	Contra-indications and general precautions	Advice for client
Onychomalacia (eggshell nails) (on-ee-chom-al-a-c-ah)	Thin weak soft nails which can look cloudy. Can be caused by illness, poor diet or stress.	Not contra-indicated. Take extra care when you are working on these fragile nails.	Treat nails carefully. Regular manicures and hand massage will help. Seek medical advice if this is a concern.

NAIL DISEASES AND DISORDERS THAT WILL PREVENT TREATMENT

The following conditions will prevent treatment. You must be able to recognise them so that you can advise your client to seek medical advice.

Disorder	Description and cause	Contra-indications and general precautions	Advice for client
Onychatrophia (atrophy) (on-ee-chat-tro-fi-ah)	**Wasting** of the nail plate. It looks dull and cloudy and might even come away from the nail bed. Caused by injury, strong chemicals or disease. **Wasting** When something is no longer healthy.	Contra-indicated. Avoid the nail plate to prevent any further damage.	Seek medical advice.
Onychomicosis/tinea unguium (ringworm of the nail) (on-i-koh-me-koh-sis)	The nail rots. The nail plate is discoloured (can vary from yellow to brown) and powdery. The nail plate has lifted. Often a build-up of discoloured tissue can be seen under the nail plate. Caused by fungus or bacteria which feeds on keratin.	Contra-indicated. Contagious.	Seek medical advice.

Disorder	Description and cause	Contra-indications and general precautions	Advice for client
Onycholysis (severe nail separation) (*on-ee-kol-e-sis*)	Severe separation of the nail from the nail bed. Nail plate looks white not pink. If you tap the surface of the nail you will hear a hollow sound.	Contra-indicated. Contagious. Check the nail very carefully to make sure it is onycholysis. Some non-contagious conditions, eg a bruise growing out or psoriasis, can also cause the nail to lift.	Seek medical advice.

HANDY HINTS

See also warts and verrucae page 27.

Analyse

The result of looking at something carefully.

Prevented

Stop something from taking place.

DISEASES AND DISORDERS AFFECTING THE CUTICLE AND SKIN

It is just as important to **analyse** the skin around the nail. Cuticles are just as important as perfect nails for beautiful hands. Hang nails are one of the most common conditions you will need to correct during a manicure. Often they can easily be **prevented**. Some nasty infections start around the base of the nail and will contra-indicate treatment. These bacterial infections can cause a lot of damage to the nail matrix.

Disorder	Description and cause	Contra-indications and general precautions	Advice for client
Hang nail	The cuticle or nail wall splits leaving a loose piece of skin. Caused by very dry or uncared for skin and cuticles that tear as the nail grows.	Not contra-indicated. Take care to avoid cross-infection as the skin is open.	Keep cuticles nourished, conditioned and pushed back to avoid tearing as the nail grows.
Pterygium (*terr-e-gee-um*)	The cuticle sticks to the nail plate as it grows forming a shield of skin. Caused by excessive cuticle growth.	Not contra-indicated. Avoid damaging the nail plate by trying to lift and push the cuticle back.	At home, treat cuticles daily to keep them nourished and conditioned. Keep the skin pushed back to avoid tearing as the nail grows.

Disorder	Description and cause	Contra-indications and general precautions	Advice for client
Onychia (*oh-nik-ee-uh*) 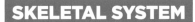	Bacterial infection of the nail fold causing the skin around the base of the nail to become red and inflamed. Pus might be visible.	Contra-indicated. Contagious.	Seek medical advice.
Paronychia (*parr-uh-nik-ee-uh*)	A bacterial infection of the cuticle. Symptoms include tenderness, redness and swelling in the infected area. A small pus-filled spot will appear if the condition is not treated.	Contra-indicated. Contagious.	Seek medical advice.
Onychocryptosis (ingrown nail) (*on-i-koh-krip-toe-sis*)	Symptoms include discomfort or pain around the side of the nail as well as redness and swelling. It is caused by poorly fitting shoes and incorrect nail care, in particular incorrect filing or cutting of the nail. It is often seen on the big toe.	Contra-indicated. Avoid the skin around the infected toenail.	Consult a podiatrist who will remove the part of the nail with the disorder. If very infected the client might need to seek medical advice.

SKELETAL SYSTEM

Bone is the hardest tissue in the human body. Bone is made from specialised cells called osteocytes which create rigid non-elastic tissue. These cells are surrounded by a matrix of collagen fibres strengthened by calcium and **phosphate**. Bones have lots of hollow spaces within their structure that serve to both make the bone light and to provide tiny spaces for blood vessels and nerves to supply the bone tissue.

Phosphate

A chemical compound containing phosphorous.

In this part of the chapter you will learn about:

- the function and structure of the skeleton
- the types of joints and the range of movement provided
- the structure of the head, shoulder, girdle, vertebral column and limb bones
- skeletal conditions that restrict treatment.

FUNCTIONS OF THE SKELETON

The skeleton has five main functions.

1 Protection – the skull protects the brain; the spine protects the spinal cord; the rib cage protects the heart and lungs.

2 Support – bones give support for the muscles of the body and give shape to the body contours and the characteristics of our face shape.

3 Movement – bones have ridges where muscles attach to allow bones and joints to provide flexible movement.

4 Formation of blood cells – all red blood cells and some of the white blood cells are made of specialised tissue called bone marrow.

5 Storage and release of certain vitamins and minerals – including calcium and phosphorous.

STRUCTURE OF THE SKELETAL SYSTEM

SHAPES OF BONE

There are 206 bones in the body and these are shaped according to the function they need to perform. There are five different shapes or types of bone:

1 long bones

2 short bones

3 irregular bones

4 flat bones

5 sesamoid bones.

Long bones

These act as levers to raise and lower limbs. They have a shaft, made of compact bone with a central canal that contains bone marrow, and two ends that have an outer covering of compact bone. Long bones contain bone marrow.

Short bones

These often form bridges and are subject to pressure type forces, eg the wrist and ankle.

Irregular bones

These often have complex shapes, eg the vertebra.

Flat bones

These bones are good for creating protective shells, eg the bones of the cranium and the sternum and scapular in the torso.

Sesamoid bones

These are often rounded bones and sit inside tendons or synovial joints, eg the patella/knee cap.

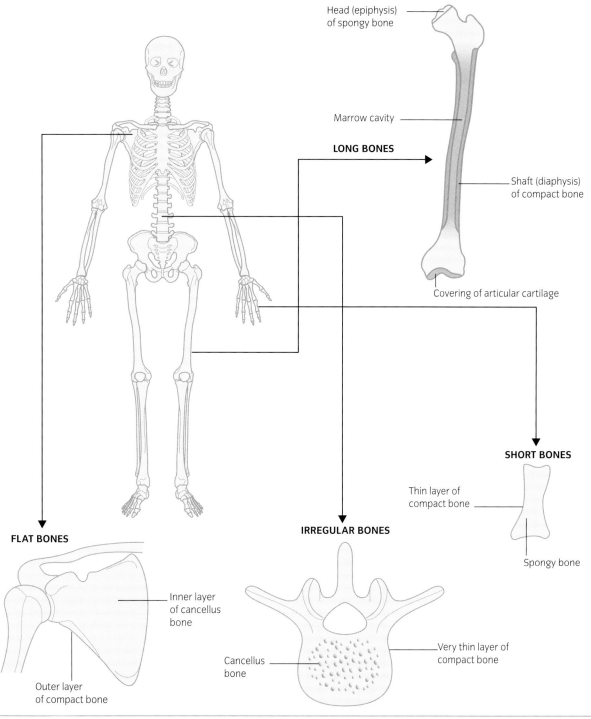

Head (epiphysis)
of spongy bone

Marrow cavity

LONG BONES

Shaft (diaphysis)
of compact bone

Covering of articular cartilage

SHORT BONES

Thin layer of
compact bone

Spongy bone

FLAT BONES

Inner layer
of cancellus
bone

Outer layer
of compact bone

IRREGULAR BONES

Cancellus
bone

Very thin layer of
compact bone

Structure of the skeletal system

JOINTS

A joint is where two bones meet. Muscles and tendons stretch across joints when they move. Joints are **classified** by their structure or by the way they move. There are three main types of joints:

1 fibrous/fixed joints

2 cartilaginous/slightly moveable joints

3 synovial/freely moveable joints.

FIBROUS/FIXED JOINTS

These joints are tight linked with a tough fibrous material and have virtually no movement, eg the skull.

Classified

Arranged or assigned to a particular category or type.

CARTILAGINOUS/SLIGHTLY MOVEABLE JOINTS

These joints are formed by a pad of tough fibrous cartilage and have no or only a limited range of movement. The pad acts as a shock absorber (eg joints between the vertebrae).

SYNOVIAL JOINTS/FREELY MOVEABLE JOINTS

As their name suggests these joints have the ability to move and they have a range of movement. The majority of joints in the body are synovial. Each bone end is covered with a smooth coating of cartilage. In the small space between the bones is a lubricating liquid called synovial fluid. Around this is a capsule to hold the joint in place. Ligaments provide stability to the joint.

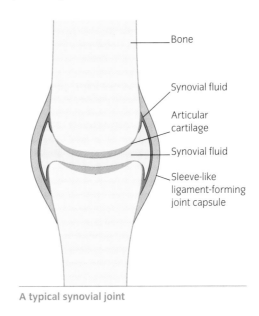

Bone

Synovial fluid

Articular cartilage

Synovial fluid

Sleeve-like ligament-forming joint capsule

A typical synovial joint

TYPES AND LOCATION OF SYNOVIAL JOINTS

Type of synovial joint	Description	Movement range
Ball and socket Intracapsular ligament Socket (pelvis) Ball (head of femur)	The rounder end of one bone fits into a neat cup-shaped cavity in another bone (eg the shoulder and hip).	Flexion, extension, adduction, abduction, rotation and circumduction. See page 54 for more details.
Hinge Humerus Radius Ulna	The convex (rounded outward) surface of the end of one bone fits in the concave surface of a second bone (or bones), eg elbow and knee. (Think of the hinge of a door.)	Flexion and extension.

Type of synovial joint	Description	Movement range
Pivot **Pivot joint** Atlas Axis	A bony projection from one joint turns within the ring-shaped socket of another. The top two cervical vertebra allow the head to turn from side to side.	Rotation.
Gliding/plane **Gliding joint** Tarsals Metatarsals	The surfaces of the bone are almost flat and glide over each other (eg **tarsals** and **metatarsals**). **Tarsals** Bones of the ankle and heel. **Metatarsals** Bones of the foot.	Range is limited.
Condyloid **Condyloid joint** Radius Scaphoid	This is a smooth rounded **projection** on a bone which sits into a cup-shaped depression on another bone (eg mandible and temporal bone, metacarpal and phalange). **Projection** A part that sticks out.	Flexion, extension abduction, adduction and circumduction.
Saddle **Saddle joint** Trapezium of the wrist First metacarpel bone of the thumb	The surfaces of the two bones that meet have both concave and convex surfaces. There is only one saddle joint in the body at the base of the thumb.	Movement range is similar to condyloid.

LIGAMENTS

Ligaments are made up of strings of connective tissue consisting of tough fibrous collagen protein. Their function is to hold bones together.

When bones are next to each other, ligaments link the bones where they meet at the joints. Some ligaments hold bones together so tightly that they can hardly move. Others are looser and allow the bones to change position. Ligaments are extremely strong. Although they sometimes tear it takes a very powerful jolt to break them.

TYPES OF MOVEMENTS OF JOINTS

Type of movement	Description
Adduction	A movement towards the body.
Abduction	A movement away from the body.
Flexion	A bending movement bringing two level joints together.
Extension	Straightening a joint ie taking two levers away from each other.
Rotation	The movement of a bone in a circle around a fixed point.
Circumduction	The movement of a limb or finger with little movement where it is attached and greater movement at the end. For example, where the finger is attached to the hand its movement is small but the finer tip can draw a large circle.

ACTIVITY

Stand up. Now go through each of the range of movements so that you are familiar with them.

STRUCTURE OF THE HEAD, SHOULDER GIRDLE, VERTEBRAL COLUMN AND LIMB BONES

BONES OF THE HEAD

The skull consists of the cranium, which encloses and protects the brain. The cranium consists of eight bones, which are fused together.

Bones of the head	Position
Frontal	Front of the cranium. One bone forming the forehead.
Occipital	One bone forming the back of the skull.
Parietal	Two bones forming the sides and roof of the cranium.
Sphenoid	One bone forming the back of the eye sockets and the middle of the cranium.

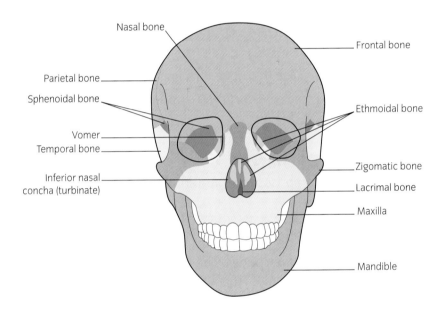

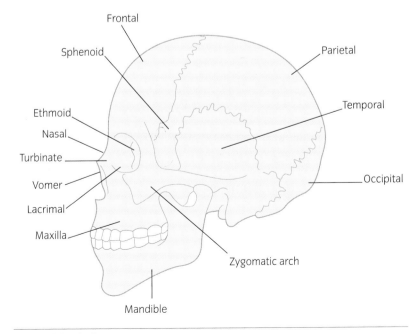

Bones of the skull

Bones of the head	Position
Temporal	Two bones forming the sides of the skull. It sits under the ears.
Ethmoid	One bone between the eye sockets forming part of the nasal cavity.

There are also 14 facial bones.

Facial bones	Position
Maxillae	Two bones forming the upper jaw.
Zygomatic arch	Two bones forming the cheekbones.
Nasal	Two bones forming the bridge of the nose.
Mandible	Lower jaw bone.
Palatine	Two bones forming the floor of the nose and the roof of the mouth.
Inferior conchae	Two bones forming the sides of the nasal cavity.
Vomer	One thin bone forming the nasal septum.
Lacrimal	Two bones forming the inner wall of the eye sockets.

VERTEBRAL COLUMN

The vertebral column comprises of 33 vertebrae bones. Of these, 24 bones are moveable.

Bones of the spine	Position
Cervical	Seven bones. The first cervical bone is called the atlas. This sits on the second cervical vertebra known as the axis. The axis allows the head to rotate and the atlas supports the position of the skull.
Thoracic	Twelve bones. The ribs are attached to the thoracic vertebra.
Lumbar	Five bones between the ribs and pelvis.
Sacral	Five fused bones between the pelvis.
Coccyx	Four fused bones that form a small tail at the base of the spine.

The functions of the vertebral column are to:

- protect the spinal cord
- provide a pathway for delicate spinal nerves to sit while being protected
- allow flexion, extension and rotation
- support the skull
- absorb shock – there are special discs which sit in between the vertebrae that absorb shock during movement to prevent tissue damage

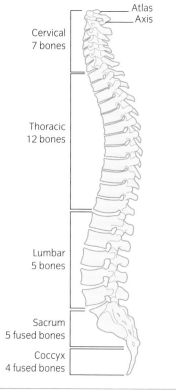

Atlas
Axis
Cervical
7 bones

Thoracic
12 bones

Lumbar
5 bones

Sacrum
5 fused bones

Coccyx
4 fused bones

The spinal column

- provide attachment for other bones, including the ribs, shoulder girdle, arms and pelvis
- provide attachment for muscles.

BONE STRUCTURE OF THE TORSO

Bones of the chest

The sternum (breastbone) is a bone that runs down the centre of the chest and connects to most of the ribs. There are 12 ribs which all connect with the **thoracic vertebra**. Only the upper seven ribs connect to the sternum at the front of the chest. They protect the internal organs of the chest.

> **Thoracic vertebra**
>
> Each of the 12 bones of the backbone to which the ribs are attached.

Thorax

The thorax is the protective cavity for the chest and includes the ribs and sternum. The sternum runs down the centre of the chest and is commonly known as the breastbone. The ribs are long flat bones that run across the sides of the chest and there are 12 pairs in total. At the front of the body they are attached to the sternum and at the back of the body they are attached to the vertebra.

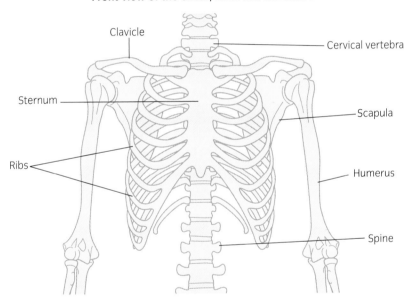

Front view of the chest, neck and shoulders

Clavicle · Cervical vertebra · Sternum · Scapula · Ribs · Humerus · Spine

Shoulder girdle

The shoulder girdle includes:

- two scapulae – the large bones at the back that look like wings
- two clavicles – the bones that sit across the shoulder
- the upper ends of the two humerus bones – the bones of the upper arm.

BONE STRUCTURE OF THE UPPER LIMBS

The arms consist of the:

- humerus (upper arm)
- ulna (forearm) – runs along the little finger side of the forearm
- radius (forearm) – runs along the side of the thumb in the forearm.

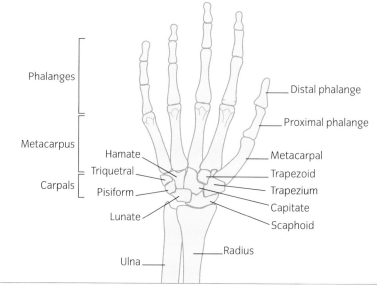

Phalanges

Metacarpus

Carpals

Distal phalange

Proximal phalange

Metacarpal

Trapezoid

Trapezium

Capitate

Scaphoid

Hamate

Triquetral

Pisiform

Lunate

Radius

Ulna

Bones of the arm and hand

Bone structure of the hands

The hands consist of:

- eight carpals (wrist): triangular, lunate, scaphoid, trapezium, trapezoid, pisiform, hamate and capitate. These eight bones form the wrist.
- five **metacarpals** (these form the palm of the hand)
- fourteen phalanges (these form the fingers).

Metacarpals
Bones of the hand.

ACTIVITY

Look at your hand. Can you make out any of the bones of the carpals?

BONE STRUCTURE OF THE LOWER LIMBS

The legs consist of the:

- femur – forms the thigh and is the longest bone in the body
- patella – the knee cap
- tibia – on the big toe side of the lower leg and commonly called the shin bone
- fibula – on the little toe side of the lower leg.

WHY DON'T YOU...
look at your bare foot. Can you make out any of the bones of the tarsals?

BONE STRUCTURE OF THE FEET

The feet consist of:

- seven tarsals (talus, calcaneus or heel bone, cuboid, central cuneiform, medial cuneiform, lateral cuneiform, navicular)
- five metatarsals (the main part of the foot)
- fourteen phalanges (forms the toes).

The ankle is formed from the talus bone and the ends at the tibia and fibula.

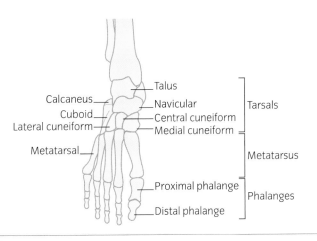

Calcaneus
Cuboid
Lateral cuneiform
Metatarsal
Talus
Navicular
Central cuneiform
Medial cuneiform
Tarsals
Metatarsus
Proximal phalange
Distal phalange
Phalanges

Bones of the foot

INDUSTRY TIP

Hammer toes occur where the second, third and fourth toe joints become deformed causing the joints to become permanently bent.

Bunions are caused by wearing high heels and poorly fitting shoes.

SKELETAL CONDITIONS THAT RESTRICT TREATMENT

Skeletal conditions can be easily overlooked as they are hidden away from view inside the body. It is important to remember that whether something is inside or not the body needs time to repair itself. The conditions below will require you to **modify** your treatment. You should not work over the area directly around a sprain or broken bone.

Modify

Making changes to your treatment.

Skeletal condition	Description and cause	Contra-indications and general precautions
Bunion	A big toe joint is displaced and inflamed. Fluid collects around the joint. Caused by repeated pressure on the side of the first metatarsal, commonly from wearing tight, poorly fitting shoes.	Not contra-indicated. Take extra care as the joint might be very tender. Massage should be very gentle.
Broken and fractured bones	A fracture is a crack or a break in the bone either across its width or **diagonally** across the bone shaft, or where the bone is shattered into small pieces. A **compound** or open fracture happens when the bone breaks through the skin's surface. Closed fractures happen when the bone is still within the body. These can cause large tissue damage in the area of the break. A greenstick fracture is where a long bone is fractured along the bone but not all the way through.	Contra-indicated. Do not treat the area until fully healed to prevent further tissue damage. **Diagonally** In a slanted direction. **Compound break** An injury where there is a break in the skin around a broken bone.
Sprains	When a ligament is overstretched or torn. A common area for sprains is around the ankle joint. A sprain can occur as the result of a fall when the full force of the body's weight is placed onto a joint.	Contra-indicated. Do not treat until it is fully healed to prevent any further tissue damage or discomfort to the client.

MUSCULAR SYSTEM

Our muscular system includes all the muscle tissue in the body. It provides movement, maintains posture and is vital for the function of the organs of the body, including the heart and digestive system.

In this part of the chapter you will learn about:

- the structure and function of the muscular system
- the three types of muscle tissue
- the action of the main muscles of the head and face, thorax, shoulder, arm, hand, lower leg and foot.

STRUCTURE AND FUNCTION OF THE MUSCULAR SYSTEM

The muscular system has several functions:

- **Movement:** Movement happens as a result of the shortening (contracting) and the lengthening (extending) of muscle tissue.
- **Posture:** Some of the muscle's fibres are always contracted even when the muscle is at rest. Otherwise the body would not be able to function. This is essential for maintaining posture. This muscle tone is weakest when we are sleeping and in a relaxed state. Muscle tone makes sure enough blood supply reaches the muscles.
- **Creation of heat:** Muscular activity creates heat in the cellular tissues.
- **Assists with blood flow and lymphatic movement:** Muscular movement squeezes the blood and lymphatic vessels which helps to assist both blood flow and lymphatic movement.
- **Protection:** Some muscles also help to provide protection for some of the abdominal organs.

TYPES OF MUSCULAR TISSUE

There are three types of muscular tissue:

1 cardiac muscle

2 smooth, involuntary muscle

3 skeletal, striated or voluntary muscle.

Cardiac muscle
This is a specialised type of muscular tissue found only in the heart.

Smooth, involuntary muscle
This is not under **conscious** control and is found in the walls of hollow organs, ie blood and lymphatic vessels, alimentary canal (digestive system), **respiratory** tract, bladder, uterus and ducts of glands.

Skeletal, striated or voluntary
Theses muscles are under conscious control. A tiny motor nerve carries messages from the central nervous system to the muscle to stimulate it into action. There are 650 named muscles in our body; 150 of these muscles are in the head and neck. Skeletal muscles make up about 40 to 50 per cent of our body weight. Each muscle is made up of thousands of long narrow cells which look like fibres. These cells are surrounded by a tough sheath.

Conscious

When you are aware of what you are controlling.

Respiratory

The system for taking in oxygen and giving out carbon dioxide, which happens in humans by breathing.

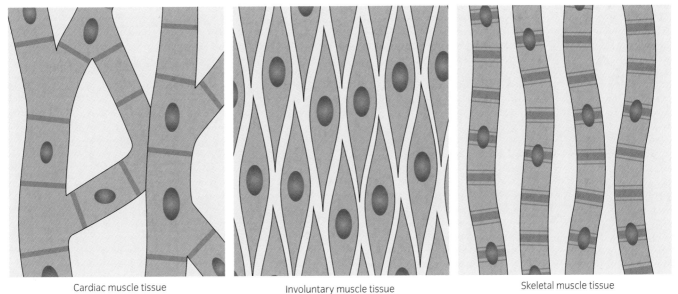

Cardiac muscle tissue

Involuntary muscle tissue

Skeletal muscle tissue

MUSCLES OF THE HEAD AND FACE

The muscles of our face **define** our facial characteristics and features. They give us expression and show our age. You will find it particularly helpful to know the location and action of each muscle during facial massage treatments.

Define

To describe or explain exactly.

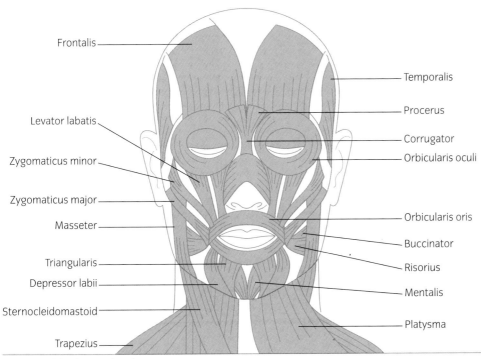

Frontalis

Temporalis

Procerus

Levator labatis

Corrugator

Zygomaticus minor

Orbicularis oculi

Zygomaticus major

Orbicularis oris

Masseter

Buccinator

Triangularis

Risorius

Depressor labii

Mentalis

Sternocleidomastoid

Platysma

Trapezius

Muscles of the face and neck

Facial muscle	Position	Action
Occipital frontalis	Forehead over frontal bone and at back of cranium over occipital bone. Two muscles are joined together by a flat tendon that stretches over the top of the skull.	Raises the brow and eyebrows. Forms horizontal frown lines or wrinkles.
Temporalis	Side of the head stretching to the mandible (jaw).	Raises the mandible during chewing.
Orbicularis oculi	Surrounds the eye socket.	Closes the eyelids.

Facial muscle	Position	Action
Corrugator	Between the eyebrows.	Depresses the forehead to frown.
Buccinator	At the sides of the cheek.	Squeezes the cheeks together during chewing.
Risorius	Runs from the corners of the mouth.	Lifts the corners of the mouth into a smile.

Facial muscle	Position	Action
Quadratus labii superioris	Sides of the upper lip.	Lifts the upper lip.
Depressor labii	Runs down the chin from the lower lip.	Pulls the lower lip down.
Procerus	Between the brows, extending down to the nasal bone.	Draws the eyebrows down in a frown.

Facial muscle	Position	Action
Nasalis	Crosses the bridge of the nose.	One part dilates and one part constricts the nostrils.
Triangularis	Outer part of the mandible.	Draws the sides of mouth down.
Orbicularis oris	Around the mouth.	Closes the mouth and pouts the lips.

Facial muscle	Position	Action
Masseter	Sides of the face.	Raises the lower jaw, help us to chew food.
Zygomaticus major	Along the cheek.	Raises the corner of the mouth into a smile.
Mentalis	Over the chin.	Allows the lower lip to pout.

Facial muscle	Position	Action
Sternocleidomastoid	Sides of the neck.	When the muscles work singularly they help to rotate the head, together they pull the head forward (chin down).
Platysma	From the chin down the front of the neck.	Draws the corners of the mouth down, lowers the mandible and maintains skin texture.

INDUSTRY TIP

If you confuse orbicularis oris and oculi, remember the i in oculi for eye.

 SmartScreen 204 Worksheet 10

MUSCLES OF THE THORAX

The thorax relates to the chest area. There are two muscles that you should know as we touch on these muscles during facial treatments.

Thorax muscles	Position	Action
Trapezius	A large diamond shaped muscle that extends from the occipital bone to the vertebra in the thoracic region.	Lifts and braces the shoulders, rotates the scapula.
Pectoralis major	Front of the chest.	Flexion, adduction and rotation of the upper arm, draws the arm across the chest.

MUSCLES OF THE SHOULDER, ARM AND HAND

It is important to be aware of these muscles during facials and manicures.

Muscles in the shoulder, arm and hand	Position	Action
Deltoid	Lies over the shoulder (like a shoulder pad).	Draws the arm backwards and forwards, abducts the arm.
Levator scapula	At the back of the neck between the cervical vertebra and the scapula.	Lifts the shoulder and rotates the scapula.
Biceps	Front of the upper arm.	Turns and flexes the forearm, flexion of the elbow.

Muscles in the shoulder, arm and hand	Position	Action
Triceps	Back of the upper arm. Extensor carpi radialis longus	Extension of the arm at the elbow.
Extensor carpi radialis longus	Covering the back of the forearm. Brachio radialis Extensor carpi radialis longus Extensor carpi radialis brevis Flexor carpi radialis Palmaris longus Flexor carpi ulnaris Flexor digitorum Thenar eminence Hypothenar eminence Extensor carpi ulnaris Extensor digitorum	Extension and abduction of the wrist.

Muscles in the shoulder, arm and hand	Position	Action
Extensor carpi ulnaris	Covering the back of the forearm.	Extends the wrist and adducts the hand.
Extensor carpi radialis brevis	Inner side of the forearm.	Extends and abducts the wrist and flexes the forearm.
Flexor carpi radialis	Front of the forearm.	Flexes and abducts the hands.

Muscles in the shoulder, arm and hand	Position	Action
Flexor carpi ulnaris	Front of the forearm.	Flexes and adducts the ulna.
Extensor digitorum	Back of the forearm.	Extends the fingers and the wrist.
Thenar eminence	A group of small muscles located in the thumb and palm of the hand.	Movement of the thumb.

Pronator quadratus

Thenar muscles

Flexor carpi ulnaris

Hypothenar muscles

MUSCLES OF THE LOWER LEG AND FOOT

There are some large muscles that give the lower leg its shape and definition. There are lots of smaller muscles that attach to different bones to flex and extend the lower leg, foot and toes.

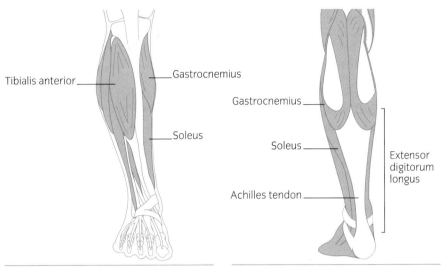

Muscles of the lower leg (front view)   Muscles of the lower leg (back view)

Muscles in the lower leg and foot	Position	Action
Gastrocnemius	Forms the bulk of the calf at the back of the lower leg.	**Plantar** flexion of the ankle, flexes the leg at the knee joint. **Plantar** Sole of the foot.
Soleus	Lies under the gastrocnemius.	Plantar flexion of the foot.
Tibialis anterior	Runs along the outside of the tibia.	Inverts the foot, flexes the foot.
Flexors of the toes – flexor digitorum brevis, flexor digitorum accessorius, flexor hallucis brevis	The lower leg and to the heel of the foot.	Flexes the toes.
Extensors of the toes – extensor digitorum brevis, extensor digitorum longus, extensor hallucis longus	The lower leg and the foot.	Extends the toes and flexes the ankle.

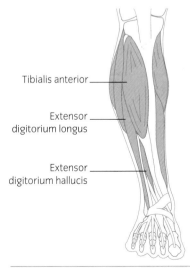

 SmartScreen 208 Worksheet 4

Muscles that flex the foot and ankle

CARDIOVASCULAR SYSTEM

The cardiovascular systemn includes the heart, blood vessels and blood cells. The blood is the transport system of the body making sure that the body is provided with the essential **nutrients** it needs to function. The blood cells play a crucial role in fighting infection and providing **immunity**.

Nutrients
Substances that help us grow.

Immunity
Being protected from a disease.

In this part of the chapter you will learn about:
- the basic structure of the cardiovascular system
- the functions of blood
- the primary blood vessels
- disorders of the cardiovascular system.

BASIC STRUCTURE OF THE CARDIOVASCULAR SYSTEM

HEART

The heart is a powerful pear-shaped muscular organ that sits in the centre of the chest, tilted at its base slightly to the left side. It is surrounded by a protective membrane called the pericardium. The pericardium is a fluid-filled cavity which prevents any friction between the heart and the surrounding tissues. The chambers of the heart vary in size according to the work being done. The atrium walls are very thin, as they only have to push blood into the ventricles. The ventricles are very thick as they have to push blood around the body.

Blood vessels of the heart
The most important blood vessels in the heart are:
- the vena cava which carries blood from the body into the right atrium
- the pulmonary vein which carries blood from the lungs into the left atrium
- the aorta which carries blood from the left ventricle to the left tissues.

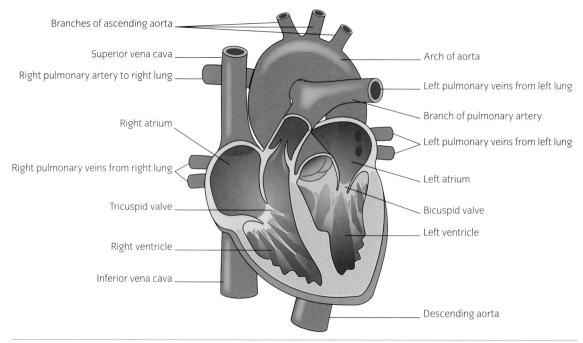

Branches of ascending aorta
Superior vena cava
Right pulmonary artery to right lung
Right atrium
Right pulmonary veins from right lung
Tricuspid valve
Right ventricle
Inferior vena cava

Arch of aorta
Left pulmonary veins from left lung
Branch of pulmonary artery
Left pulmonary veins from left lung
Left atrium
Bicuspid valve
Left ventricle
Descending aorta

Structure of the heart

FUNCTIONS OF BLOOD

Our blood can be described as our life force, making sure our cells have all the essential supplies they need and keeping **micro-organisms** at bay.

The blood has several essential functions. These functions can be divided into two main areas:

- transportation
- protection.

TRANSPORTATION

The erythrocytes transport oxygen attached to **haemoglobin** from the lungs to the body's cells and return carbon dioxide from the cells to the lungs for **elimination**. Hormones and enzymes are transported from their cells of production to their target organs and tissues.

The blood supplies nourishment to the cells. Nutrients are absorbed from the small intestine into the bloodstream and transported to where they are needed.

The circulation removes waste products from the cells and surrounding tissues. These waste materials are transported via circulation to the liver to be prepared for removal, and to the kidneys for excretion.

PROTECTION

Cells in the blood defend the body against **invasion** of micro-organisms and their toxins. They achieve this by:

- the phagocytic action of neutrophils and monocytes
- the presence of **antibodies** and **antitoxins**.

Clotting prevents the loss of any further body fluid and blood cells when the tissues are injured.

The blood helps to maintain the body temperature. Chemical activity in the cells and tissues produces heat. This heat makes the blood warm as it circulates. If the body produces too much heat the blood vessels near the surface of the body dilate and heat is lost by radiation, **conduction**, **convection** and the evaporation of sweat. If the external temperature is cold, the superficial blood vessels constrict to prevent heat loss.

COMPOSITION OF BLOOD

Blood accounts for 7–9 per cent of our total body weight and we have approximately 5.6 litres of this red viscous liquid flowing around our body. Around 55 per cent of blood is plasma and the other 45 per cent is made up from the different blood cells. The volume and **concentration** of our blood must be kept within narrow limits to maintain **homeostasis.**

Micro-organism

A very small living thing that can only be seen through a microscope.

Haemoglobin

A protein that gives red blood cells their colour. Their main function is to transport oxygen from the lungs to the body tissues.

Elimination

Getting rid of something.

Invasion

Entering uninvited.

Antibody

Also called immunoglobulin. Proteins produced by the body attach to micro-organisms and help to destroy them. They neutralise antigens.

Antitoxins

Antibodies that the body forms in response to a specific toxin with the capability of neutralising the toxin.

Conduction

Heat or electricity being passed from one object to another.

Convection

Movement of heat through a gas or liquid.

Concentration

Amount of.

Homeostasis

The body needs to maintain a constant state of internal balance. If one or more of the body's systems gets out of balance, ill health and disease can occur.

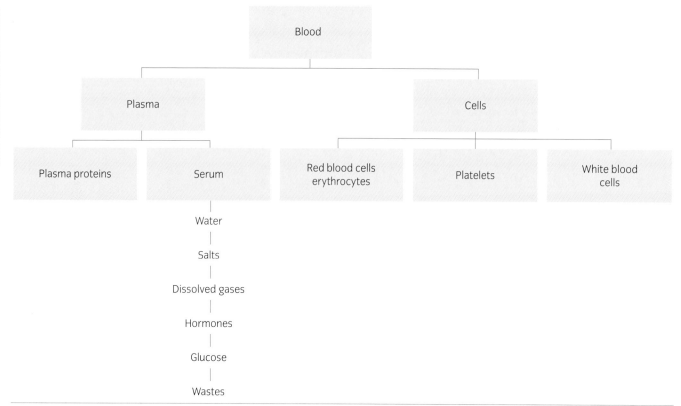

Composition of blood

Erythrocytes
Circular cells with a biconcave surface and no nucleus.

Molecule
The smallest amount of a substance.

Anticoagulant
A substance that prevents blood clotting.

Phagocytes
These help the body to dispose of unwanted matter, such as dirt and dead body cells. They engulf the matter and then digest it in a process called phagocytosis.

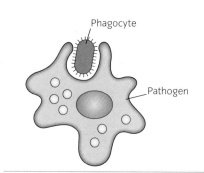

A phagocyte

Erythrocytes/red blood cells

Red blood cells account for 45 per cent of all blood cells .They contain the **molecule** haemoglobin that combines with oxygen to allow it to be transported around the body. Red blood cells are manufactured in the bone marrow of the short bones (ribs) and in the ends of the long bones.

White corpuscles – leukocytes

Leukocytes account for 1 per cent of the blood. They vary in size, shape and function.

Granulocytes are formed in the bone marrow. They develop into three different specialised cells, each having a specific function in response to injury and inflammation:

- eosinophils protect the body against foreign pathogens
- basophils contain an **anticoagulant** and histamine
- neutrophils are attracted to the site being invaded by micro-organisms and ingest foreign particles and damaged tissue through a process called **phagocytosis**.

Agranulocytes

These account for 25 to 50 per cent of all leukocytes. There are two types.

Monocytes

These cells are also formed in the red bone marrow. There are two different monocytes. One is phagocytic that engulfs germs. The other is a macrophage that has an important function in inflammation and immunity.

Lymphocytes

Lymphocytes circulate within the blood and are also found in lymphatic tissue. Unlike other blood cells they are developed in the lymphoid tissue as well in the red bone marrow. Larger lymphocytes play an essential role in immunity and help the body to recover. Lymphocytes respond to specific **antigens** and produce antigens. Antigens and antibodies work together. There are two different lymphocytes, each having a distinct function.

- **T-lymphocytes** combat and destroy cells containing antigens
- **B-lymphocytes** are involved in the production of the antibodies that neutralise antigens.

Antigen

Something that provokes an immune response against itself.

Plasma

Plasma is a transparent very pale yellow fluid. If you remove all the blood cells from the blood, this is what is left. Plasma is composed of many important elements including:

- water
- blood proteins
- salts and minerals, eg sodium chloride
- food substances, eg amino acids, glucose, fats
- waste, eg urea, uric acid
- gases, eg oxygen, carbon dioxide, nitrogen
- enzymes
- antibodies
- hormones
- antitoxins.

Thrombocytes/platelets

These are small fragments in the blood and play an essential role in blood clotting. When a blood vessel is damaged the blood vessels constrict and the thrombocytes stick to the damaged wall and form a thread-like mesh to prevent any further blood escaping.

ACTIVITY

Discuss with your tutor or manager what effect you think poor circulation will have on a client and how this might be noticed during a treatment. What treatments do you think will be beneficial and why?

BLOOD VESSELS

The blood vessels are our transport system and are responsible for transporting blood around the body, carrying blood from the heart to the tissues and back to the heart again.

ARTERIES

Arteries are blood vessels that carry oxygenated blood away from the heart (with the exception of the pulmonary artery). The oxygen the blood is transporting gives it a bright red colour. Arteries are designed to withstand the high pressure **exerted** from the blood as it is pumped from the heart. They vary in size but all have thick walls consisting of three layers of tissue. The middle layer is a thick layer of muscle. Eventually arteries become smaller and become arterioles, finally feeding into capillaries.

Artery   Capillary   Vein

Structure of blood vessels

Exerted

Apply pressure.

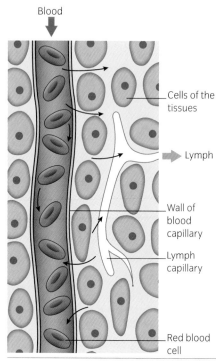

Blood

Cells of the tissues

Lymph

Wall of blood capillary

Lymph capillary

Red blood cell

Capillary exchange

CAPILLARIES

Capillaries are the smallest blood vessels and create a large network of blood vessels. They link the smallest arteries carrying blood from the heart back to the smallest venules to return blood back to the heart. The capillary walls are only a single cell layer thick, which is semi-permeable. Substances such as oxygen, vitamins, minerals, water and amino acids are easily able to move from the capillaries into the surrounding tissues to become tissue fluid to nourish and feed the cells. Substances such as carbon dioxide, cellular waste and water pass back into the capillaries to be removed. This simple process is known as capillary exchange. Blood cells and large substances, such as plasma proteins, remain in the capillaries and cannot move out into the surrounding tissue, unless the blood vessels are damaged.

VEINS

Veins are the blood vessels that transport blood to the heart and carry deoxygenated blood (with the exception of the pulmonary vein). The blood is dark purplish red in colour as it is not now carrying rich oxygen supplies. The walls of the veins are much thinner than the walls of the arteries and have less muscle and elastic tissue. Muscular movement and breathing help to move blood along the veins in the body and the blood is not under pressure unlike the blood flow in the arteries. Most veins contain special valves and these prevent blood flowing back along the vein. The smallest veins are called venules.

PRIMARY BLOOD VESSELS

You need to be familiar with the location of each of the blood vessels in the following tables.

Head, face and neck

The following blood vessels supply and remove blood from the tissues in the head, face and neck.

Primary blood vessels in the head, face and neck	Position
Common carotid artery	Starts at the aorta and travels up either side of the neck. The vessels divide to become the internal and external carotid arteries.
External carotid artery	Travels up the side of the neck to the base of the skull where it divides into smaller vessels which branch off to supply the brain, eyes, forehead and nose.
Internal carotid artery	Travels up the inner side of the neck where it divides into smaller vessels which branch off to supply the **superficial** tissues of the head and neck. **Superficial** On the surface; not deep or penetrating.
External jugular vein	Starts at the jawline and travels down in front of the sternocleidomastoid and behind the clavicle where it joins the subclavian vein.
Internal jugular vein	Begins in the middle of the cranium and travels down the neck behind the sternocleidomastoid and behind the clavicle where it joins the subclavian vein.

ACTIVITY

If you put your hand to your neck and press gently along the line of the sternocleidomastoid muscle with two fingers, you will feel the pulse of the carotid artery.

Forearm, wrist and hand

Primary blood vessels in the forearm, wrist and hand	Position
Brachial artery Brachial artery	Runs down the inner (medial) side of the upper arm, past the elbow where it divides into the radial and ulna arteries.
Radial artery Radial artery	Travels down the ulnar side of the forearm to cross the wrist and into the hand.
Ulnar artery Ulnar artery	Travels down the radial side of the forearm down over the wrist and into the palm of the hand.

ACTIVITY

If you put your hand on the inside of your wrist and press gently with two fingers, you will feel the pulse of the radial artery.

Lower leg, ankle and foot

Primary blood vessels in the lower leg, ankle and foot	Position
Femoral artery	Begins at the ligament in the groin and travels down the front of the leg. It then runs **medially** across the thigh where it finishes in the popliteal space and becomes the popliteal artery.
Anterior tibial artery	Travels from the tibia and fibula. It lies on the tibia and runs across the ankle joint.
Posterior tibial artery	Runs down the back of the leg and turns medially to the sole of the foot where it becomes the plantar artery.
Saphenous vein	The great saphenous vein is the longest vein in the body. It begins halfway up the top of the foot, travels up the medial side of the tibia and inner side of the thigh. It joins the femoral artery in the groin. The small saphenous vein starts behind the ankle joint. It travels up the back of the leg and joins the deep popliteal vein at the back of the knee.
Femoral vein	In the groin.

Medially

In the middle.

WHY DON'T YOU...
find your pulse in your wrist or neck. Compare your pulse with other colleagues and discuss your findings.

Venous return

The blood flow back to the heart via the veins.

Adjust

Changing or adapting.

Continually

To keep doing something over and over.

DISORDERS OF THE CARDIOVASCULAR SYSTEM

The following medical conditions might require you to adapt or modify your treatment so it is important you are familiar with each of the following conditions.

BLOOD PRESSURE

Blood pressure is the force or pressure the blood exerts on the walls of the blood vessels in which it is contained. Normal blood pressure is dependant of several factors including:

- the function of the heart
- the blood volume
- the elasticity of the artery walls
- the **venous return**.

Hypotension/low blood pressure

If blood pressure is too low, the vital organs will not be able to function properly. Some people, when they get up quickly, suffer with postural hypotension which is a sudden drop in blood pressure as the body **adjusts**. This can make someone feel very light headed or faint. The easiest way to avoid this is to make sure that clients get up or sit up slowly or in stages.

Hypertension/high blood pressure

If the blood pressure is **continually** too high there is an increased risk of damage to the blood vessels and a risk of internal bleeding. High blood pressure is quite common as a person gets older and is often associated with hardening of the artery walls. When there is internal bleeding in the brain it is known as a stroke. There is a slightly higher risk of the client bruising more easily when they have high blood pressure. Always make sure that their high blood pressure is kept at the same level with medication before carrying out any treatments.

Varicose veins

The veins in the legs contain valves to prevent the blood flowing backwards. If one of these valves stops functioning properly, the blood will collect in the vein and, during muscular movement, it will seep into the surrounding tissues. The veins become swollen. It is a good idea to raise the legs regularly if this is a problem to help the blood flow return. It is also important not to apply pressure over the varicose vein to avoid further pressure on the already weak valve. Areas where varicose veins are visible should not be waxed or massaged.

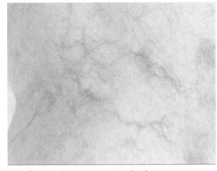
Swollen varicose veins in the legs

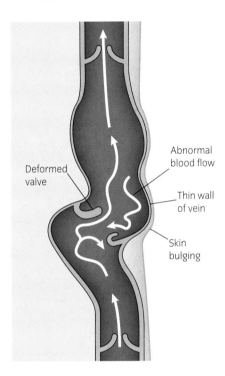

Deformed valve

Abnormal blood flow

Thin wall of vein

Skin bulging

Erythema

You should look for erythema following many of your treatments. It can be a sign of increased circulation from an **effective** massage or from skin trauma following waxing or eyebrow shaping. Erythema is a reddening of the skin caused by **congestion** of the tiny capillaries near the skin's surface through increased blood flow. Erythema can also be an **adverse** reaction and might be a sign of an allergic reaction. Usually if this is the case, the client will experience other symptoms, such as irritation or tingling.

Effective
Most successful or proven.

Congestion
Overfilling the capillaries with blood.

Adverse
Unpleasant, difficult or harmful.

Bruising

A bruise is caused by damage to the blood vessels allowing the blood to flow freely into the surrounding tissues. This makes the skin tissue look blue, black or yellow. A bruise is usually caused by a sharp blow or too much pressure exerted on the body. Some people are more prone to bruising than others. There are also some medical conditions that cause people to bruise more easily. Bruised tissue should be avoided until the body has had a chance to fully repair to prevent any further blood vessel damage.

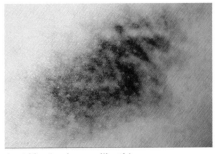
Avoid bruised areas like this

LYMPHATIC SYSTEM

The lymphatic system is a network of lymphatic vessels and lymphatic organs that stretches throughout the entire body. It provides transportation of nutrients to the tissues and drains excess fluid from the spaces between cells. The lymphatic system is one-way; it returns fluid to the bloodstream but cannot collect lymph from the bloodstream.

In this part of the chapter you will learn about:

- the basic structure of the lymphatic system
- the function of the lymphatic system
- the location of the major lymph nodes in the head and neck
- diseases and disorders of the lymphatic system
- lymphatic contra-indications
- other contra-indications that will prevent or restrict treatment.

BASIC STRUCTURE OF THE LYMPHATIC SYSTEM

Lymph is a pale milky-coloured fluid that consists of approximately 95 per cent water and lymphocyte cells. Lymph is also known as tissue fluid and it bathes the tissues of the body. It is formed from plasma seeping out of our blood capillaries. Lymph also contains additional substances that are too large to pass through blood capillary walls (eg debris from areas of infection and cells damaged by disease).

Transfer
Sent to or shared with.

As tissue fluid, lymph acts as a means of **transferring** nutrients, such as food, oxygen and water and collects up waste, such as urea and carbon dioxide. It creates the essential environment cells we need to survive.

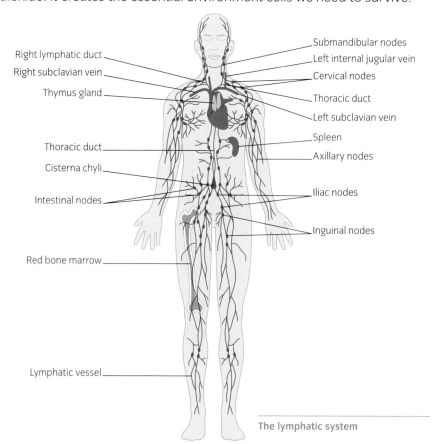

Right lymphatic duct
Right subclavian vein
Thymus gland
Thoracic duct
Cisterna chyli
Intestinal nodes
Red bone marrow
Lymphatic vessel

Submandibular nodes
Left internal jugular vein
Cervical nodes
Thoracic duct
Left subclavian vein
Spleen
Axillary nodes
Iliac nodes
Inguinal nodes

The lymphatic system

Most tissue fluid returns to the bloodstream via the blood capillary walls, but the rest becomes lymph and enters the lymphatic system.

The lymphatic system is made up of the following:

- lymphatic capillaries
- lymphatic vessels and lymphatic fluid (lymph)
- lymph nodes or glands
- the **adenoids**
- the tonsils
- the thymus
- the spleen.

LYMPHATIC CAPILLARIES

Lymphatic capillaries are located throughout the body. They start as tubes with a dead end **projecting** into the tissues. Their structure is similar to blood capillaries, in that they are composed of a single layer of cells. Their walls are more **permeable** and allow larger particles, such as cell debris and proteins, to be absorbed. They differ from blood capillaries in that blood capillaries have a venous and an arterial end, whereas lymphatic capillaries do not.

LYMPHATIC VESSELS

These vessels have thin **collapsible** walls and are similar to veins in structure. The lymphatic system, unlike the circulatory system, does not rely on the heart to pump the fluid along. Lymph is pushed towards the heart by the contraction of muscles nearby. Lymphatic vessels have many valves that prevent the backflow of lymph and make sure that the lymph moves in the right direction. The lymphatic vessels gradually get larger and eventually form two large ducts called the thoracic duct and the right lymphatic duct. The right lymphatic duct drains lymph from the right half of the head, neck, right arm and thorax. The thoracic duct drains lymph from both legs, the pelvic and abdominal cavities, the left half of the head, neck, thorax and left arm. Lymph is then returned to the bloodstream via the subclavian veins.

LYMPH NODES

Lymph nodes are often referred to as lymph glands, even though glands usually **secrete** and lymph glands do not. Lymph nodes vary in size with some as small as a pinhead and larger nodes the size of an almond. These nodes are in carefully planned locations throughout the body. Some are nearer to the surface and are called superficial, others are positioned deep in the tissues.

Lymph nodes are made up of **reticular** and lymphatic tissue that is enclosed inside a tough **fibrous** capsule. Each node contains a network of fibres and white blood cells called lymphocytes. Lymphocytes produce antibodies that destroy micro-organisms. These cells work to filter and clean the lymph before it is returned to the venous bloodstream.

Adenoids
Lymphoid tissue found at the back of the throat.

Project
Extend or reach down into.

Permeable
Porous, leaky.

Collapsible
Able to break down.

Secrete
To release a substance from a cell or gland.

Reticular
Layer of the dermis.

Fibrous
Containing fibres.

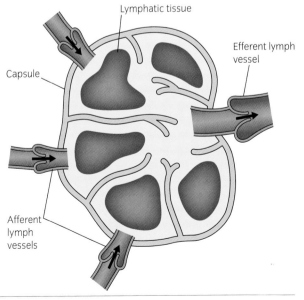

A lymph node

TONSILS

The tonsils are a mass of lymphatic tissue. There are two tonsils at the back of the roof of the mouth, and a small pair of tonsils at the base of the tongue. They help to protect the throat and airways from infection. Together with the adenoids they produce antibodies against **ingested** or inhaled organisms attempting to enter the body through the nose or mouth.

FUNCTION OF THE LYMPHATIC SYSTEM

The main function of the lymph nodes is to filter lymph and prevent infection. The lymphatic system has a crucial role in immunity, producing T- and B-lymphocytes and antibodies in the lymph nodes.

Lymphatic vessels called **lacteals** collect **microscopic** molecules of fat from the small intestine. The fat then travels through the lymphatic system and is slowly emptied into the bloodstream.

LOCATION OF THE MAJOR LYMPH NODES IN THE HEAD AND NECK

There are many lymph nodes located throughout the body. The main lymph nodes are in the neck, armpit, breast, abdomen, groin, pelvis and behind the knee. The main nodes of the head, face and neck are illustrated below.

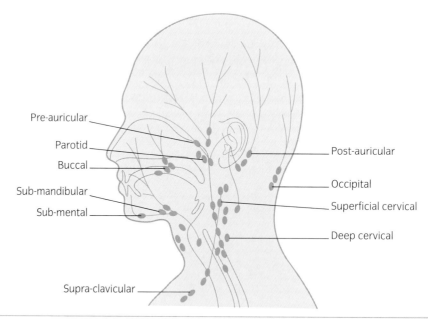

The major lymph nodes of the head

Ingested
When something is brought into the body through the nose or mouth.

Lacteals
Special lymphatic capillaries that lie inside projections of intestinal tissue called villi that cover the walls of the small intestine.

Microscopic
Something that can only be seen through a microscope.

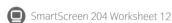 SmartScreen 204 Worksheet 12

DISEASES AND DISORDERS OF THE LYMPHATIC SYSTEM

It is important that you have a basic understanding of some of the common conditions. Insurance companies expect you to carry out a full consultation before starting any treatment and, if necessary, to refer your client to a medical practitioner. Many conditions can be treated with care and treatments can be **modified** providing the client's medical practitioner has been consulted. However, some conditions are contra-indicated. You should be familiar with the location of the main lymphatic

Modified
Changing or adapting.

nodes or glands of the body so that you can advise your client correctly should you suspect that their glands are swollen. Swollen glands can be an early sign that an infection is present.

ACTIVITY

Discuss with your manager or tutor what signs you will see if a client has a problem with their lymphatic system. What benefits will certain beauty treatments have for the lymphatic system?

LYMPHATIC CONTRA-INDICATIONS

The lymphatic system's role in immunity and health means that any condition that a client has that has an impact on the lymph system should be given time to recover.

Lymphatic contra-indication	Description and cause	Contra-indications and general precautions	Advice for client
Swollen glands	Inflamed, tender lymph nodes are usually a sign that the body is fighting an infection. The nodes might swell even before the effects of the infection are felt (eg glands in the neck might become tender and sore even before a sore throat is experienced).	The condition causing the swollen glands might be contagious. If the body is fighting an infection it should not be treated to allow the body to heal. Pressure over swollen nodes could affect the natural **filtering** of pathogens, forcing them through the nodes rather than being dealt with within the node itself by the lymphatic tissue.	Rest and recovery.

ACTIVITY

Discuss with your tutor what might happen if you were to treat a client with swollen glands or diagnosed lumps.

Filter
Method of allowing some but not all substance through.

OTHER CONTRA-INDICATIONS THAT WILL PREVENT OR RESTRICT TREATMENT

There are many contra-indications that you will come across so it is important that you have a basic understanding of some of the common conditions. Insurance companies will expect you to carry out a full consultation before starting any treatment and the client should be referred to a medical practitioner before treatment if necessary. There are many conditions that can be treated with care and the treatment can be modified providing the client's medical practitioner has been consulted first. There are some clients, however, that should not be treated while they have the condition.

Contra-indication	Description and cause	Contra-indications and general precautions	Advice for client
Influenza (flu)	Flu is caused by a virus that is spread by airborne infected droplets. It can be caught by direct contact with an infected client or colleague. Symptoms include feeling very unwell, aching, headache and a high temperature. Other symptoms might include a runny or blocked nose, watery eyes, sneezing, catarrh and a sore throat. There can also be a stomach upset with gastric flu.	Yes as this is a very contagious virus.	Go home and rest.
Cancer	Cancer is a broad term that is given to over 200 different types of the disease. Cancer is classified according to the organ where it has started. Each cancer has different symptoms depending on the organ or part of the body affected. Cancer is caused by **uncontrolled** abnormal cell growth and is known as a malignant growth. Sometimes this growth is localised to a specific area (primary cancer); on other occasions the cancer can spread to different parts of the body (secondary cancer). **Uncontrolled** Not controlled.	We avoid treating these clients because their **immune system** is under attack and because of the side effects they might be experiencing from their treatment. Whether you can treat a client is dependent on a variety of factors. Initially, the client should be considered contra- indicated until they have sought advice from their medical practitioner. There is a theory that massage can spread cancer cells but this is highly unlikely and not proven. **Immune system** The system that protects the body from micro-organisms.	Suggest the client seeks medical advice before considering any treatment.

Contra-indication	Description and cause	Contra-indications and general precautions	Advice for client
Epilepsy	Epilepsy can be described as uncontrolled, electrical activity in the brain. This change in activity can lead to a simple vacant expression with a lack of response or a grand mal seizure, which is when the individual becomes partially unconscious and suffers twitching and uncontrollable movements. Epilepsy often has no known cause but it can be triggered by a brain injury or a chemical imbalance. Some epileptics have seizures that are caused by flashing lights which is known as photo sensitive epilepsy.	Not generally a contra-indication, however, you might want to refer the client to their medical practitioner for advice. If the client's condition is controlled and they know what triggers their seizures, so that they can avoid the trigger, there is no reason why they should have safe treatments like a facial, manicure or pedicure. As a therapist you need to decide whether you can cope with the possibility of an epileptic client having a seizure. This might be a frightening experience but if you are aware, prepared and take the right precautions you can treat these clients.	Suggest the client seeks medical advice before considering any treatment.
Type 1 diabetes **Glucose** A type of sugar that the body uses for energy. **Amino acid** The building blocks that make proteins. **Fatty acid** The building blocks of fat. **Deficiency** Something lacking. **Metabolism** Process in the body that uses food for growth and energy.	This is a condition caused by a disorder of the pancreas gland. The pancreas is responsible for producing the hormone insulin. Insulin's main function is to lower the levels of **glucose**, **amino acids** and **fatty acids** being carried in the blood. In type 1 diabetes the body suffers a severe **deficiency** or total absence of insulin and is unable to control the **metabolism** of carbohydrates (sugars) and fat. Type 1 diabetes is treated with insulin injections.	There is no cure and diabetes can have many long-term side effects on many of the systems of the body. This is why diabetic clients should be treated with caution. If the client knows that they have problems with skin sensitivity (ie they are having tests to see if they can feel different sensations) you should not treat them until they have consulted their medical practitioner. As a therapist you need to be aware of some of the complications that can occur as the treatment might need to be adapted or restricted. A diabetic might develop changes to the small blood vessels which become weakened and blocked. The nerves might become affected causing numbness or pins and needles in the hands and feet, both of which will also reduce their sensory perception. This will particularly affect treatments, such as pedicures and leg waxing.	Suggest the client seeks medical advice before treatment if you feel this is appropriate to the treatment the client is wishing to have.

Contra-indication	Description and cause	Contra-indications and general precautions	Advice for client
Type 2 diabetes	This is the most common form of diabetes and about 90 per cent of diabetics are type 2. There are a variety of causes but the most common is obesity. Insulin secretion might be below or above normal levels. Treatment might include changes to diet and the use of drugs to help control the condition. In some cases there might still be the need for insulin injections to control the symptoms.	There is no cure and diabetes can have many long-term side effects on many of the systems of the body. This is why diabetic clients should be treated with caution. As a therapist you need to be aware of some of the complications that can occur as the treatment might need to be adapted or restricted. A diabetic might develop changes to the small blood vessels which become weakened and blocked. The nerves might become affected causing numbness or pins and needles in the hands and feet both of which will also reduce their sensory perception.	Ask the client to seek medical advice before treatment if you feel this is appropriate to the treatment the client is wishing to have.

CHEMOTHERAPY

Chemotherapy is the use of drugs to destroy cancer cells. There are lots of different drugs that can be used. The drugs can be administered as tablets or intravenously through a vein. Chemotherapy has a wide range of side effects depending on the drug being used to treat the cancer. Often more than one drug is used. Avoid treating clients that are having chemotherapy because their immune system is under attack and because the side effects they might be experiencing from their treatment can be quite unpleasant. They are more at risk from catching infections as their immune system is under a lot of stress. Advise them to wait until the chemotherapy treatment is over before they have beauty treatments.

ACTIVITY

Discuss with your manager precautions you might need to take when treating an epileptic client. What procedures might you put in place?

UNIT SUMMARY

Now you have reached the end of the chapter, check the following list to see if you feel confident in all the areas covered. If there are still any areas you are unsure of, go back over them in your book and ask your manager for additional support:

- the skin
- the hair
- the nails
- the skeletal system
- the muscular system
- the cardiovascular system
- the lymphatic system.

TEST YOUR KNOWLEDGE

Use the questions below to test your knowledge of anatomy and physiology to see how much information you have retained. These questions will help you to revise what you have learnt in this chapter.

Turn to page 601 for the answers.

1. Which **one** of these vitamins is made in the skin?
   a) Vitamin A
   b) Vitamin B
   c) Vitamin C
   d) Vitamin D

2. What is the name of the chemical released by the body that causes vasodilation?
   a) Histamine
   b) Erythrocyte
   c) Macrophage
   d) Pathogen

3. Which **one** of the following is not found in the acid mantle?
   a) Urea
   b) Water
   c) Sweat
   d) Sebum

4. The outer most layer of the epidermis is called the stratum _____
   a) germinativum
   b) granulosum
   c) lucidum
   d) corneum.

5. Which **one** of the following is produced by fibroblasts?
   a) Histamine
   b) Collagen
   c) Pathogens
   d) Papillae

6. Meissner's corpuscles are nerve endings that are able to sense which one of the following?
   a) Pressure
   b) Pain
   c) Touch
   d) Temperature

7. The depth of skin colour is dependent on which of the following?
   a) How melanin is structured
   b) More active melanocytes
   c) The amount of melanin in the melanosomes
   d) How melanosomes are distributed

8. Which **one** of the following is a bacterial infection?
   a) Impetigo
   b) Shingles
   c) Milia
   d) Urticaria

9. What is psoriasis often caused by?
   a) Bacteria
   b) Virus
   c) Fungus
   d) Stress

10. Which **one** of the following is the name given to a fungal infection of the feet?
    a) Tinea capitis
    b) Tinea pedis
    c) Tinea ungium
    d) Tinea corporis

11. What is the outer layer of the hair called?
    a) Medulla
    b) Shaft
    c) Cortex
    d) Cuticle

12. What is pediculosis capitis another name for?
    a) Ringworm
    b) Head lice
    c) Split ends
    d) Dandruff

13. Which part of the nail structure can be affected by prolonged exposure to water?
    a) Nail bed
    b) Matrix
    c) Nail plate
    d) Cuticle

14. Which **one** of the following is the correct term for severe nail separation?
    a) Onychophagy
    b) Onychocryptosis
    c) Onycholysis
    d) Onychomicosis

15. Which **one** of the following bones of the skull forms the cheek?
    a) Maxilla
    b) Palatine
    c) Zygomatic arch
    d) Lacrimal

16. How many cervical bones are there?
    a) 4
    b) 5
    c) 7
    d) 12

17. Which **one** of the following is a characteristic of veins?
    a) They carry oxygenated blood
    b) Blood flow is under pressure
    c) The vessels have a thick layer of muscle
    d) The vessels have valves

18. Which **one** of the following is involved in the blood clotting process?
    a) Thrombocytes
    b) Leukocytes
    c) Erythrocytes
    d) Granulocytes

19. Which area does the thoracic duct not drain lymph from?
    a) Both legs
    b) Abdominal cavities
    c) Neck and left arm
    d) Thorax and right arm

20. Which **one** of the following muscles draws the sides of the mouth down?
    a) Orbicularis oris
    b) Triangularis
    c) Quadrates labii superioris
    d) Zygomatic major

21. Which **one** of the following muscles causes the vertical wrinkle between the eyebrows?
    a) Frontalis
    b) Corrugator
    c) Orbicularis oculi
    d) Nasalis

22. Which **one** of the following muscles is located on the back of the forearm?
    a) Flexor carpi radialis
    b) Flexor carpi ulnaris
    c) Extensor digitorum
    d) Extensor carpi radialis brevis

23. Where are the buccal group of lymphatic nodes located?
    a) In the cheek
    b) Behind the ear
    c) In front of the ear
    d) Under the chin

24. Which **one** of the following types of blood cells is responsible for transporting oxygen to the cells and tissues?
    a) Leukocytes
    b) Granulocytes
    c) Erythrocytes
    d) Thrombocytes

25. Which **one** of the following is a bone found in the foot?
    a) Cuboid
    b) Lunate
    c) Scaphoid
    d) Hamate

LEGISLATION

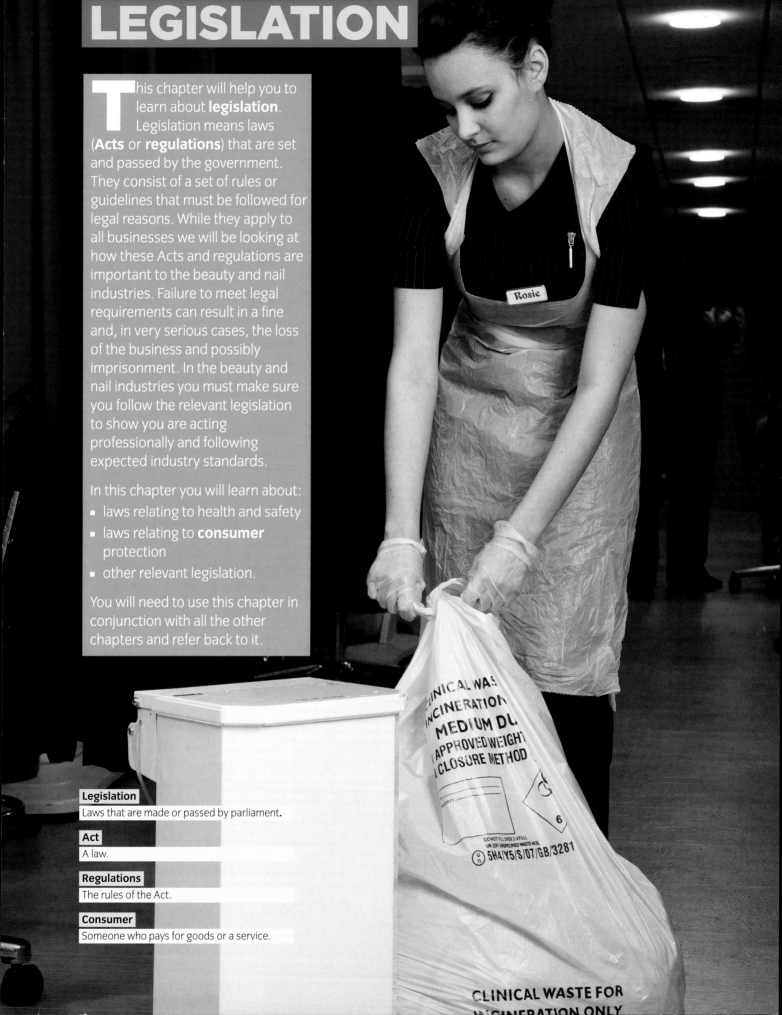

This chapter will help you to learn about **legislation**. Legislation means laws (**Acts** or **regulations**) that are set and passed by the government. They consist of a set of rules or guidelines that must be followed for legal reasons. While they apply to all businesses we will be looking at how these Acts and regulations are important to the beauty and nail industries. Failure to meet legal requirements can result in a fine and, in very serious cases, the loss of the business and possibly imprisonment. In the beauty and nail industries you must make sure you follow the relevant legislation to show you are acting professionally and following expected industry standards.

In this chapter you will learn about:

- laws relating to health and safety
- laws relating to **consumer** protection
- other relevant legislation.

You will need to use this chapter in conjunction with all the other chapters and refer back to it.

Legislation
Laws that are made or passed by parliament.

Act
A law.

Regulations
The rules of the Act.

Consumer
Someone who pays for goods or a service.

LAWS RELATING TO HEALTH AND SAFETY

In this part of the chapter you will learn about the:

- Health and Safety at Work Act 1974
- Workplace (Health, Safety and Welfare) Regulations 1992
- Provision and Use of Work Equipment Regulations 1998
- Local Government Miscellaneous Provisions Act 1982
- Control of Substances Hazardous to Health Regulations 2002
- Electricity at Work Regulations 1990
- Fire Precautions Act 1971 and Fire Precautions (Workplace) Regulations 1997
- Personal Protective Equipment (PPE) at Work Regulations 1992
- Manual Handling Operations Regulations 1992
- Reporting of Injuries, Diseases and Dangerous Occurences Regulations 1995
- Health and Safety (First Aid) Regulations 1981
- Health and Safety (Display Screen Equipment) Regulations 1992.

ACTIVITY

Use this table to help you remember the initials of some of the legislation you must learn.

Initials	Legislation name in full
HASAWA	Health and Safety at Work Act
COSHH	Control of Substances Hazardous to Health
PPE	Personal Protective Equipment at Work Regulations
RIDDOR	Reporting of Injuries, Diseases and Dangerous Occurrences Regulations
PUWER	Provision and Use of Work Equipment Regulations
EAWR	Electricity at Work Regulations
DPA	Data Protection Act
DDA	Disability Discrimination Act.

HEALTH AND SAFETY AT WORK ACT 1974

The Health and Safety at Work Act (HASAWA) regulates the workplace to make sure that safe working practices are being followed and maintained. It covers all aspects of health, safety and welfare at work. It identifies the responsibilities of both the employer and the employee (including people who are self-employed).

No-one in the workplace should knowingly endanger the health, safety and welfare of the employee, employer or client or interfere with or misuse any equipment or products provided. The HASAWA includes guidelines and rules on:

- hygiene, cleanliness and disposal of waste
- heating, lighting and ventilation
- work facilities and maintaining a safe and healthy work environment
- providing a safe working environment
- fire exits and firefighting equipment
- safe storage
- manual handling.

ACTIVITY

Discuss with your tutor how the salon would be affected if the guidelines and rules of the HASAWA were not followed. What could happen?

THE MAIN LEGISLATION UNDER THE UMBRELLA OF THE HASAWA

The HASAWA is an umbrella for all other legislation relating to health and safety in the workplace.

EMPLOYER'S RESPONSIBILITIES

Under the HASAWA, your employer is not just responsible for the health and safety of its clients but also the staff and any visitors (such as product representatives, area managers and tradespeople). Your employer must:

- maintain the workplace and make sure it is safe to work in
- give staff appropriate training and supervision
- keep access and exit points clear and free from hazards at all times
- provide a suitable working environment and facilities that comply with the HASAWA
- make sure the salon's health and safety systems are reviewed and updated.

EMPLOYEE'S RESPONSIBILITIES

Your responsibilities under the HASAWA are to yourself, your colleagues and your clients. You must:

- maintain the health and safety of yourself and others who might be affected by your actions
- work together and communicate with your employer about health and safety issues, so your employer can keep within the law.

Who is the person responsible for reporting health and safety matters? YOU are! If you see a health and safety problem, you must deal with it or report it. Everyone is responsible for putting it right.

WORKPLACE (HEALTH, SAFETY AND WELFARE) REGULATIONS 1992

The Workplace (Health, Safety and Welfare) Regulations require everyone in the workplace to help maintain a safe and healthy working environment. You and your employer should follow **environmentally friendly** working practices.

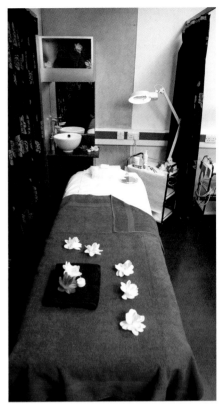

Work areas must be clean and tidy

SmartScreen 202 Worksheet 1

Environmentally friendly
Safe for or good to the environment.

EMPLOYER'S RESPONSIBILITIES

Your employer's responsibilities under the regulations are to:

- maintain equipment and the workplace
- regulate temperatures
- make sure working conditions and size and shape of the room suit the number of staff employed
- make sure there is sufficient lighting and ventilation
- make sure all walkways are clear of hazards
- provide **sanitary conveniences** and washing facilities
- provide drinking water and facilities for staff to rest, eat meals and change clothing
- provide secure areas or lockers for employees' clothing and property.

Sanitary conveniences

Clean toilets and washrooms free from infection.

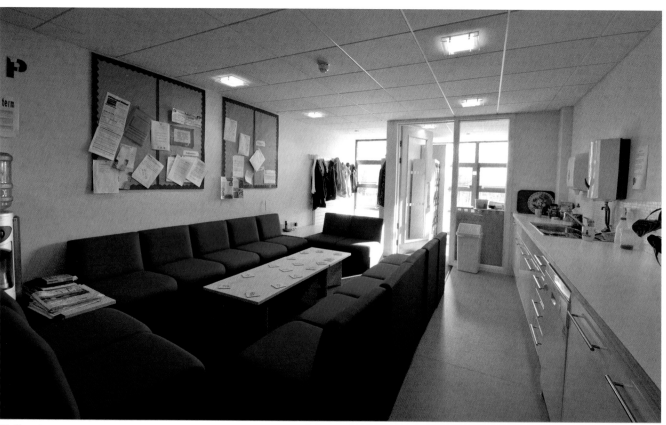

Staff rest room

EMPLOYEE'S RESPONSIBILITIES

Your responsibilities under the regulations are to:

- make sure all doors, fire exits and stairways are kept free of **obstructions** and hazards
- make sure you know the fire **evacuation** procedure
- prevent infection and **contamination** by keeping the salon's workstations, mirrors, floors, gowns, towels, equipment and tools clean
- keep the salon tidy to prevent accidents, such as tripping over trailing electrical wires
- clean up spillages immediately to prevent slippery surfaces
- make sure all lights above the stairways and at fire exits are working
- report any problems that you are unable to deal with to your employer.

Obstruction

Something that blocks your path.

Evacuation

Leaving the area because of fire.

Contamination

The presence of something unwanted that might be harmful.

PROVISION AND USE OF WORK EQUIPMENT REGULATIONS 1998

The Provision and Use of Work Equipment Regulations (PUWER) require that all the equipment in the salon (both new and second-hand equipment) must be used for its intended purpose only and kept in good working condition.

EMPLOYER'S RESPONSIBILITIES

Your employer's responsibilities under the regulations are:

- to provide you with training to use the equipment as it is intended
- to make sure that the equipment is properly built and fit for use.

EMPLOYEE'S RESPONSIBILITIES

Your responsibilities under the regulations are:

- to make sure you know how to use the equipment in the salon properly and safely
- to use equipment only for its intended purpose (eg do not use a warm wax heater for heating paraffin wax).

Greenhouse gas emissions

The release of gases into the atmosphere that absorb infra-red radiation. These gases contribute to the greenhouse effect and global warming.

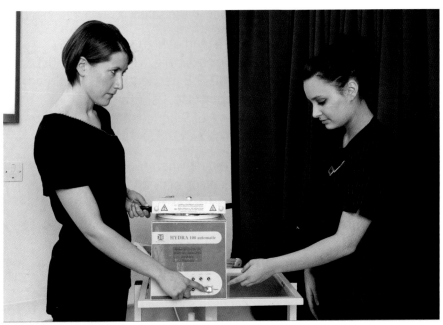

Therapist instructing a colleague

LOCAL GOVERNMENT MISCELLANEOUS PROVISIONS ACT 1982

The Local Government Miscellaneous Provisions Act requires all businesses to be registered with the local authority, first so that the government knows they exist and second so they can be **monitored** and regulated. Your employer must make sure they take the relevant steps to register for the services they are offering.

A business must show that its standards meet the rules and regulations set out in the local council's **by-laws**. By-laws are a set of local laws that deal with local issues and tell a business how it must act with regards to health and safety, hygiene and cleanliness. Specific by-laws relate to specific business practices (eg ear piercing and electrolysis). Some councils have a downloadable copy of their by-laws on their website.

Monitor

Keeping an eye on.

By-law

A local council rule.

Ingestion

To take food into the mouth and digestive system.

Absorption

The process whereby nutrients enter the bloodstream via the stomach or intestines.

Inhalation

To breathe in.

Identified

Recognised or pointed out.

Accessible

Easy to access.

Alternative

A different possible choice.

Fire retardant

A chemical used to slow down the spread of fire.

Incinerate

To burn something to ashes.

Environment

This can be both the natural world around us as well as the things that have an affect on you.

This Act also gives local authorities the power to inspect business premises and to act if something falls below the required standard. The owner can be fined or the business shut down if the issues are serious.

CONTROL OF SUBSTANCES HAZARDOUS TO HEALTH REGULATIONS 2002

Various chemicals are seen as hazardous (eg cleaning substances and bleach). The Control of Substances Hazardous to Health (COSHH) Regulations identify dangerous chemicals. Hazardous substances can enter the body through **ingestion**, **absorption** or **inhalation**. A hazardous substance in the workplace can put a person's health at risk and cause disease or injury, such as asthma, cancer or dermatitis.

Hazardous substances must be **identified** by specific symbols which you should be able to recognise. All suppliers must legally provide guidelines on how their materials should be stored and used. All products identified as hazardous must by law be listed and a COSHH risk assessment must be **accessible**. (This can be obtained from the manufacturer.) Be aware that substances which seem to be harmless can be hazardous if used or stored incorrectly. A risk assessment should be carried out for each substance used in the salon.

Low-risk products should be used instead of high-risk products wherever there is an **alternative**. For example, a low-risk product would be tinting peroxide (10 volume or 3 per cent) that had already been diluted and packaged for the purpose. Using a higher concentration of peroxide (30 volume or 9 per cent) that needed to be diluted in the salon would be high risk.

Under COSHH you must make sure that any hazardous substances are stored, handled, used and disposed of correctly and safely. The best way of remembering this is by following **SHUD**:

- **S**torage: in a locked cupboard at room temperature when not in use, ideally this cupboard should also be **fire retardant**.
- **H**andling: wear appropriate personal protective equipment (PPE) such as gloves, mask and apron.
- **U**sage: according to the manufacturer's instructions or workplace guidelines.
- **D**isposal: make sure you dispose of all hazardous waste in a hazardous waste bag; the local authority or a private company will collect the waste and **incinerate** it. This usually consists of tissues, cotton wool and wax strips that have been in contact with bodily fluids (eg blood).

The manufacturer's instructions will explain how to store, handle, use and dispose of the chemicals or substances. The local by-laws will tell you how to dispose of them, be considerate to the **environment** and follow the local authority's guidelines on waste and refuse. Your salon's policy will explain where to store and mix the chemicals and where to dispose of them in the workplace.

EMPLOYER'S RESPONSIBILITIES

Your employer's responsibilities under the regulations are:

- to make sure COSHH health and safety information sheets are available for substances and chemicals in the workplace
- to make sure chemicals are **disposed** of according to local by-laws and with respect to the environment.

Disposal

The action of getting rid of something that is no longer wanted or needed.

EMPLOYEE'S RESPONSIBILITIES

Your responsibilities under the regulations are:

- to follow SHUD
- to read and follow the manufacturer's instructions, local by-laws and your salon's policy
- to know where to find the COSHH information sheets.

WHY DON'T YOU...
make a list of all the items in your salon that would come under COSHH – everything from washing powder to peroxide. Ask your tutor or manager to check your list.

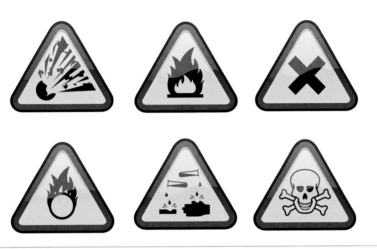

Hazard labels

ELECTRICITY AT WORK REGULATIONS 1990

The Electricity at Work Regulations (EAWR) require all electrical **appliances** to be used with caution and handled correctly. Electrical equipment must be *maintained in a condition suitable for use*, checked and tested on a routine basis.

Appliance

A device or piece of equipment made to perform a specific task.

EMPLOYER'S RESPONSIBILITIES

Your employer's responsibilities under the regulations are to make sure that all electrical equipment:

- is in a safe working condition
- is portable appliance tested (PAT) by a qualified electrician at least once a year (some appliances might need checking more frequently). This means anything that has a cable and a plug must be tested. A record must be kept. Insurance companies require all electrical equipment to be routinely tested
- is visually checked by salon employees routinely and frequently.

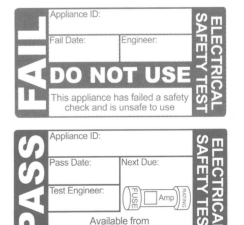

PAT testing stickers/labels

EMPLOYEE'S RESPONSIBILITIES

Your responsibilities under the regulations are to:

- not use electrical appliances until you have been trained
- use appliances correctly and to switch them off after use
- carry out routine visual checks. These could be done in the morning when equipment is switched on or at the end of the day when equipment is switched off. You must check any electrical appliance you use for faults or problems (eg frayed or loose cables or flexes, broken plugs or damage to the external casing)
- not overload plug sockets
- report any faults immediately to your supervisor or manager and to label the item as faulty. The label should be clear and secure. Write down what the problem or fault is and include the date. Remove the equipment from the working area if possible until it can be repaired or disposed of
- not use faulty equipment.

WHY DON'T YOU...
make a list of the electrical checks that a therapist should carry out routinely. Discuss the list with your tutor or manager.

ACTIVITY

Can you see evidence of PAT testing having taken place in your salon? What date did it take place? When is the next test due?

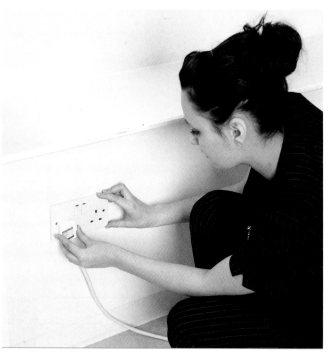

Therapist checking a plug

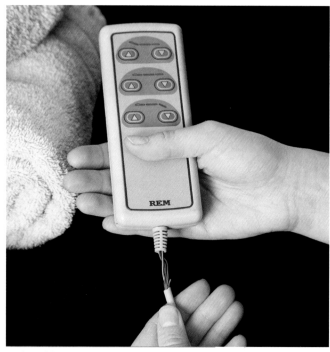

Faulty wiring

FIRE PRECAUTIONS ACT 1971 AND FIRE PRECAUTIONS (WORKPLACE) REGULATIONS 1997, AMENDED 1999

The Fire Precautions Act and the Fire Precautions (Workplace) Regulations require all premises to have basic standards of fire prevention and control and an **emergency exit route**.

Every business must carry out a fire risk assessment which should be reviewed annually or following any changes. It assesses how to prevent a fire and in the event of a fire how to control it.

Emergency exit route
The safest route by which staff, clients and visitors can escape a building.

A fire safety risk assessment must:

- identify fire hazards
- identify people at risk
- evaluate, remove or reduce risks and protect staff, clients and visitors from risk
- record, plan, inform, instruct and train staff
- be reviewed.

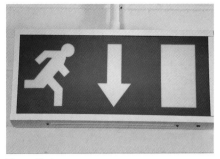

Fire exit sign

EMPLOYER'S RESPONSIBILITIES

Your employer's responsibilities under the Act and the regulations are to:

- carry out a full fire risk assessment, even if the workplace is covered by a fire certificate
- make sure all fire exits are unlocked, have fire exit signs and are easy to access
- train staff in fire evacuation procedures so that they know what is expected if there is an emergency – procedures should be practised so that all staff know what to do
- supply suitable fire-fighting equipment, such as fire extinguishers and fire blankets and to make sure they are maintained.

EMPLOYEE'S RESPONSIBILITIES

Your responsibilities under the Act and the regulations are to:

- know where the fire extinguishers and blankets are located in the salon
- know which fire extinguishers can be used on different fires
- know the evacuation procedure and where the safe meeting point is for salon staff and clients.

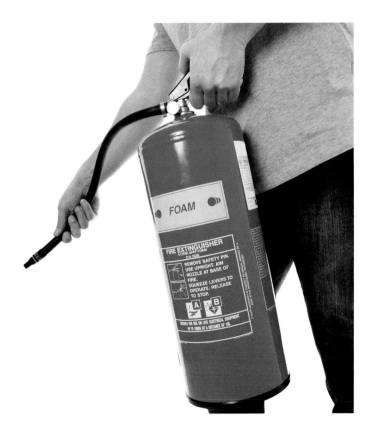

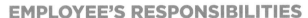

HANDY HINTS

Further information on which extinguishers can be used on different fires can be found in Chapter 202, pages 158–159.

PERSONAL PROTECTIVE EQUIPMENT (PPE) AT WORK REGULATIONS 1992

Gloves, aprons, masks and eye protection for salon employees as well as your uniform and shoes all come under the Personal Protective Equipment (PPE) at Work Regulations. Protective equipment used for the client is not covered by these regulations. It is important that you wear the appropriate PPE to protect yourself from harm when you are working with chemicals and to minimise cross-infection.

EMPLOYER'S RESPONSIBILITIES

Your employer's responsibilities under the regulations are to:

- supply free of charge any PPE required for you to carry out your job
- maintain supplies of PPE so that they are always accessible
- train staff how to use PPE appropriately (eg to use gloves when waxing but not when giving a client a manicure)
- carry out risk assessments and to recommend when to use PPE.

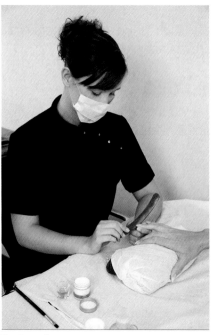

Dust mask

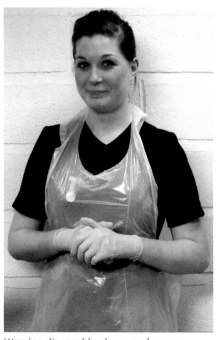

Wearing disposable gloves and apron

WHY DON'T YOU...
make a list of all the occasions when you know you will need to wear PPE and what PPE you will need. Review the list with your tutor or manager.

EMPLOYEE'S RESPONSIBILITIES

Your responsibilities under the regulations are to:

- wear PPE when you are mixing, handling and using chemicals or substances
- report any shortages of PPE to the relevant person so that additional stock can be ordered.

MANUAL HANDLING OPERATIONS REGULATIONS 1992

You are sometimes required to move equipment and stock around the salon and this is called manual handling. Always follow the Manual Handling Operations Regulations. There are correct ways to lift objects so you do not injure yourself.

According to the Health and Safety Executive (HSE), more than a third of all injuries resulting in over three days' absence from work are caused by manual handling. A recent survey showed that over 12.3 million working days are lost each year due to work-related **musculoskeletal disorders** that have been caused or made worse by poor manual handling.

Musculoskeletal disorders
Muscle and bone disorders.

ACTIVITY

Write a list of problems or disorders that might affect a therapist's muscles and bones if they do not follow manual handling guidelines.

EMPLOYER'S RESPONSIBILITIES

Your employer's responsibility under the regulations is to carry out risk assessments on all employees for manual lifting to make sure they are able to lift boxes and other heavy objects without causing injury.

EMPLOYEE'S RESPONSIBILITIES

Your responsibility under the regulations is to always ask yourself: 'Can I lift this?' If the answer is 'no', then don't! Ask for help. If the answer is 'yes', remember to bend your knees and keep your back straight. Lift the weight with your thigh muscles not your back and keep the item you are lifting close to your body. Even if a box is light, you should ask for help if it obscures your view.

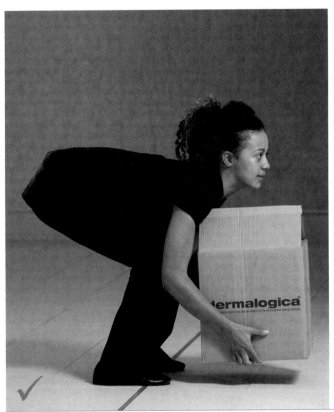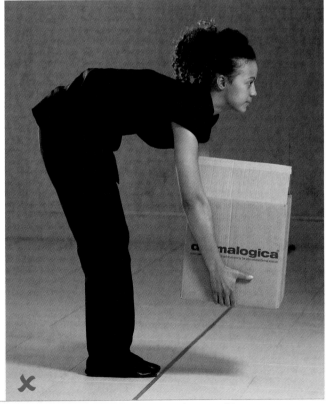

The picture on the left shows the correct lifting technique; the lifting technique on the right is incorrect. This technique will put pressure on the spine and could lead to injury.

REPORTING OF INJURIES, DISEASES AND DANGEROUS OCCURRENCES REGULATIONS 1995

The Reporting of Injuries, Diseases and Dangerous Occurrences Regulations (RIDDOR) require the following occurrences to be reported to the HSE immediately by telephone and then in writing within ten days of the incident:

- injuries (eg falls) sustained by you, your colleagues, clients or visitors in the workplace that result in three or more days off work
- major injuries, such as amputation, dislocation, fractures (not fingers or toes), loss of sight and any other eye injuries
- any work-related incident where a person has had to spend more than 24 hours in hospital
- accidents and injuries sustained from violence in the workplace
- death in the workplace
- diseases, such as **occupational** dermatitis or work-related asthma
- dangerous occurrences (eg a gas leak) even if they occur outside working hours and no-one is injured.

EMPLOYER'S RESPONSIBILITIES

Your employer's responsibility under the regulations is to report any of the above **occurrences** and make sure that information about the occurrence has been recorded.

EMPLOYEE'S RESPONSIBILITIES

Your responsibilities under the regulations are to:

- report any work-related diseases to the person responsible for health and safety
- prevent any work-related diseases by wearing PPE
- report any accidents or injuries that happen to you at work
- prevent accidents or injuries by following safe working guidelines and maintaining a tidy environment.

ACTIVITY

Which work-related diseases might you be exposed to? Make a list. Discuss your list with your manager and colleagues.

HEALTH AND SAFETY (FIRST AID) REGULATIONS 1981

The Health and Safety (First Aid) Regulations apply to all workplaces in Great Britain – including those with fewer than five employees and those with self-employed staff. The regulations require the protection of everyone in the workplace by making sure risk assessments are carried out to prevent accidents and injuries at work. It is **advisable** that at least one person has undertaken first-aid training.

ACTIVITY

Find out who your first aider is and how to contact them.

Occupational
Relating to a job.

Occurence
Something that happens.

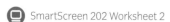 SmartScreen 202 Worksheet 2

HANDY HINTS
Make sure you know where the business keeps their health and safety policies as these should all be accessible.

Advisable
Suggested that you should.

HANDY HINTS
Know where your first-aid box is kept just in case you need to access it.

A basic first-aid box or container should include:

- a leaflet giving general guidance on first aid (eg HSE's leaflet *Basic advice on first aid at work*)
- 20 individually wrapped sterile plasters (assorted sizes), appropriate to the type of work (**hypoallergenic** plasters can be provided, if necessary)
- two sterile eye pads
- four individually wrapped triangular bandages, preferably sterile
- six safety pins
- two large sterile individually wrapped unmedicated wound dressings
- six medium sized individually wrapped unmedicated wound dressings
- a pair of disposable gloves.

The appointed person should check the contents of the first-aid container frequently and make sure it is restocked if anything is used. They should make sure the safe disposal of items when they reach their expiry date.

EMPLOYER'S RESPONSIBILITIES

Your employer's responsibilities under the regulations are to:

- take immediate action if employees are injured or taken ill at work
- consider providing a first aider
- choose an appointed person to be responsible for first-aid arrangements
- provide a well-stocked first-aid container
- make sure all staff know who the appointed first aider is (if appropriate).

EMPLOYEE'S RESPONSIBILITIES

Your responsibilities under the regulations are to:

- avoid taking any unnecessary risks that might put you or others in danger
- report to your appointed person any first-aid supply shortages
- record any accidents in an accident book. Make a note of who had the accident, the date and time of the accident and what action was taken. Record the name of any witnesses and who else was present at the time of the accident. The accident book should be kept in a central location in the salon.

HEALTH AND SAFETY (DISPLAY SCREEN EQUIPMENT) REGULATIONS 1992

The Health and Safety (Display Screen Equipment) Regulations protect the health of people who work with display screen equipment (DSE). This includes computer workstations or visual display units (VDU) (ie computer screens). It applies to people, such as salon receptionists, who use display screen equipment for long periods at a time as part of their job. It does not apply to occasional use, such as making appointments. Long-term use is often associated with neck, shoulder, back or arm pain, fatigue and eyestrain. Display screen equipment work is not risky but users need to follow good practice, such as setting up their workstations well and taking **periodic** breaks.

Hypoallergenic
Products that do not contain any or many of the known allergens.

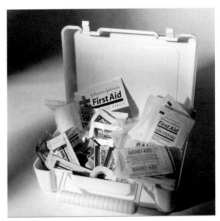
First-aid box

HANDY HINTS
Make sure you know where the accident record book is kept.

HANDY HINTS
Don't worry about the year that an Act is given, it is the content that is important.

HANDY HINTS
Everyone has a duty of care so follow your salon's rules and guidelines when you are treating clients.

Periodic
A set period of time.

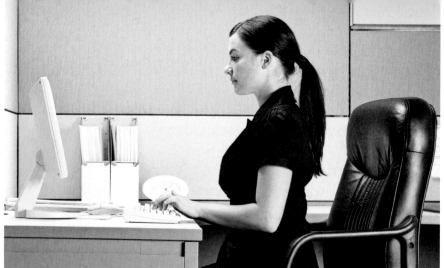

Good posture when sitting

EMPLOYER'S RESPONSIBILITIES

Your employer's responsibilities under the regulations are to:

- carry out risk assessments on new workstations or make changes to current workstations
- re-assess workstations if staff suffer from any discomfort
- train employees in good practice for working with display screen equipment
- plan scheduling of work, regular breaks and changes of activity
- pay for employees to have eyesight tests if required.

EMPLOYEE'S RESPONSIBILITIES

Your responsibilities under the regulations are to:

- make sure you maintain good posture. Keep your back straight when you work and do not slouch. Keep your feet flat on the floor when sitting
- take regular breaks if you are using display screen equipment for long periods of time and to change activity. If you are a receptionist change to a different task, such as dusting the reception area
- organise your desk space effectively
- keep your 'mouse arm' straight and rest it lightly on the mouse
- use a wrist support
- keep your keyboard close to your body and not to overstretch
- adjust the screen or lighting position where possible to suit your personal needs.

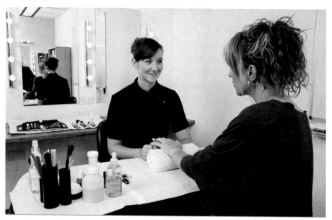

The therapist and client must be comfortable

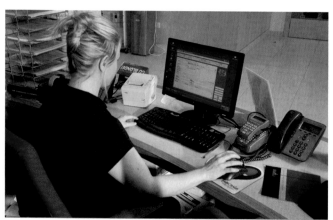

Supporting posture is important when sitting

LAWS RELATING TO CONSUMER PROTECTION

In this part of the chapter you will learn about the:

SmartScreen 201 Worksheet 3

- Data Protection Act 1998
- Consumer Protection Act 1987
- Consumer Protection (Distance Selling) Regulations 2002
- Supply of Goods and Services Act 1982
- Sale of Goods Act 1979
- Sale and Supply of Goods Act 1994
- Trade Descriptions Act 1968 and 1972
- Prices Act 1974.

DATA PROTECTION ACT 1998

Clients give you their personal information, such as their address and phone number, because they trust you and the salon to use it correctly. Clients' information must be protected and you must always follow the Data Protection Act.

The Information Commissioner's Office is the UK's independent authority set up to uphold information rights in the public's interest. It sets the rules for the Data Protection Act, which protects people's rights to confidentiality and privacy. When completing client record cards and taking contact details at reception, you must make sure you follow the requirements of the Data Protection Act. Under the Data Protection Act, businesses must register if they keep client data on a computer. There are several principles to the Data Protection Act.

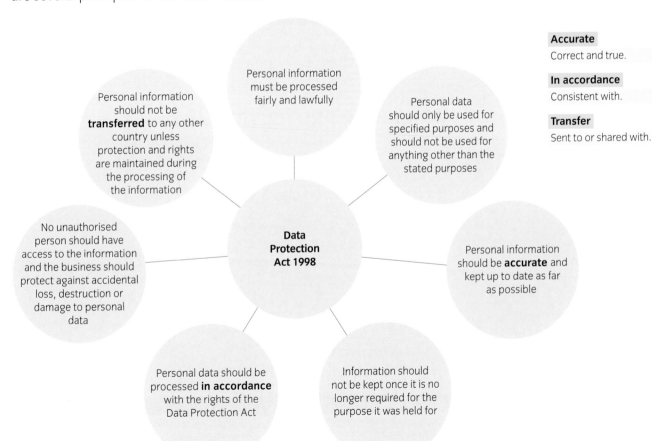

Accurate
Correct and true.

In accordance
Consistent with.

Transfer
Sent to or shared with.

Third party

Another person who is not directly involved but has connections with the business.

Gross misconduct

Very bad, unacceptable behaviour.

Retail price list

Unethical

Immoral or unacceptable behaviour.

Negligent

Failing to take proper care.

EMPLOYER'S RESPONSIBILITIES

Your employer's responsibilities under the Act are to:

- only keep information that is needed for the business
- keep records as accurate as possible and up to date
- dispose of information carefully (eg shred paper documents) when it is no longer required
- never pass on any information to a **third party**
- limit access to records to only those employees who need it for their work.

EMPLOYEE'S RESPONSIBILITIES

The Data Protection Act protects you and all the data stored about you whether it is held on paper or on a computer. This includes medical and dental records, bank records and employment and college records. You have a right to access this information if and when you want to and you should expect it to be kept confidential. Remember this and be professional with any information you record regarding any individual.

You must keep records as accurately as you can and keep information confidential. You must not pass on any information about your clients to a third party, whether that is personal details, services that they have had or products that they have bought.

Failing to keep client confidentiality could mean losing clients and gaining a poor reputation. A client could sue the business in which case the guilty employee could be given a warning or lose their job for **gross misconduct**.

INDUSTRY TIP

Never give clients personal information, such as your address or phone number. It is **unethical** and might put you at risk. Your contract of employment might also forbid this – for example, to prevent staff from encouraging clients to have their treatments done privately in their homes.

CONSUMER PROTECTION ACT 1987

In the salon, we are exposed daily to different products and we have a right to expect those products to be as safe as possible. The Consumer Protection Act safeguards staff and clients from products that do not reach a reasonable level of safety.

It is now possible to sue a supplier even without proof of the supplier being **negligent** under the Sale of Goods Act (see page 109). A therapist using the product in the salon can sue if a product is faulty (even though your employer purchased it).

The Consumer Protection Act also covers:

- misleading prices, services or facilities
- price comparisons
- inaccurate conditions attached to the price.

HANDY HINTS

Do you know where to find the product price lists, if there is a price query?

EMPLOYER'S RESPONSIBILITIES

The employer's responsibilities under this Act are to:

- have clear prices for products and services. The client should be able to tell exactly how much something will cost
- not make false claims about a product or service nor mislead a client
- not attach conditions of sale for either a product or service that are inaccurate or misleading.

EMPLOYEE'S RESPONSIBILITIES

Your responsibilities under the Act are to:

- give clients clear prices for products and services
- be honest when you are promoting or selling a product or treatment. Do not say a product or treatment does something if it does not.

CONSUMER PROTECTION (DISTANCE SELLING) REGULATIONS 2002

The Consumer Protection (Distance Selling) Regulations make sure that when goods are purchased over the phone, off the Internet or by mail order the consumer has the right to receive a refund. If there was a delivery charge this must also be refunded. However, costs **incurred** by the client to return the item are not included.

Incur
Acquire or come into.

If you need to return something you must check the contract information, which will include the name and address of the supplier, a description and details of the goods or services and the price paid.

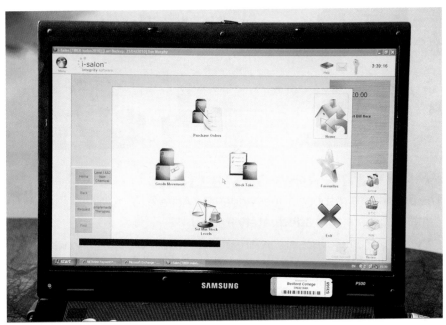

Controlling stock electronically

EMPLOYER'S RESPONSIBILITIES

The employer's responsibilities under the regulations are:

- to give clients a refund if they are unhappy with a product but not to cover the cost of the postage to return the item
- to display **contractual** information on the website with clear terms and conditions of sale.

Contractual
Information agreed in a contract.

EMPLOYEE'S RESPONSIBILITIES

Your responsibility under the regulations is to offer and process a refund if a client wants to return a product.

SUPPLY OF GOODS AND SERVICES ACT 1982

Services, faulty goods and materials provided with those services or treatments are covered within the Supply of Goods and Services Act. The Act makes sure that:

- a service is carried out with skill and reasonable care
- a service is carried out within a reasonable amount of time
- a service meets what it claims to do
- the charge for the service is reasonable
- any goods supplied in the course of the services are of a satisfactory quality and fit for the purpose
- a consumer has the right to have goods replaced, repaired or compensated if they are of poor quality or are not fit for the purpose for which they have been supplied.

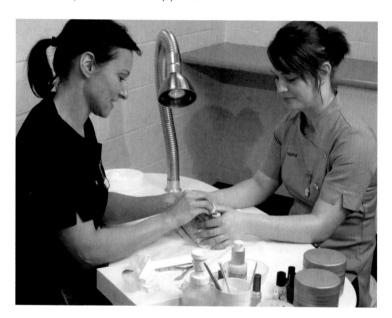

EMPLOYER'S RESPONSIBILITIES

The employer's responsibilities under the Act are to:

- make sure staff are **adequately** trained
- make sure employees are aware of their responsibilities and what is expected of them during their working hours
- charge a reasonable price for a service
- have clear treatment/service times and to make sure therapists know and work to the treatment/service times
- state exactly what a treatments does
- make sure that the goods that the business supplies are of a good quality and fit for the purpose they are sold for
- replace products which are faulty or not fit for the purpose for which they were sold
- **compensate** a client if a service is of a poor quality.

Adequate

To a suitable or acceptable standard.

HANDY HINTS

Always check that the products you are using are in date. If they are out of date let your manager know so that the product can be replaced.

Compensate

To get your money back.

EMPLOYEE'S RESPONSIBILITIES

Your responsibilities under the Act are to:

- carry out services professionally with skill and care and to only offer those treatments for which you are trained
- charge a reasonable price for services
- know and work to the service times of the salon
- only state what a treatments does (do not make up information)
- only retail products of a good quality and fit for the purpose for which they are being sold
- refer any complaint regarding faulty goods or services to a manager to action a refund or compensation.

SALE OF GOODS ACT 1979 AND SALE AND SUPPLY OF GOODS ACT 1994

The Sale of Goods Act and the Sale and Supply of Goods Act cover consumer rights including:

- goods being of satisfactory quality
- the conditions under which goods might be returned after purchase
- whether the goods are fit for their intended purpose
- goods being free from faults or defects.

If these are not followed the consumer has the right to a replacement or refund.

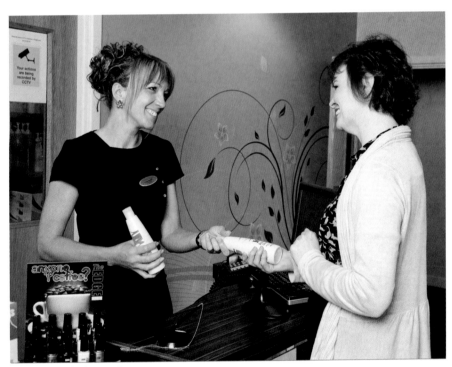

Explaining a faulty product

EMPLOYER'S RESPONSIBILITIES

The employer's responsibilities under the Acts are to:

- check that goods being ordered are of a satisfactory condition and free from faults
- have a clear conditions of sale policy that states when products can be returned.

Expectations
A strong belief that something will happen.

EMPLOYEE'S RESPONSIBILITIES

Your responsibilities under the Acts are to:

- check stock being delivered for damage or faults and to make sure it meets **expectations**
- check stock before retailing to make sure it is in good condition and has not passed its shelf life
- accept returns within the return period and to offer a replacement or refund.

TRADE DESCRIPTIONS ACT 1968 AND 1972

The Trade Descriptions Act prevents services or products:

- being falsely described or false claims being made
- giving false information, including quality, price or purpose
- being falsely advertised, displayed or described.

EMPLOYER'S RESPONSIBILITIES

The employer's responsibility under the Act is to make sure that all staff are properly trained and understand the products they are using and the services they are giving.

EMPLOYEE'S RESPONSIBILITIES

Your responsibilities under the Act are to:

- describe treatment and products accurately. You need to know your product information well so that you can do this
- not make any false claims about a treatment or product.

ACTIVITY

Make a list of the different ways products could be priced incorrectly or advertised to give a misleading impression. Discuss with your colleagues.

ACTIVITY

Discuss with your colleagues offers that you have been interested in only to discover hidden costs. How did it make you feel?

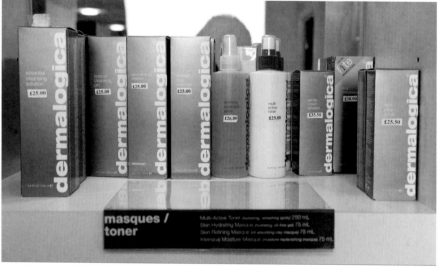

Retail products with prices displayed

PRICES ACT 1974

The Prices Act requires the price of products or services to be displayed clearly. A treatment price list needs to be visible and product prices need to be clearly marked either on the item or on the shelf where they are displayed.

OTHER RELEVANT LEGISLATION

In this part of the chapter you will learn about the:

- Equality Act 2010
- Employers' **Liability** (Compulsory Insurance) Act 1969
- Copyright, Designs and Patent Act 1998.

Liability
Responsibility for something that has been done wrong.

EQUALITY ACT 2010

The Equality Act lays down laws to prevent discrimination against anyone on the grounds of:

- race or ethnic origin
- sexual orientation
- marriage or civil partnership status
- pregnancy
- religion
- beliefs
- age
- disability.

The Equality Act includes the:

- Sex Discrimination Act 1975
- Race Relations Act 1976
- Race Relations Act 1976 (Amendment) Regulations 2003
- Equal Pay Act 1970
- Disability Discrimination Act 2005
- Employment Equality Regulations.

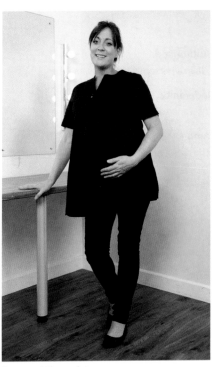

Pregnant therapist

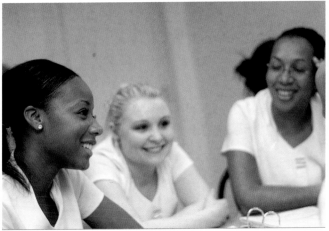

Beauty and nail therapy is multicultural

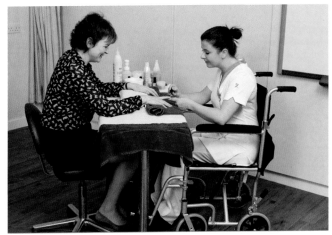

Disabled therapist at work

Victimisation

When a person is treated less favourably than others.

Harassment

Unwanted behaviour towards someone.

Authorised

When a person or company has official power.

Indemnity

Insurance against damage or loss.

Ambience

The surroundings of a place.

The Equality Act applies to both the employer and the employees within a business so it is important that everyone understands the effects of not adhering to it as they could be held liable. The Act includes protection against intimidation and bullying through **victimisation** and **harassment**.

EMPLOYERS' LIABILITY (COMPULSORY INSURANCE) ACT 1969

If a business has employees it must have employers' liability insurance to comply with the Employers' Liability (Compulsory Insurance) Act. If an employee becomes injured or ill as a result of their work they have the right to claim compensation from their employer. Employers must have adequate insurance to cover any possible insurance claims. Most business would be unable to pay a claim so insurance is taken out to cover potential payments. The insurance must be with an **authorised** insurance provider. It might be part of a wider insurance package to meet the other liabilities, such as professional **indemnity** and public liability insurance.

COPYRIGHT, DESIGNS AND PATENT ACT 1998

Music being played in the salon can help to create the right atmosphere and **ambience**. Music can create an upbeat feel to a room or help listeners to feel calm and relaxed. In order to play music in the salon you need to hold a special licence to comply with the Copyright, Designs and Patent Act.

When we play music (even the radio in the staff room) it becomes a public performance. Your employer must purchase a licence from the Performing Rights Society Ltd (PRS) in order to play music in the salon using a radio, TV, CD or MP3 player. The PRS works on behalf of artists, writers and publishers to collect and distribute a fee for a licence as royalties.

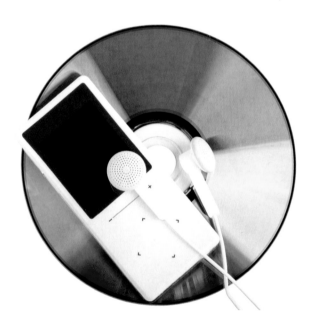

Use the questions below to test your knowledge of legislation to see how much information you have retained. These questions will help you to revise what you have learnt in this chapter.

Turn to page 601 for the answers.

1. How does the Data Protection Act protect the public?
   a) It limits the number of treatments available
   b) It ensures the right to confidentiality
   c) It makes sure all staff are treated fairly
   d) It limits access to clients' records

2. Who is responsible for providing personal protective equipment in the workplace?
   a) Receptionist
   b) Employee
   c) Employer
   d) Colleague

3. Which **one** of the following provides guidelines for the storage of chemicals?
   a) Control of Substances Hazardous to Health (COSHH) Regulations
   b) Personal Protective Equipment (PPE) at Work Regulations
   c) Provision and Use of Work Equipment Regulations (PUWER)
   d) Health and Safety (First Aid) Regulations

4. Which **one** of the following is a responsibility of the employer in relation to the Health and Safety (First Aid) Regulations?
   a) To give all staff members a first-aid leaflet and ask them to read it
   b) To take immediate action if an employee is taken ill at work
   c) To make all staff pay for a first-aid course
   d) To provide PPE and a first-aid container

5. Which **one** of the following types of behaviour is harassment?
   a) Being assertive
   b) Hostility
   c) Delegating
   d) Giving instructions

6. The Consumer Protection Act protects the client from:
   a) special offers
   b) misleading prices
   c) sales prices
   d) cheap products.

7. The Equality Act prevents discrimination against anyone on the grounds of:
   a) working hours
   b) religious beliefs
   c) annual leave
   d) the minimum wage.

8. Falsely describing or making false claims about a product are prevented by which Act?
   a) Supply of Goods and Services Act
   b) Trade Descriptions Act
   c) Prices Act
   d) Consumer Protection Act

9. Which **one** of the following Acts states that the price of a product or service must be clearly displayed?
   a) Trade Descriptions Act
   b) Consumer Protection Act
   c) Supply of Goods and Services Act
   d) Prices Act

10. The Performing Rights Society (PRS) licence gives you the right to play music in the salon on:
   a) an MP3 player
   b) any device
   c) a CD player
   d) an Android phone.

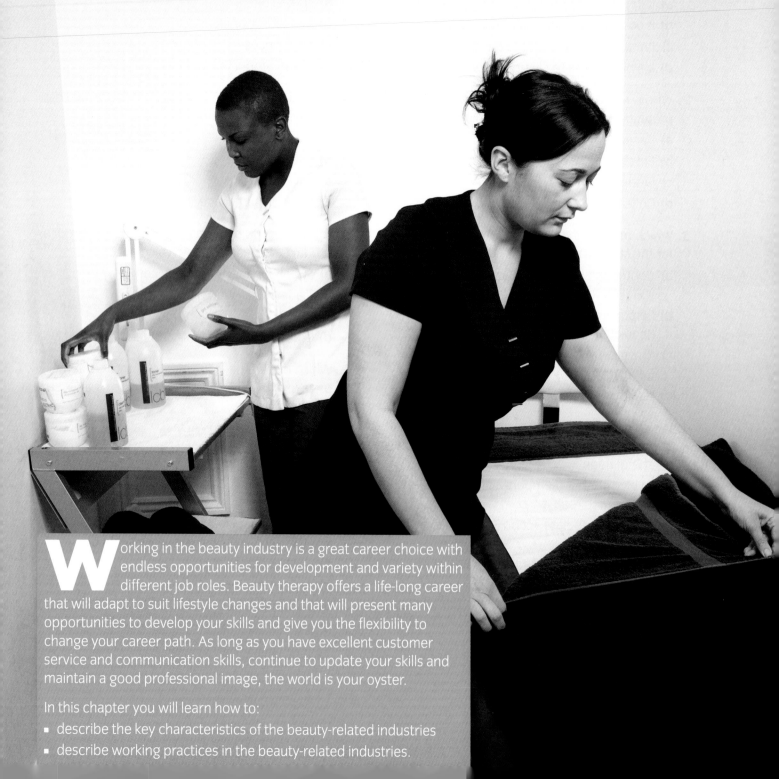

201
WORKING IN BEAUTY-RELATED INDUSTRIES

Working in the beauty industry is a great career choice with endless opportunities for development and variety within different job roles. Beauty therapy offers a life-long career that will adapt to suit lifestyle changes and that will present many opportunities to develop your skills and give you the flexibility to change your career path. As long as you have excellent customer service and communication skills, continue to update your skills and maintain a good professional image, the world is your oyster.

In this chapter you will learn how to:

- describe the key characteristics of the beauty-related industries
- describe working practices in the beauty-related industries.

KEY CHARACTERISTICS OF BEAUTY-RELATED INDUSTRIES

In this part of the chapter you will learn about:

- qualifications within beauty therapy and nail services
- career opportunities and occupational roles within beauty-related industries
- employment characteristics of beauty-related industries
- developing and promoting a professional image
- continuing professional development (CPD)
- professional organisations within the beauty-related industries.

There are five main beauty-related industries:

- beauty therapy
- massage therapies
- spa therapies
- nail services/nail technology
- make-up/media make-up.

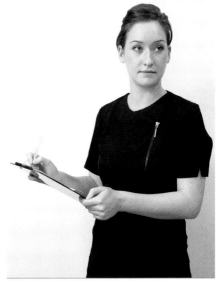

Beauty therapist

QUALIFICATIONS WITHIN BEAUTY THERAPY AND NAIL SERVICES

Each qualification will offer a different range of **generic** and technical treatment units depending on the qualification route and level. Some of the units will be **mandatory** and are therefore needed to achieve the qualification and others will be optional. Have a look at City & Guilds' website (www.cityandguilds.com) for details of which units appear in which qualifications.

Generic
General, not specific.

Mandatory
Mandatory units are units that you must cover in order to achieve your qualification.

VRQ stands for Vocationally-Related Qualification. VRQs are preparation for work qualifications that involve training towards a practical qualification. VRQs aim to help build and develop employment skills within a particular vocation or industry. The Level 2 qualifications that this book relates to are VRQs.

NVQ stands for a National Vocational Qualification. It is a work-based qualification that is designed to measure competency in a specific professional role. NVQs are assessed in a realistic work environment and are commonly part of an apprenticeship route to gain a qualification.

LEVEL 1 QUALIFICATIONS AND RESPONSIBILITIES

At Level 1, the therapist is taught about the hair and beauty industry and they learn some basic treatment routines. There is an opportunity to explore the industry and learn some basic techniques on a Level 1 training programme.

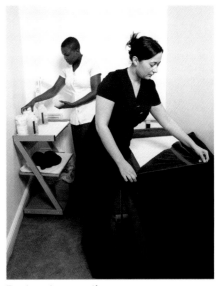

Treatment preparation

LEVEL 2 QUALIFICATIONS AND RESPONSIBILITIES

At Level 2, there is the opportunity for extending knowledge and skills and learning a range of the more popular beauty treatments. At Level 2, the therapist works in a junior capacity developing into a therapist or nail technician when they have gained some experience. The Level 2 therapist learns and carries out treatments on the face (including the head and the scalp), the lower arms and the lower legs. In addition, they are responsible for maintaining the treatment and retail areas, offering treatments and carrying out reception duties.

At Level 2, therapists and nail technicians can gain employment, however it is limited and the expected level to gain is Level 3.

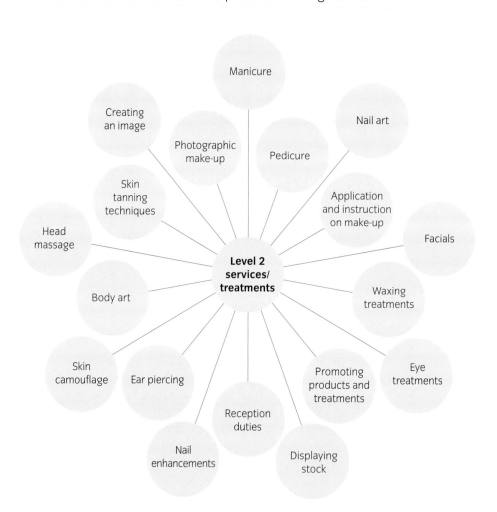

Mentoring
To give advice and guidance to less experienced members of staff.

LEVEL 3 QUALIFICATIONS AND RESPONSIBILITIES

At Level 3, more specialised treatments and massage therapies are studied, such as full-body treatments. At Level 3, the therapist or nail technician should be looking to take on a more supervisory role, coaching or **mentoring** more junior members of staff.

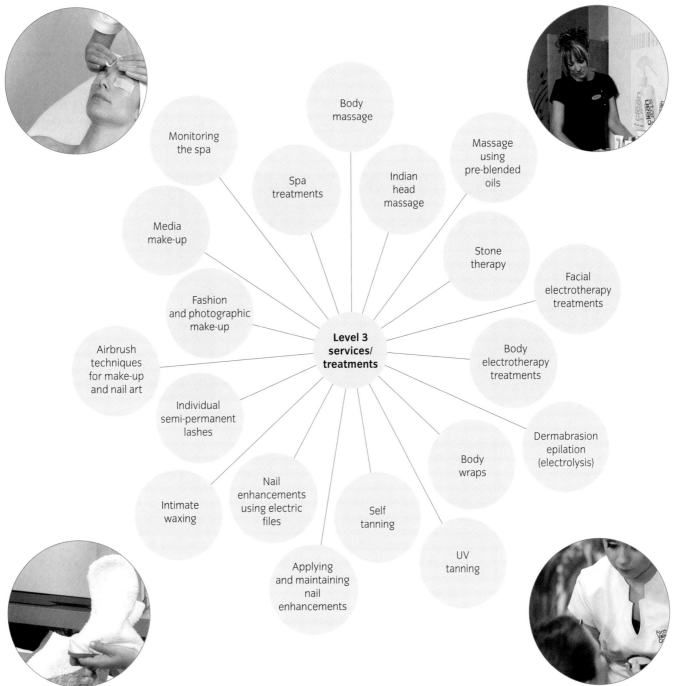

Level 3 services/treatments

- Body massage
- Monitoring the spa
- Spa treatments
- Indian head massage
- Massage using pre-blended oils
- Media make-up
- Stone therapy
- Facial electrotherapy treatments
- Fashion and photographic make-up
- Body electrotherapy treatments
- Airbrush techniques for make-up and nail art
- Individual semi-permanent lashes
- Dermabrasion epilation (electrolysis)
- Body wraps
- Intimate waxing
- Nail enhancements using electric files
- Self tanning
- UV tanning
- Applying and maintaining nail enhancements

LEVEL 4 QUALIFICATIONS AND ABOVE

There are a few therapists who choose to study to degree or foundation degree level. Foundation degrees start at Level 4 in the first year of study with Level 6 being achieved upon completion of the qualification. Before being accepted onto a degree course, students will be required to demonstrate that they have achieved a certain level of study.

CAREER OPPORTUNITIES AND OCCUPATIONAL ROLES WITHIN BEAUTY-RELATED INDUSTRIES

BEAUTY THERAPIST

A beauty therapist will offer a selection of beauty therapy treatments working on the face, body, hands and feet. If they qualify to Level 3, they will also be able to offer a range of full-body treatments. Some of these treatments might involve the use of electro-therapy equipment.

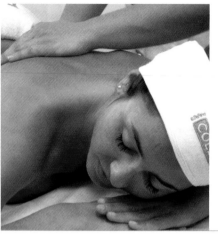 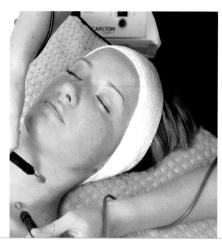 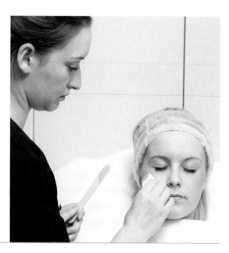

Beauty therapy services at Level 3

Destination spas

These are places where you can go for a longer stay with the aim of helping you to develop a healthier lifestyle through healthy cuisine, a physical activity programme, relaxing spa treatments and education on wellbeing. They are often located abroad.

Tranquil

Peaceful.

A beauty therapist can choose to work in a variety of employment settings including a salon, a spa (including **destination spas** and hotel spas) and on cruise ships.

A spa therapist will tend to provide more holistic, slimming and detoxifying treatments. They will spend a lot of their treatment time performing massage treatments (both on the face and the body). A spa is a large establishment usually offering both spa treatments and water therapies to complement the spa treatments. Destination spas are based in more luxurious and **tranquil** settings (often abroad) and offer longer-term stays.

Life as a beauty therapist on a cruise liner is quite demanding. Therapists often specialise in certain treatments, such as massage, electro-therapy treatments or nail enhancements and generally work long hours. They often earn their wage through commission on the treatments and products they sell. On the other hand, they get to travel the world, meet lots of interesting people and see some fantastic places.

INDUSTRY TIP

The term 'beautician' is occasionally used to refer to a therapist who just works on the face, hands and feet.

INDUSTRY TIP

Health farms are now generally known as spas. Traditionally, health farms were seen as somewhere to go and stay to try and lose some weight, eat healthily and have treatments to assist with the process. Spas today are seen more as a luxurious place where you can go to relax and de-stress.

MAKE-UP ARTIST

A make-up artist specialises in creating an image through the use of make-up techniques and hairstyles. As a result, they might also be qualified in hairdressing and wig making. A make-up artist might specialise in make-up techniques for photographic make-up or application of prosthetics and theatrical make-up. They will work in a variety of settings, including photographic studios (for still images), film

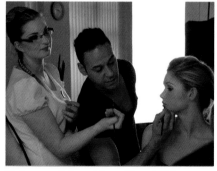

Make-up artist working with a stylist

THE CITY & GUILDS TEXTBOOK

sets (for films, adverts and music videos), various locations for weddings or special event work, backstage at fashion shows, fashion studios and backstage for theatre productions.

NAIL TECHNICIAN

A nail technician specialises in nail treatments and nail enhancements. They often work with a variety of systems – including gel, acrylic, fibreglass, tip and overlay and nail sculpturing (a freehand nail enhancement technique). They might also work with coloured enhancements or 2D and 3D nail art. Many nail technicians work in nail bars or studios rather than in beauty salons. Nail technicians need to practise their skills regularly to make sure they provide a quick, efficient and cost-effective service.

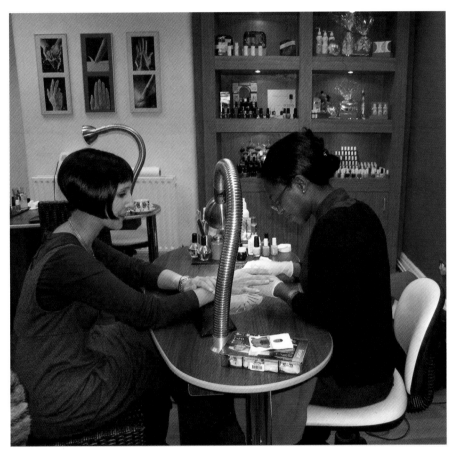

Nail technician at work

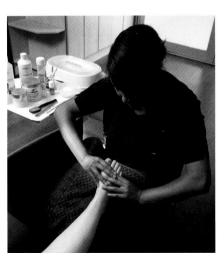

Massage therapist

COMPLEMENTARY THERAPIST

A complementary therapist specialises in **holistic** treatments, including body massage, reflexology and aromatherapy. They might work **independently** or within spas or within the healthcare sector (in clinics or hospices) where they work alongside medical practitioners and nurses to offer complementary care alongside medical care.

Holistic
Looking at the body as a whole.

Independently
On your own, not part of a spa.

COSMETIC OR BEAUTY CONSULTANT

A cosmetic or beauty consultant will work in a department or a specialist cosmetics store. They will have a lot of knowledge of a particular skin care or make-up range that they will be responsible for retailing and advising customers on.

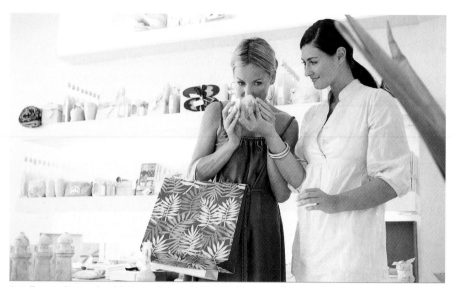

Retail consultants should always be ready to help find exactly what the customer is looking for

RECEPTIONIST

The reception is the focal point of any business and the receptionist is the client's first point of contact with the salon. Receptionists are responsible for maintaining the reception area, meeting and greeting clients, making appointments, taking telephone calls or picking up emails, relaying message to colleagues, filing or monitoring treatment information, organising treatment rooms and taking payments.

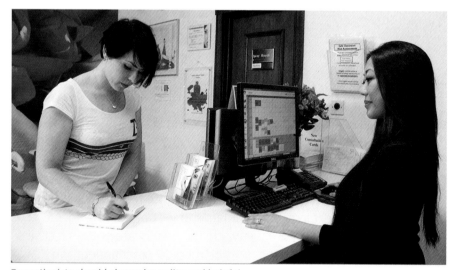

Receptionists should always be polite and helpful

SPECIALIST ROLES WITHIN THE BEAUTY-RELATED INDUSTRY

When qualified, therapists might decide to specialise in a specific area. For example, a beauty therapist could specialise in permanent hair removal using techniques, such as electrolysis, IPL and laser treatments.

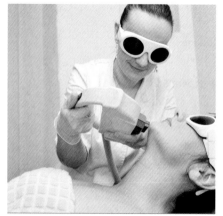

Laser treatment is one area a therapist can specialise in

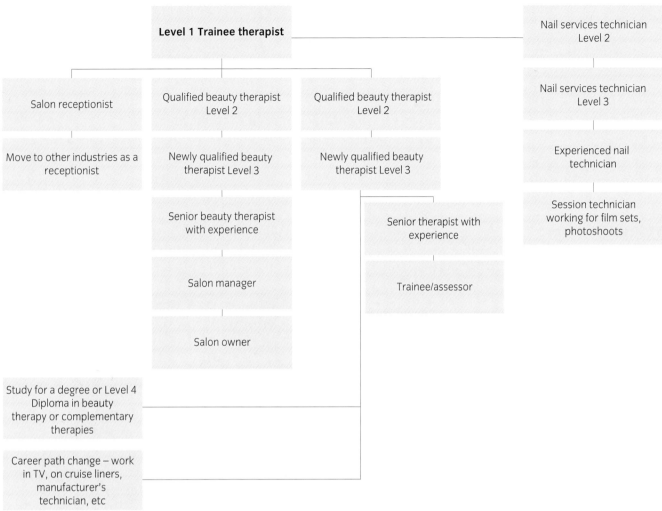

| Level 1 Trainee therapist | | | Nail services technician Level 2 |

Flowchart boxes:

- **Level 1 Trainee therapist**
- Nail services technician Level 2
- Salon receptionist
- Qualified beauty therapist Level 2
- Qualified beauty therapist Level 2
- Nail services technician Level 3
- Move to other industries as a receptionist
- Newly qualified beauty therapist Level 3
- Newly qualified beauty therapist Level 3
- Experienced nail technician
- Senior beauty therapist with experience
- Senior therapist with experience
- Session technician working for film sets, photoshoots
- Salon manager
- Trainee/assessor
- Salon owner
- Study for a degree or Level 4 Diploma in beauty therapy or complementary therapies
- Career path change – work in TV, on cruise liners, manufacturer's technician, etc

The different career pathways within the beauty-related industries

There are some practitioners who choose to train and specialise in one area (eg a manicurist, a masseuse, an aromatherapist, a reflexologist). The more specialised you are, the harder it is to establish a career since by only offering a limited choice of treatments, it takes a long time to build up a **client base**.

Client base

Clients that visit a salon or therapist regularly.

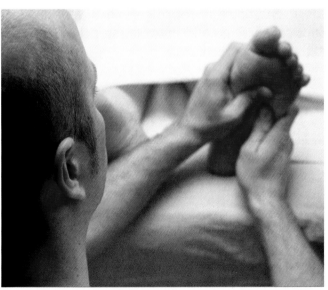

A reflexologist might specialise in one or more complementary therapies

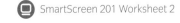
SmartScreen 201 Worksheet 2

OTHER OCCUPATIONAL ROLES WITHIN BEAUTY-RELATED INDUSTRIES

For some roles it is essential that some job experience has been gained before starting the role. This is because the experience and knowledge will help you to perform the role with more proficiency and confidence.

Sales representative or area account manager

A sales representative or area account manager will work for a product, equipment or manufacturing company, such as Decleor, CACI, Jessica (Gerrard International) or Bare Escentuals. The role involves travelling around the country (or a region) visiting salon owners or managers to tell them about the company's products. Some are office based. The role also includes **business development**, managing business accounts, organising stock orders and arranging promotions. Sometimes these roles involve **cold-calling** new salons to generate new business.

Business development

Identifying new business opportunities, such as attracting new customers or identifying new sales opportunities.

Cold-calling

Contacting a new customer or business for the first time without an appointment.

It is important that a sales representative is knowledgeable about all their products

Salon or spa manager

The salon or spa manager is responsible for managing the day-to-day running of the business. They need to be experienced, organised and able to **delegate** work to ensure the smooth running of the business. Their role might include supervising staff, controlling stock levels and daily cashing up at the end of the working day.

Delegate

Passing work to someone else.

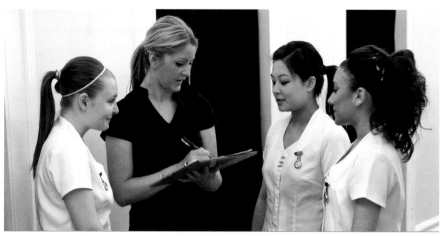

A manager must be able to direct and motivate a team

THE CITY & GUILDS TEXTBOOK

Salon owner

The salon owner owns the business and has overall responsibility for the day-to-day running and success of the business. The business could be one that has been started from scratch or it might have been bought as a **going concern**. It might also be a **franchise**. The owner can employ people to help with the running of the business, including therapists, a receptionist, a bookkeeper and an accountant. The salon owner is responsible for making the sure the salon runs smoothly, for example by making sure there is enough stock and that the bills are paid.

Going concern
An existing business that is making a profit.

Franchise
This is where an individual or group of salons have been given the right to trade under an **established** brand and market that company's goods or services. An example of a franchise in the beauty industry is Saks. The advantage of buying a franchise means that you are using an established business format and brand and will therefore have access to support systems and business expertise from the company that owns the franchise.

Established
Found on/in.

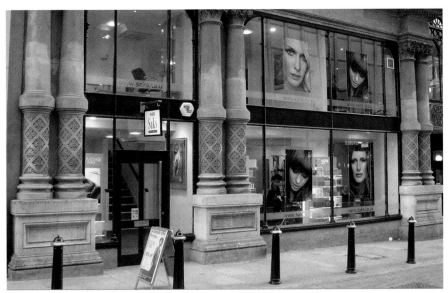
A large high street hair and beauty salon

Recruitment consultant

A recruitment consultant works for a specialist recruitment company or agency and matches job vacancies to suitable candidates. The recruitment company might carry out **trade testing** on candidates.

Trainer

A trainer works with a specific company to train therapists or nail technicians in treatment techniques and/or product knowledge. The trainer might be based at the company's head office and train there or provide on-site training at a salon or business.

Trade testing
This is an activity that businesses use to see whether your skills are good enough for the job. For example, you might be asked to carry out a nail polish application, a half-leg wax and a facial massage.

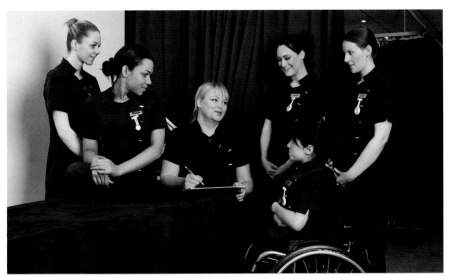
A trainer can provide on-site training in treatment techniques

Teacher, lecturer or assessor

A teacher passes on their knowledge and experience to others. Teachers might have knowledge and experience in several different treatments or be a specialist in a particular treatment. If teachers are to deliver effective lessons and practical sessions, they need to do a lot of planning.

Teachers, lecturers and assessors are employed by private training providers and further or higher education colleges.

A tutor or lecturer might also have the additional role of being an assessor. An assessor observes candidates in a practical salon environment and provides feedback on treatments, written assignments and tests. Assessors must have occupational experience and expertise in the areas that they are assessing so that they can make informed judgements (against **criteria** given to them by the **awarding organisation**) of the learners' work.

Criteria
Standards that you are measured against.

Awarding organisation
The body that awards qualifications if certain criteria have been met.

A Quality Assurance Coordinator needs to be able to observe and judge assessments

EMPLOYMENT CHARACTERISTICS OF BEAUTY-RELATED INDUSTRIES

As a therapist there are a variety of ways in which you can be employed. You can be:

- full-time
- part-time
- permanent
- on a contract
- freelance
- self-employed.

FULL-TIME EMPLOYMENT

Full-time employment means that you are likely to be contracted to work between 37 and 40 hours a week. Your contract will state the hours that you work and your terms and conditions. You might work set hours or on a shift pattern (eg working four days and then having two days off).

INDUSTRY TIP

Shift patterns are common in businesses that are open seven days a week to make sure the opening hours are fully covered by staff.

The employer that you work for will deduct the tax and national insurance payments you are required to make from your pay and this will be detailed on your wage slip.

PART-TIME EMPLOYMENT

Part-time employees, as the term suggests, work less hours per week than full-time employees. Part-time employees typically work between 15 and 29 hours per week. They usually have set hours (eg every Saturday and one evening per week) but this can be flexible.

Full-time and part-time employees can either be permanent employees or employed on a contract.

PERMANENT EMPLOYMENT

You will have a contract that states that you work for the company on a permanent basis. Your contract will outline how much notice you need to give should you choose to leave the company. Your contract works both ways and it will also state what notice the company needs to give you should it decide that you are not carrying out your duties or meeting the terms and conditions of your contract or in cases of redundancy.

CONTRACT WORK

This type of employment will mean that you are employed for a specific contract over a specific period of time. The period of time that you will be working for the company will be specified in the contract. You are not a permanent member of staff but have the same minimum rights as a permanent member of staff for the period that you are employed. You might be full- or part-time.

FREELANCE

A freelance therapist is usually self-employed and is usually paid a fee. They arrange and schedule their own work. Make-up artists and nail technicians are often freelance and might carry out a specific make-up or photographic session on a fee basis.

SELF-EMPLOYED

As a self-employed therapist, make-up artist or nail technician you could work independently as a freelancer but you could also work for someone in a self-employed capacity. For example, you could rent a room within a salon. However, there can **potentially** be some legal issues with doing this so before you did this you would need to look into it carefully to understand clearly who is responsible for what within the business. This type of employment can be flexible but it does mean that you are responsible for paying your own tax and National Insurance and there might not be a constant stream of work. You will also be required to take out your own insurance cover for your work activities.

DEVELOPING AND PROMOTING A PROFESSIONAL IMAGE

When both working in the salon and representing the business externally, it is important that you present a professional image and promote yourself positively.

HANDY HINTS

Information about careers in beauty therapy can be found from a variety of sources – the Internet, journals, textbooks, e-books, podcasts, your college or training provider and professional organisations, such as Habia. You can also find career information at your local Connections office and at www.careersadvice.direct.gov.uk.

Potentially
Possibly.

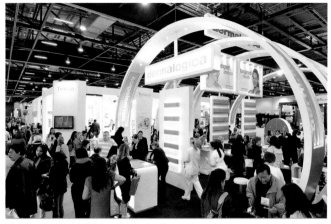

Visiting large exhibitions is useful for seeing developments and trends

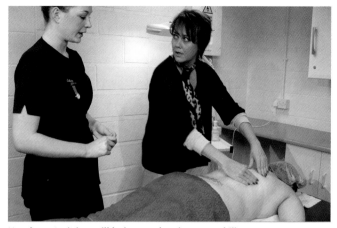

Hands-on training will help you develop new skills

PERSONAL DEVELOPMENT

Opportunities for personal development include:

- shadowing senior therapists
- attending exhibitions
- participating actively in training courses
- carrying out product and treatment demonstrations
- participating positively in promotional events, such as holding open evenings
- learning new skills or treatments
- watching demonstrations of new products and techniques on DVDs, podcasts and even shopping channels
- reading trade journals
- participating in network meetings (if you belong to any associations).

CONTINUING PROFESSIONAL DEVELOPMENT (CPD)

It is important to grow both professionally and personally within your career. CPD enables therapists to learn and practise new treatments and to keep up to date with and develop the latest techniques. It also helps to prevent work from becoming stale, mundane and boring. Adding new skills is a good way to increase business by adding new services to the treatment menu. It also enables you to be confident in your treatment techniques and product knowledge which will help you to perform your job better.

The best form of CPD is training. Many salons will send their employees on training courses, especially if they use a particular range of professional products. When a salon agrees to use and stock a company's product range, the company might require the salon to send its employees on their training course. This is to make sure the products are used correctly and in the way that the company wants them to be used. Some salons will also carry out their own training in the salon to make sure that their team of therapists is trained in carrying out treatments to the standard required by the salon.

HANDY HINTS

Learn from others by having a treatment from a colleague or at another salon. Learn from the experience. Was it a good or poor customer experience? Did you learn something new that you are going to try out?

INDUSTRY TIP

Professional training is essential for keeping employees motivated and up to date with the latest trends and techniques.

INDUSTRY TIP

Employees should be trained professionally not just by another member of staff. You want to make sure they are being taught accurately and correctly.

INDUSTRY TIP

If you work on your own, training events offer an ideal networking opportunity as you can meet other therapists and exchange ideas.

PROFESSIONAL ORGANISATIONS WITHIN BEAUTY-RELATED INDUSTRIES

SmartScreen 201 Worksheet 1

There are many different organisations within the beauty-related industries giving you plenty of career opportunities:

- salons
- hotels
- fitness and leisure providers
- cruise liners
- health spas
- manufacturers
- suppliers
- industry-led bodies
- awarding organisations
- professional membership organisations.

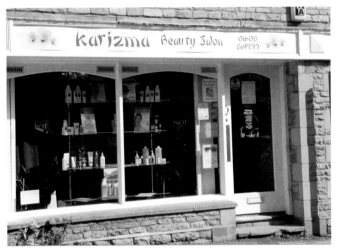

A smaller high street salon can still offer a range of services and products

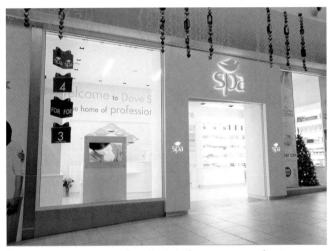

Day spas are an easy way for clients to have a pamper day or individual treatments

SALONS

Salons can take many different forms, from a simple treatment room based in the therapist's home to larger salons that have several treatment rooms and large spacious retail areas. A hairdressing salon or a chemist could also have a beauty therapy treatment room.

HOTELS

In addition to traditional facilities, some hotels also have salons or spa facilities within the hotel. Hotels that do not have on-site salons might be able to recommend beauty therapy services in the local area to their guests.

FITNESS AND LEISURE PROVIDERS

Fitness and leisure providers offer facilities to promote and encourage fitness and health. These typically include a swimming pool and a gym. They might also have an on-site salon.

CRUISE LINERS

Cruise liners are floating hotels. They offer a range of facilities including beauty therapy and hairdressing salons. Cruise liners provide an

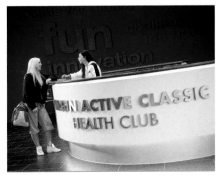

Large health clubs can offer a wide range of services

opportunity for the therapist to travel the world while working. Therapists are expected to be qualified to Level 3 before they can work on a cruise liner. Usually therapists sign a contract for a period of time (typically 9 months) and on a certain cruise route (eg Mediterranean or Caribbean). Since there will be people from a variety of backgrounds and nationalities working together on a cruise liner, there is usually an intense course of training that takes place before starting work to make sure that all therapists perform treatments in the same manner and to the required standard.

HEALTH SPAS

Today, the term spa is commonly used to mean somewhere that provides luxurious pampering treatments. However, it used to mean somewhere that had water facilities. Spas are **lucrative** businesses with more and more clients wanting a bit of luxurious pampering. They provide beautiful surroundings where clients can go for a day or short break to relax and unwind and be pampered with luxurious signature treatments. Destination spas are becoming increasingly popular with people who want a longer relaxing break. Spas usually offer a range of treatments. They also have wet areas, such as steam baths, hydro pools, wet treatment areas and a relaxation room. There might be less well-known therapies to try out.

MANUFACTURERS

Manufacturers design and make equipment for businesses. The manufacturer may sell this product themself or through a third party. They usually provide training to show salons how to use their equipment and will send out someone to fix it if anything goes wrong. See below for a summary of the benefits manufacturers can offer:

Lucrative
Profitable and makes money.

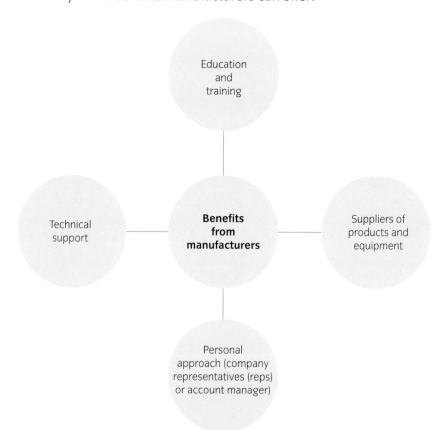

- Education and training
- Technical support
- **Benefits from manufacturers**
- Suppliers of products and equipment
- Personal approach (company representatives (reps) or account manager)

SUPPLIERS

There are two types of product suppliers:

- **Specific brand suppliers** supply a specific brand or product. For example, Inline supplies overalls and work wear. Some branded suppliers might offer **exclusivity** which means that only one business in an area will be permitted to use and retail their products. Some suppliers offer an account facility which means that you can order the goods and pay for them within 30 days of receiving them.
- **General suppliers** supply a range of essential **consumables** and products, such as wax, couch roll and cotton wool. Examples of general beauty therapy suppliers are Salon Direct, Essential Beauty Supplies and Salon Serve. They will offer more than one brand of the same product, for example they will offer waxing products from both Hive and Gigi.

INDUSTRY-LED BODIES

Habia is the Hairdressing and Beauty Industry Authority. They are an industry-led body and have information about the standards for hairdressing, barbering, beauty, nails and spa treatments.

Habia also offer support and advice to:

- salons by providing them with guidance on employment law and health and safety legislation
- employees by offering them advice on where to access suitable qualifications, training and centres delivering qualifications and by supplying support manuals
- to learners by providing advice on career pathways and a place from which to purchase books for their courses.

AWARDING ORGANISATIONS

The main awarding organisations within the beauty therapy industry are:

- City & Guilds (the biggest for the hair, beauty and nail industries)
- VTCT (Vocational Training Charitable Trust)
- ITEC (International Therapy Examination Council)
- BABTAC (British Association of Beauty Therapy and Cosmetology)
- Edxecel.

These organisations work closely with Habia to create qualifications based on the National Occupational Standards (NOS).

PROFESSIONAL MEMBERSHIP ORGANISATIONS

These organisations offer an industry **forum** and other services to their members often in return for a membership fee. The services that they offer include insurance cover, access to network meetings, recruitment services, professional products and journals. The main organisations in addition to those already listed above are:

- FHT (Federation of Holistic Therapists)
- The Beauty Guild
- British Institute and Association of Electrolysis
- International Spa Association.

Exclusivity
Offering products to one salon only.

Consumables
Items that need to be replaced.

WHY DON'T YOU...
take a look at the Habia website: http://www.habia.org.uk.

Forum
A place where members can exchange ideas and views.

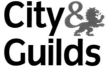
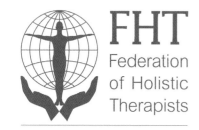
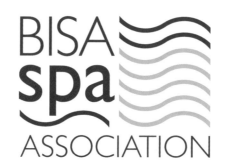
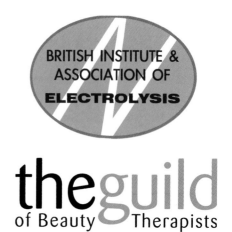

Awarding organisations and associations can be recognised by their logos

KNOW THE WORKING PRACTICES ASSOCIATED WITH BEAUTY-RELATED INDUSTRIES

HANDY HINTS

Research from Princeton University has shown that it takes only one tenth of a second for us to make up our minds about people, so we need to create a good first impression.

INDUSTRY TIP

The easy way to win over a client is with a genuine smile – it shows you are interested.

Judgemental
To form opinions about another person's behaviour or conduct. These judgments might be incorrect but are based on your personal opinions or values.

In this part of the chapter you will learn about:

- personal presentation
- employment rights and responsibilities.

PERSONAL PRESENTATION AND CREATING A GOOD FIRST IMPRESSION

People are **judgemental** and tend to form opinions about one another when they first meet, so it is essential that the first impression is a positive one. You only get one chance to make a good first impression!

Be prepared and look the part. Demonstrate a professional smart image; this will give both you and the client confidence. There is a lot of truth in the saying, 'dress the part to play the part'. If you went to see a nurse and they were wearing a scruffy uniform, with dirty finger nails, greasy hair and they were chewing gum, how would you feel? Would you feel confident?

ACTIVITY

Working in small groups, discuss an experience you have had where the first impression was negative and left you feeling disappointed, let down or irritated. Your experience could be about a visit to a hairdresser, a salon, a spa, a department store or a restaurant. Write down five points that you felt created the poor first impression.

ACTIVITY

Think of some professionals that have to wear a uniform and write down what the uniform tells you about their profession. Do you think that if they wore everyday clothes it would make you feel differently about them? What problems do you think could occur from not wearing a uniform as a beauty therapist or nail technician?

Many followers of trends and fashion feel that fashion trends should be carried across into the industry. You might love your image and look but will the majority of your clients? Your image needs to represent your industry and create a positive first impression as this is the one that will last.

When greeting clients for the first time, always introduce yourself. Make sure your client knows your name as it will help them relate to you on a more personal level. Always wear a name badge as it gives you identity and by giving the client your name in this way, you will become their point of contact. Therefore, if you make a good impression, the client will ask for you again if they want further treatments or advice.

DRESS CODE

There are many choices for uniform styles and colours. The photos below show a selection of the different types of uniforms available. It is important that any salon dress code is adhered to to maintain a professional or corporate image. Uniforms should always be clean, free of creases and fit well. You might also be required to wear flesh-coloured tights if you are wearing a skirt or dress.

ACTIVITY

Working in small groups, discuss an experience you have had where the first impression was positive. Write down five points that you felt created this positive first impression.

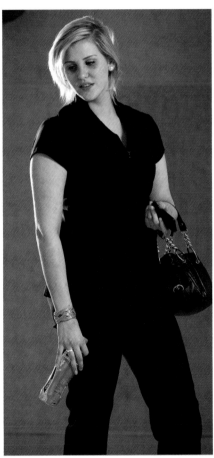

If you present an unprofessional image, clients will think you will treat their service the same

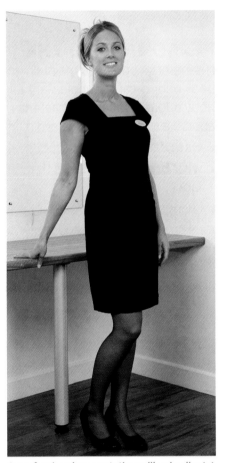

A professional presentation will gain clients' confidence

WHY DON'T YOU...
look at the image above on the left. Write down the ways in which the therapist in the picture could improve their professional appearance.
You are booked into have a luxury spa treatment with this therapist; how does that make you feel?

WHY DON'T YOU...
write down how the therapist in the photo above on the right creates a professional image. How does this therapist make you feel about having a treatment with her? Of the two pictures, which one would you prefer to have your treatment with?

 SmartScreen 201 Worksheet 5

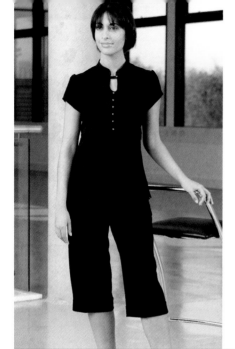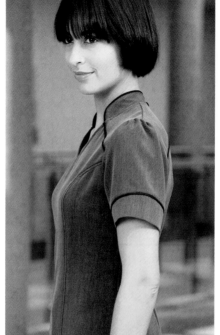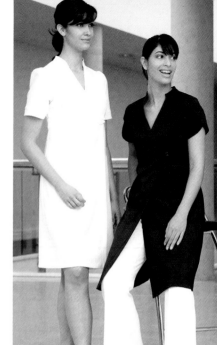

Workwear can come in lots of styles to fit the salon image and for comfort

PERSONAL HYGIENE

It is important that you maintain good personal hygiene as unpleasant body odours can be unpleasant for both clients and work colleagues. Bad body odour is caused by bacteria breaking down sweat from the apocrine sweat glands. To avoid any possible problems with body odour:

- wash daily
- wear **breathable** fabrics that help stop the growth of bacteria on the fabric.
- change your clothes daily
- use a deodorant to reduce any odour by **inhibiting** the growth of bacteria or an antiperspirant which will reduce the size of pores so that the body sweats less
- avoid wearing strong or heavy perfumes as these can be **overpowering**
- avoid eating strong-smelling foods, such as garlic, that will come out through your skin pores when you are working
- think about when you smoke – smoke often clings to clothing and hands and is unpleasant when working in **close proximity** with clients.

ORAL HYGIENE

Bad breath can be caused by:

- strong foods (eg onion, garlic)
- smoking
- digestive problems
- tooth decay and gum disease.

To avoid bad breath:

- brush your teeth regularly – morning and evening
- use dental floss regularly
- visit the dentist regularly
- avoid eating foods that will make you and your breath smell
- don't smoke.

INDUSTRY TIP

The nose tires of an odour after about 20 minutes and so you might not be able to smell your perfume any more, but those around you will!

Breathable

Allows air to the skin and lets sweat evaporate.

Inhibiting

Preventing.

Overpowering

Too strong.

Close proximity

Being close or very near to someone.

INDUSTRY TIP

To freshen your breath, suck a mint rather than chew gum as this looks unprofessional.

INDUSTRY TIP

Chewing gum actually creates excess stomach acid as your stomach is preparing for food and so this can make your breath smell.

HAIR CARE

To create a smart image, your hair should be **secured** away from your face and neck.

- If your hair is long, keep it tied back.
- Use a hair band or hair clips to stop stray hairs hanging down that might come into contact with the client's skin, oils or worse still, wax – this is not hygienic and can distract the client.
- Shampoo and condition your hair regularly.

Secured
Fixed firmly.

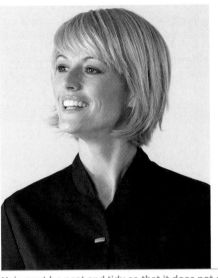 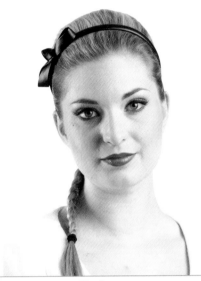

Hair must be neat and tidy so that it does not get in your way and look messy

FOOT CARE

The importance of taking care of your feet cannot be underestimated – some 90 per cent of people have some sort of foot condition.

- Wear clean socks, tights or stockings (preferably cotton or breathable **synthetic** fibres) and change them daily.
- Wash your feet daily and dry them well – particularly between the toes.
- Cut your toenails straight across to avoid ingrown nails.
- Wear correctly fitting shoes that are:
  - enclosed (ie no open-toed shoes) and secure on your feet to avoid accidents
  - leather to allow your feet to breathe
  - low healed (no higher than 5 cm) to support your posture.
- Wear arch supports if required.
- Treat **infectious** conditions.

Poor-fitting footwear will encourage a range of foot problems, including blisters, corns, ingrown toenails, bunions, fallen arches (flat feet) and all sorts of postural problems – as posture starts with the feet.

Synthetic
Not made naturally.

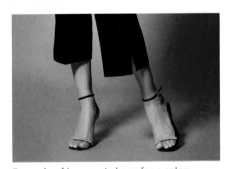

Example of incorrect shoes for a salon. These are heels and not enclosed

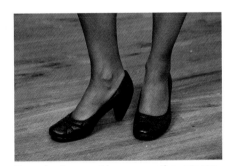

These heels cannot be worn as they are too high

HAND AND NAIL CARE

Your hands are your tools. If you damage them then you will not be able to perform your job properly and so it is essential to take excellent care of your tools.

- Keep your nails short and well-manicured to prevent scratching the client. It also makes it easier to keep your nails clean.

Infectious
Another word for contagious; catching.

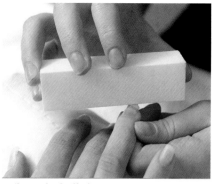

Nails can be buffed to a natural healthy shine

Acceptable
Suitable or satisfactory.

- Wash your hands and dry them well before and after each client.
- Apply hand cream often.
- Remove jewellery and watches when you are working. Sharp edges could scratch your client and products can get caught in jewellery. It is **acceptable** to wear small stud earrings and a wedding band.
- Cover cuts with waterproof plasters.
- Be aware of hand odours (eg from smoking and food).
- If there are any warts on your hands, these should be treated. Keep them covered with a waterproof plaster until they have gone.

ACTIVITY

Label the picture with the labels on the right.

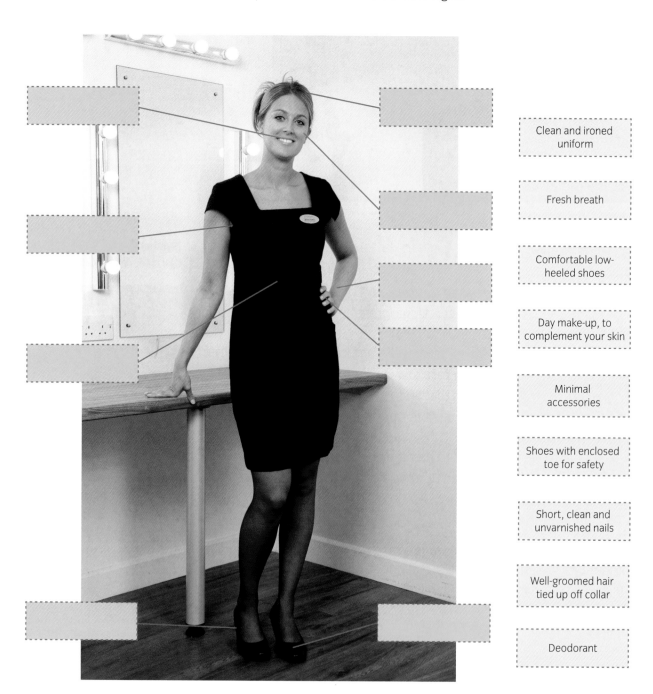

Clean and ironed uniform

Fresh breath

Comfortable low-heeled shoes

Day make-up, to complement your skin

Minimal accessories

Shoes with enclosed toe for safety

Short, clean and unvarnished nails

Well-groomed hair tied up off collar

Deodorant

EMPLOYMENT RIGHTS AND RESPONSIBILITIES

As an employee, it is essential to know your employment rights and responsibilities to make sure that:

- there is no discrimination within the workplace
- you understand the requirements of your contract
- you have a basic understanding of employment law.

EMPLOYMENT RIGHTS ACT 1996

This Act outlines the rights that most employees should have in relation to their work. It includes the requirement for a contract of employment.

Contract of employment

This is a **legally-binding** document given to each employee that sets out their rights, **entitlements** and conditions of employment. It is a legal requirement that every employee receives a contract of employment within 2 months of beginning work. It is often sent to you with the formal letter offering you the job so that you can check the conditions of employment before accepting the job. It is in the interest of both the employer and employee to make sure that the contract is agreed and signed and kept safe. A contract of employment must include:

- your name
- the company's or employer's name, their business address and the address of your workplace (this might be different if you are working for a large organisation)
- the date that employment began/begins
- your job title
- the type of contract you are on (eg full-time, part-time or contract, etc.)
- the responsibilities of the job
- your hours of work and hours of the business
- your notice period
- any holiday entitlement (including details about holiday pay and holiday restrictions, such as holiday might not be permitted over the Christmas period)
- the length of your probationary period
- salary information (how much you will be paid, when you will be paid (eg monthly) and how you will be paid (eg by BACS)
- Sick pay entitlement and injury terms and conditions (including how you are expected to notify the company if you are to be absent)
- details of the company's disciplinary and grievance procedures.

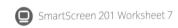

SmartScreen 201 Worksheet 7

Legally binding
Something that must be followed according to the law.

Entitlements
The basic things, by law, that must be provided to an employee (eg a contract, sick pay etc).

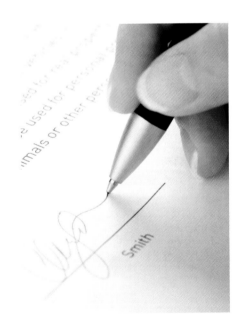

In addition and, if applicable, your contract might also include information about:

- targets
- the company's bonus scheme
- the company's pension scheme
- any company benefits (eg staff discount)
- training agreements (eg some training costs might have to be paid back to the employee if the employee leaves the company within a certain time frame)
- company property, such as a uniform policy, as some companies might provide a uniform that you are required to wear
- working for the competition or a radius or restrictive clause limiting where you can work, should you leave the business
- security measures and procedures
- data protection
- special leave, such as compassionate leave or leave needed for carer's responsibilities.

WORKING TIME REGULATIONS 1998

The Working Time Regulations aim to improve health and safety in the workplace by setting guidelines about working hours that businesses should follow. These guidelines make sure that both the employer and employee know what they are entitled to and cover:

- working hours
- holiday or annual leave entitlement
- regular rest breaks.

Working hours

An adult over the age of 18 cannot be forced to work over 48 hours a week averaged over 17 weeks. The law is different for workers under the age of 18. Workers under 18 might not normally work more than 8 hours a day or 40 hours a week.

Holiday or annual leave entitlement

All full-time workers are entitled to 5.6 weeks paid annual leave (including bank holidays). If you work part-time, this is worked out based on the hours you work. The business might set some restrictions around when you can take your holiday. For example, you might be required to take holidays at certain times of the year when the business is quiet and you might not be allowed to take holiday during busy periods (eg over Christmas).

Regular breaks

Regular breaks include lunch, tea and other short breaks during the day that might be paid or unpaid. Each employee is entitled to a 20-minute break when they have worked 6 hours. Under 18s are entitled to a 30-minute break if they have worked four-and-a-half hours or more.

 SmartScreen 201 Worksheet 6

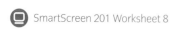 SmartScreen 201 Worksheet 8

THE NATIONAL MINIMUM WAGE ACT 1998

The majority of workers in the UK are entitled to be paid at least the National Minimum Wage (NMW). If your employer does not pay you at least the minimum wage, they are breaking the law. The minimum wage should not include tips or bonuses. There are different levels of the National Minimum Wage depending on your age or if you are an apprentice. There are four levels:

- the main rate for workers aged 21 and over
- the 18–20 rate
- the 16–17 rate for workers above school-leaving age but under 18
- the rate for apprentices under 19 or 19 and over in the first year of their apprenticeship.

If you are of school age, you are not entitled to NMW and you will also find some of your employments rights will be different.

ACTIVITY

Using the Internet, find out what the National Minimum Wage is for each of the following age categories:

- workers aged 21 and over
- workers aged 18–20
- workers aged 16–17
- apprentices aged 16–18 and in the first year of an apprenticeship
- apprentices aged 19 and over and in the first year of an apprenticeship.

You are not entitled to the National Minimum Wage if you are self-employed, a volunteer or are doing work experience. You are also not entitled if you are participating in certain government schemes at pre-apprenticeship level.

HANDY HINTS

For the most up-to-date rates on the National Minimum Wage refer to the government website – www.direct.gov.uk. The website also contains telephone numbers for pay and work rights' helplines for confidential help if you are being underpaid.

HANDY HINTS

Refer to the chapter on Legislation (pages 91–113) to find out more about legislation related to employment.

WHY DON'T YOU...

check the following website for the current minimum wage: http://www.direct.gov.uk/en/Employment/Employees/TheNationalMinimumWage/DG_10027201.

Use the questions below to test your knowledge of Chapter 201 to see how much information you have retained. These questions will help you revise what you have learnt in this chapter.

Turn to page 601 for the answers.

1. Which **one** of the following is a treatment that you would only carry out if you were training at or qualified to Level 3?
   a) Leg waxing
   b) Micro-dermabrasion
   c) Ear piercing
   d) Eye treatments

2. Which **one** of the following is classed as a Level 4 treatment?
   a) Reflexology
   b) Aromatherapy
   c) Intense pulse light (ILP)
   d) Electrolysis

3. Which **one** of the following is the best form of CPD to undertake?
   a) Reading trade journals
   b) Attending a trade exhibition
   c) Completing an industry training course
   d) Watching a training video

4. Which **one** of the following best describes the reason for completing CPD?
   a) To learn new techniques to meet industry trends
   b) It builds your confidence and experience
   c) It gives you the opportunity to learn new skills and therefore helps to increase business by adding new services to the salon
   d) It enables the therapist to perform their job efficiently

5. Which **one** of the following statements about the National Minimum Wage is true?
   a) The National Minimum Wage includes tips and products for personal use
   b) The National Minimum Wage includes treatment bonuses
   c) There are three different levels of National Minimum Wage depending on your age
   d) An employer who does not pay at least the National Minimum Wage is breaking the law

6. An employee who is under 18 is entitled to:
   a) a 20-minute break for each shift that lasts at least 6 hours
   b) a 30-minute break if they work four-and-a-half hours or more
   c) a 20-minute break if they work four-and-a-half hours or more
   d) a 30-minute break if they work at least 6 hours.

7. What is a contract of employment?
   a) A formal letter offering you a job before you start your employment
   b) A legally-binding document setting out an employee's rights, entitlements and conditions of employment
   c) Guidelines that make sure that both the employer and employee know what they are entitled to
   d) A policy that states that you work for the business on a permanent basis

8. Which **one** of the following best describes the occupational role of a beauty consultant?
   a) Carries out a range of Level 3 full-body treatments
   b) Manages the reception area, the appointment system and meets and greets clients in a salon
   c) Advises on skin care and make-up for a specific product range
   d) Applies theatrical and photographic make-up

9. When should you be given a contract of employment?
   a) Before starting work
   b) Within 2 months of starting work
   c) Within 6 months of starting work
   d) Within 12 months of starting work

10. Which **one** of the following best describes how a beauty therapist should maintain personal hygiene?
    a) Wear breathable fabrics, wash daily, wear deodorant and brush your teeth
    b) Wash regularly
    c) Wear a light fragrance
    d) Keep your nails short and do not wear nail enamel

CASE STUDY: HELLEN WARD

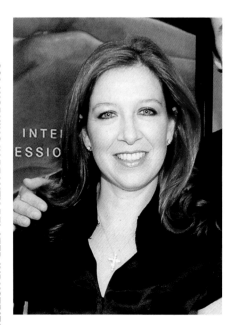

Having originally trained as a hairdresser upon leaving school at 16, I progressed up the ranks of the company from Salon Manager, then Regional Manager to General Manager of Harrods Hair & Beauty Salon before opening my own business with my husband Richard nearly 20 years ago. Now I run one of the largest independent hair and beauty salons and brands in the country, and I lecture at business seminars, educate salon owners, write a monthly column for a beauty magazine and now I have written three books for City & Guilds as part of the 'Ultimate Salon Management' series – *Getting Established, Managing Finances and Team Performance* – which is part of the Level 4 diploma in Salon Management and Advanced Techniques in the hair and beauty sector.

Salon life is like no other – fun, varied, exciting and never, ever dull. Our industry is unique – where else could one person be able to create such a diverse career? My role encompasses accounting, management, brand development, marketing, PR, HR, journalism and now I'm an author, too! The talented therapists that I am lucky enough to work with never cease to amaze me with their skill sets. They have a unique ability to make people feel better about themselves through the treatments and services they conduct, which is immensely rewarding and hugely empowering. A career in our growing sector (we employ nearly 1 per cent of the UK's workforce) is a great choice, and with its ever-growing diversity it offers a multitude of opportunities to branch out into and develop your hidden talents under one fabulous umbrella.

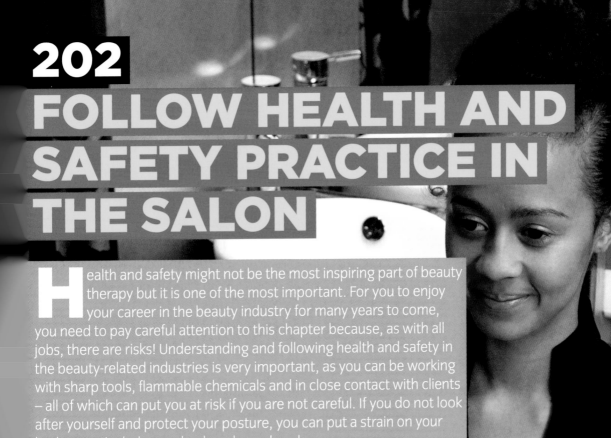

202
FOLLOW HEALTH AND SAFETY PRACTICE IN THE SALON

Health and safety might not be the most inspiring part of beauty therapy but it is one of the most important. For you to enjoy your career in the beauty industry for many years to come, you need to pay careful attention to this chapter because, as with all jobs, there are risks! Understanding and following health and safety in the beauty-related industries is very important, as you can be working with sharp tools, flammable chemicals and in close contact with clients – all of which can put you at risk if you are not careful. If you do not look after yourself and protect your posture, you can put a strain on your body – particularly your back and your hands.

In this chapter you will learn about the health and safety information and requirements that will be important to you when working in the industry. In this chapter you will learn how to:

- maintain health, safety and security practices
- follow emergency procedures.

You will need to keep referring back to this chapter as you work through the other chapters in the book to ensure the wellbeing of yourself and those around you.

HEALTH AND SAFETY LEGISLATION

In order to make sure you are following health and safety regulations, you need to be familiar with all the legislation that are relevant to the workplace. This information can be found in the Legislation chapter on pages 91–113. Make sure you have a good understanding of each Act and how it will affect you in the workplace. The Acts you should be familiar with are:

- the Health and Safety at Work Act (HASAWA)
- the Personal Protective Equipment (PPE) at Work Regulations
- the Workplace (Health, Safety and Welfare) Regulations
- the Manual Handling Operations Regulations
- the Control of Substances Hazardous to Health (COSHH) Regulations
- the Provision and Use of Work Equipment Regulations (PUWER)
- the Electricity at Work Regulations (EAWR)
- the Reporting of Injuries, Diseases and Dangerous Occurrences Regulations (RIDDOR)
- the Fire Precautions Act
- the Health and Safety (First Aid) Regulations
- the Health and Safety (Display Screen Equipment) Regulations.

SmartScreen 202 Worksheet 1

MAINTAIN HEALTH, SAFETY AND SECURITY PRACTICES

In this part of the chapter you will learn about:

- codes of practice and workplace policies
- hazards and risks
- personal protective equipment (PPE)
- protecting your hands
- hygiene and infection control
- disposal of salon waste.

CODES OF PRACTICE AND WORKPLACE POLICIES

In everything we do in life there are right and wrong ways of doing things so, to make sure we do things correctly, we have to follow rules. In the workplace, these rules could be official UK laws or your salon's rules.

CODES OF PRACTICE

A **code of practice** is a set of written guidelines for members of some professions or occupations. These guidelines provide best-practice guidance on behaviour and the standards expected within the profession. HABIA, who is the standard-setting body for the beauty therapy, nails and spa industries, has written codes of practice for all of these industries, including codes of practice for:

HANDY HINTS

You must make sure you are familiar with all the legislation that is listed in the Legislation chapter of this book (see pages 91–113).

Code of practice

A written set of rules/guidelines for everyone in the profession to follow.

- beauty therapy
- nail services
- waxing services.

Professional organisations that you might choose to belong to will have their own codes of practice.

A code of practice will include guidance on:
- dress codes for the salon
- hygiene control
- operational procedures
- salon safety.

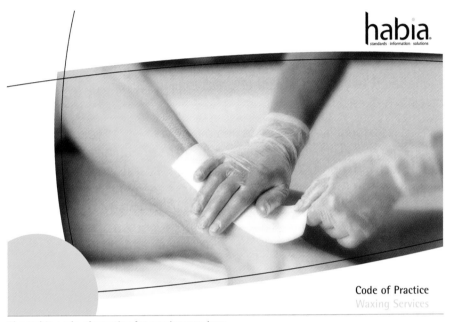

The Habia code of practice for waxing services

WORKPLACE POLICIES

Workplace policies are rules put in place by a business specifically for its employees. Policies might include:
- how you should meet, greet and treat clients
- how to behave in the salon
- how you must maintain the salon's hygiene and **interior**
- how to dispose of the salon's waste
- booking annual leave
- the salon's appeal and grievance procedures
- the salon's procedures for dealing with emergencies.

Workplace policies
The individual rules in your salon.

Interior
The design and decoration of the inside of the salon.

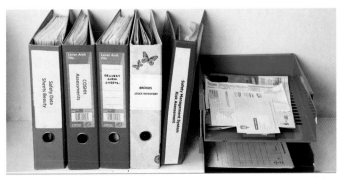

It is important to keep documents neatly stored and easily accessible

Negligence

Lack of proper care or attention.

Conduct

The way in which you behave in the workplace.

 SmartScreen 202 Worksheet 4

Equality

Treating people equally regardless of any difference in race, religion or gender, etc.

Diversity

Showing a great deal of variety.

Identified

Recognised or pointed out.

 SmartScreen 202 Worksheet 5

HANDY HINTS

Refer to the Legislation chapter on pages 91–113 for further details on relevant laws.

ACTIVITY

If you work in a salon, from memory list as many of your workplace's policies as you can. If you do not work in a salon, list your college's or training provider's workplace policies – both will be very similar.

Conduct

One of your workplace's policies is likely to relate to **conduct**. Your conduct should reflect the standard expected of you in the salon and reduce the risk of harm to yourself and others. You are representing your salon and the image you give of yourself has an impact on the whole business. Always act professionally, speak politely to visitors and clients and promote **equality** and **diversity** for all.

HAZARDS AND RISKS

Almost anything can be a hazard in the salon and it is your responsibility, along with your employer, to prevent these hazards from becoming risks to the safety of yourself and others. Maintaining a clean and tidy salon helps to reduce hazards.

A risk assessment is a process carried out by your employer or manager where workplace activities are reviewed and any potential risks are **identified** and reported. A health and safety risk assessment will include COSHH (see page 96) and a fire risk assessment. A risk assessment should be carried out and updated regularly. You should be familiar with the content of a risk assessment report so that you are aware of the potential hazards in your workplace and what you should do to reduce the risks.

- **A hazard** is anything with the potential to cause harm, such as a wax heater that has been left on.
- **A risk** is the likelihood that a hazard will cause some sort of harm to someone or something – for example, cleaning a wax heater that has been left on could result in the person cleaning it being burnt.

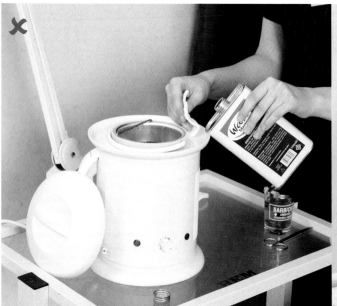
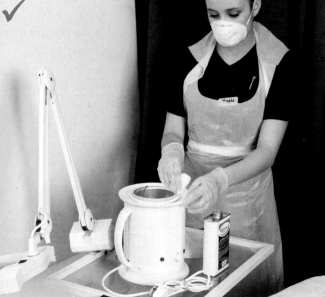

It is good practice to keep equipment clean but remember to unplug electricals and wear gloves when you are using chemicals

According to the Health and Safety Executive's (HSE) website (www.hse.gov.uk), the most common hazards found in the workplace are:

Hazard	Causes of accidents	Risk
Chemicals	■ **Exposure** during handling ■ Spillages ■ Splashing	■ Burns ■ Eye injuries
Electricity	■ Poorly maintained electrical equipment	■ Electric shock ■ Burns
Manual handling	■ Repetitive and/or heavy lifting ■ Bending and twisting ■ Exerting too much force ■ Handling bulky or unstable loads ■ Handling in uncomfortable working positions	■ Fractures ■ Sprains and strains
Slip-and-trip hazards	■ Uneven floors ■ Trailing cables ■ Obstructions ■ Slippery surfaces due to spillages ■ Worn carpets and mats	■ Fractures ■ Lacerations ■ Sprains and strains
Working at heights	■ Overreaching or overbalancing when using ladders ■ Not using suitable steps or ladders to work at height	■ Head injury and loss of consciousness ■ Spinal injury ■ Fractures ■ Sprains and strains

HAZARDS THAT MIGHT OCCUR IN THE SALON

Not all hazards are easily fixed. Some might need to be referred to a more senior person, such as a manager to organise a repair – for example, a loose floor tile or a loose shelf that is at risk of coming away from the wall. While you might be able to remove the shelf to reduce the risk, it is unlikely you will be in a position to fix or replace the shelf.

Exposure

To have contact with something, such as a harmful chemical.

ACTIVITY

What is wrong with the equipment in the photo?

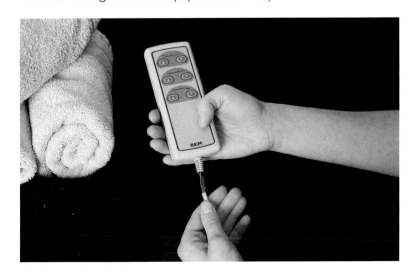

INDUSTRY TIP

It is your duty to ensure the health and safety of yourself and others who might be affected by your actions.

INDUSTRY TIP

When you are working in the salon, always use safe methods of working and follow health and safety rules and regulations.

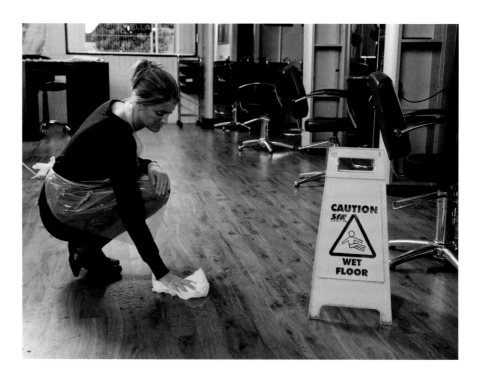

Hazards that might need to be referred to a more senior person

ACTIVITY

Complete the table below by identifying the potential hazards in the salon that you can deal with and those that must be referred to someone more senior. How would you control each of the potential hazards listed in the table to reduce risks?

Potential hazards in the salon	My responsibilities within my job role and workplace policies	How I would control and reduce the potential risk to safeguard myself, my colleagues and my clients?	Who I should report health and safety matters to when they are outside my limits of authority
Faulty electrical equipment	Label, report and remove the item from the salon.	Visually check all electrical items prior to use. Do not use items that are faulty and follow warning signs.	Inform the salon manager.
Trailing wires			
Spillages			
Chemicals			
Obstructions to access and **egress** **Egress** An exit or way out.			
Loose floor tiles			

PERSONAL PROTECTIVE EQUIPMENT (PPE)

Not only does your uniform give you a professional identity in the beauty salon or in a retail sales area but it is also a piece of protective workwear. Your shoes should be secure to prevent slips and trips and ideally your toes should be enclosed (ie no open-toed shoes) as this will also protect your feet from injury.

Some PPE for the employee should be supplied by the employer. As a beauty therapist or nail technician, your employer should provide:

- disposable powder-free and latex-free gloves
- aprons
- particle masks
- eye protection.

DISPOSABLE POWDER-FREE AND LATEX-FREE GLOVES

There are some treatments where it is **advisable** to wear disposable gloves to protect your the hands, prevent staining to your hands and more importantly to avoid cross-infection. Gloves should ideally be nitrile or PVC and should be powder free. Latex should also be avoided in case the therapists or clients are allergic to latex. Gloves should be worn during waxing treatments. It is a personal choice to wear a pair of disposable gloves when you are checking the feet for contra-indications or when you are applying an eyelash tint.

Removing disposable gloves

When you wear gloves, it is important that you remove them correctly. The top of the glove should be pulled back on itself to avoid contact with the contaminated surface and to avoid the contaminated surface of the glove being exposed in the waste bin. The glove is almost turned inside out with one glove inside the other before being disposed of. Gloves should not be reused.

Advisable
Suggested that you should.

INDUSTRY TIP
Do not think that wearing the gloves alone is all the protection you need.

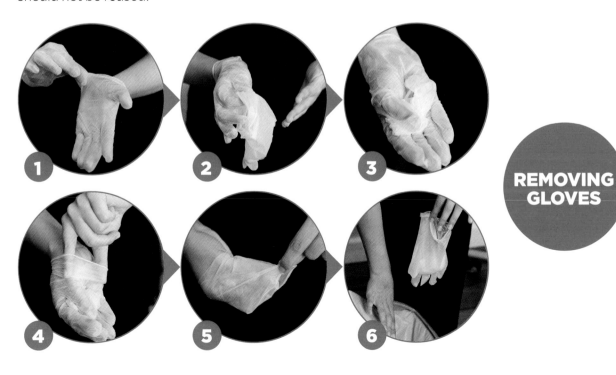

REMOVING GLOVES

INDUSTRY TIP

Avoid choosing products containing latex (eg disposable gloves and latex media make-up products) since there is a high risk that people are allergic to it. Synthetic gloves, such as nitrile gloves, are preferable. Nitrile gloves are slightly thicker and fit better than vinyl.

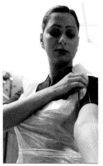
Apron

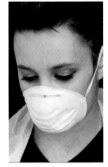
Mask

Limited

Restricted in size or amount.

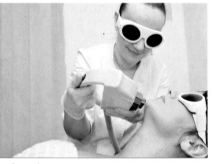
Safety glasses

Decanting

To pour from one container into another.

When you have removed your gloves, you should wash your hands. Your hands are warm and will have been perspiring inside the glove creating the ideal environment for breeding bacteria.

APRONS

An apron might be worn during certain treatments to protect your clothes from damage and spillages – for example, when you are waxing, carrying out a pedicure or applying body art.

PARTICLE MASKS

If you suffer from asthma or allergies, it is advisable to wear a particle mask when you are filing nail enhancements. Particle masks will also give you protection when you are working with fine sprays and airbrushing, such as nail art, media make-up or body art. You might also choose to wear a mask to provide some protection against cross-infection if you or the client has a cold. Be aware though that most face masks will give only **limited** protection or provide protection for a limited period of time only.

EYE PROTECTION – SAFETY GLASSES

There are very few occasions when eye protection is worn in the salon. You might choose to wear safety glasses when clipping nails (both natural and nail enhancements) to prevent nail clippings from flying into your eyes. Eye protection should however be worn when you are handling chemicals (eg when **decanting** from larger professional containers to smaller ones for salon use) to prevent chemicals from entering the eyes or when you are checking water chemicals in a spa.

PROTECTING YOUR HANDS

Hand washing

One simple procedure that many therapists neglect is thorough hand washing. This is one of the easiest and most effective ways of maintaining hygiene and minimising any risk of cross-infection.

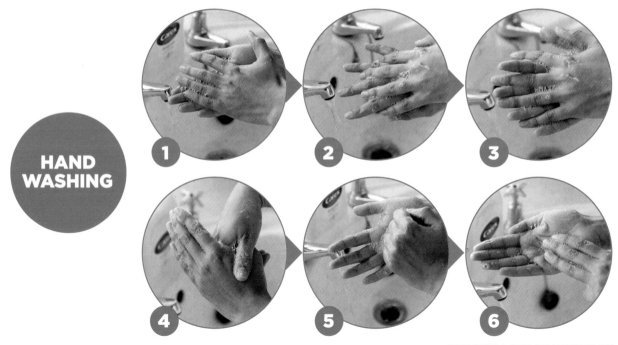

HAND WASHING

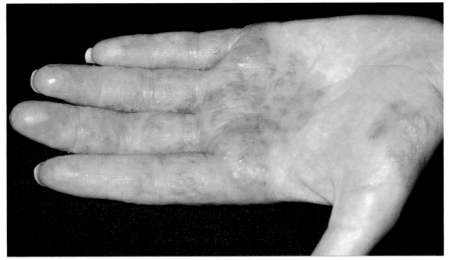
It is important to protect and look after hands to prevent dermatitis

DERMATITIS

It is important to protect your hands to avoid occupational **dermatitis**. Dermatitis can happen when your skin comes into contact with **substances** that can irritate it and cause allergies. Each person's skin will react differently to substances and dermatitis can occur at any time in your career. Beauty therapists are particularly **prone** to **occupational** dermatitis because of the need to wash their hands constantly to maintain hygiene. Their hands are also in contact with a variety of different products which might become irritants after **prolonged exposure**. Dermatitis is not contagious to others but it can spread on your own skin. Although it is most commonly found on the hands, it can appear on the face, lips and arms and can cause irritation to the eyes. The good news is that it can be avoided.

INDUSTRY TIP

Keep a tub of aqueous lotion handy in the salon – any pharmacist will be able to supply it. It is great for both cleansing your hands if they are very dry and as a barrier/moisturiser to protect your hands from moisture loss.

Dermatitis

An inflammation of the skin caused by a reaction to a substance that has irritated the skin. It is fairly common on the hands of beauty therapists. It results in red, dry, itchy and cracked skin and is caused by the use of certain chemicals.

Substance

A chemical.

Prone

Likely to suffer from.

Occupational

Relating to a job.

Prolonged

Happening for a long time.

Exposure

Open to the elements.

HANDY HINTS

Follow these *four* simple steps to healthy hands:

1 Wear non-latex, powder-free disposable gloves for waxing, mixing tint, tanning treatments and when you are using latex products in media make-up.
2 Dry your hands thoroughly after washing them.
3 Moisturise your hands regularly.
4 Check your hands regularly for signs of contact dermatitis. If you notice any signs of dermatitis, let your salon manager know and seek further advice from a pharmacist.

HANDY HINTS

See page 26 in the Anatomy and Physiology chapter for information on how to recognise dermatitis.

INDUSTRY TIP

Dermatitis can stop your career and can be painful and uncomfortable so you must look after your hands and always follow the steps to healthy hands.

HYGIENE AND INFECTION CONTROL

The importance of maintaining salon hygiene cannot be stressed enough. You must protect yourself and your clients. Failure to follow basic hygiene practices can be **disastrous** to a business. Poor personal hygiene can be off-putting to clients and colleagues. Failure to maintain hygiene standards in the salon can lead to **cross-infection** and potentially a client suing if the infection is serious enough. Failure to follow basic hygiene practices and standards can lead to a poor reputation and loss of business.

It is essential that the cleanliness of both the staff and salon is maintained throughout the day. This will make sure that a professional image is presented to your clients and that you maintain a high standard of infection control.

Disastrous

Causing a disaster; major problem.

Cross-infection

To pass an infection from one person to another – both directly and indirectly.

HANDY HINTS

Review page 132 in Chapter 201 about personal hygiene.

WHY DON'T YOU...
make a list of all the things you need to consider every day to make sure you are maintaining your personal hygiene throughout the day. When you have completed your list, look back at Chapter 201 (page 132 on personal hygiene) to see if you have remembered everything.

In order to ensure a high standard of hygiene and infection control in the salon you need to:

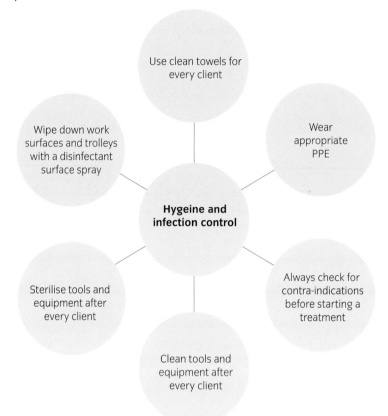

HANDY HINTS

More information on micro-organisms can be found in the Anatomy and Physiology chapter (pages 1–90).

Spore

A tiny reproductive cell.

Salmonella

A type of **bacterium** that causes food poisoning. It can be transferred between people.

Bacterium

The singular of the word bacteria.

Organic matter

Natural.

Secrete

Release.

Enzymes

Proteins that speed up chemical reactions.

Decompose

To decay or rot.

Candida

A fungus that naturally occurs on the skin, in the gut and the mouth. However, it can cause infections, such as thrush.

MICRO-ORGANISMS

Good hygiene practices should kill or at least temporarily remove micro-organisms. Micro-organisms happen naturally and can be found inside and outside our bodies and in the environment around us. Some are important to our health; others are harmful and can cause disease. There are *four* types of infections caused by micro-organisms:

- bacterial infections
- fungal infections
- viral infections
- infestations.

Bacterial infections

Bacteria are single-celled organisms that come in different shapes and sizes. They exist as **spores**. Under suitable conditions – warm and moist environments – bacteria can multiply very quickly. In their spore state, bacteria are more difficult to kill. Examples of bacterial infections include impetigo, acne vulgaris, conjunctivitis and **salmonella**. Most bacterial infections can be treated with antibiotics.

Fungal infections

Fungi include moulds and yeasts. Fungi feed on **organic matter** and are naturally occurring on human skin. They **secrete enzymes** that break down the organic matter so that it dissolves. Nutrients are released as the organic matter **decomposes** and these can then be absorbed by the fungi. Fungi produce spores. Examples of common fungal infections include tinea corporis (ringworm), tinea pedis (athlete's foot), **candida** and thrush.

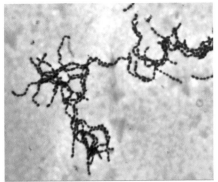

Bacterial infection

Fungal infection – tinea pedis

WHY DON'T YOU...
make a list of all the contagious infections that would prevent a client from having a treatment. You might want to refer to the Anatomy and Physiology chapter (pages 1–90).

INDUSTRY TIP

Staphylococcus aureus is a type of bacterium that occurs naturally on the skin and in the nasal passages. It causes skin infections, such as boils and impetigo.

Viral infections

Viruses are tiny **infectious** agents that multiply in the cells of other living organisms. Examples of viral infections include warts, herpes, influenza (flu), hepatitis and HIV/AIDS.

Infestations

Infestations are caused by tiny insects and include pediculosis capitis (head lice) and the scabies mite. They are described as parasites because they live off the blood of their host.

Infectious

Another word for contagious; catching.

INDUSTRY TIP

Always cover any cuts or open wounds with a waterproof covering or dressing to prevent **cross-contamination**.

Cross-contamination

Passing unwanted and harmful infections to others through direct or indirect contact.

INDUSTRY TIP

Poor standards of health and hygiene can cause concern to your clients, spread germs and allow cross-contamination.

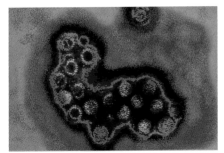

Viral infection

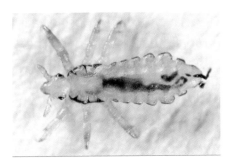

Head lice – pediculosis capitis

ACTIVITY

Make a general list of all the contra-indications you can think of. Put a cross against all those that would prevent you from carrying out a treatment and a tick against those that would restrict a treatment and require the treatment to be modified.

INDUSTRY TIP

It is always advisable *not* to treat anyone who is unwell. If you catch an infection, it will mean that you might not be able to work and not all employers will pay for time off sick.

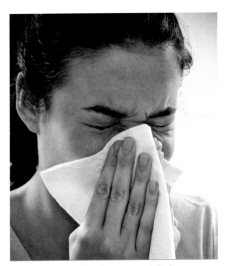

Catch sneezes in a tissue to minimise cross-contamination

HOW INFECTIONS AND INFESTATIONS ARE TRANSMITTED

Infections and infestations can be transmitted by:

- **Direct contact** – micro-organisms are passed on from person to person through direct contact with an infected person.
- **Indirect contact** – micro-organisms can be passed on by contact with contaminated equipment, such as towels, spa baths and dirty tools.
- **Inhalation** of **airborne** organisms into the **respiratory** system through the nose and mouth – this is how coughs and colds are transmitted.
- **Ingestion** – micro-organisms on contaminated food are swallowed or eaten. We can also **ingest** micro-organisms by putting dirty hands into our mouth or having contact with dirty cups or glasses.
- **Injection** – micro-organisms can be transmitted when the skin is pierced either **accidently** (eg during electrolysis) or **intentionally** (eg when the ears are pierced).

METHODS USED FOR MAINTAINING HIGH STANDARDS OF HYGIENE

Sterilisation

Sterilisation is the total removal or destruction of *all* living micro-organisms, including their spores. An object is either sterile or it is not! Within 20 minutes of sterilising an object, bacteria will already be well-**established** again on the surface.

Sterilisation is done by using heat:

- **Moist heat** – steam or boiling water. Steaming using an autoclave is the most practical method.
- **Dry heat** – the item is baked using a high heat, for example in a glass bead steriliser which uses dry heat to heat the tips of small metal items (such as tweezers).

Autoclave

Using heat is the most **effective** method of sterilisation. Using an autoclave is the only **acceptable** method of sterilisation. An autoclave is a piece of equipment that heats water under pressure to around 126°C. The steam created is used to sterilise equipment (usually small metal tools). The sterilisation cycle takes about 20 minutes plus cooling time. Before putting anything into the autoclave, it should be wiped over with an alcohol-based product (eg surgical spirit) or washed (if it is not metal) in hot soapy water. This is to make sure that the equipment is clean and free from grease before sterilisation. Anything left on the surface of the equipment will prevent the equipment from being properly sterilised.

The autoclave is only suitable for small pieces of equipment that can tolerate high temperatures. The only metal that should be put in the autoclave is stainless steel, as the moist **atmosphere** in the autoclave will cause other metals to rust over time.

Glass bead steriliser

This is a small **insulated** heater that contains hundreds of tiny glass beads. The beads are heated to very high temperatures of between

Sidebar glossary

Airborne
Transported by the air.

Respiratory
The system for taking in oxygen and giving out carbon dioxide, which happens in humans by breathing.

Ingest
To take in as food.

Accidentally
Happening by accident.

Intentionally
Happening on purpose, deliberate.

 SmartScreen 202 Worksheet 6

Established
Found on/in.

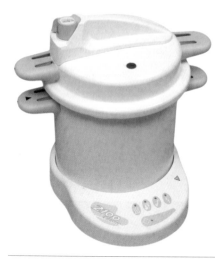

An autoclave uses moist heat

Effective
Most successful or proven.

Acceptable
Suitable or satisfactory.

Atmosphere
In the air.

Insulated
Covered with material to reduce heat loss.

190°C and 300°C. The beads sterilise by intense, dry heat. Glass bead sterilisers, because of their size, have limited use as they can only sterilise items that are inserted into the beads. This means that a glass bead steriliser is only suitable for small metal tools, such as tweezers. Although tools are not totally **immersed** in the beads, the heat is so hot it still sterilises the whole item. You must be very careful when you are removing items from the heat by using a special pair of insulated tweezers to avoid burning. The disadvantage of glass bead sterilisers is the **tarnishing** of metal over periods of time. They are rarely used in salons now because they are not cost-effective due to their limited use.

Disinfection

A disinfectant is a chemical agent that destroys micro-organisms but not usually bacterial spores. Disinfection is less effective than sterilisation. Methods of disinfection might be used to prepare tools for sterilisation (eg wiping over tweezers with surgical spirit to remove grease) but should not be relied on to maintain high levels of hygiene control.

Sanitisation and disinfection can be carried out by the use of:

- **UV (ultraviolet) radiation** – ie a UV cabinet
- **chemicals** – eg Barbicide.

UV cabinet

This is a small cabinet into which objects can be placed on a wire tray. When the door is closed the objects are exposed to UV rays. Only the surface areas of objects that the rays come into contact with will be sanitised. This means that the items need to be turned after about 20 minutes. It is therefore not an effective method for treating tools with crevices or unexposed areas. UV cabinets are often referred to as disinfectors as they are incapable of complete sterilisation.

UV cabinets are ideal for the storage of sterilised instruments to keep them sterile, or for keeping items in a clean atmosphere (eg make-up brushes and sponges). It is important that wet items are not placed in the UV cabinet.

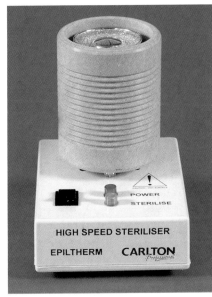

A bead steriliser uses dry heat

Immersed
Covered by completely.

Tarnishing
Making metal less bright or dull.

Sanitisation
Sanitisation means to make **hygienic** and clean by the destruction of the majority of micro-organisms. The working environment, including tools and equipment (such as trolleys and workstations), should be sanitised daily as it is essential that the environment is as healthy and as germ free as possible.

Hygienic
Clean.

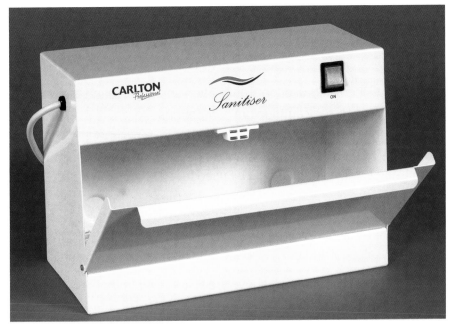

A UV cabinet uses UV radiation

WHY DON'T YOU...
make a list of tools or equipments that you can put into a UV cabinet and the tools that you can't.

Chemicals used for sanitisation and disinfection

Chemicals are a commonly used method of sanitisation. Chemicals can be placed in small jars into which tools, such as tweezers or cuticle nippers, can be placed. They can also be placed in worktop sterilisers that are larger jars or trays with lids to completely immerse the tools. Chemical solutions are only effective if they are used according to the manufacturer's instructions. They must be diluted, disposed of and replaced exactly as stated in the manufacturer's instructions. Items that are placed in the solution must be cleaned before placing them in the solution and they must be fully immersed. If the item is not fully immersed then the equipment cannot be fully sanitised and it will only be disinfected.

Common branded chemical products include Barbicide, Marvicide and Sterilsafe. Chemical solutions normally come in a concentrated form which needs to be diluted correctly before use. Chemical solutions lose their effectiveness over time with items continually being placed in the liquid and removed. As a result they must be changed regularly to maintain their sanitisation properties.

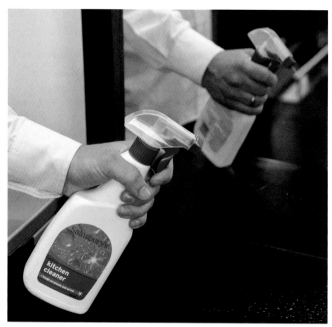

Sprays are useful for sanitising surface areas

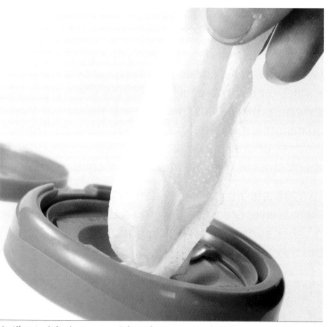

Antibacterial wipes are quick and easy to use for cleaning small tools

Examples of chemicals used for sanitisation and disinfection are:

- **QUATS** – quaternary ammonium compounds
- **hypochlorite** – a form of chlorine (eg Milton Sterilising Fluid)
- **bleach** – most bleach contains chlorine which makes it unsuitable for sanitising equipment. It should be used for cleaning toilets, surfaces, sinks, etc
- **glutaraldehyde** – an organic compound (eg Cidex)
- **alcohol** – available in a number of forms including surgical spirit, isopropyl alcohol and ethyl alcohol. It is suitable for wiping tools.

Not all of the chemicals listed above are suitable for immersing equipment in as some might cause metals to **corrode**. Always follow the manufacturer's instruction and guidelines.

Corrode

To destroy or damage slowly by chemical reaction. This can be seen as rust on a metal tool.

ACTIVITY

With a colleague, make a list of the advantages and disadvantages of each of the following methods of sterilisation and sanitisation:

- an autoclave
- a UV cabinet
- chemical solutions.

MAINTAINING SALON HYGIENE AND INFECTION CONTROL

To avoid the risk of cross-infection within the salon environment, equipment and surfaces must be cleaned regularly.

- Clean all work surfaces (ie trolleys, units and basins) at least once a day use using a recommended product. Avoid scouring products as these can cause scratches on the surface which can then hold micro-organisms, dirt and grease.
- Dispose of all waste as you produce it by placing it straight into a covered bin containing a bin liner. Avoid direct contact with any waste. When disposing of bin liners into an external waste collection bin, make sure you tie up the dustbin liners.
- Sterilise all equipment before and after each use using an appropriate method.
- Wash bowls and dishes with hot soapy water after use.
- Change towels after each client
- Cover couches with couch roll which should be disposed of and replaced after every client.

INDUSTRY TIP

Do not mix bleach with other cleaning products as it will react and give off poisonous fumes.

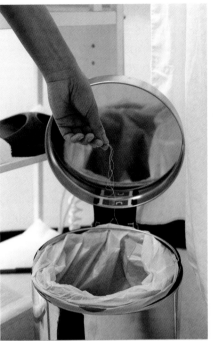

Waste should be disposed of immediately and never left on work surfaces

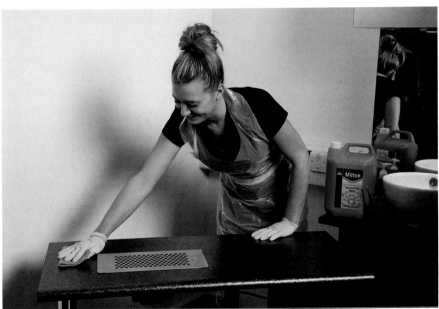

Keeping the salon clean is important

SmartScreen 202 Worksheet 7

Examples of how to maintain salon hygiene

Tools and equipment	Liquid disinfectant (chemical)	Autoclave (heat)	UV cabinet (UV radiation)	Other methods
Towels and gowns	No	No	No	Wash in a washing machine at a temperature between 60°C and 95°C
Tweezers, scissors, comedone extractors, cuticle nippers and cuticle knives	Yes – chemical solutions, sprays and wipes can be used	Yes	Yes	
Sponges	Yes – but caution should be taken to make sure all the disinfectant solution is removed to avoid any possible skin sensitivity	No	No	These can be washed and soaked in a mild solution of Milton Sterilising Fluid. However, it is recommended that sponges are used only once and thrown away or given to the client to use at home
Wooden and plastic-handled make-up brushes and mask brushes	No	No	Yes	Items should be washed first with hot soapy water or sprayed with a special brush sanitiser
Work surfaces, trolleys, washbasins, salon floor and chairs	Yes – sprays, wipes and suitable cleaners	No	No	

Environmentally friendly

Safe for or good for the environment.

DISPOSAL OF SALON WASTE

In the salon plenty of waste will be created during a working day that must be disposed of in a safe and **environmentally friendly** manner. Always follow local by-laws as well as the manufacturer's instructions for the disposal of products and other waste. Salons and businesses will have set days for refuse collection and will rent larger commercial waste bins for their waste disposal.

Any waste that is not contaminated with blood can be disposed of with the general rubbish. Some treatments can produce contaminated (clinical) waste that might have blood on and this needs to be disposed of in a particular way. Check with your refuse removal company for guidance as to how to dispose of specific salon waste. It is recomemended that materials, such as wax strips, are placed into a second bin liner before placing in an external bin for collection.

There are five categories of clinical waste but only the first *two* are relevant to the beauty industry:

- **Group A – high risk** – any items containing human tissue – including contaminated tissues, cotton wool, cloths and items used to mop up blood spots from waxing or comedone extraction – and any waste materials that pose a risk to staff handling them.
- **Group B – high risk** – **sharps** – **microlances** and electrolysis needles. These should be disposed of in a special sharps container and again removed by specialist collectors.

It is recommended that general salon waste should be disposed of as follows:

- Leftover products, such as masks and massage oil, should be wiped out of the container with tissue and placed in a refuse bin. These products should not be washed down the sink as they collect in the pipes and block the drains.
- Any food waste *must* be placed in the staffroom waste bin, with a lid on, to avoid smells.
- Very small quantities of unused chemicals might be rinsed down the sink with plenty of cold water to dilute the product. Always follow the manufacturer's instructions for the products you are using and the COSHH datasheets to make sure you do not harm the environment or cause a hazard.
- Contaminated waste, such as used plasters, must be disposed of carefully in a contaminated waste bin, with a lid on, to avoid the spread of micro-organisms.
- Ideally, packaging from products (ie plastics, cardboard and paper) should be recycled if facilities exist. Recycling signs on packaging are generally colour coded to help identify where and how you can recycle them.
- Broken glass, such as **ampoules**, should be wrapped in paper, secured and placed in a waste bin.

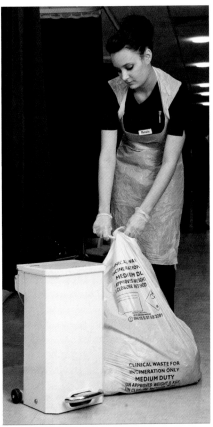

Bin bags should be tied securely

Sharps

This refers to any sharp object that might have become contaminated during use and includes electrolysis needles and microlances.

Microlance

A tiny probe used to remove whiteheads (milia) after steaming during a facial treatment.

Ampoule

A small sealed glass capsule containing a liquid.

 SmartScreen 202 Worksheet 8

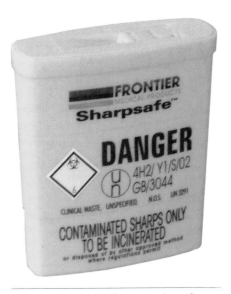

A sharps container is for contaminated needles

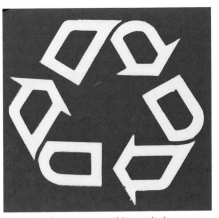

Recycle where you see this symbol

INDUSTRY TIP

If you break anything in the salon that is glass and that is not contaminated, it should not go in a sharps bin as this is for contaminated waste only. Broken glass should be cleared away carefully and wrapped in newspaper to make sure there are no sharp edges exposed that could cause harm. It is also a good idea to write on the package that it contains broken glass so that it is not opened by someone accidently. It should then be placed in a separate dustbin liner to keep it secure before disposing of it in the normal waste bin.

FOLLOW EMERGENCY PROCEDURES

In this part of the chapter you will learn about:

- fire safety and fire-fighting equipment
- first aid
- reporting and recording accidents
- gas safety
- fire and emergency procedures
- security of belongings.

FIRE SAFETY AND FIRE-FIGHTING EQUIPMENT

The most widely used fire extinguishers in salons contain water or carbon dioxide (CO_2). Currently all fire extinguishers come in red cylinders and can be identified by a coloured label. The types of extinguishers found in the beauty-related industries are listed in the table below. The table explains how they should be used, how they work and their limitations.

Type of extinguisher	How it can be identified	What is it used for?	How it works	Limitations
 Water extinguisher	Red label and a thin hose	Class A fires involving wood, paper, hair and textiles	Water cools and smothers the fire and extinguishes the flame and heat source.	▪ Do not use on electrical fires as you might get an electric shock and water can cause an electrical fire to get larger and spread. ▪ Do not use on oil fires as water is heavier than oil and sinks to the bottom. It can also create a blast of steam causing the fire to spread.
 Foam extinguisher	Cream label and a thin hose	Class B fires involving flammable liquids (except cooking oils)	As the extinguisher is mainly water based with a foaming agent, the foam floats on top of the burning fluid and breaks the contact between the flames and the fuel's surface.	▪ Do not use on electrical fires as you might get an electric shock and the fire might spread. ▪ Do not use on chip-pan fires as the oils get extremely hot and might explode if the foam extinguisher is used.

Type of extinguisher	How it can be identified	What is it used for?	How it works	Limitations
Carbon dioxide (CO₂) extinguisher	Black label and wide nozzle	Class C fires involving electrical fires and flammable gases	CO_2 does not burn and it replaces the oxygen in the air. Fire needs oxygen to burn; CO_2 suffocates the fire by removing the oxygen.	▪ Not good at cooling fires. ▪ The extinguisher horn gets very cold and can cause 'freeze' burns and blisters so it must not be touched when in use.
Dry powder extinguisher	Blue label and a thin hose	Class C fires involving electrical fires and flammable liquids	Dry powder helps to reduce the chemical reactions needed for the fire to continue.	▪ Not good at penetrating into appliances, so electrical fires might reignite. ▪ Not very good at cooling the fire down.
Fire blanket and wet chemical extinguisher*	Blanket	Class F fires involving cooking fats. Also to be used to wrap around people if their clothes are on fire	Suffocates the flames by removal of the oxygen while the person is wrapped or the item is covered.	▪ The person or item it is covering needs to be left to cool, to prevent reignition when the person is unwrapped or the item is uncovered and exposed to oxygen.

NB The guidance above is for use within the salon and not general use.

*Wet chemical extinguishers can also be used for fires involving cooking fats, but these are not required in the hairdressing environment.

ACTIVITY

Draw a simple sketch of the floor plan of your salon. Add the location and type of fire extinguishers available.

WHY DON'T YOU...
find out the emergency procedures for your workplace.

 SmartScreen 202 Worksheet 3

Assistance

Action of helping someone.

Casualty

A person who has been injured.

FIRST AID

First aid is the first **assistance** or treatment given to a **casualty** before the arrival of an ambulance or qualified person. The aims of first aid are to:

- preserve life
- prevent the injury or condition from becoming worse
- promote recovery.

The first aider's tasks are to:

- assess the situation to find out what has happened
- deal with any dangers to oneself or the casualty
- get help if needed
- deal calmly with the injury or condition
- arrange for further care or treatment.

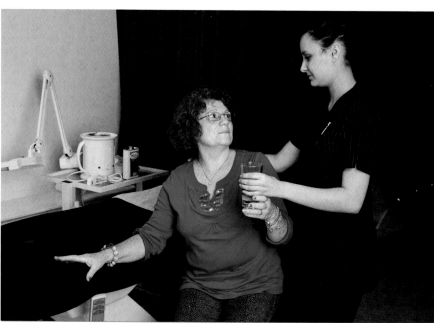

If a client feels unwell, sit them down and reassure them

The minimum first-aid provision on any work site is:

- a suitable well-stocked first-aid box
- an appointed person to take charge of first-aid arrangements.

FIRST-AID BOX

All salons must have a first-aid box. This should be located in an easily accessible and visible position. Modern first-aid boxes are green with a white cross. The box should be kept closed to keep the contents free from dust and moisture.

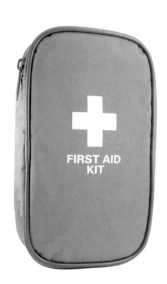

REPORTING AND RECORDING ACCIDENTS

The reporting and recording of accidents, injuries and emergencies in your salon is very important. Your employer must always be informed if someone has been injured, had an accident or something has happened in the salon that could lead to accidents or injuries. Under RIDDOR (Reporting of Injuries, Diseases and Dangerous Occurrences Regulations), it might also be a legal requirement for your employer to report the accident or incident to the Health and Safety Executive (HSE).

PROCEDURES FOR REPORTING AND RECORDING ACCIDENTS

It is a legal requirement for all staff to know where the first-aid box and the accident book are stored. Your employer should explain where these are, who is responsible for maintaining the contents and how to complete the accident book.

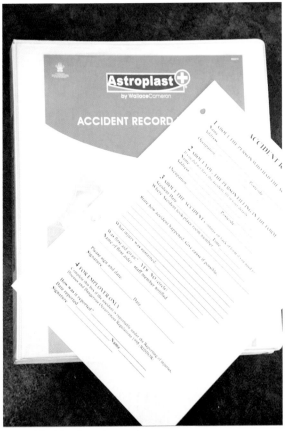

An accident book and record

If an accident occurs in the salon, always make sure that:

1 you look after the injured person
2 you inform your employer or line manager as quickly as possible and make sure that the accident is written up in the accident book immediately.

The salon's accident book must be kept in a safe place and every member of staff must know where this is. Any accidents, even a cut to a therapist's finger, must be reported in the accident book.

You need to record the following information:

- the date and time of the incident
- the name and address of the person involved
- the name and address of any witnesses
- a clear description of the details (eg a cut from manicure scissors to the therapist's third finger on her left hand, resulting in a small bleed).
- the treatment given or whether none was required.

WHY DON'T YOU...
add to your salon diagram from earlier the locations of the first-aid box and accident book.

INDUSTRY TIP

Always make sure the accident book is located in a central, easy-to-locate position. The reception is a good place to keep it.

INDUSTRY TIP

The accident book can be reviewed by the Health and Safety Executive and environmental health officers when they inspect premises, so make sure all entries are professionally recorded.

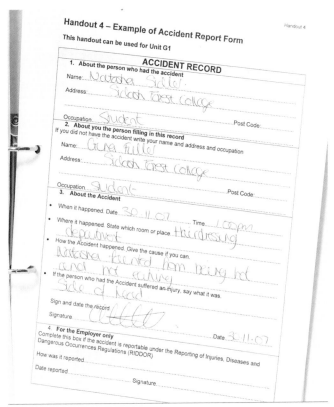

Records should be legible

Appliance

A device or piece of equipment made to perform a specifc task.

 SmartScreen 202 Activity assignment 2

INDUSTRY TIP

The salon should have regular practices of emergency procedures to make sure everyone is familiar with what they are expected to do and where they must go.

WHY DON'T YOU...

add to your plan of the salon the fire exits and assembly meeting point.

Evacuate

Leaving the area because of fire.

 SmartScreen 202 Revision cards

GAS SAFETY

Some salons might use gas for central heating, hot water and cooking facilitates. Gas **appliances** must only be fitted and maintained by qualified engineers. There must be adequate ventilation to avoid any problems with a build-up of gases (carbon monoxide).

A common cause of gas leaks is a pilot light on an appliance or boiler going out. If you smell gas follow these guidelines:

- do not smoke or use a naked flame
- do not turn on or off any electric switches
- open window and doors to ventilate the area
- check pilot lights
- turn off the gas at the mains supply (usually by the meter) if the source of the leak cannot be found
- telephone for emergency assistance from an engineer.

FIRE AND EMERGENCY PROCEDURES

If you discover a fire or any other emergency in the salon, you should raise the alarm in a calm and safe manner, notify other staff and **evacuate** clients to the assembly point. Employees and staff should not collect anything other than what they have with them. Dial 999 and ask the operator for the fire service. Give the salon's address and describe the current situation. No-one should re-enter the building until the emergency services have said it is safe to do so.

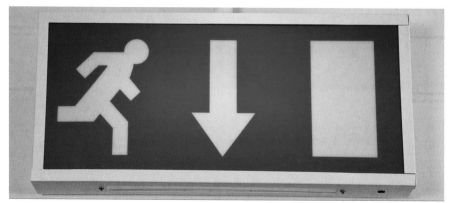

Emergency exit sign

SECURITY OF BELONGINGS

Your salon should make sure they protect clients' and staff's personal belongings, salon equipment and the reception area, such as the till point and the products on display. They must also protect client and salon records by following the requirements of the Data Protection Act (DPA).

MAINTAINING THE SALON'S SECURITY

Each salon will have a different policy for maintaining the security of its premises, its stock and the safety of its staff and clients. Some salons might have a shutter that covers the salon's door and windows when it is closed for the day. Others might have a buzzer or video-entry system which allows entry to **authorised** clients and salon visitors only. The majority of salons will have a front door that allows access and entry to all; this is best kept closed for your personal safety and the safety of

Authorised

When a person or company has official power.

those around you. If the reception area is not **permanently** manned, the door should have some sort of device that lets you know when someone has entered the salon. This could be a quiet buzzer or bell that rings when the door is opened, a pressure mat that buzzes when stepped on or simple wind chimes that jingle when the door is opened.

To prevent **breaches in security**, you must follow your salon's security policy. This could include:

- storing minimal cash in the till – all other cash should be kept in a safe with limited access
- keeping the till drawer locked at all times and the key removed when the receptionist leaves the reception area
- tidying away the salon equipment and not leaving expensive items, such as full containers of products, on display where there is no staff to keep an eye on them
- keeping staff's personal belongings in a locker or secured in staff-only areas
- making sure clients keep their personal belongings in view and with them at all times
- displaying retail stands away from the entrance door or in a glass display cabinet with doors that can be locked to make access more difficult
- making sure that clients' records are stored away and not left lying around in the salon.

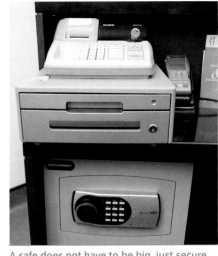

A safe does not have to be big, just secure

Permanently

Always.

Breaches in security

Breaking a security policy.

SmartScreen 202 Worksheet 9

> **INDUSTRY TIP**
>
> Avoid leaving the reception area unattended.

> **INDUSTRY TIP**
>
> Mirrors which help you to see into blind spots are really useful.

> **INDUSTRY TIP**
>
> If you need to remove a client's jewellery for a treatment, make sure it is somewhere within their view. If you are doing a treatment, such as a facial, where this is not possible, ask the client to place their jewellery in their handbag. Alternatively, you could get your client to place it in their shoe if it is enclosed. As soon as they go to put their shoe on it is there and it is also out of view.

> **INDUSTRY TIP**
>
> For security purposes, make sure all records that need to be destroyed or any letters with personal details on are always cross-shredded and not just thrown away in a bin.

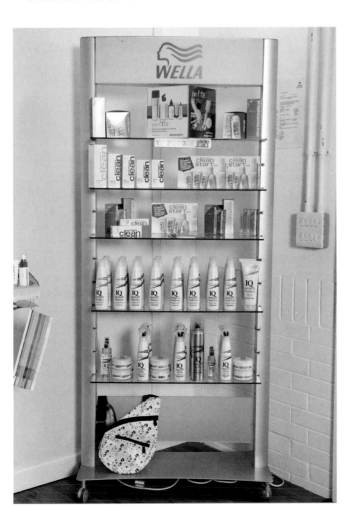

Displays should be clean and tidy

TEST YOUR KNOWLEDGE

Use the questions below to test your knowledge of Chapter 202 to see how much information you have retained. These questions will help you revise what you have learnt in this chapter.

Turn to page 601 for the answers.

1. Which **one** of the following sentences best defines the term hazard?
   a) Something that reduces the risks in the workplace
   b) Something with the potential to cause harm or injury
   c) Anything that might eliminate damage at work
   d) Anything that must be reported under RIDDOR

2. What action should be taken when hearing the fire alarm?
   a) Collect your personal belongings and leave the building
   b) Finish off the treatment you are carrying out and wait to be called to leave the building
   c) Take your client and leave the building quickly and calmly by the nearest fire exit
   d) Leave the building by the main entrance only and close the door

3. Which **one** of the following pieces of fire-fighting equipment should be used on electrical fires?
   a) A fire blanket
   b) A foam fire extinguisher
   c) A water fire extinguisher
   d) A carbon dioxide fire extinguisher

4. Which **one** of the following will a code of practice *not* give guidance on?
   a) Salon dress code
   b) Hygiene and infection control
   c) Salon evacuation procedures
   d) Salon safety

5. What is the most common cause of work-related injuries?
   a) Manual handling
   b) Slips and trips
   c) Electric shocks
   d) Chemical burns

6. Which **one** of the following is a hazard that would need to be referred to a manager?
   a) A trailing cable
   b) An overloaded socket
   c) A loose stair carpet
   d) A spilt liquid

7. Which **one** of the following is the main reason for wearing enclosed shoes in the salon?
   a) To follow fashion trends
   b) To protect the feet
   c) To prevent trips and slips
   d) To follow the salon's dress code

8. Which **one** of the following is a disadvantage of using a UV cabinet?
   a) Items must be dry before being placed in the cabinet
   b) It is only suitable for metal tools
   c) It is only suitable for plastic tools
   d) Items must be turned during the sanitisation process

9. Which **one** of the following should be placed in a yellow refuse bag?
   a) Cotton wool from a facial
   b) Contaminated waxing strips
   c) Disposable make-up brushes
   d) Wooden orange sticks

10. Which **one** of the following best describes a risk assessment?
    a) A process in which work activities are reviewed
    b) A list of risks that might occur in the salon
    c) A process that is carried out to meet health and safety requirements
    d) A list of hazards that can occur in the salon

CLIENT CARE AND COMMUNICATION IN BEAUTY-RELATED INDUSTRIES

Client care makes up a large part of the service that a client receives so it is important that you know how to treat clients and how to communicate with them. Clients should be made to feel special and that during the time they are in the salon they have your full attention.

Communication is a way of passing on, receiving and responding to information. Good communication skills are essential as part of client care since they can make the difference between a poor service and an excellent one. Poor communication often leads to confusion, misunderstanding and, more importantly, mistakes. You should listen to the feedback you are given from clients, managers, assessors and colleagues and evaluate your own personal performance. It is important to review your performance continually to make sure you are giving the best service and care that that you can.

In this chapter you will learn how to:

- communicate with clients
- provide client care.

HANDY HINTS

You will need to keep referring back to this chapter as you work through the other chapters in the book to make sure your clients and customers have the best professional experience that you and your salon have to offer them.

INDUSTRY TIP

You should know about who does what job roles within your workplace, including who is responsible as the manager, receptionist, senior therapist/nail technician.

Multimedia materials

Materials that can be interactive, such as websites, audio and DVDs.

Good communication will be very important to you in your chosen career within the beauty-related industries. You should take care to talk to your clients and colleagues in a respectful way that earns their trust.

In this part of the chapter you will learn about:

- legislation relating to client care
- methods of communication
- the consultation process
- personal space.

LEGISLATION RELATING TO CLIENT CARE

You will need to make sure you have a good understanding of the legislation relating to client care. This information can be found in the Legislation chapter on pages 91–113. Make sure you have a good understanding of each Act and how it will affect you in the workplace. The Acts you should be familiar with are:

- the Data Protection Act (DPA)
- the Supply of Goods and Services Act
- the Consumer Protection Act
- the Sale of Goods Act.

METHODS OF COMMUNICATION

The way we communicate can be divided into *three* categories:

- **verbal communication** – the spoken word or sounds we make, such as laughing or sighing
- **non-verbal communication** which includes:
  - body language and gestures (eg the way you act, eye contact, shaking your head, crossing your arms, waving and turning away)
  - written communication (eg emails, text messages, letters, leaflets, magazines, promotional materials and **multimedia materials**)
- **listening skills** – you can show the client you are really listening to them by maintain good eye contact, leaning forward slightly, tilting your head slightly to one side or nodding as they give you information.

Using visual aids can also help you to communicate more effectively with your client. These can be useful during the consultation process so that clients can see the finished result of their treatment or service.

In the salon, spa, nail studio or on set, the majority of communication is face to face with people. However, there is a growing trend for the use of electronic communication, by means of email and text messaging, for communicating in writing. It is important to be aware of the effect distance can have on communication.

During conversation, only 7 per cent of what we are communicating comes from the words we use, 38 per cent comes from the tone of voice you use to say the words and 55 per cent comes from your body language or non-verbal communication. You can therefore see how important it is that you pay attention to your tone of voice when communicating over the phone. The tone of your voice will say far more than the words you use.

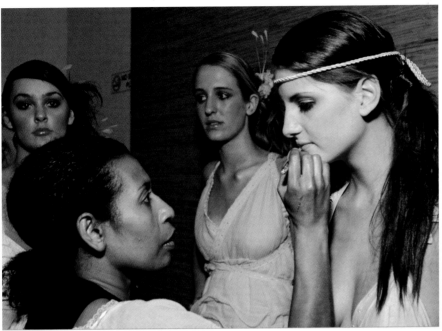
Always be aware of the tone of your voice during treatments

VERBAL COMMUNICATION

How we communicate verbally is important. Some tips for good communication are:

- **Speak clearly with a soft tone of voice** – do not speak too loudly otherwise you might disturb other clients and do not speak too softly because you will not be heard properly.
- **Avoid jargon and slang** – for example, the client might not know what a comedone is but they will know what a blackhead is.
- **Address the client directly by name whenever you can** – this lets the client know that you are talking to them and also makes them feel that they are getting personal service.

Questioning skills

Questioning is a type of verbal communication and it is important to use the right question in order to get the answer you need. The type of question you will use will be determined by the information that you need to find out from your client.

Open questions

Open questions can be used to start a conversation or find out information and allow the client to give you a more detailed response. Examples of open questions include:

- How would you describe your skin?
- Can you tell me about the outfit you will be wearing for your special occasion?

SmartScreen 203 Handout 1

WHY DON'T YOU...
make a list of some open and closed questions you might use during a consultation.

Confirm
To accept or agree something.

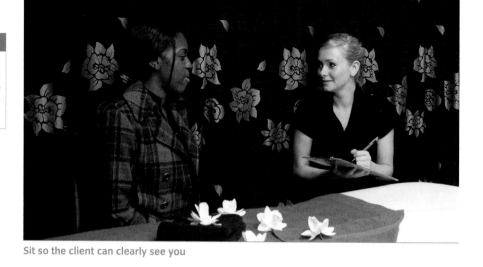
Sit so the client can clearly see you

However, during a consultation, a therapist is likely to use the words tell, explain and describe to start a sentence to draw out more information from the client – for example:

- **Tell** me about your skin.
- **Explain** exactly what your medication is for.
- **Describe** to me the outfit you will be wearing for your special occasion.

Avoid asking unclear questions as these will give unclear answers and not necessarily the response you need (eg 'Do you have an appointment?' 'No, I would like to buy a voucher'). Avoid questions that are likely to get a one-word answer, such as ok and alright (eg 'How are you today?' 'OK!' or 'How did you get on with the moisturiser?' 'Alright'). One-word answers will show that your questioning technique is not direct enough to get the information you are trying to gain.

Closed questions
Closed questions are used to:

- get a short response (ie 'yes' or 'no') and **confirm** information (eg 'Is that warm enough?')
- close a conversation or shorten it when clients are talkative (eg 'Is there anything else I can help you with today?').

ACTIVITY

Play charades with a group of your colleagues. Each person in the group should take one of the following situations and act it out. The other people in the group should then guess the situation from the body language:

- The therapist is running late and only has 30 minutes to complete the treatment. Is there another therapist that can do the treatment?
- A client is angry as the therapist only took 45 minutes to complete an hour-long facial.
- A client wants a replacement for a product that she has reacted badly to.
- A replacement therapist is trying to explain to a client that she is carrying out the treatment today instead of her usual therapist as her usual therapist has just gone home sick and there was no time to call her to let her know.
- Try completing a consultation without saying a word!
- Give a client aftercare advice following a facial.

Check your answers with your tutor.

NON-VERBAL COMMUNICATION

Body language

Body language is a large part of non-verbal communication. Body language helps other people to interpret what you are thinking. Your body gives messages through:

- gestures (eg a thumbs up or waving)
- movements of your arms and legs (eg crossing your arms or your legs and fidgeting)
- nodding your head
- facial expressions (eg frowning or smiling)
- eye contact (eg staring (which can be aggressive) or a lack of eye contact (which can show **nervousness**))
- your posture (ie how you carry yourself).

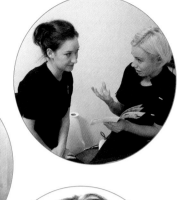

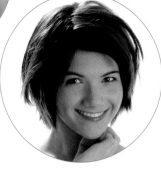

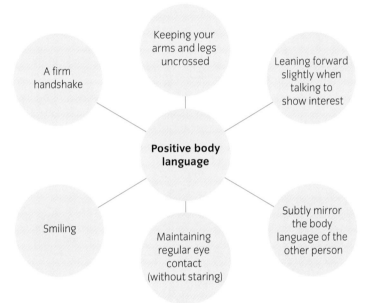

Positive body language:
- A firm handshake
- Keeping your arms and legs uncrossed
- Leaning forward slightly when talking to show interest
- Subtly mirror the body language of the other person
- Maintaining regular eye contact (without staring)
- Smiling

Nervousness

Feeling anxious or worried.

> **INDUSTRY TIP**
>
> Good posture shows confidence; poor posture shows a lack of confidence or disinterest.

Look for the following positive body language from your client as a sign that they are happy, relaxed and hopefully enjoying their treatment:

- relaxed body language – arms uncrossed and sat or laid comfortably
- smiling
- looking sleepy (or actually going to sleep during a relaxing treatment)
- good eye contact with you when they are not having a relaxing treatment, such as a make-up or nail treatment.

Look out for the following negative body language from your client as a warning sign that they are nervous, **disinterested**, defensive or, in the worst case, want to leave the salon:

- leaning back or away from you
- crossed legs
- crossed arms
- a lack of eye contact
- the client keeps looking away.

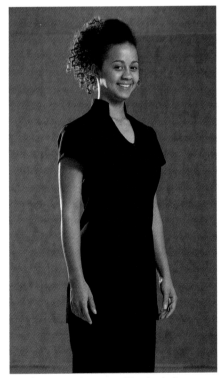

Good posture shows positive body language

Disinterested

Lack of interest.

Aggressive

Angry or attacking behaviour.

Intimidating

Threatening or frightening.

Disdain

The feeling that you do not need to be bothered about someone or something.

 SmartScreen 203 Worksheet 1

INDUSTRY TIP

Reading body language is like reading words in a sentence. You must look at all the body language to make sure you are not misinterpreting what is being said.

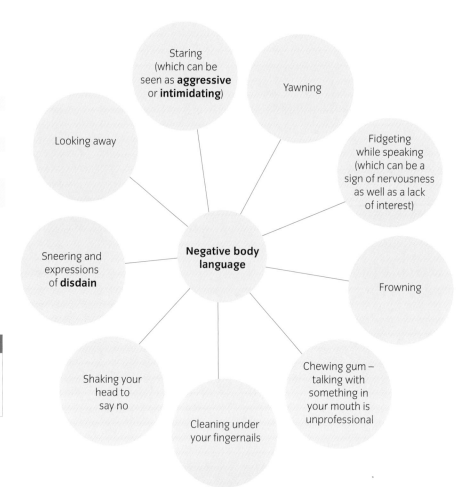

Staring (which can be seen as **aggressive** or **intimidating**)

Yawning

Looking away

Fidgeting while speaking (which can be a sign of nervousness as well as a lack of interest)

Sneering and expressions of **disdain**

Negative body language

Frowning

Shaking your head to say no

Cleaning under your fingernails

Chewing gum – talking with something in your mouth is unprofessional

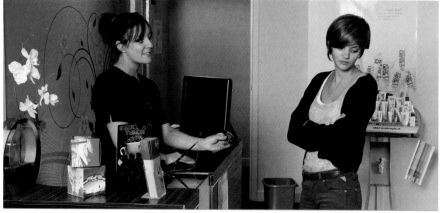

If you see negative body language, you need to stop and ask yourself why

Written communication

There are a number of different ways that we can communicate in writing. Written communication can be:

- by email
- by text message
- by letter
- on consultation forms and record cards
- through leaflets and promotional materials (eg appointment cards and price lists)
- through magazines and trade journals
- through multimedia – this includes the Internet, websites, audio and DVDs that are used to promote the salon.

It is important that anything that is written and sent out on behalf of the business is checked for spelling and grammar. It is important that promotional material gives a positive image of the business. Often promotional materials will contain the salon's **logo** and pictures of treatments that the salon offers. It is important that the information and images used are true and accurate so that you do not make any false claims or show false images of treatments you do not offer.

Logo
A symbol or small design that represents a business and is used on all its products.

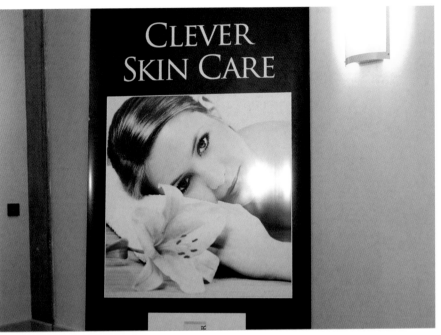

Marketing material with correct spellings

HANDY HINTS

The Data Protection Act relates to information that is stored electronically. Remember that it is important that any information that you hold electronically about your clients is stored in line with the requirements of the Data Protection Act. Further information on the Data Protection Act can be found in the Legislation chapter on pages 105–106.

INDUSTRY TIP

If you know that spelling is not your strong point, keep a small dictionary handy in the salon. Always use the spell check facility on your computer before sending anything.

HANDY HINTS

Refer to Chapter 205 to find out more about promotional materials and the written word.

Record cards

Record cards provide details of the treatments that a client has had. It is important that this information is accurate, easy to read and can be understood by someone else who might need to access these records. There are always occasions when clients will need to be contacted (eg if a therapist is off sick) so it is important to make sure you have correct contact details. It is also useful to refer to previous treatment information. You can also include images on a client's record card to show things visually. For example, if a client has had a consultation for a facial, you could draw an image of a face on their consultation card and illustrate it to represent what you have seen. You could use lines to show where there are thread veins and dots to show where there might be comedones. For a make-up application you could use the make-up on the record card to create a colour record of the treatment.

ACTIVITY

Think back to the last time you were in a salon or nail studio and make a list of all the different types of written communication you saw. Compare your list with a colleague's list to see if they have listed anything else.

Clients often have the same treatment regularly or ask for the same finish as last time (eg they might want the same nail varnish colour). If you have made an accurate note of this on their record card you can make sure you use the same colour. It is often difficult to remember details mentally so a quick note on a record card is always useful. Detailed records are also essential in case a member of staff is absent and the client's records need to be accessed and read by someone else.

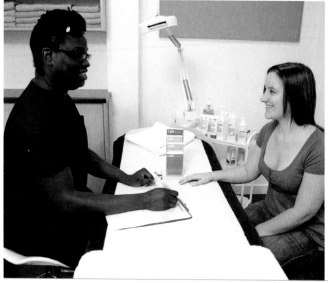 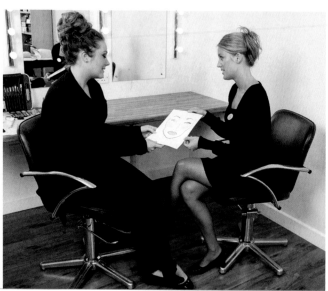

Record cards need to be clear so that clients and colleagues can read them

Text messages and emails

Text messages and emails are often used by a business. Text messages are sent to remind clients of appointments and email is being used more frequently by businesses to let clients know about offers and to send newsletters.

Remember if you are communicating by text or email on behalf of your salon or spa to check the message for spelling and grammar. It will look unprofessional if you make spelling errors. Make sure that messages have the right tone so that they are friendly and polite. You might need to check with a manager before sending any messages on behalf of the business if you do not have permission to do so. For messages sent by email to a number of customers, make sure that you keep the recipients' email addresses private by using the bcc address line.

INDUSTRY TIP

We tend to read what we expect to see. This is why it is easy for errors to occur. Read your message out loud to check that it reads correctly.

INDUSTRY TIP

Never send a message when you are angry. You can write the message but wait until you are in a better mood before checking it and sending it. It is better to write things when you have a clear head as you can be more objective and express your thoughts with more clarity.

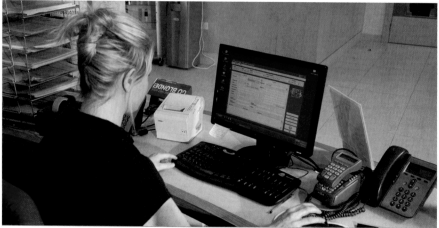

Many salons now use electronic communication

LISTENING SKILLS

When you are giving client care, it is essential that you listen to them. Demonstrate to the client that you are actively listening to what they are saying and give them time to ask questions. You can show that you are actively listening by nodding, leaning in slightly to show interest if you are sitting or by tilting your head. You can also respond in agreement to what they are saying with 'yes' or 'ok' and ask closed questions to confirm what they have said to you. This shows the client you are interested and that what they have to say is important.

In order to check your understanding a good tip is to repeat back the important points of the conversation with the client.

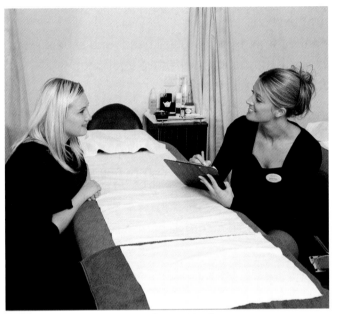

Give your clients 100 per cent of your attention

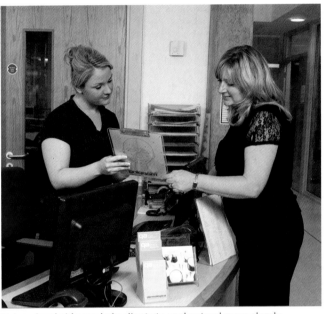

Using visual aids can help clients to understand more clearly

VISUAL AIDS

There is a lot of visual supporting material in the salon that you can use when you are discussing a treatment with your client to help explain to the client what you are doing. You can show the client the products you will be using and encourage them to touch and feel the products and sample them. When applying make-up, you can put some of the colour on the record card to help with recording the details of the treatment. You can also let the client hold the make-up item so that they can have a closer look. Many product companies produce promotional material to support their products and treatments. Refer to this material so that clients have a visual image of the end result of the treatment.

ACTIVITY

Make a list of all the visual aids you can think of that you have access to. Write a brief summary of when and how you would use each of the visual aids that you have listed.

ACTIVITY

What is your favourite product that you use? Why is it your favourite product? Write a list of the features and benefits of the product. Then take part in a role play with a colleague to sell this product.

CONSULTATION PROCESS

The purpose of the consultation is to provide the client with the correct and most suitable treatment. During the consultation, you should:

- record important or key information
- assess whether the treatment is suitable for the client
- explain the treatment process
- provide an opportunity to discuss the treatment with the client and for the client to ask any questions
- ask the client about their treatment priorities, needs and expectations
- make sure you are providing a safe and effective treatment
- establish a **rapport** and build confidence.

The very first consultation that you have with a new client will always be more in-depth than later consultations. When the client returns for future treatments, a shorter **review** consultation should still be performed and the treatment plan amended according to the client's needs.

INFORMATION THAT NEEDS TO BE RECORDED

At the first consultation, you should record all of the client's details including their:

- full name
- address
- contact number – landline (home or work) or mobile
- email address.

It is important that that your writing is **legible** so that other colleagues are able to read it. There will always be occasions when a client might need to be contacted by someone else – for example, if you are off sick and a colleague needs to stand in. It will be really unhelpful if they cannot read the client's details.

Check with the client that they are happy to be contacted on the phone number they have given you. If you are using postal addresses and email addresses for sending your promotional information, you should check at the consultation whether the client is happy for you to contact them with this information.

During the consultation, you will also need to record details of:

- any contra-indications to the treatment
- the treatment plan.

Contra-indications

A contra-indication is a reason why a treatment cannot be carried out. It might be a contra-indication that prevents the client from being treated at all or one that might require the treatment to be restricted or modified.

INDUSTRY TIP

Do not be **complacent** – regular clients still need to be treated with exceptional client care if you want them to keep coming back.

Complacent

Being oversatisfied with your own work or achievements.

Rapport

A close relationship between two people in which they understand one another's feelings and attitudes.

Review

Assessing or examining something, eg your skills or behaviour.

Legible

Easy to read.

INDUSTRY TIP

If you are worried about your spelling or if the client has an unusual name, ask the client to complete just this section of the record card. Most people will not object to being asked to do this.

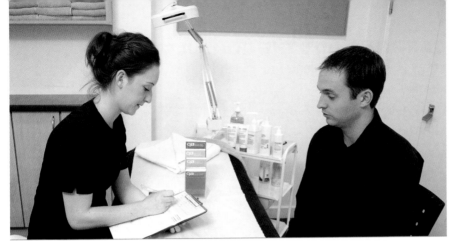

Make sure you record the information from your consultation

INDUSTRY TIP

Make sure you read questionnaires from product companies before you ask clients to complete them. You need to know their content in case the client has questions..

Ask the client if they have any contra-indications that might be relevant to the treatment. The client should sign and date the consultation card or questionnaire to confirm that the information is accurate.

If you discover the client has a contra-indication that prevents the treatment they are requesting, you must tactfully tell them that the treatment cannot go ahead and explain why. If the client has disclosed a medical condition you can refer to the condition. Advise the client that you do not want to make their condition worse. Suggest that they seek medical advice. You can, if appropriate, recommend an alternative treatment where possible.

Seeking medical advice

When you suggest that a client seeks advice, remember this is not a referral it is just a recommendation. You are not qualified to make a diagnosis and so it is important that you recommend that the client sees a professional who is qualified to make a diagnosis.

A medical practitioner will *not* give you approval to treat a client (since they do not want to be held responsible if anything goes wrong) but they can advise the client whether or not they should have the treatment. You can ask their GP to sign a letter to say that they are not aware of any medical reason why the client cannot have the treatment. Unfortunately GPs will charge even to sign a letter and this puts most clients off.

If the client has a contra-indication that will just require the treatment to be adapted or an area to be avoided, you must make sure you clearly explain this to the client before the treatment starts.

The treatment plan

Before you begin any treatment you should discuss the client's expectations of their treatment. Let the client know you have a few quick questions to help find out exactly what to focus on throughout the treatment. Remember, you must ask the client what they want from the treatment as this might be quite different from what you can see as being the obvious treatment.

Some clients might be having a course of treatments and might have unrealistic expectations after one treatment. It might require several treatments to achieve the result they want or it might be that they will never achieve the result they want. It is important that you are honest but tactful and make the client aware of this.

HANDY HINTS

See Chapter 205/213 for some further advice on fulfilling client needs.

 SmartScreen 203 Handout 3

CARRYING OUT THE CONSULTATION

When you greet the client:

- smile
- say hello
- introduce yourself
- confirm the treatment
- complete a consultation form
- ask your client to sign the form
- sign the form yourself.

Ideally, you should sit next to the client for the consultation rather than sitting either side of a couch or desk. This is because the couch or desk acts as a barrier to the conversation.

To recap on earlier parts of this chapter, as part of your consultation you should:

1 use questioning skills
2 observe the client and make a mental note of their body language
3 let the client tell you their treatment needs
4 use visual aids where appropriate.

During the consultation, remember to follow the Data Protection Act and the salon's policy for client confidentiality. This means you must store information securely and only take information that is required for the purpose or the service. Clients have the right to take legal action against the salon if their personal information is not kept confidential and in line with the Date Protection Act.

SmartScreen 203 Handout 2

PERSONAL SPACE

Personal space is an area around the human body that an individual will regard as their own. The size of this space can vary between individuals. Invading this space can lead to someone feeling very uncomfortable and possibly anxious. As therapists we step into this personal space regularly during our treatments so it is important that you are aware of how it might make people feel.

INDUSTRY TIP

In 1966, an academic, Edward Hall, identified four different zones of personal space – three of which are relevant to your work as a beauty therapist:

- **Intimate distance** is up to 45 cm from the person – this might involve personal contact and is reserved for our most intimate relationships.
- **Personal distance** is between 45 cm and 120 cm – at this distance we are comfortable to interact with close friends and people that we trust.
- **Social distance** is between 120 cm and 3.7 m and is used for formal, business and impersonal interactions, such as when first meeting a client.

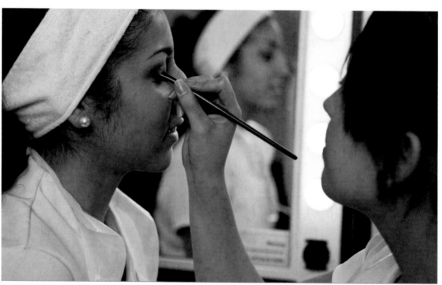

During treatments you will be working within a client's personal space

ACTIVITY

Get into pairs. Stand so that you are back to back with your partner (ie intimate distance). Then stand so that you are nose to nose. How do you feel? What do you want to do?

Now stand about 45 cm apart (personal distance). How do you feel now?

Now stand 1–3 m apart (social distance). How do you feel?

WHY DON'T YOU...
think of occasions when someone has made you feel uncomfortable because they have been too close.

PROVIDE CLIENT CARE

There are plenty of practical things you can do to improve your client's experience in the salon. You must never forget that the customer has lots of choice and they can easily go to another salon if they do not like the level of care you are giving them.

In this part of the chapter you will learn about:

- client comfort
- professionalism
- client feedback
- dealing with complaints and problems.

CLIENT COMFORT

SALON TEMPERATURE

The ideal working temperature is about 18°C but can range from 15.5°C to 20°C. Temperatures in a salon should be slightly higher as clients are often required to remove some clothing for certain treatments. It is therefore important that the client is warm so that they are able to relax.

INDUSTRY TIP

When we relax our body temperature drops so it is important to make sure when your client is relaxing that they are kept warm. Offer them a blanket if necessary.

HUMIDITY

Humidity is the amount of water vapour or 'dampness' in the air. When the air can hold no more water it is said to be saturated. The higher the temperature the more water vapour it can hold. If the water content cools it forms condensation. Too much condensation in a salon atmosphere can create problems with damp.

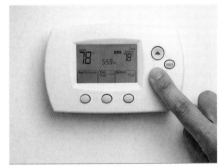

Thermostats should be used to keep temperatures constant

VENTILATION

Ventilation is when fresh air replaces stale air. The air in the salon should ideally be changed every 3–4 hours to prevent a build-up of stale air. Keeping fresh air flowing by ventilating the salon also helps to prevent tiredness. The salon should be ventilated by:

- natural ventilation (eg opening doors or windows to allow new air to circulate)
- controlled ventilation (eg fans and vents)
- artificial ventilation (eg electric extractors or fans).

It is important to ensure the correct level of ventilation in the salon. Overventilating an area can cause drafts and loss of heat and result in

INDUSTRY TIP

A thermostat is a small device for controlling temperature that is usually found on the wall in a central area. It monitors the temperature and cuts off the electric current to the heating when a pre-set temperature is reached. This helps to keep the salon at an even temperature.

clients and employees feeling chilly or uncomfortable. On the other hand, if an area is not adequately ventilated:

- micro-organisms can build up and increase the risk of cross-infection
- the atmosphere can become warm and stuffy
- carbon dioxide can build up and make employees feel **lethargic** and tired
- condensation can collect making the atmosphere damp.

Lethargic
A lack of energy.

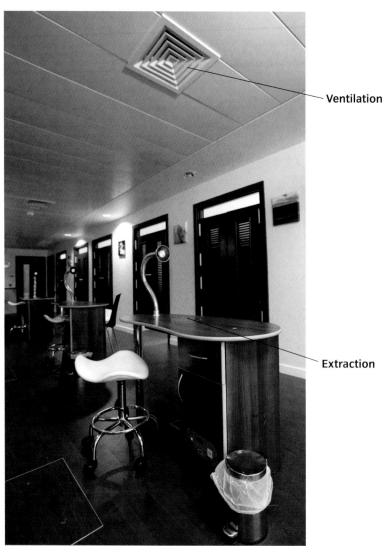

Ventilation

Extraction

An example of a nail station with ventilation and extraction

AIR CONDITIONING

Some salons are lucky enough to have air conditioning. These systems are very effective but are expensive to install. An air-conditioning system:

- controls temperature – it is effective for keeping the temperature of the salon warm when it is cold outside and cool when it is hot outside
- controls humidity – it adds moisture to the air or dries the air as necessary
- filters out dust and dirt.

LIGHTING

Suitable lighting is crucial in a salon. The right lighting helps to create a good environment and atmosphere. Poor lighting can result in poor visibility meaning an unsatisfactory service for the client if you cannot see what you are doing. It can also lead to eyestrain and headaches. There are several factors to consider when choosing appropriate lighting.

- Lights need to be positioned so that they do not create shadows or glare.
- Lights need to be positioned so that they are not in your line of focus.
- If possible, lights should be adjustable.
- You will need different types of lights for different treatments (eg bright lighting for waxing and subtle lighting for a facial).

INDUSTRY TIP

Magnifying lamps are great for giving direct lighting to a small area for close inspection.

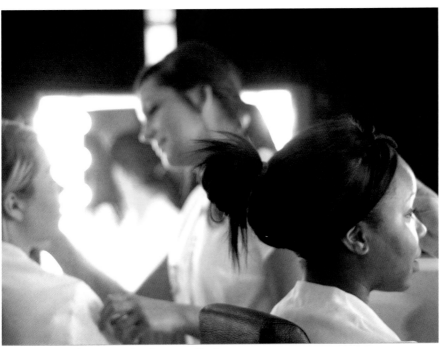

Good lighting is key to good make-up application

PROFESSIONALISM

It is extremely important to be professional at all times when you are working in any beauty-related environment. The definition of professional is to some degree subjective (ie we have a personal view on what it means to us).

You should behave professionally at all times and with all the people you have contact with – colleagues, clients and any other people you might have contact with during your working day (such as company representatives, delivery people and amenities agents (ie people who come to read the meters)). They should all be treated with the same respect.

Behaving professionally lets people know you are a trustworthy person. It also demonstrates your ability to perform your job in a professional manner which in turn gives confidence to the people you deal with.

WHY DON'T YOU...
Write down what the word professionalism means to you and how you can make sure you are being professional.

Use the spider diagram to help you recognise professional behaviour.

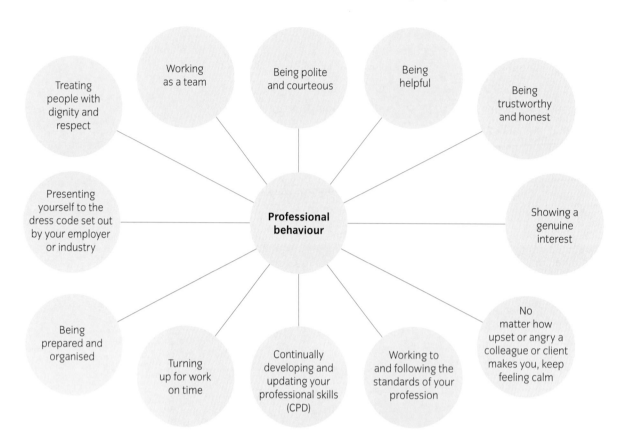

Unprofessional behaviour includes negative behaviour and attitudes. Use the spider diagram to help you recognise unprofessional behaviour.

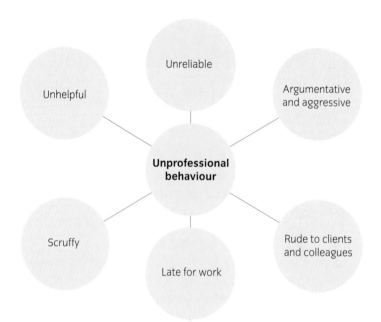

Over a period of time you might get to know some of your clients really well. It can then become difficult to keep the conversation from becoming too familiar and personal. Remember to keep a balance and to keep the main conversation focused on the client and their treatment.

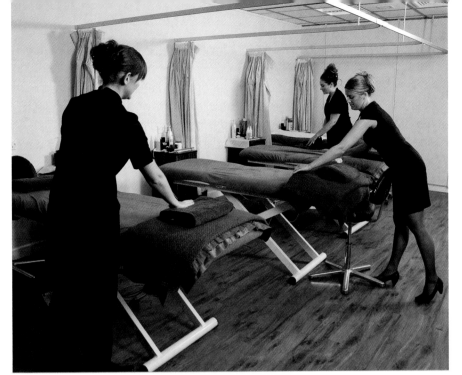
Keeping the salon tidy is essential for professional presentation

MAKING EACH CLIENT FEEL SPECIAL

Every client should be treated as an individual. They should be given devoted service time. They are paying for you to look after and advise them during their treatment time. They are not expecting you to be distracted by your phone or by other colleagues. They are paying for you to focus on them. Remember you are their 'therapist' and they come to you so that you can listen to them and give them advice, not for an hour's chat about *your* personal life. This means that the conversation you have is about *them*. The client does not want to spend their treatment time listening to you talk about yourself.

Here are some tips to make the client feel special and show that you care.

- Always make sure any new client knows your name – introduce yourself as soon as you greet the client.
- Address the client by name when you are giving them any instructions or when you are checking on them during treatment.
- Give the client your full attention.
- Always tell the client what you are doing so that they know.
- Give the client the opportunity to ask questions and the opportunity to let you know if they want you to change anything, such as massage pressure.
- At regular intervals during the treatment, check that the client is comfortable. Monitor the client's body language and react to any changes (eg if the client begins to look cold offer them a blanket).
- Protect the client's clothing.
- Give the client beneficial hints and tips during the service.
- Always give the client proper aftercare and home care advice to follow at home. Make sure you give them advice as to what they should do should a contra-action occur. Make sure they know that they can contact you if they have any queries.

INDUSTRY TIP

A common error that many therapists make is to forget about providing aftercare advice when a client comes in regularly. Client care must be on-going and consistent.

- Recommend to your client when they should have their next service if appropriate and when to book.
- Make accurate notes on the client record card about the service or treatment and also about things the client likes or dislikes (eg a client might prefer to sit up slightly during a facial and hates to be laid flat). The information on the record card can help you to prepare your work area for their next treatment.
- Go the extra mile. What else can you do for a client to make their treatment extra special and one to remember? It can be something as simple as offering them their favourite fruit tea or a hot water bottle in the winter.
- If you tell the client you are going to do something, do it. For example, if you say you will give them a sample, give them one. If you say you are going to call them back, call them back.

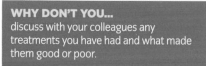

WHY DON'T YOU...
discuss with your colleagues any treatments you have had and what made them good or poor.

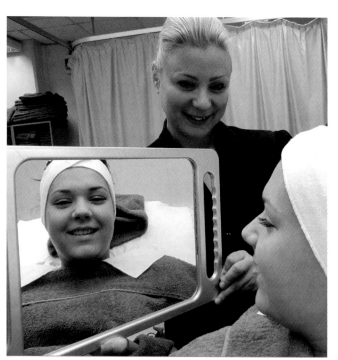

Give the client the chance to see the finished result

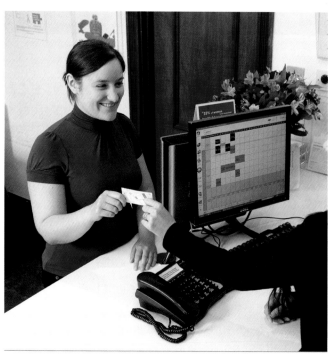

Always confirm appointment details back to the client and give an appointment card for reference

ACTIVITY

Have you had any treatments or appointments with a doctor, nurse or therapist where they have failed to introduce themselves? How did this make you feel?

ACTIVITY

Watch the following clip on YouTube which shows John Cleese demonstrating how not to give instructions!

http://www.youtube.com/watch?v=pXw7LYWNi5E

CLIENT FEEDBACK

Asking for client feedback helps you to:

- evaluate the effectiveness of a treatment or service
- understand how a treatment or service can be improved
- improve continually by learning from your experiences.

It is important to gain feedback from the client. When you have completed a treatment you should seek confirmation from the client that they are satisfied with the finished result.

Do not be frightened or nervous about asking clients about their treatment. Ask open questions rather than closed ones that will just get a one-word answer (eg 'yes' or 'OK'). You want feedback to be constructive to help you improve. If the client is happy with their service hopefully they will come back and ask specifically for you. Always thank the client for their feedback whether it is negative or positive.

INDUSTRY TIP

If you are using a questionnaire to gather feedback and want it to be objective, get someone else (who has not given the treatment) to carry out or collect the questionnaire. Clients are more likely to complete a questionnaire if they feel it is being given to them by a different individual.

METHODS OF GATHERING FEEDBACK

Ideally, you should use a range of methods for gathering feedback as different information can be gained from each method.

Verbal questioning

You can gain feedback by asking clients questions. Keep your questions concise and to the point (eg 'What did you enjoy most about your treatment today?' 'Is there any part of your treatment that you would like to be different if you had this treatment again?'). Verbal feedback gives quick and instant answers; you do however have to rely on the client being truthful and not just being polite. You can respond to verbal feedback accordingly.

Observation

What was the client's body language like during their service? If they were having a relaxing treatment did they look relaxed? Visibly, did they appear to enjoy their treatment? Observation will give you instant feedback. In many cases, it will allow you to respond to the client without them having to say anything to you.

Written questionnaires

These are very popular and give the client a short list of questions to answer. The questions can require a short answer, a written response or a series of boxes to be ticked with a 'yes' or 'no' response. Some questions try to gain more detail and might ask clients to rate a treatment or service using a sliding scale (ie poor, satisfactory, good, excellent and above expectation). Many businesses offer an incentive, such as a monthly prize draw, to encourage clients to complete questionnaires.

SmartScreen 203 Worksheet 3

INDUSTRY TIP

One way of evaluating your customer care and quality of service is to review how many of your clients come back as repeat business – especially for regular services. Repeat business is usually a positive sign, however, there is always room for improvement no matter how good you think you are.

POSITIVE FEEDBACK

We always focus on the negative aspects of feedback but responding to positive feedback is just as important. When a client pays you a compliment always make sure you thank them. If the person the feedback relates to is not present, it should always be passed on as praise is always lovely to hear.

DEALING WITH COMPLAINTS AND PROBLEMS

When a problem comes up, it is best to deal with it with a positive **attitude**. Being positive will help you to be objective and **constructive** in thinking of ways to deal with the problem. It might be that they have a **justified** complaint so you should listen carefully to what they are saying. However, some clients might be rude and get very vocal, especially if they are not getting their own way. Remain polite and calm no matter how you really feel.

IDENTIFYING THE PROBLEM

You need to allow the client to express their concern or complaint. Not all clients shout and get angry when they are unhappy with a treatment. This usually only happens when a client is not getting the response that they are looking for. Listen carefully and show that you are interested and are taking the complaint seriously. At this stage, you need to identify exactly what the complaint or problem is. If the problem relates to a treatment or personal performance, the issue should be dealt with tactfully and positively, making sure that the exact problem is addressed.

DEALING WITH THE PROBLEM

The business should have a set procedure that should be followed when dealing with customer complaints. Depending on the nature of the complaint, you might be able to resolve the problem yourself – for example, the client might have returned with a faulty product that can be easily replaced. The flow chart below gives a suggested course of action for dealing with a problem so that a positive outcome can be achieved.

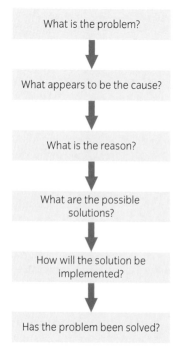

Attitude
The way you think or feel.

Constructive
Fix or find an answer to.

Justified
Reason for an action or idea.

INDUSTRY TIP
If the client who is angry is standing up, take them somewhere where you can both sit down (so that you are at the same level as them) and discuss their complaint.

If you are unable to **resolve** the complaint yourself, you should refer the client to a senior member of staff or manager. Depending on the nature of the complaint, or if the client becomes **agitated**, it might be a good idea to move the client into a quiet area away from the main reception if you can. You do not want other clients to be aware you have a problem. Before going to get a more senior member of staff or your manager, be sure to excuse yourself and explain to the client that you are going to get another member of staff to help them.

If the complaint is about another therapist, do not pass comment or **criticise** them in public and in front of the client. This could cause ill feeling among your colleagues and you also cannot **assume** your colleague's actions were wrong.

ACTIVITY

How would you deal with the situation in the photo below?

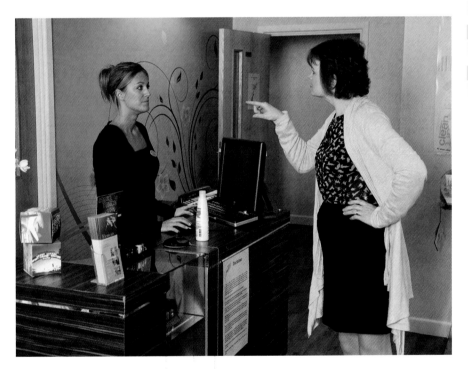

When you are dealing with a complaint, remember the following dos and don'ts:

Do...	Don't...
be truthful about the situation	lie
see the problem from different viewpoints (eg the therapist's and the client's)	lose your temper
be positive	forget the objective – what is the problem?
deal with problem if you can or go get a senior member of staff or manager	ignore the situation as this can cause further tension and anger
be assertive	be aggressive or defensive

INDUSTRY TIP

Think of dealing with an angry client like opening a shaken-up bottle of fizzy drink. Let them say what they need to say and then hopefully the fizz will settle down. You can then discuss the situation and come to a resolution.

INDUSTRY TIP

Some businesses might have a person who is responsible for dealing with complaints. This person could be a manager, the receptionist, a senior therapist or a technician.

Resolve
To find a solution or answer.

Agitated
Irritated or stirred up.

Criticise
To point out a fault.

Assume
To believe that something is true.

INDUSTRY TIP

Role play is an excellent way of practising possible situations. It gives you an opportunity to gain experience in dealing with situations and gets you used to your salon's procedures.

 SmartScreen 203 Worksheet 4

ACTIVITY

In groups of four, carry out a role play of the situations below giving feedback to one another. Decide as a group on the best environment in which the situation might occur. One person should be the therapist and one person the manager. The other two people should observe and make notes about whether the situation was dealt with positively or negatively. You might like to use the flow chart on page 184 to help you.

Situation 1

A client has complained about a treatment stating that they felt the therapist was disinterested and had rushed the treatment. They also felt that the therapist's personal presentation represented the salon poorly.

Situation 2

A client has openly praised her therapist in the reception area in front of other clients saying that the facial she had just received was the best one she had ever had. She is a regular client to the salon and the therapist is new.

LEARNING FROM MISTAKES

Being able to learn from a bad experience is as valuable as the satisfaction of a positive outcome. When something goes wrong, take the time to review the situation and assess what you can learn from it.

ACTIVITY

Working in small groups, discuss experiences where you have received feedback that was either negative or very positive. This could be feedback from a treatment that you have given or feedback on a piece of work that has been marked or feedback on inappropriate behaviour.

- Write down *three* points that you felt were positive or negative about the feedback.
- Write down *three* emotions you felt from the experience.
- Write down *three* ways in which the experience could have been improved.

TEST YOUR KNOWLEDGE

Use the questions below to test your knowledge of Chapter 203 to see how much information you have retained. These questions will help you revise what you have learnt in this chapter.

Turn to page 601 for the answers.

1. During a conversation, what percentage of what we are communicating comes from the tone we use?
   a. 7 per cent
   b. 38 per cent
   c. 55 per cent
   d. 100 per cent

2. Which **one** of the following is considered to be a type of multimedia communication?
   a. A consultation
   b. A DVD
   c. A poster
   d. A price list

3. Which **one** of the following is an example of negative body language?
   a. Staring
   b. Giggling
   c. Nodding
   d. Waving

4. Which **one** of the following is an example of negative behaviour?
   a. Being efficient
   b. Being proactive
   c. Being argumentative
   d. Being assertive

5. When you give instructions you should:
   a. stand beside the person
   b. use technical abbreviations
   c. write them down
   d. speak clearly and not rush.

6. Which **one** of the following is an example of an open question?
   a. What is your skin care routine?
   b. Is this what you use on your face?
   c. Do you use this product on your skin?
   d. You can use this product on your skin

7. In relation to the storage of record cards, the Data Protection Act applies to records that are:
   a. stored in an electronic database
   b. stored in a filing cabinet
   c. stored in a reception area
   d. stored in a lockable cabinet.

8. A client complains that they were sold a moisturiser that had already been opened. Who should the client be referred to?
   a. The receptionist
   b. Another therapist
   c. The product company's representative
   d. The salon manager

9. Which **one** of the following would not be required on a consultation card?
   a. The client's mobile number
   b. The client's marital status
   c. The products used during the treatment or service
   d. Any contra-indications to treatment

10. Where is the best place to carry out a consultation?
   a. In the main reception
   b. In the relaxation room
   c. In a treatment room
   d. In the retail area

CASE STUDY: PAMELA LINFORTH

Without a doubt, beauty therapy is the best industry to be in. I have enjoyed every job I have been lucky enough to have throughout my career. The great thing about being a beauty therapist is the variety of jobs and the opportunities that are open to you.

I have worked in salons, clinics and spas before going on to qualify as a teacher. Working in a large FE college and then running an academy led onto training in human resources and I am now a company director at Ellisons, the leading supplier to the hair and beauty industry in the UK.

The best thing is the great people you get to work with. Colleagues are caring, fun and committed to doing a good job. Clients are enthusiastic and enjoy their treatments, coming back again and again until they become firm friends. In surveys, beauty therapy always comes out as being one of the happiest jobs to be in and no wonder. I would not change what I have done and I always encourage people to train as beauty therapists and join our dynamic, busy and growing industry.

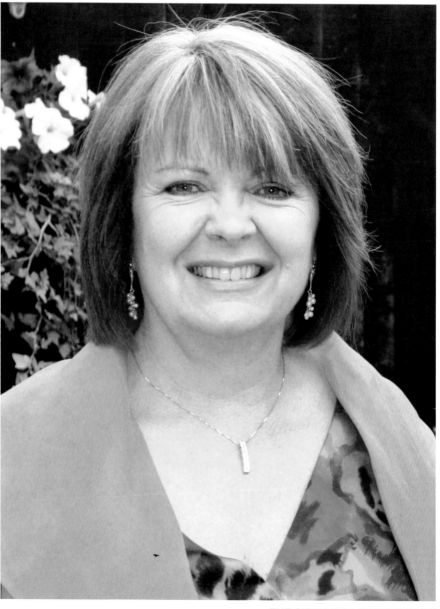

PROMOTE PRODUCTS AND SERVICES/ DISPLAY STOCK

It is important that you have the skills that salons and clients want. Salons are offering an increased range of treatments, services and retail products to provide more choice and to increase profit margins. Being able to promote your salon's services and products effectively enhances business. It is vital that you are aware of the latest services and product ranges and understand how these could benefit both your clients and the salon. If you are successful you will benefit from this knowledge with higher earnings.

In this chapter you will learn how to:

- promote products and services to the client
- prepare the display area
- maintain and dismantle the display area.

Competition between salons is tough. Clients will choose a salon that offers the best value for money, a range of services and excellent customer care. Your salon must be competitive. It must hold onto its existing business as well as encourage new trade. Eye-catching, exciting and enticing display showcases are one of the main ways to increase a salon's retail sales. It is vital that your salon's display of stock is attractively and artistically exhibited.

These chapters will be used in conjunction with other chapters to make sure professional practice and health and safety requirements are followed and that the wellbeing of yourself and your clients is maintained.

HANDY HINTS

You need to review and develop your basic communication skills. Refer back to Chapter 203, pages 166–176.

 SmartScreen 205 Worksheet 1

INDUSTRY TIP

It is important that your appearance and personal presentation reflect the image of the salon. You must always dress professionally and maintain your personal hygiene. Review Chapter 201 for further information – see page 132.

PROMOTE PRODUCTS AND SERVICES TO THE CLIENT

The keys to successful selling are a confident knowledge of what you are selling and good communication skills.

In this part of the chapter you will learn about:

- communication skills
- knowledge of products and services
- features and benefits
- principles of selling
- stages of the sales process
- methods of payment
- principles of finance
- principles of marketing and publicity
- promotions.

Communication is a two-way process involving speaking *and* listening. Listening carefully is very important.

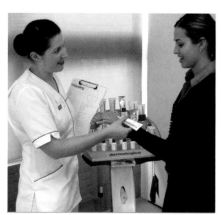

Touch, feel and smell essential retail products

SmartScreen 201 Worksheet 5

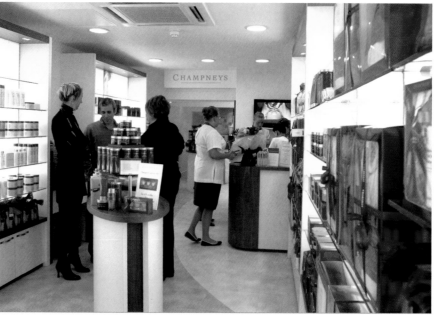

An attractive retail area will draw clients in

COMMUNICATION SKILLS

You should acknowledge a client within 30 seconds of them walking into the reception or retail area of your salon. Something as simple as 'hello' with a smile and direct eye contact is all that is needed. You might not necessarily be able to respond to them if you are dealing with another client or if you are on the phone but it shows the client that they are important to you and that you are aware they are present.

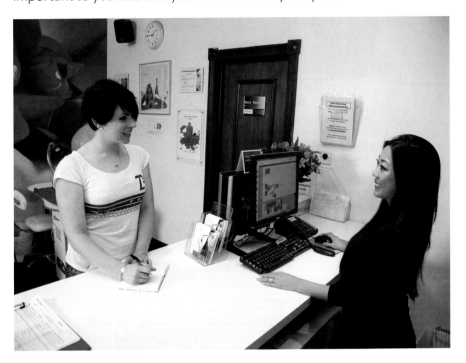

INDUSTRY TIP

People buy people first! If the client likes and trusts you they will be more likely to buy from you.

INDUSTRY TIP

Making recommendations and selling products and treatment is part of good customer service; selling the wrong product or service or trying to force a sale is poor service and likely to result in a lost client.

INDUSTRY TIP

Try to spot opportunities throughout your working day when you can naturally promote additional services. For example, if you are shaping a client's eyebrows, would the client benefit from an eyebrow tint? If a client comments that her skin is dry, match her need and recommend a hydrating facial or a suitable moisturiser.

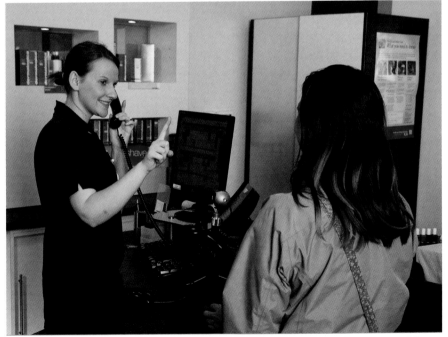

If you are on the phone, make eye contact with the client, smile and signal that you will be with them shortly

Remember, the client has walked into your business because they are interested in something you have. This might be a product, treatment or a voucher. Adopt a positive mental attitude; if you are cheerful, upbeat and positive about what you are doing, the client is more likely to buy from you. A therapist who is negative and miserable will put off a client.

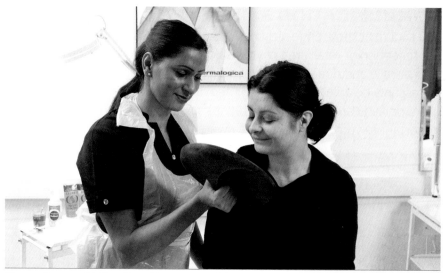

Always discuss with the client thier treatment objectives

VERBAL COMMUNICATION

Use of language

When you communicate with clients and make suggestions for buying products or for trying a new service or treatment, your use of language is very important. Always make sure you use non-technical words. Give your clients clear, accurate advice about the benefits of trying new products, services or treatments. Do not forget to advise clients of the benefits of repeating a service or treatment on a regular basis so that they get maximum results. Also follow up a product that a client has used before so that you can encourage and promote regular sales.

Tone of voice

Your tone of voice should be soft and confident. Do not shout. Be careful not to come across as demanding or intimidating. Have a calm, assertive voice and deliver clear, accurate and relevant facts for your client to make an informed decision.

Open and closed questioning techniques

When you are discussing new services, treatments or products with your clients, you need to give them as much accurate information as they need to make an informed decision. Open questions start with 'why?', 'what?', 'when?' and 'how?'. Use open questions first to get lots of information from your client about their requirements. Closed questions have 'yes' or 'no' answers. Use closed questions to confirm your client's agreement.

Examples of open questions

- What moisturiser do you currently use on your face?
- How do you find the product works for you?
- Why did you choose these products?

Examples of closed questions

- Would you like to purchase the hydra-flora nectar de fleur moisturiser that we discussed today?
- Shall I book you in for a super-**hydrating** facial for your next appointment?

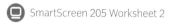 SmartScreen 205 Worksheet 2

Hydrating
To increase moisture.

ACTIVITY

Look at the questions below. Which are open questions? Which are closed questions?

- When was your last manicure?
- How do you get on with your current cleansing product?
- If you use this nourishing cream on your cuticles before you go to bed at night you will find it helps to soften and maintain the condition of your cuticles. Would you like to purchase one today?
- Would you like to buy the advanced serum that we discussed as well?

NON-VERBAL COMMUNICATION

Listening techniques

Non-verbal communication includes your listening skills. You must listen carefully to what your client says. Repeat back to the client what has been discussed and nod regularly so your client knows you are paying attention and considering their requests.

Body language and facial expressions

Your facial expressions and body language give away a lot of information. You need to use positive body language and avoid the tell-tale signs of negative body language. This works both ways – watching your client's body language will tell you how your client is feeling and whether or not they are interested in the services and products you are suggesting.

> **HANDY HINTS**
>
> Look at Chapter 203 for more information on non-verbal communication.

 SmartScreen 203 Worksheet 1

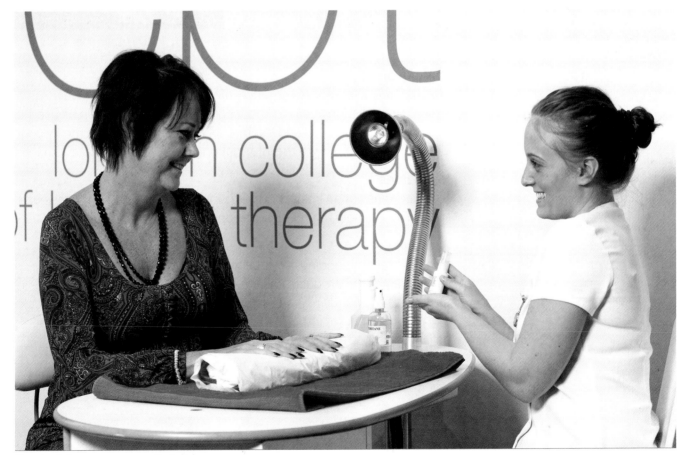

Keep body language open and relaxed

VISUAL AIDS

Visual aids are items you can use to help get information across to clients more clearly.

Colour charts

You can use a nail colour chart prior to a manicure or pedicure to help clarify the colour choices, or make-up charts prior to a make-up application to show the range of colours available.

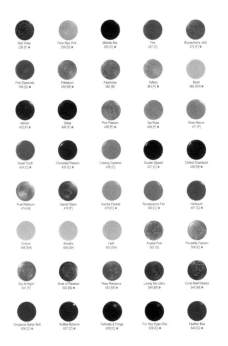

Colour charts show clients your available colours for nails

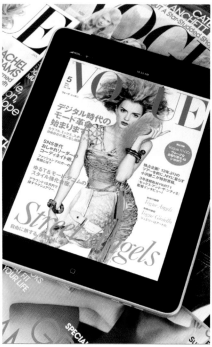

Use magazines for inspiration

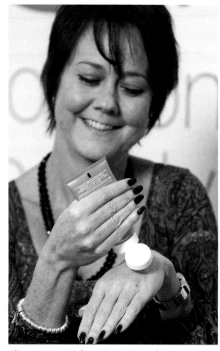

Clients may wish to try out products

Leaflets and flyers

Manufacturers sometimes produce information leaflets that give detailed information about a product or treatment. These can be used to support your services and treatments and can be taken home by your client so they can refer to the information later.

Magazines

Use magazines or an image portfolio when you are discussing make-up ideas. This will help to provide ideas and inspiration.

Packaging

If you are recommending any retail products, let your client see, hold, feel and smell the products you are suggesting. Manufacturers spend thousands of pounds researching what attracts clients to the visual look of a product's packaging. Showing the client the actual product might help you to close a sale.

Testers

Use make-up testers for colour matching and discussing colour themes.

WHY DON'T YOU...

put together a collection of looks for different events – for example, a bridal day, a prom or a wedding. Include different face shapes and colour themes. Put your collection into a presentation folder. Show your folder to your clients to give them ideas. This will show your clients you are thinking about different options and are open to both traditional looks and fashion trends.

INDUSTRY TIP

Even if there is a record of previously purchased services or products, do not assume your client will not be interested in new ideas. It could be that they are waiting for someone like you to make a suggestion.

RECORD CARDS

The client's record card can be a very useful visual prompt. It will give you a comprehensive record of the client's history and the services that they have had before and might want to have again. The record card might also indicate a particular service that was not viewed positively. You might be able to see a record of the client's purchases to indicate whether your client might be interested in purchasing products.

KNOWLEDGE OF PRODUCTS AND SERVICES

You will need a thorough knowledge about the full range of services and retail products available in your salon in order to promote them effectively to your clients. Although you might not personally be able to offer every treatment that the salon offers, you might need to advise your client about other available treatments. It is your responsibility to know which staff members carry out which services and when they are available. Armed with this information you will be able to offer the best service and make future recommendations to your clients. You do not want your client to come into the salon just once, you want them to return regularly.

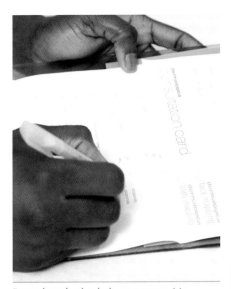

Record cards also help as a prompt to remind you which questions to ask

ACTIVITY

From memory, make a list of all the treatments and services your salon offers. Now make a list of all the types of products you think your salon sells (eg cleansers and toners). Check your answers with your salon manager.

ACTIVITY

Find out whether any therapists or technicians in your salon offer specialist treatments or services, and ask them to show you how to do them.

INDUSTRY TIP

Your continuing professional development (CPD) should include training on new or forthcoming products. It is important that you are up to date in your knowledge of salon services offered. In Chapter 201, page 126 you will find further information about CPD.

USING PRODUCTS AND SERVICES THAT ARE NEW TO THE CLIENT

To be able to sell and recommend additional or new services and products, you need to know what is available and how your clients can benefit from them. It is important that you have good product and service knowledge to make sure:

- the client gets maximum benefits from purchasing your recommendations
- you give accurate advice and information
- you effectively promote the products and services the salon offers
- you follow the Sale of Goods Act and the Trade Descriptions Act.

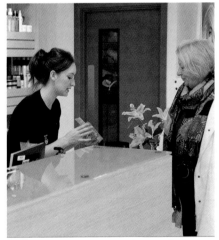

Always give clients instructions on how to use products

INDUSTRY TIP

Keep a record of when your client purchased a product and put a rough date as to when they will need to replace it. You can then prompt them to replace their products at the appropriate time. You will also be able to check they are using the product correctly and confirm the benefits of using the product regularly. This will demonstrate good client care as your client will know you are thinking about their needs and following up your recommendations.

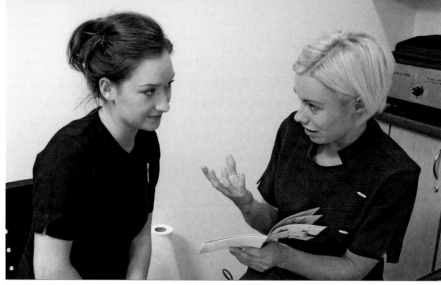

It is important to have excellent product knowledge

Profit

The amount of money made from the sale of a treatment, product or service after the costs of carrying out the treatment or service or the costs of buying the product have been taken away.

Turnover

The money that a business takes from products, services and treatments over a set period of time before the costs of carrying out the treatment or service or the costs of buying the product have been taken away.

Personal targets

Goals given to individuals for them to work towards and hopefully achieve.

Reputation

The opinion that people have about a person or business.

Professional

The standard of work by, or presentation of, someone who is working in a particular profession.

Image

The public face of a person or business.

Stability

To be steady.

Benefits of promoting products and services to you and the salon

The diagram below shows how promoting products will benefit both you and your salon.

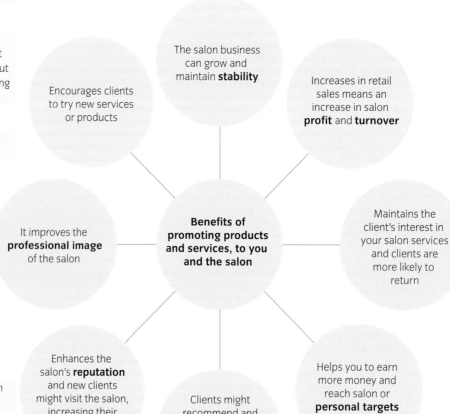

SERVICES AND PRODUCTS AVAILABLE IN YOUR SALON

Services available in your salon

To identify which services are available in your salon, a good place to start is the salon price list or menu. The price list will contain all the services and treatments available and how much they cost. Try to learn the salon treatment prices off by heart and always keep a copy of the price list to hand. You should be able to remember and think of reasons why your clients would benefit from these services or treatments.

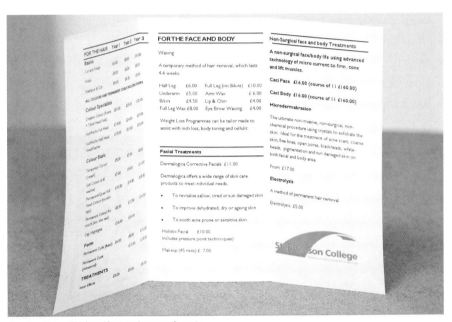

A price list will identify services and costs

> **INDUSTRY TIP**
>
> Keep your own personal copy of the salon price list and make notes on it. You can write notes, such as treatment timings and, if certain therapists offer specialist treatments, until you know these off by heart.

> **INDUSTRY TIP**
>
> If you are unfamiliar with any of the services offered in your salon, ask a colleague or your manager to explain them to you or ask to observe a treatment taking place – better still would be to experience the treatment yourself.

Products available in your salon

You should also look at the retail product price list and make sure you are familiar with all the products available to your clients and their costs. Make sure you are up to date and aware of all the skin care, nail care and make-up ranges and treatments available for each skin type and condition.

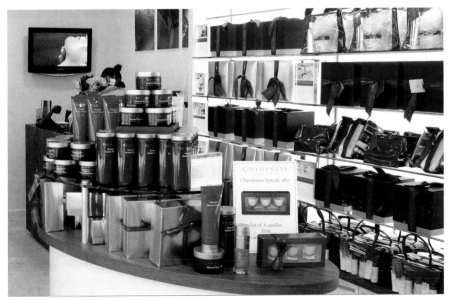

Retail areas should be well-stocked

Features

The things that identify a particular product (eg the ingredients within the product).

Benefit

An advantage of a product, service or treatment.

Characteristics

Qualities or features of a product, service or treatment.

WHY DON'T YOU...

list the products in your salon that you are not familiar with and ask for some product knowledge training on them.

INDUSTRY TIP

Use your salon's products so that you are familiar with their application and texture. Products sell better if you are able to recommend them personally.

INDUSTRY TIP

If your salon will allow you to, take a tester home occasionally and use a product that you might not normally use – this will help to improve your product knowledge.

FEATURES AND BENEFITS (FABS)

Encouraging your clients to buy retail products and to try new services will be beneficial to you, the salon and, most importantly, to your client. When you promote your salon's services and products, you should be able to explain the **features** and the **benefits**.

FEATURES

A feature is either a description of a product or treatment (eg the texture of a cream) or a **characteristic** of the product or treatment (eg it has a pump dispenser or a special, active ingredient). Features include:

- what it does
- how long it will last
- how to use it
- how much it costs
- what ingredients it contains.

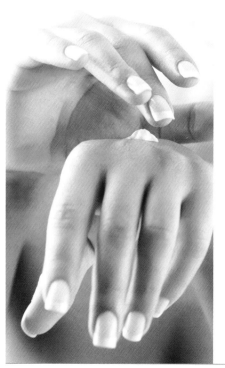
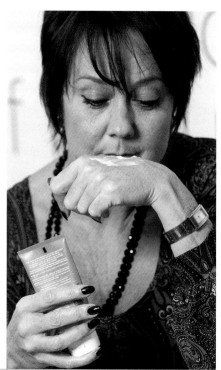

Clients should be able to touch and smell products

BENEFITS

The benefits are the advantages to your client of using the product or having the treatment. For example, the product or treatment:

- gives the skin a healthy glow
- is anti-ageing
- will improve the condition of the skin
- defines the eye shape
- gently shapes the nail
- softens and conditions cuticles.

The benefit is the most important point. You will need to personalise the benefits for each client. If the client is having a service or treatment, you must find out during your consultation what their needs are. If the client is just interested in products, you need to ask them appropriate questions and then tailor your product suggestions specifically to their needs. You can then promote the product by explaining how it is of value to them.

ACTIVITY

Write a list of features and benefits for each of the following products:

- cream blusher
- red nail polish
- cuticle oil
- eye make-up remover
- after-wax oil.

Now find an example of each product from your salon's range. Write down the features and benefits for each item. How does the information compare?

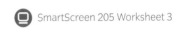 SmartScreen 205 Worksheet 3

FEATURES AND BENEFITS OF SOME COMMON PRODUCTS AND SERVICES

Look at the table below for the features and benefits of some common products and services. Remember that the products you use will have different features and benefits – these are only to give you ideas about the information you can look for.

Service/product	Features	Benefits
Cleansing milk	■ A light, silky cleanser to gently cleanse the skin. ■ It has a pump dispenser. ■ This will last about 3 months if you use it twice a day.	■ The pump dispenser gives you just the required amount of cleanser. ■ It gently cleanses all impurities. ■ It removes make-up. ■ Lavender is soothing.
Alcohol-free toner	■ A gentle toner for all skin types. ■ It comes with a flip cap. ■ It has a light aroma.	■ It has a flip cap that allows easy pouring and avoids spillage. ■ It refreshes the skin. ■ It revives the skin. ■ It removes all traces of leftover cleanser. ■ It allows the acid mantle to breathe. ■ It balances pH levels.

Service/product	Features	Benefits
Moisturising cream	■ A light but rich cream to hydrate all skin types. ■ It is available in a 50 ml or 40 ml tub. ■ It comes with a small dispensing spatula so that you only take an economical amount of product. ■ It will last approximately 4 months.	■ It instantly hydrates the skin. ■ It leaves skin feeling supple and soft. ■ It protects the skin and complexion from pollution. ■ It moisturises and promotes water circulation in the skin.
A one-hour luxury facial	■ Each facial uses professionally-selected products to fulfil the needs of a demanding skin. ■ Concentrated ingredients deep cleanse and hydrate the complexion. ■ A one-hour relaxing treatment with effective results.	■ It deep cleanses the skin to remove impurities and leave the skin soft and glowing. ■ It envelopes the skin in a range of products suitable for the skin type and condition to achieve maximum results. ■ Massage relaxes the muscles and creates a feeling of wellbeing. ■ It increases the circulation giving the skin a healthy glow.

INDUSTRY TIP

Whenever you recommend something, always recommend it positively, eg 'I have a *fantastic* cream to treat your congested skin' or 'I have the *perfect* moisturiser for you'.

BENEFITS OF PROMOTING PRODUCTS, SERVICES AND TREATMENTS TO CLIENTS

The following diagram shows the benefits of promoting products and services to your clients.

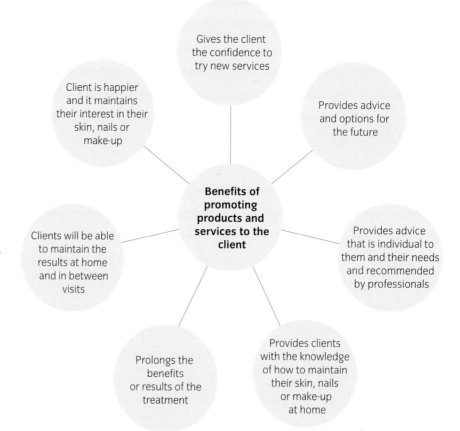

Gives the client the confidence to try new services

Client is happier and it maintains their interest in their skin, nails or make-up

Provides advice and options for the future

Benefits of promoting products and services to the client

Clients will be able to maintain the results at home and in between visits

Provides advice that is individual to them and their needs and recommended by professionals

Prolongs the benefits or results of the treatment

Provides clients with the knowledge of how to maintain their skin, nails or make-up at home

ACTIVITY

Look at your salon's services or treatment menu. Write one feature and one benefit for each service. Make a note of any services you are not sure about and discuss these with a colleague or your salon manager.

ACTIVITY

- Andrea has a newborn baby and has very little time to spend on her nails. Her nails have been poor since having the baby but she likes her nails to look groomed. Which services and products would you recommend to her and why?
- Angela is a new client and has stated that her main concern is her congested skin. Her skin is very irritated. Which services and products would you recommend to her and why?
- Hannah has her school prom coming up in 2 months' time. Her parents have given her a salon voucher for £150. Which services and products would you recommend to her and why?

PRINCIPLES OF SELLING

Selling is not just about selling products but also about giving customer service and selling additional or further treatments. Many therapists and nail technicians feel uncomfortable selling a product but have no problem selling a treatment. This is because they know the treatment inside out but not the products they use. Selling is a process and while they might not come naturally, selling skills can be acquired. Having a team that can sell confidently will make a big difference to a salon's profits.

UP-SELLING

Up-selling can be applied to treatments, services or products. When you up-sell you are recommending a product or service that isn't directly linked to a client's needs or expectations but that will enhance their salon experience. Up-selling increases a salon's profits and offers clients alternatives. Clients are often unaware of alternative or additional treatments or products that might suit them and this is a good way to introduce them. Always give them the benefits of the different or additional product or services and tell them how much extra it will cost. Remember, up-selling is not just about increasing profits and meeting targets, it is also about client care.

INDUSTRY TIP

Remember these tips for successful selling:

- have good communication skills
- listen to what your client wants and needs
- explain the product or treatment in clear, simple terms
- avoid jargon
- use open and friendly non-verbal communication
- build a rapport – get chatting with the client
- be enthusiastic – you must believe in what you are trying to sell
- have a positive mental attitude (PMA)
- believe in yourself
- avoid hard selling.

ACTIVITY

Think of other examples where you could up-sell and try putting them into practice.

WHY DON'T YOU...

make a list of your salon's retail products. Write one feature and one benefit for each of them.

 SmartScreen 205 Worksheet 4 and Worksheet 5

INDUSTRY TIP

Always use positive words when selling the benefits of something:

'what I can do is …'

'me'

'I'

'we'

'yes'

'successful'

'now'

'recommended'

'you can be confident that …'

'immediately'

'results'

'money-saving'

'time-saving'

'easy'

'new'

'safe'

'proven'

'I will'

'I can'

'immediate'

'it is quicker for you …'

'powerful'

'I am positive that …'

'thank you!'

INDUSTRY TIP

An example of up-selling might be if a client came in for anti-ageing moisturiser and you told her about an SPF and a new moisturiser that is both anti-ageing and contains SPF.

INDUSTRY TIP

If you have a client booked but have some free time after the treatment, invite the client to upgrade their treatment – this is called up-selling.

HARD SELLING

We have all experienced hard selling. It makes us feel uncomfortable and puts us under pressure. Hard selling is when someone is pushy and does not consider the client's needs; they just want to make the sale or reach their target. We all hate having a superb treatment only to be pressurised into buying a product before we leave. This is off-putting and might make the client reluctant to return. If the client says 'no' or is not interested, you must accept this and not keep pushing them to buy something.

ACTIVITY

Discuss with a colleague occasions when you have experienced a hard sell. How did it make you feel? What was the outcome? Did you make a purchase? What was the reason for your decision?

STAGES OF THE SALES PROCESS

The diagram below shows the stages of the sales process.

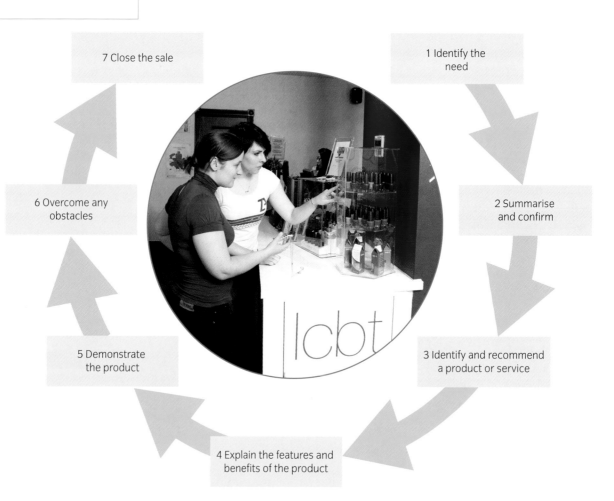

7 Close the sale

1 Identify the need

6 Overcome any obstacles

2 Summarise and confirm

5 Demonstrate the product

3 Identify and recommend a product or service

4 Explain the features and benefits of the product

IDENTIFYING THE NEED

Think:

- Am I asking the right questions?
- What do I need to know?

To sell well, you need to understand what the client sees as a priority. It is not necessarily what you think their priority or need is. Try to engage your client and let them do the talking.

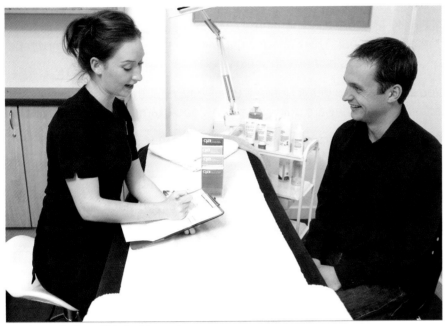

Good consultation will indentify need

If you ask a client whether they follow a skin care routine, they might say 'yes' but this will neither tell you whether they are using the right products, nor whether they are using them correctly or regularly. It is better to ask direct, targeted questions so you can recommend the products you know will benefit them.

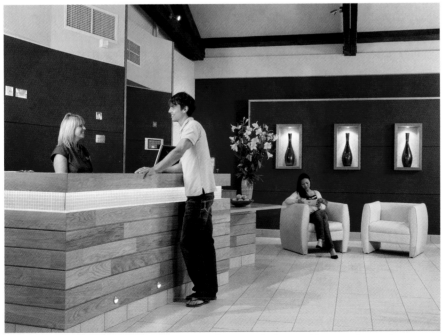

Receptionists also need to be aware of identifying need when making appointments

Using open questions

Remember to use open questions to get your client talking.

- First, you need to find out why they are in the salon and what they want their treatment to achieve. You need to find out what their main concern is. Ask: 'What is your number one priority from your treatment today?'
- Next, you need to find out why they have that concern. For example, if they are concerned about dry skin, say: 'Why do you think your skin is dry?'
- Finally, ask your client what they would like you to focus on during their treatment. Think about what will benefit your client the most and give them results they can see or feel.

You should aim to get your client to tell you what their problem is and admit to what they are doing wrong. A good example is:

Therapist:	'What is your main priority from your facial today?'
Client:	'My skin is very spotty.'
Therapist:	'Why do you think your skin is spotty?'
Client:	'I'm not sure I am using the best products for my skin. I use facial cleansing wipes as they are quick and easy.'

At this point you can match a treatment or product to meet your client's priorities and needs. They have admitted they have a problem rather than being told they have one.

Below is a poor example where the therapist tells the client what the problem is:

| Therapist: | 'Your skin is very spotty, it must be the facial wipes you use – they are cheap and nasty.' |

How would you feel if a therapist said this to you? Defensive? Upset?

Talk to your client before, during (if appropriate) and especially after a treatment. During a treatment explain to your client what you are doing, what you are using and why – even if they have been in for the same treatment before. A manicure or pedicure is approximately one hour of quality time to offer advice and to **educate** your client into good habits. There is no need to give them a running commentary – just summarise what you are going to do and why.

INDUSTRY TIP

Some treatments (eg a massage) are meant to be relaxing and your client might feel annoyed if you keep talking to them.

Educate

Teach.

INDUSTRY TIP

Familiarity can become a problem with regular clients. Do not forget the importance of discussing the treatment process rather than personal topics. Remember, people love to talk about themselves; it is the client's time and they are paying you. The conversation should focus on your client, not you!

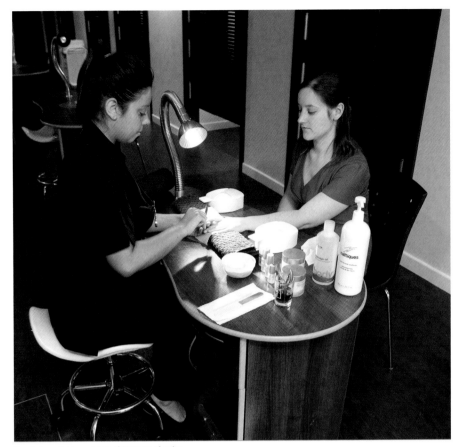
Explain what you are doing and why

SUMMARISING AND CONFIRMING

Before continuing, summarise and confirm what your client has said. Keep the information brief and simply highlight the important points without elaborating.

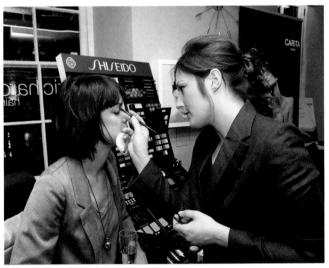

Summarise and confirm to check understanding

Talk to the client to explain your technique

By summarising and confirming what has been said, you will show you are interested and, more importantly, have been listening. Look for confirmation from the client that what you have said is correct – this might be a nod or a 'yes'. Then check using a closed question, such as: 'Is that right?'.

INDUSTRY TIP

Remember: people do not buy a thing, they buy the benefits of a thing!

INDUSTRY TIP

Avoid using a sales pitch that sounds as if it has been learnt from a sheet or that sounds as if the same information is given to every client.

INDUSTRY TIP

If your salon is on a high street, there is always potential for clients to walk in and look for products and treatments – be prepared.

INDUSTRY TIP

If your client would like to commit to a service that you personally do not offer, invite the relevant salon team member to join your discussion to offer further advice and guidance. Let the person responsible for the service take over the conversation and book the client for the relevant service.

Tactile

To touch and feel.

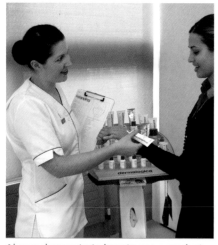

Always demonstrate how to use a product

IDENTIFYING AND RECOMMENDING A PRODUCT OR SERVICE

When you have all the necessary details from the client and have confirmed that you have understood them correctly by summarising and confirming, you should be able to confidently recommend products and treatments that will suit your client's needs. This is why it is essential to know your treatments and products inside out.

EXPLAINING THE FEATURES AND BENEFITS OF THE PRODUCT OR SERVICE

Now you have consulted with the client and established their needs, you need to match their needs to the benefits of the products and treatments you are going to recommend. Do not sell on price, sell on benefit. You *do not* know how much the client can afford. For example:

Therapist:	'What is your main priority from your facial today?'
Client:	'My skin is very spotty.'
Therapist:	'Why do you think your skin is spotty?'
Client:	'I'm not sure I am using the best products for my skin, I use facial cleansing wipes as they are quick and easy.'
Therapist:	'So your main priority is that your skin is spotty which might be because you are not using the best products for your skin. We will work on this during your facial treatment and I can make some recommendations to you to help improve the spotty skin.'

DEMONSTRATING THE PRODUCT

If you are selling a product rather than a service or treatment, it is now time to demonstrate the product. Remember to involve the client in the process as the **tactile** part of selling is important. Let the client hold the product so that they already feel they own it. Let them look at the product. Talk about the product and how to use it and give your client instructions about the product. Use 'you' when you give your instructions and recommendations (eg: 'You use this twice a day, about a pea size amount, to make your skin feel silky smooth.'). After a few minutes, take the product back. Psychologically, your client has taken hold of something to own it and now you have taken it away. This encourages a feeling of wanting the product.

INDUSTRY TIP

Link-selling means selling more than one product from a range. They are usually products that complement each other. It could be that the product 'links' to the clients' needs expressed during a treatment or there are two products that 'link' together (eg a cleanser and toner, a base coat and red nail varnish or an eyebrow pencil and eyebrow brush).

INDUSTRY TIP

Often manufacturers select suitable products and put them together in a bonus set to help promote products. This helps to link-sell items.

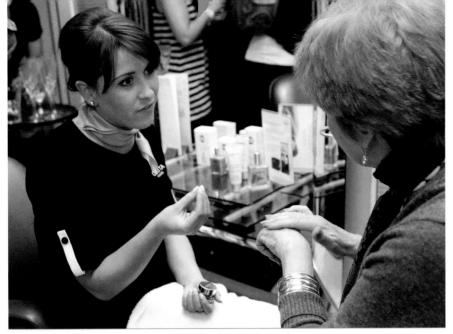
Explaining the benefits to a client can make them interested

OVERCOMING OBSTACLES

It is likely that some clients will be unsure about suggestions you make; be prepared for this and have an answer ready. If you know your products really well you can match products to your clients' needs perfectly. Be positive when a client is unsure; it shows the client you are paying attention. You are aiming to hear the client say 'yes'. If the client says 'no' or they are not interested you must accept this. The client might not purchase today but they might go home and think about the benefits and purchase the product or book the treatment next time they come to the salon.

Obstacles
Something which is in your way and is making it difficult to achieve something.

ACTIVITY

You and your colleagues should regularly test each other on your product knowledge. You can share information if one of you has used a product or had a particular treatment and the other has not.

Objections

Try to find out what the client is thinking and why have they raised an objection. If it is a real objection, you can then address their concern. It is a good idea to think about this and some possible responses you can give. Common objections include:

- I cannot afford it.
- I am not convinced it will work.
- I have not budgeted for this.
- I have been using facial wipes for years, why should I change?
- I would like to compare the price with another range.
- I want to think about it.

You can show you agree with your client's thoughts and reasoning without agreeing with their actual objection, eg: 'I used to think the same but since I have been using the cleanser I have discovered...' or 'Some of our clients thought that too but once they'd had the treatment they thought the results were brilliant'.

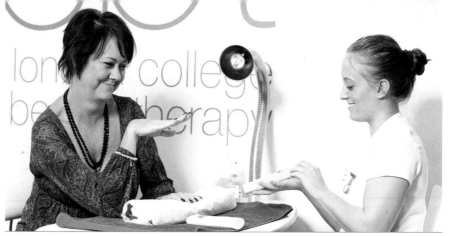
If a client says 'no' firmly, then accept it

In order to gain your client's commitment to using additional services or purchasing products, you will need to identify any factors that might influence their decision. These factors could be:

- uncertainty due to lack of knowledge
- the cost of the services or products
- the manufacturer's advice
- past experience
- advertising material.

Uncertainty due to lack of knowledge

If your client is unsure about whether to commit to the service or products you are advising, then you will need to find out the reason why. Make sure that your client has a thorough understanding of why they would benefit from the products or from having a regular service or treatment. Make sure you give clear and accurate information and always give your client guidance on how to use products and maintain services to give them the confidence to commit to them.

The cost of the services or products

Always make sure you give the exact price to the client and explain any offers that are available. Your client will want to know what the cost will be when the special offer ends if they want to continue using the product or having the service. Never assume that your client can or cannot afford the service or product; let them make the decision.

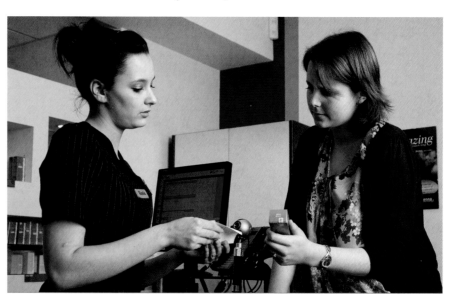
Clients should always be clear how much products cost

Manufacturer's advice

Always encourage your clients to read the product labels and the manufacturer's instructions. Your clients might want to read the ingredients if they have any allergies or they might decline purchasing the products if they have been tested on animals, contain animal products or certain ingredients, such as **parabens**. Always make sure that you follow the manufacturer's instructions and check for contra-indications or medical reasons as to why your client should or should not commit to certain services or products.

Past experience

If a client has previously used the services you are suggesting, make sure you ask why they stopped using them; was it for financial reasons or were they disappointed with the results? Of course, it might be that your client just wanted a change. When you know their reasons you will be able to offer suitable advice about how, or why, things might be different this time.

Parabens

A chemical used in products to act as a preservative. It is now common for products to state whether they are paraben free as they are chemicals that should be avoided.

ACTIVITY

Which of the above objections could you easily overcome and which would be difficult? Write down some reasons why you feel like that.

INDUSTRY TIP

If it is a regular client, plant the seed of suggestion. If you talk about a product or treatment in casual conversation, your client will take the idea or suggestion away and think about it. It is amazing how regular clients will remember and come back to book a treatment you have suggested or a product you have recommend. You also have an opportunity to follow up your recommendations, to remind clients and to get them to think about your advice further.

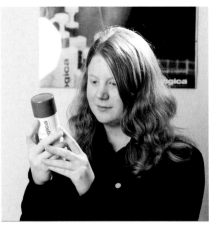

Ingredients should be clearly labelled

Advertising material

Most companies will market their products to promote them and this will include promotional flyers and posters. These can be used to support the information that you are giving a client and to give more scientific facts and detail. You should use these if you have access to them as they make excellent visual aids and are a good source of information for the client to take away should they be unsure.

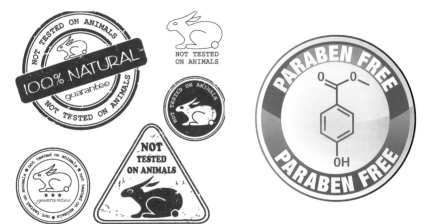

Examples of facts found on products

INDUSTRY TIP

Make sure you keep copies of any articles that feature your products. If you see them in a magazine highlight or circle them so that the client is drawn to the article if they pick the magazine up.

INDUSTRY TIP

If the client is concerned about price or commitment or if a product will suit their skin, offer them a sample to try.

CLOSING THE SALE

There are many ways to close a sale. Closing the sale is simply asking the client to make the sale or book the appointment (eg: 'Would you like to take one of the cleansers I have recommended?' or 'Would you like to book an eye treatment with your next facial?').

However, there is a difference between closing the sale and helping someone make a decision. When your client shows that they are ready to proceed – this might be by displaying positive buying signals or indicating their satisfaction – it is time to close the sale. Most therapists fail to close the sale due to a fear of being rejected or hearing the word 'no'. Remember, it is only a word and it is not personal.

ACTIVITY

A client is saying 'no' to you firmly. Write down what you would say to the client and discuss your responses with your manager. How do you want the client to feel when they leave?

Signals to look for that a sale is possible

The following are examples of signals a client might use to show they are interested in what you are saying. If you handle it well, these are opportunities that should lead to a retail sale or treatment booking. The client:

- asks about what you are using and wants more information
- comments they like the smell or feel of a product
- sees the benefit of a product during use (eg lotion after wax, exfoliant during self-tanning)
- asks for a sample
- picks up products for a closer look
- studies leaflets
- asks 'How much?'
- agrees positively with the recommendations you have given
- has relaxed body language (ie smiling, good eye contact)
- asks to try the product.

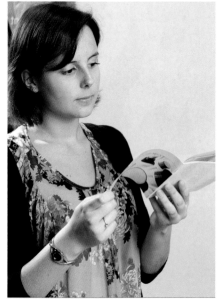

Flyers are useful for clients to take away information or instructions

INDUSTRY TIP

Avoid mentioning money in 'pounds'. If an item costs £16.90 say: 'This is sixteen ninety'. It still has a value but not a monetary one. Without mentioning the word pounds, we create a different association. The emphasis is now on the item, not how much it costs.

INDUSTRY TIP

Do not defend the price of your products and treatments, sell the benefits.

INDUSTRY TIP

If you have paid for something you value it and will be more likely to appreciate and look after it than something you have been given for free.

Closing the sale

Smile, maintain eye contact, then ask for the sale and stay silent. The silent pause is uncomfortable for many but it lets your client think and respond. Do not start talking again – your client needs to speak first. The longer the silence the more likely the sale! Some examples of questions to close the sale are:

- Would you like to take the small or large size?
- Would you like to book the standard manicure or the deluxe manicure?
- Would you like to pay by cash or card?
- Would you like to take the cleanser and toner?

INDUSTRY TIP

If you are giving your client two options, always put the option you want to sell (the better or bigger option) second. Try it!

INDUSTRY TIP

Be wary of clients who just want samples. Make a note on the record cards of all samples you give and do not give clients the same sample again. If they were going to buy it, they would have bought it!

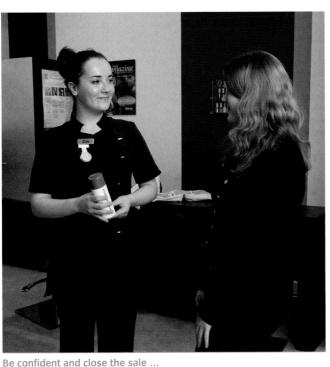
Be confident and close the sale ...

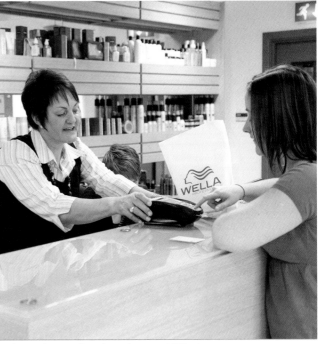
... then ask your client how they would like to pay

ACTIVITY

Many therapists find closing the sale the hardest part of the sales process. You will find it helpful to practise and to carry out role plays closing the sale. Carry out role plays of the following situations with a colleague:

- A client has had a make-up application for a special occasion and you have recommended that the client purchases a lipstick. How would you recommend the benefits and close the sale?
- A client is objecting to a moisturiser you have recommended as it is too expensive. What alternatives can you offer this client to work towards a sale?

HANDY HINTS

Make sure you review the legislation that relates to selling in the Legislation chapter.

INDUSTRY TIP

You must not tell lies! It is important that you are truthful with your client about the products and services, their features, benefits and costs. You might lose your client when they find out the truth, the salon might get a bad reputation and you could also face legal action under the Sale of Goods Act.

INDUSTRY TIP

Samples are given as promotional material by most companies depending on the amount of products you order. Some product companies charge for them.

METHODS OF PAYMENT

When you have successfully secured the sale, you will need to determine the method of payment your client wishes to use. Many salons will accept the following methods of payment.

CASH

Coins and notes from the Bank of England are **legal tender** for payment in the UK. Businesses might also accept Scottish and Northern Irish notes and coins and legal tender from Jersey and Guernsey. The notes usually need to be processed through a bank rather than passed onto another client.

DEBIT CARDS

When a client uses a debit card, the salon is paid within a day or two. The client's money leaves their bank account immediately and is transferred to the salon's account a couple of days later.

CREDIT CARDS

Credit card companies authorise payments to the salon and then request their client's payment at a later date – normally on a monthly basis.

CHEQUES

Cheques are used in place of cash. The client writes a cheque for the money and gives this to the business. The business then banks the cheques and the bank processes the payment from the client's account to the salon's account. Cheque guarantee cards are being withdrawn and cheques will gradually be used less and less.

VOUCHERS

Vouchers are normally purchased by a customer and given as gifts to others. The client with the voucher uses it as an alternative to cash.

PROCESSING THE SALE

When a sale has been closed or treatment has been completed, the sale needs to be processed. You salon might use a simple small cash tin or a complex computerised till.

Legal tender

Coins and notes that are legal to use as payment in the country in which they are being received.

HANDY HINTS

Unit 216, pages 252–258 will guide you through different methods of payment and how these should be processed.

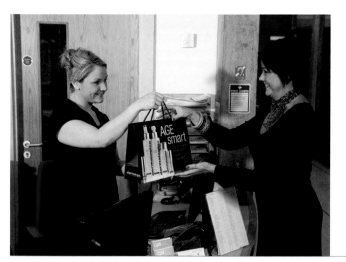
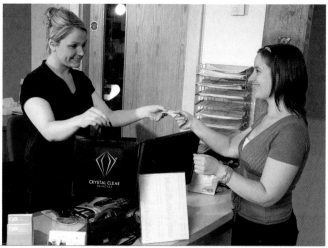

Complete your sale with a smile and a 'thank you'

PRINCIPLES OF FINANCE

For a salon to succeed it must be profitable. The charge for treatments, services and products must be calculated carefully. If this is not worked out to give the correct **profit margins**, the treatment or sale could make the salon a loss.

The owner or manager of the salon should know:

- how much each treatment or product brings into the business. Is the treatment popular or booked rarely? Does the product sell well or get discarded due to lack of interest?
- how much profit there is on each treatment
- how much each treatment costs to carry out, ie the cost in products and consumables used and staff wages.

Profit margin

The total amount of profit divided by the amount of sales. The profit margin is shown as a percentage.

WHY DON'T YOU...
practise your selling techniques on your colleagues.

HANDY HINTS

For further information on how to take payments and check for authenticity, refer to Chapter 216, Salon reception duties.

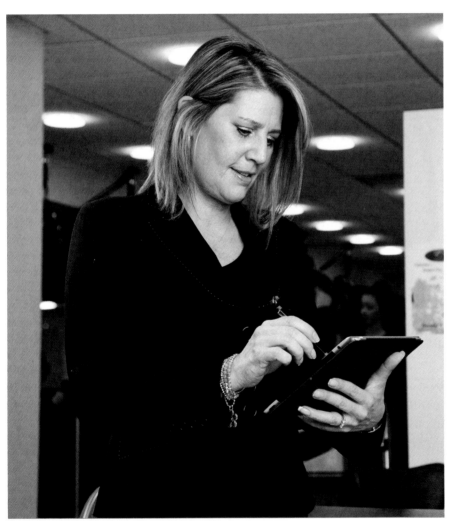

Keeping accounts up to date is very important

FIXED COSTS

These are costs that remain constant and change only slightly within the business. They do not change regardless of how many clients are treated or if the salon is open or closed. They include:

- wages
- **rent** or **mortgage**
- rates (taxes paid by the salon to the local council for local services)
- general overheads (eg gas, electric, refuse collection).

Rent

A regular amount of money paid to an owner in return for being able to use the building or equipment.

Mortgage

A loan from a bank or building society used to buy a property.

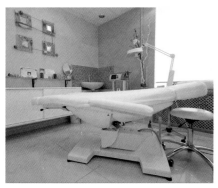

Equipping a treatment room can be expensive

Consumable items

Items that can only be used once, for example: cotton wool, couch roll, spatulas.

WHY DON'T YOU...
make a list of items used during a pedicure or facial treatment that are consumables.

A business should set aside money for its fixed costs and the easy way to do this is to calculate the costs and divide them into monthly payments to make sure this amount is put aside. A wise salon owner or manager would set up monthly direct debits to keep the costs manageable.

To work out the salon's costs and profit margins, the owner needs to work out how much the fixed costs are.

VARIABLE COSTS

These are costs that can vary depending on their use. These will include stock, retail products and **consumable items**.

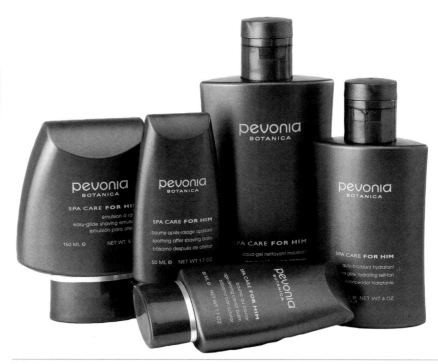

Retail products are examples of consumable items

NET AND GROSS

In business, there are two important terms that are used when looking at costs:

- **Gross** – an amount before costs have been taken into consideration. The amount a client pays for a treatment is gross.
- **Net** – the amount left after all deductions or costs have been taken away.

VALUE ADDED TAX (VAT)

Value Added Tax (VAT) is a government tax that is charged on most goods and services within the UK. Business with a turnover of £70,000 or more over 12 months have to register the business for VAT.

VAT is charged when a VAT registered business sells products or services to another business. When a VAT registered business buys goods or services they can claim back the VAT they have paid on products or services.

INDUSTRY TIP

It is important that special offers or discounts are agreed with the management before offering them to clients as you could be giving away the profit margin.

INDUSTRY TIP

Some wholesalers display their stock at the net price (ie without including the VAT). The extra cost of the VAT is added when you pay for the goods.

PRINCIPLES OF MARKETING AND PUBLICITY

Marketing is the use of various methods to get your business and its message across to potential or existing clients. It is also a way of generating good publicity and **public relations**. Marketing should be cost-effective and aim to make the business more profitable. Businesses should set a budget for marketing and publicity and include this in their annual expenditure. Without publicity how will clients know you exist?

Marketing tools include:

- advertising (eg in journals, magazines, newspapers)
- editorials (articles in magazines endorsing the business) and press releases (a piece of text that tells the customer about the benefits of a product or service)
- promotional events (eg open evenings, launches, taster sessions)
- commercial radio broadcasts
- emails, text messages
- direct mailing, direct marketing (advertisements that are posted to potential or existing clients at home)
- leaflets, flyers, **traffic stoppers**
- websites, social networking sites (eg Facebook).

None of these are guaranteed to work and it is important that you do some research and test the different methods to see what works best for your business.

Public relations
Establishing and maintaining goodwill between a business and its clients.

Traffic stopper
A leaflet that is given to passing customers (eg in a high street or shopping mall).

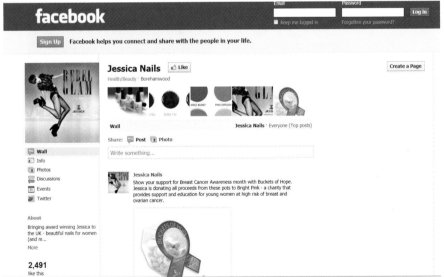

Social media can be an effective marketing tool if managed well

ACTIVITY

How do you think social networking sites (eg Facebook) could benefit a salon? What potential disadvantages might there be? Write down your ideas.

INDUSTRY TIP

A salon loses around 10 to 15 per cent of its regular clientele a year through relocation, staff changes and sadly death. Keep this in mind as businesses always need to grow to make up for this loss.

ADVERTISING

Advertising material can grab someone's attention and entice them to buy items they do not even need. Manufacturers spend thousands of pounds on advertising so always make sure you promote services and products professionally and creatively in your salon.

Generally speaking, manufacturers will provide salons with promotional advertising materials for their products. This makes sure that the advertising is accurate and uniform across all salons.

Advertising materials can take the form of:

- wall posters
- suspended window posters
- banner stands
- pop-up stands
- leaflets.

These should be displayed in key areas of the salon as well as near to the product display.

Alongside the manufacturers' advertising materials you could promote the stock in your salon with additional images or photos. Alternatively, you could use DVDs of the products' features and benefits played on a PC or flat-screen TV in the salon's waiting areas.

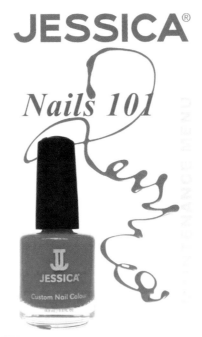

Advertising helps to make clients aware of products

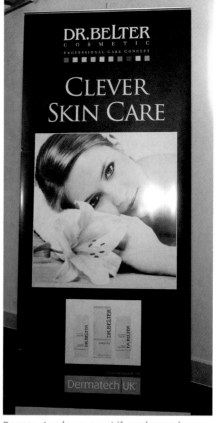

Banner stands are great if you have a large space to fill

Press advertising

Press advertising is used to increase awareness. Different types of print can be used depending on the market you are aiming to attract. You could use local newspapers or magazines, such as local directories. These often work if the advert is being included as part of a special promotional event (eg Valentine's Day or Mother's Day). During this type of promotion the reader is more likely to be drawn to the advert as they might be looking for ideas for the event.

Regular advertising will create familiarity but might not produce instant results and is best when used as part of a long-term marketing plan. Regular advertising is more competitive in cost than a single advert. Small regular advertisements will often be more productive by increasing recognition over a period of time rather than using one large advertisement.

Planning an advertisement

Plan your advertising around what the salon needs. Set up a plan so that you know what the salon is doing during the coming year and plan your promotions and offers around this.

Start by considering what you want to advertise. Do you want to raise the salon's profile, attract new clients or launch a new treatment or product?

Do lots of research and look at different types of advertising and their rates. Ask if there are any deals, such as booking a series of advertisements. Find out exactly where your advertisement will be placed within the publication as this will also affect the cost.

Use a voucher to see how successful the advertisement has been (eg a tear-off slip for the client to bring in when having the treatment). Keep a record of the number and date of slips returned so you can see over what period of time the slips are returned.

EDITORIALS AND PRESS RELEASES

An editorial is written by somebody important outside the business. It is someone else's word that the salon is great. Some editorials can be free and so are useful to include in any marketing strategy.

A press release is when you send a piece of news to the media. This news could be an announcement or piece of newsworthy information. The information could relate to a person, event, product, treatment or service. The article aims to generate interest and to raise public awareness of the business.

PROMOTIONAL EVENTS

These are specific events to promote a new treatment or product. They could be used to open a new business. These events can be used for publicity, such as a charity event, or in conjunction with other businesses, such as a bridal fair. The event might include taster sessions where the clients can try out new products or treatments and usually includes demonstrations and gifts or special offers to reward the clients for attending.

> **INDUSTRY TIP**
>
> Statistically the best place for an advert is in the bottom right-hand of the right-hand page.

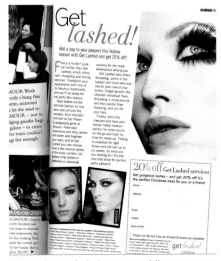

Press releases help increase public awareness

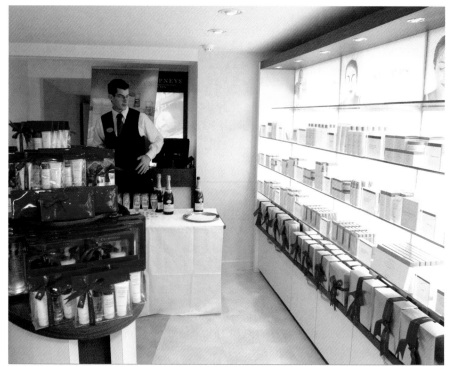

Promotional events are great social events for promoting new treatments and products

These events can be linked with newspaper editorials to raise the salon's profile.

COMMERCIAL RADIO

Radio advertising can be very powerful if done well. However, it can be costly. It aims at a **captive audience**. You can advertise on or sponsor commercial local radio. It can be a good tool for generating new business.

EMAIL

Email is an easy way to keep in touch with clients. Start by setting up an email contact list. Specific group contact lists can be made when all the main contacts have been entered. Groups with similar needs can be set up (eg clients who have had a particular treatment). When you send an email flyer or newsletter, all the contacts you have selected for that group will receive the email. You must enter the required group contact in the Bcc box (*not* the To box) as clients' email addresses are confidential and therefore must not be seen by other recipients.

DIRECT MARKETING OR DIRECT MAIL

Direct marketing means sending promotional mail directly to existing or prospective clients. A successful mail shot should bring around a one to two per cent return (this means one to two per cent of the total profit is won by a successful campaign). This might not seem much but consider how much this worth over the year. A client's average spend is around £350 a year so two new regular clients will bring the salon a £750 increase in **annual revenue**.

Captive audience

A group of people who are already gathered for another purpose. They are then exposed to information that they are not specifically gathered to hear.

Annual revenue

The money the business makes in a year.

This is a good method of marketing and advertising for small businesses as it can be specifically targeted both to the chosen market as well as a campaign or offer.

Direct marketing could be by post, the Internet or by text message. It can target existing clients or it can be sent out to increase awareness of your salon. Direct mailing includes leaflets and flyers dropped door to door. These are more effective if they are dropped individually rather than with other leaflets.

LEAFLETS, FLYERS AND TRAFFIC STOPPERS

These are all leaflets that aim to promote the business and can be used in a variety of ways. They can be used within the salon for promotions, handed directly to clients in the street or posted through doors in residential areas. They can be any size but are typically A5 or A6.

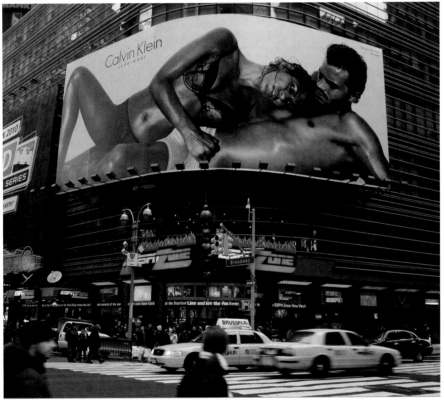

Example of a traffic stopper

INDUSTRY TIP

It is worth paying a bit more to get a professional designer to help you design a leaflet, brochure or flyer. They will have good ideas as to what works and it can be a costly exercise if the leaflet does not make the impact you want it to.

INDUSTRY TIP

A6 is the size of a postcard – an easy size to pop into a handbag or through a door.

WEBSITES AND SOCIAL NETWORKING SITES

Electronic media is very powerful. Most clients are now more likely to search the Internet for a local salon or to research a treatment. Few clients will now use a directory, such as *Yellow Pages*, to find out information; they will use *Yell.com* instead.

A website can give more information than a simple advertisement. It can show a map of the location, images to represent the salon (eg of the interior) or logos of product brands that the salon uses. It can also provide links to other websites.

Advertisements and promotions can be placed quickly on websites and social networking sites. They still need to be planned carefully and checked to make sure they are accurate. Businesses that intend to use social networking sites or websites need to make sure that the information shown is kept up to date. A website displaying old offers will not help you increase business and will not impress potential clients.

ACTIVITY

Write down a list of businesses you have searched for on the Internet over the last month. What did you do last time you could not find a contact number?

PLANNING A MARKETING CAMPAIGN

When producing a marketing campaign, you need to:

- consider the mailing list - will you post it or use the Internet?
- create something that is clearly presented and powerful to the eye – it should be uncluttered as less is more!
- test the campaign by sending it to a small group of people first to see if it is going to work and changing it if necessary before running the main campaign
- evaluate the results – if possible use a method, such as a return slip, to see how effective the campaign has been and keep a record of the results. The return slip could be a discount voucher or treatment offer on production of the tear-off slip.

PROMOTIONS

The aim of a promotion is to boost sales of a product or treatment service by using a short-term marketing activity.

PRICE PROMOTIONS

A price promotion aims to increase sales and should make up for any discount given. They include:

- buy-one-get-one-free offers
- three-for-two offers
- up-selling by offering a more deluxe treatment for the same price as a standard one.

INDUSTRY TIP

To make websites work successfully they need to be set up so that search engines, such as Google, can link to your website. It is worth finding someone to do this for the business to make sure the salon's website can be found by potential clients who do not have the web address.

WHY DON'T YOU...

use a search engine such as Google and see if you can find local beauty salons, nail studios or make-up consultants in your area. How do their adverts compare? For each website, list five features that you liked, found useful and found easy to use. Now list five features you thought were difficult to use or that you would not have included on your own website if you were designing one. Discuss you answers with your manager.

Careful planning is key to success

INDUSTRY TIP

Always ask new clients how they heard of you and keep a record. This will help you to plan your marketing strategy more effectively when you know what is working.

INDUSTRY TIP

A loss leader is a promotion that does not make any profit and aims to bring new business into the salon.

Complimentary promotions include something for free and include:

- a complimentary gift with treatment or purchase
- loyalty vouchers or incentives. This could be a simple card that is stamped after payment for a treatment or purchase, eg collect stamps for nine facials and get a complimentary tenth facial.

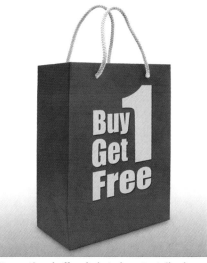

Promotional offers help to boost retail sales

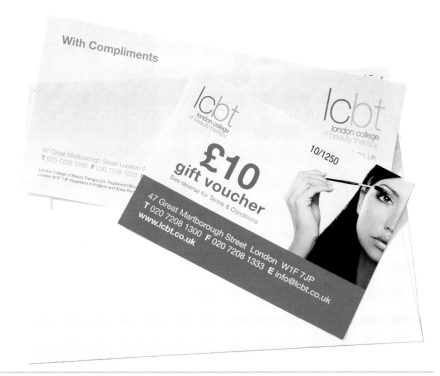

Vouchers make an excellent gift

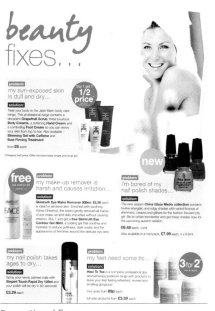

Promotional flyer

PREPARE THE DISPLAY AREA

Displaying stock effectively is another way of encouraging clients to buy products at your salon. If you can get creative and make a really eye-catching display, you are well on your way to making a sale!

In this part of the chapter you will learn about:

- safety considerations
- organising a display
- the purpose of a display
- setting up the display
- making the display eye-catching.

SAFETY CONSIDERATIONS

SAFE WORKING AND HYGIENIC PRACTICES

When displaying and dismantling the salon's stock, you must follow all the relevant health and safety regulations and keep all areas clean and tidy.

INDUSTRY TIP

Both you and the salon are bound by legislation and must adhere to the rules of several sets of regulations and Acts to make sure your client's rights are protected when you are selling retail products, equipment and services.

221

Dismantle

To take something apart.

When you start a display area or change or **dismantle** a current one, you should choose a suitable time of your working day in which to do so. Make sure that you do not disrupt the daily running of the salon or block any exits or walkways as you unpack boxes, load the shelves or dismantle a display.

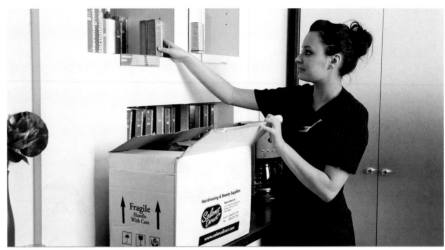

Dismantle displays carefully

COSHH AND DISPLAY AREAS

The manufacturer's instructions will give you guidance on how to store, handle, use and dispose of the substances that are considered hazardous. Your local by-laws will tell you how to dispose of the substances and their packaging to suit the environment and how to follow the local authority's guidelines on waste and refuse. Your salon's policy will explain where to store the substances and how to dispose of them.

When planning your display, you need to consider the products and how the display area might affect them. A product that might appear quite harmless can become extremely hazardous in the wrong conditions. For example, the manufacturer's instructions might state to avoid high temperatures. Displays in a sunny window will get very hot behind the glass and the heat could cause the product to become faulty.

ACTIVITY

Make a list of all the legislation that affects retail and promotion in a salon.

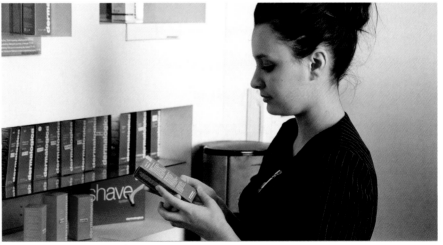

Regularly check stock is in date

PERSONAL PROTECTIVE EQUIPMENT (PPE)

Clean and prepare the display area and get items ready for the display. It is a good idea to wear gloves to protect your hands when you clean and restock retail areas.

MANUAL HANDLING OPERATIONS REGULATIONS

When stocking the shelves with products and equipment, you will need to move boxes of products around the salon. This is called manual handling. Remember to lift boxes correctly so you do not injure yourself. Follow the Manual Handling Operations Regulations 1992.

Please refer to the Legislation chapter for more information.

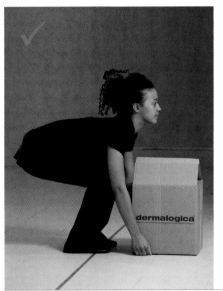

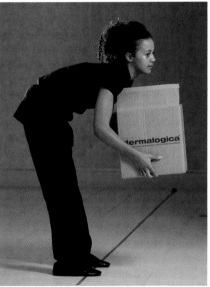

The picture on the left shows the correct lifting technique; the lifting technique on the right is incorrect. This technique will put pressure on the spine and could lead to injury

If you have several small items to carry from the unpacking area to the display area use a suitable container, such as a box or bag, to carry them rather than carrying them individually. Otherwise items might get dropped, damaged or broken.

When stocking shelves, you must also make sure that you do not overreach. If you have to stretch to reach a higher shelf you should stand on a step or stepladder. Never stand on tables (a table might tip up or break) or on salon chairs (they might swivel as you stand). You must always consider your safety and never put yourself at risk of injury. Be sensible and safe at all times to avoid injuries.

ORGANISING A DISPLAY

It might be a good idea to plan the time you organise the display area, whether this is to put it together or to take it apart. First thing in the morning or last thing at night (before the salon closes for the day) are often good times.

HANDY HINTS

Look back at Chapter 202 to refresh your knowledge of PPE.

INDUSTRY TIP

It is a good idea to wear cotton gloves or disposable gloves when you are dusting as dust can dry out your hands. It is surprising how dirty displays can get, especially if the salon is located next to a busy road.

HANDY HINTS

You can find more detailed information about the Manual Handling Operations Regulations in the Legislation chapter on page 100–101.

INDUSTRY TIP

The spine is not perfectly straight but has three distinct curves. When we bend and lift items it places additional pressure and stress on the spine.

INDUSTRY TIP

Sprains and injuries caused by lifting can usually be prevented.

SmartScreen 213 Worksheet 4

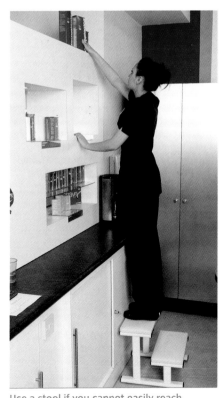

Use a stool if you cannot easily reach

If you are stocking a salon reception or waiting area, make sure that all surfaces are wiped clean with a suitable cleaning product or disinfectant spray. If you are updating or maintaining a display area, always make sure the stock displayed is clean and dust free.

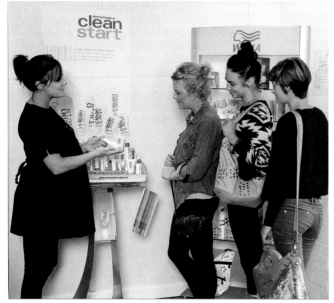

Retail areas need to be attractive to create interest

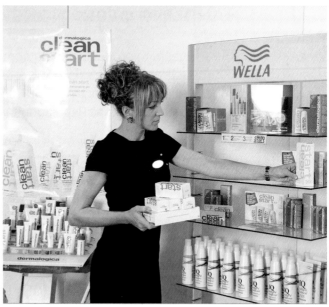

Keep displays organised

PURPOSE OF A DISPLAY

When you enter a shop, whether this is a clothing store, a department store or a perfume counter, a lot of thought will have gone into creating eye-catching displays.

It is important that your display creates impact and attracts your clients' eyes. Equally, if the display area is untidy, unattractive or too busy then the purpose of the display is lost and the client might not buy anything.

Displays should be planned before they are put into place. Think about what the purpose of the display is and what you are trying to achieve. Displays are all about increasing product awareness and sales. Your display might be a seasonal display to support salon treatments (eg summer make-up or sun preparation and protection products). Your display could be to launch a new treatment or product. When you know the purpose of the display, you need to consider what materials you will need to put the display together.

The diagram below summarises the three main purposes of salon display areas.

INDUSTRY TIP

You can create a dramatic display to promote a new product by creating a solid colour background and placing the item on a raised area. Include a small shelf talker giving the key points – positive phrases to raise clients' interest, the product's benefits and the cost without using the pound (£) sign.

 SmartScreen 213 Worksheet 1

INDUSTRY TIP

If you are stocking a lockable cabinet, take care if you need to leave the doors open and bend down to collect new stock – mind your head on the corners of the cabinet doors!

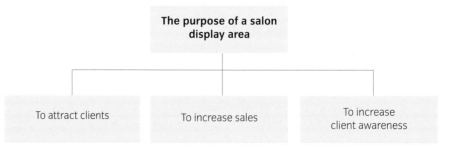

The purpose of a salon display area

To attract clients | To increase sales | To increase client awareness

ATTRACTING CLIENTS

An effective window display can attract new clients into the salon and keep regular clients interested and loyal to the business. If clients are spending a lot of money having professional salon treatments, they often want to invest in maintaining the benefits. Although purchasing retail is an additional cost, the client often sees it as important to get the best results.

An eye-catching display looks attractive and presents a professional image. It should tempt the client to either test the product or generate interest so that the client wants to find out more.

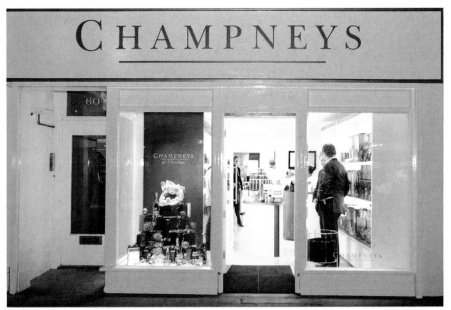

An attractive window will encourage clients to look

INDUSTRY TIP

Clients who come in with a voucher are a perfect retail opportunity. Someone else has paid for their treatment so hopefully they will be more open to invest in products if you establish and match their needs.

INDUSTRY TIP

Not all salons have the advantage of a front window or large window to create an attractive promotion and entice clients in. These businesses have to work harder using internal visual displays.

INCREASING SALES

Promoting products and services to your clients is good for the clients and also financially beneficial to the salon and staff members. Most businesses rely on retail to boost their profitability and will set commission targets to help achieve this.

Selling should not be something to dread, it should be embraced. Encourage clients to benefit from purchasing products or courses of treatments so that they get maximum results.

INCREASING CLIENT AWARENESS

People are naturally inquisitive; we cannot resist looking at an attractive display area or taking the opportunity to try something new (eg a spray of perfume or a smear of lipstick on the back of the hand to see the colour). Clients like to be able to touch and feel products and this tactile part of promotion should not be underestimated.

Promoting treatments, services and products should become natural with a little experience. To be successful you need to be confident, and good product and treatment knowledge is essential for this. Remember, you are the expert and the client wants and needs your guidance. Products will not sell themselves and no matter how stunning your display is, you also need to draw your client's attention to the display or promotion.

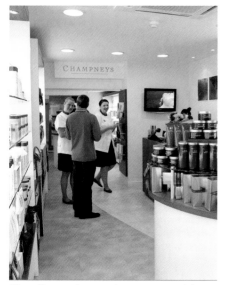

Give offers and promotions a seasonal theme

 SmartScreen 213 Worksheet 2

Special offers and promotions

If the salon has a receptionist they should also be responsible for making clients aware of the current seasonal promotions, special offers or new products. Your receptionist should encourage clients to test or sample new products and be able to talk positively about them. If your salon does not have a receptionist then this is down to you. Be quite casual and approach the client by asking if they have seen your latest promotion or seasonal offer and then telling them briefly about it. Then ask the client if they would like to know more.

If the promotion is to launch a new product which is suitable for and will benefit your client, bring the product into the conversation as you approach the promotional area. Ask the client if they would like to sample or test the product. Do not let the client feel they are being pressurised or that you are being too pushy – accept that they are not interested today.

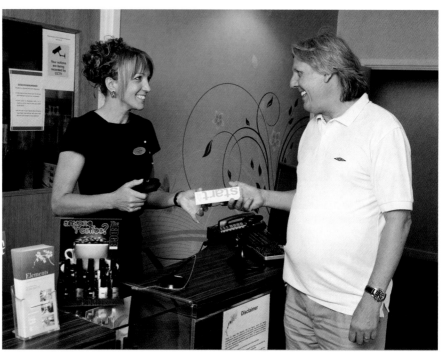

Keep retailing relaxed and friendly

SETTING UP THE DISPLAY

First, you need to know where your display is going to be located. Is it a fixed position display area or a temporary promotional display? The display needs to be in a prominent place. The products need to be accessible; clients need to be able to pick up a product and take a closer look. If promotional products are all located in inaccessible positions, such as in locked cabinets or behind closed doors, the client might be put off and an impulse buy will be lost.

FIXED POSITION DISPLAYS

Fixed position displays are likely to be:

- new showcases or displays in the salon
- an update of an existing showcase or display.

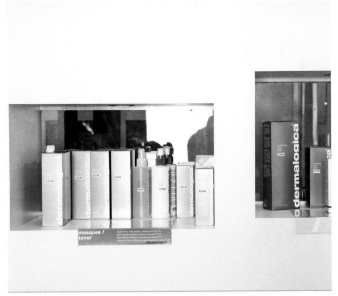

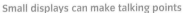

Small displays can make talking points

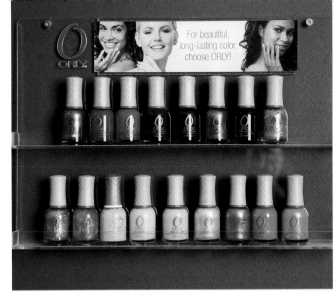

Products need to be accessible

TEMPORARY DISPLAYS

Temporary displays might advertise special offers, seasonal offers, new products or launches. They are likely to be displayed in a main area, such as reception.

NEW DISPLAY AREAS

When setting up a new display area, you will need to consider:

- the stock and equipment you require
- whether you need materials to enhance the display
- the principles behind the display
- your theme (if you have one)
- the colours you are working with
- the advertising materials you have or need.

If you have been supplied with some promotional or advertising materials from the manufacturer, you need to decide where to position these to make sure you maximise access to the display and the number of potential sales.

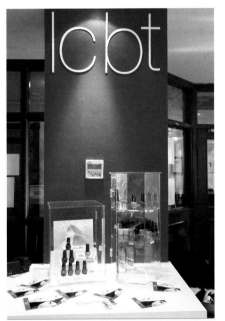

Keep product focus; displays should be uncluttered

CATEGORISING

When you have decided on the location of your display, you will need to categorise your items. If you are selling more than one manufacturers' brand you will most likely group the products from each brand together. These will be placed in the general retail area. Even general stock should be moved regularly to create new interest.

Themes

Your promotional display might follow a theme, such as a seasonal offer. Whatever theme you choose, make sure the display is not too fussy or overcrowded. Clients could be put off picking up a product if they think the surrounding products might have a 'domino effect' and all fall over.

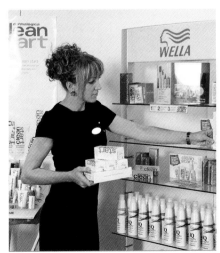

Keep displays fresh

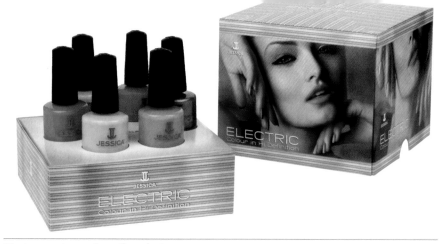

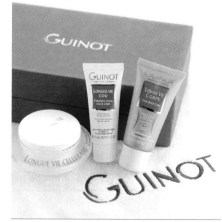

Displays made up of small products

Gift sets sell well at Christmas

 SmartScreen 213 Worksheet 3

MANUFACTURERS' PROMOTIONAL PACKAGES

Some brands and manufacturers will provide the business with special promotional packages or launches that include the retail products, testers, promotional materials and displays, such as heavy-duty cardboard display cases, testers, banners and flyers.

When launching new products, manufacturers might supply samples that can be given to clients to try the product. If this is the case, always make sure you explain to the client how to use the product rather than just letting them take the sample. If they do not use it properly they might not get the result expected and be put off.

TYPES OF DISPLAYS

Depending on what your salon already has in place, you could display your stock in a cabinet or showcase, or you could display your stock in glass or acrylic cubes that can be built up, stacked in various ways or suspended from the ceiling.

Depending on the value of the stock, you might choose to limit the amount of stock on display or secure some of it in restricted-access cabinets (eg cabinets with solid lockable doors at the bottom and a glass or wooden front area for display).

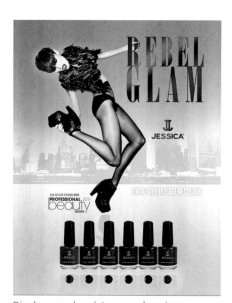

Displays can be pictures and posters

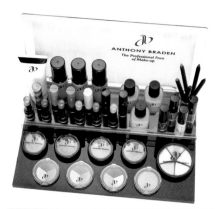

Some displays have specific permanent layouts

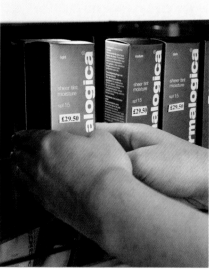

Products should be neatly arranged

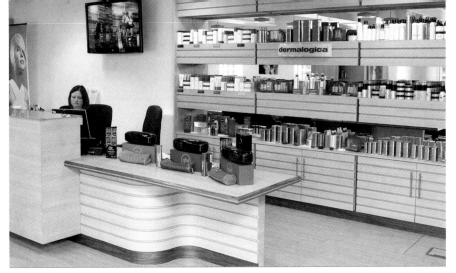

Retail areas need to be well-stocked

Tester stands

Tester stands are extremely beneficial for many salon products, such as make-up, skin and nail care. Some tester stands can be quite large and so need to be located carefully. They should be in an area where they can be easily accessed by both the therapists and clients. They can take up a lot of room in smaller salons but clients love the opportunity to try out and feel products. These stands mean that essential products are always accessible for you to be able to demonstrate the correct use and benefit of a product or show the true make-up colour or nail colour.

ACTIVITY

At some point you will have the opportunity of going to an exhibition. Take a good look at how these companies display their products. View their stands both from a distance and close up.

ACTIVITY

Go to a large department store and look at how the companies display their general stock and their promotional stock. Look around and make notes on what you found most eye-catching.

MAKING THE DISPLAY EYE-CATCHING

It is vital that the display is attractive and eye-catching if you want to increase your sales. You must make sure that you promote all services and treatments in your retail area even if you are focused on a particular promotion.

When you think you have finished creating your display, always ask other people for their opinion and take any constructive criticism on board. You want the display to be effective, so if one person does not like it, your clients might not either!

At the close of business, make sure the retail displays are lit up so they can be seen by passing trade. Remember to protect the environment where possible and use energy saving bulbs.

INDUSTRY TIP

Look at your display from close up and from a distance. If it is in a window area, go outside and look at the display from a distance. What impact does it have?

INDUSTRY TIP

Tester stands should be kept clean, free of dust and tidy so that clients feel confident about the salon's hygiene.

WHY DON'T YOU...

search on the Internet for companies that design displays; this will give you some inspiring ideas.

INDUSTRY TIP

Remember, when products are out of sight they will also be out of a client's mind. It might seem obvious but do not expect something to sell if it is shut away in a cupboard.

INDUSTRY TIP

Never make assumptions about your client's ability to pay for a product. Recommend something without emphasising the price. If you tell the client it is expensive or a lot of money, you will put them off. It is not about the value of the product to you but the value of the product for your client.

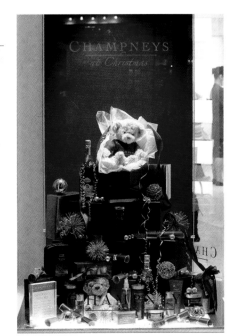

Seasonal themed displays should be eye-catching

INDUSTRY TIP

When you have finished your display, walk out of the salon and return to check it with fresh eyes. Always check the display from different angles and viewpoints.

ACTIVITY

Can you think of a display about which you were very critical? Write down three reasons why. What lessons have you learnt from this display? What would you avoid when putting your own display together?

ACTIVITY

Choose one of themes below:

- summer protection
- school prom
- luscious lips
- happy nails.

Design a mood board to detail your ideas for a display. Make sure your mood board shows all the items you will need.

MAINTAIN AND DISMANTLE THE DISPLAY AREA

In this part of the chapter you will learn about:

- maintaining the display area
- dismantling the display area.

MAINTAINING THE DISPLAY AREA

The display should be kept tidy and free of dust, Check the stock at regular intervals and, if stock is low, add additional stock if available.

MONITORING THE STOCK

Stock monitoring software

Some salons have PCs with specialised software that can monitor the sales and stock balances of products and equipment as well as tracking appointment bookings.

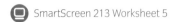

SmartScreen 213 Worksheet 5

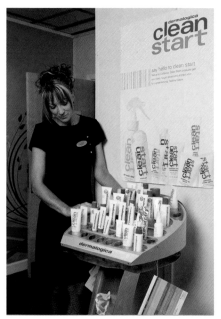

Regularly dust and tidy displays

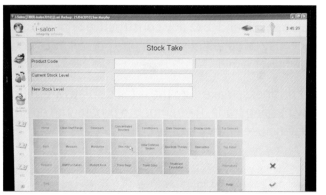

Stock levels should be monitord regularly

This software can help you to keep a stock record and to check on the sales of and demand for products. If you use this type of software, you should be able to assess which products are popular and selling well. This will make sure you have enough stock. You will also be able to identify poor sales or unpopular products. From these reports, your salon can either decide to actively promote poor selling items or choose not to stock these items in future.

Barcode scanners, hand-held scanners or swipe machines can be used at the point of sale. They read the barcode on the stock item and enable the software to track this data.

INDUSTRY TIP

Computer software can be useful for monitoring stock but most software only calculates full stock quantities so they do not always give you an accurate stock value. For more accurate stock checks, especially for the end of the salon's financial year, it is still necessary to undertake a precise stock check recording part quantities and not just full or unused stock so that the business knows exactly what stock value it has.

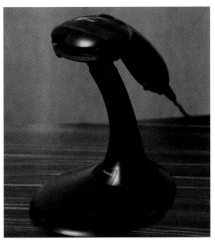

Scanner device

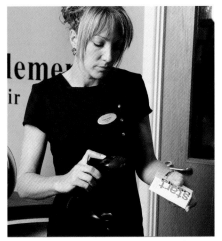

Scanners recognise bar codes on products

Stock inventory

It is ultimately the manager's responsibility to check the security and levels of the stock but the manager might **delegate** this responsibility to another person, such as the receptionist.

Delegate
To give someone a job or duty to do for you or on your behalf.

Promotional display stock

Stock that is taken specifically for promotional displays should be recorded so that it can be checked in addition to normal stock.

Delivery notes

When stock arrives direct from manufacturers or wholesalers, it should arrive with a delivery note or picking note. (Some companies send the invoice with the stock.) Check the stock received and mark it off the delivery note as it is removed from the packaging. Check that the correct amounts have been received and that the goods are undamaged. When you know you have received the correct amount of stock, you can update the salon's stock records. The stock can then be priced ready for display.

Missing or damaged stock

Any **discrepancies** between the order and the stock received should be noted on the delivery note and given to your manager or individual responsible for the stock. The company that sent the goods should be notified of any damaged or missing stock within 24 hours of delivery otherwise they might refuse to send or replace stock. Many companies will only accept returns if the correct procedure has been followed. The stock to be returned must be accompanied by special paperwork that details who the stock is from and the reason for the return.

Discrepancy
The difference between two things that should be the same.

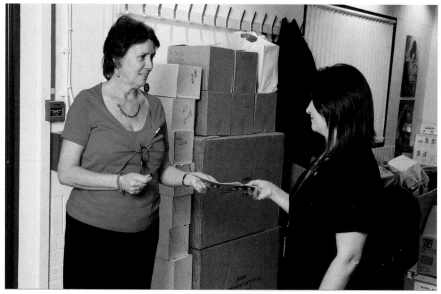

When a delivery has been checked, pass the delivery note onto the person who monitors the stock

Inventory
A list, record or catalogue of items.

SECURITY OF STOCK

When you have completed your stock **inventory**, any reductions in stock levels should be from sales only. Small items are often irresistible to thieves and items small enough to fit into pockets or handbags might be too tempting for some. This costs some businesses a great deal of money in lost revenue and can be very frustrating.

To make sure you are not losing any stock through theft, you could:

- check the stock levels on the displays regularly (at least monthly for general stock and for promotional displays more frequently)
- keep bags (both staff and clients') away from any display areas
- store any additional stock supplies away from the staff room areas in a designated lockable cupboard
- keep displays close to or behind the reception areas and away from exits and entrances
- place empty dummy containers on display where possible – these can often be obtained from the product company
- remove products from boxes if they are more expensive items and store the products in a secure location and just leave the box on display
- keep stock displays in busy areas in lockable cabinets or in cabinets that are not easy to open – child locks on cabinets can also be a deterrent.

ACTIVITY

Design a stock inventory list for your salon. Estimate how many of each item you think you should have in stock and then check against the current stock levels. Compare this list with your manager's list to identify how close your estimate was.

Commission targets are dependent on the stock inventory being accurate, as well as items sold in the salon, so any loss of stock could stop staff achieving their commission targets.

STOCK ROTATION

Stock must be rotated carefully. Place new stock at the back so that older stock moves to the front and is sold first. All products have a **shelf life**. Most products have a 2-year shelf life but some have a very short shelf life so you should always be familiar with the manufacturer's instructions for each product. If the product has not been sold by the end of its shelf life, it should be written off as old stock and disposed of. Products that have gone past their shelf life will have lost some of their benefits as the ingredients might have deteriorated over time or even have gone off.

Shelf life

The period of time that the product has to be sold by.

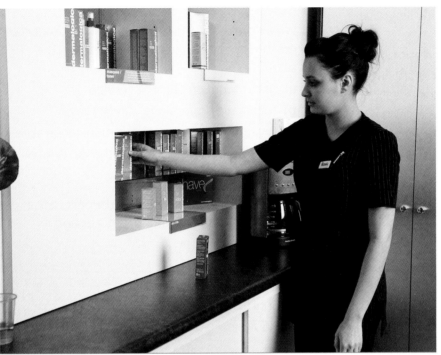

Old stock should be at the front and new stock placed behind

Most products now carry a symbol on the back showing a container with an open lid with a number in it. The number indicates the length of time that the product should be used for after the container has been opened.

DISMANTLING THE DISPLAY AREA

At some point the display will need to be dismantled. This might simply be a case of removing items from a shelf, cleaning the area and replacing the stock. It could, however, involve a larger display with items that will need to be taken apart. Make sure you do this when it is quiet to avoid any disruption and always follow the manufacturer's instructions.

 SmartScreen 213 Worksheet 5

Use the questions below to test your knowledge of Chapter 205/213 to see how much information you have retained. These questions will help you revise what you have learnt in this chapter.

Turn to page 601 for the answers.

1. Which **one** of the following techniques can be used to show that a therapist is listening closely and sensitively to others?
   a) They use relaxed and casual body language, ask lots of questions and smile
   b) They maintain eye contact and respond to questions both verbally and non-verbally
   c) They interrupt other people's conversation to show that they are listening
   d) They ask the client to complete a questionnaire

2. Which **one** of the following is most important when retailing products to clients?
   a) A sound knowledge of the products
   b) Being able to talk easily
   c) Using body language
   d) Using technical jargon

3. Which **one** of the following best describes why the client's needs must be identified?
   a) To promote any salon offers that are running
   b) To match them to the most suitable services
   c) To offer a professional service
   d) To advise on retail products

4. Which **one** of the following outlines the employee's legal responsibilities when promoting products and services?
   a) Descriptions must be honest and accurate
   b) The price of products and services must be displayed prominently
   c) Alternative services and products must be described
   d) Price comparisons with other local salons must be displayed

5. Which **one** of the following states why visual aids are helpful when promoting products and services?
   a) They give the client something to focus on
   b) The client has something to take away with them

c) They help confirm and clarify any suggestions
   d) They give a written format to the consultation process

6. Which **one** of the following is the most important reason for communicating effectively in the salon?
   a) To carry out an efficient service
   b) To behave professionally in the salon
   c) To show a high level of communication skills
   d) To make sure accurate information is given and received

7. Which **one** of the following is a benefit to the employee when promoting services and products?
   a) Repeat business
   b) A professional image
   c) Shorter working hours
   d) Additional experience

8. Which **one** of the following is a feature rather than a benefit of a treatment?
   a) A description of the treatment
   b) What it does
   c) What value it has to the client
   d) Why the client should use it

9. The benefit of a product should always be:
   a) a description of the product
   b) the ingredients it contains
   c) the container it comes in
   d) personalised to the client.

10. Which **one** of the following is a negative buying signal from a client?
    a) Asking for a product sample
    b) Looking closely at a product
    c) Asking about cost
    d) Looking away

11. Which **one** of the following statements is covered under the Supply of Goods Act?
    a) The service must be carried out with reasonable care and skill
    b) Personal Information must not be disclosed to a third party
    c) Goods must be fit for the purpose for which they are sold
    d) Products must not be described misleadingly

12. Which **one** of the following should not be used to close a sale?
    a) Would you like to take the 30 ml or 50 ml jar?
    b) Which of the products that I have recommended would you like today?
    c) Would you like the regular pedicure or the deluxe pedicure?
    d) Would you like to take this product next time you are in?

13. Hard selling will:
    a) make a client want to buy a product
    b) make a client feel uncomfortable and pressured
    c) help you reach your target
    d) make a client think you are knowledgeable.

14. Which **one** of the following statements explains what marketing is?
    a) Getting your salon's message across to clients
    b) The budget set aside for publicity and promotion
    c) Using strategies to increase business profits
    d) The annual expenditure for the salon's publicity

15. Which **one** of the following is an example of direct marketing?
    a) Traffic stoppers
    b) A press release
    c) An advert on commercial radio
    d) Emailing a flyer

I started my career on board a cruise ship with Princess Cruises. I started out as a therapist and within a year I had become a manager.

When back home I wanted to remain involved in beauty therapy as it is always changing and therefore remains exciting. I started to work for Decleor as an in-store Account Manager. This opened up a whole new avenue of salon and spa skin care. Over the course of a couple of years I worked my way up the corporate ladder to the position of Regional Manager. I have covered several areas of the country and currently I cover the South of England.

My role is always challenging, exciting and rewarding. I get to meet salon and spa owners as well as the therapists working with them who are constantly striving to be the best they can be and to achieve the goals they set themselves. Seeing them succeed and know that I have contributed to that success is rewarding in itself. You never know what each day will bring but you can always guarantee it is never the same two days in a row.

I do not think you could ever tire of working in the beauty therapy industry. It is constantly changing with new technology, trends and vision appearing daily. It comes with many rewards, including working with fantastic people and helping people to get fantastic results. There are also many avenues that you can follow and therefore I truly believe there is a career path to suit all.

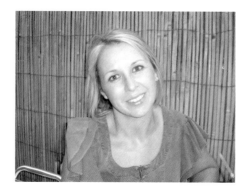

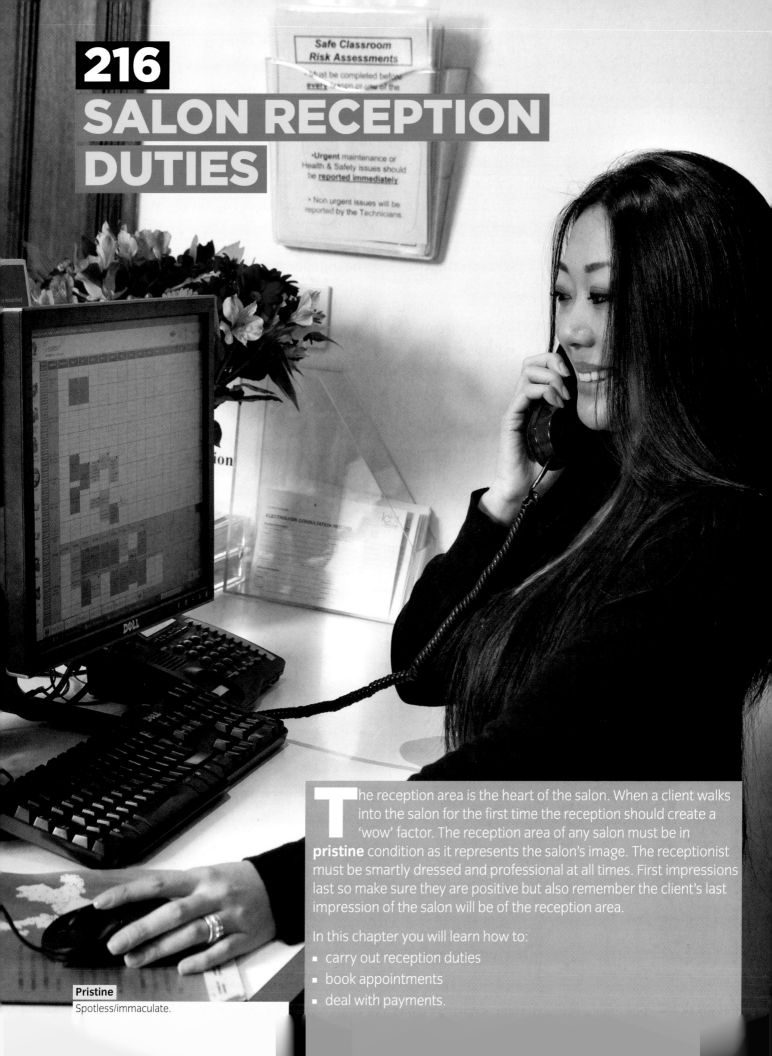

216
SALON RECEPTION DUTIES

Safe Classroom
Risk Assessments

• Must be completed before
every lesson or use of the

• Urgent maintenance or
Health & Safety issues should
be reported immediately

• Non urgent issues will be
reported by the Technicians

The reception area is the heart of the salon. When a client walks into the salon for the first time the reception should create a 'wow' factor. The reception area of any salon must be in **pristine** condition as it represents the salon's image. The receptionist must be smartly dressed and professional at all times. First impressions last so make sure they are positive but also remember the client's last impression of the salon will be of the reception area.

In this chapter you will learn how to:

- carry out reception duties
- book appointments
- deal with payments.

Pristine
Spotless/immaculate.

CARRY OUT RECEPTION DUTIES

The receptionist has lots of important responsibilities to make sure that the salon runs smoothly and clients are kept happy. The general duties of a receptionist will include some, if not all, of the following:

- dealing with enquiries and bookings
- meeting and greeting clients
- solving problems at reception, such as services running late or clients arriving late
- answering the telephone
- maintaining the salon's **hospitality** and offering refreshments to clients
- providing information about the salon's services and retail products
- checking emails and text messages
- organising the salon's post and distributing it to the relevant people
- taking messages and passing them onto the relevant people
- maintaining communication between clients and salon staff
- handling payments and promoting the sales of retail products
- preparing client record cards – if paper record cards are used the receptionist will get these out ready for the therapists to see and these might also be put with the client list.

All these duties rely on the receptionist having excellent communication skills and providing excellent customer service and client care.

In this part of the chapter you will learn about:

- maintaining the reception area
- communicating and behaving at reception
- taking messages correctly.

Hospitality

Welcoming guests in a friendly way.

HANDY HINTS

Look back at Chapter 205/213 for more information on creating and maintaining a good display area.

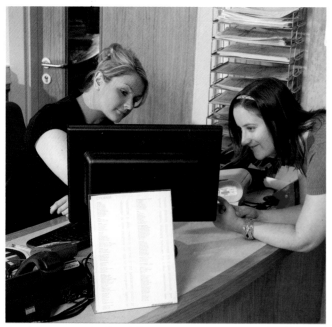

Excellent communication skills are essential

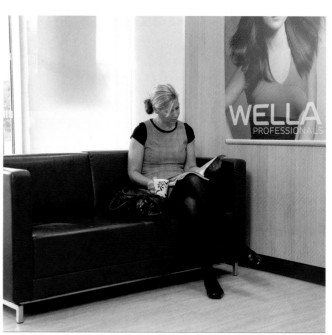

A relaxing waiting area helps clients to unwind

MAINTAINING THE RECEPTION AREA

Throughout the day, the receptionist should:

- keep the reception area clean and tidy
- maintain stationery and retail stock.

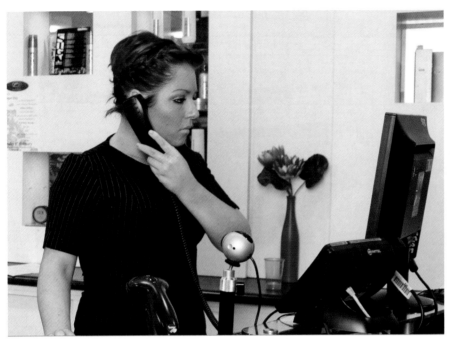

Answering telephone enquiries is part of a receptionist's role

A CLEAN AND TIDY RECEPTION AREA

As a receptionist you must make sure that the salon is always well-presented and shows a professional image of the salon as it will be the first area that the clients will see when they enter the salon. You must always make sure that the seating area is clean, tidy and welcoming.

Throughout the day, tidy up any magazines and clear away any used cups or glasses. The receptionist should also dust and tidy the area when it is quiet to make sure that the surfaces and floor in the reception area are kept clean.

INDUSTRY TIP

Keep copies of current magazines and try to get copies of magazines or journals containing articles related to the products you stock so that you can make sure that when clients are reading magazines you can highlight the products to promote them. Some brands will notify you of up-and-coming advertisements or promotions.

INDUSTRY TIP

Make sure your male clients are catered for too by having a small selection of men's magazines.

INDUSTRY TIP

Have a promotional folder, containing articles related to the products you retail and treatments you offer, for clients to read through while they wait.

ACTIVITY

Visit two salons in your area – you could go in to pick up a price list – and compare their reception areas. Put your responses into a table like the one below.

Salon 1		Salon 2	
Positive	Negative	Positive	Negative

Use the following questions to help you complete the table.

- How did the receptionist greet you?
- What did you find attractive about the reception area?
- What would you have changed?
- Did you find anything off-putting?
- Was the reception clean and tidy?

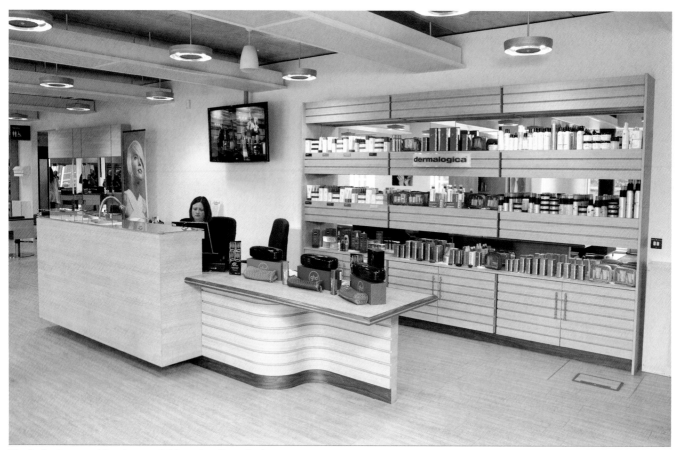

Stock displays must be clean and tidy and well-stocked

MAINTAINING STOCK

There are two areas of stock that the receptionist needs to maintain:

- the stationery stock
- the salon's retail stock and stock displays.

Stationery stock

As the receptionist you are responsible for making sure that the stationery levels are maintained. This will help the salon to run smoothly and effectively.

You should:

- make sure there are plenty of sharpened pencils for writing appointments into the appointment book and a good pencil rubber for making any cancellations or amendments
- monitor the appointment book, if it is paper based, to make sure there are enough pages left for making future appointments
- make sure a notepad or message pad and pen are to hand for taking phone messages
- make sure there are enough price lists, appointment cards, promotional flyers and product leaflets and notify the salon manager when these are running low
- keep general levels of stationery stocked up, such as making sure there are spare staples and a staple gun for attaching receipts to record cards where necessary. Post-it™ notes are also very handy to keep in supply.

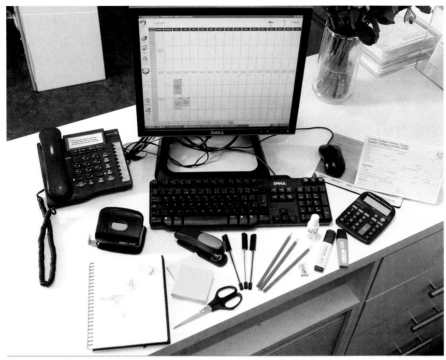

Some of the types of stationery you will need to have to hand

HANDY HINTS

Further detailed information about stock and displays can be found in Chapter 205/213.

The salon's retail stock and stock displays

The receptionist will be in charge of making sure that the retail display is clean, tidy and well-stocked. The shelves should be kept tidy and the stock should be pulled forward so that the displays are neat and the products are easily accessible. Any gaps or stock required should be noted and given to the person responsible for ordering stock.

COMMUNICATING AND BEHAVING AT RECEPTION

EFFECTIVE COMMUNICATION

Effective salon communication starts with the receptionist. This will ensure the smooth running of the salon and make sure that the therapists work effectively and efficiently.

HANDY HINTS

Look back at Chapter 203 to help you with your communication techniques.

- When communicating with clients, you must be polite at all times.
- Always speak clearly.
- Face the client if you can when you talk to them as this helps you to be understood more clearly.
- If your client is confused or English is not their first language, you might need to adapt your language style to suit their needs and the situation.
- Avoid using technical jargon as clients might not understand. Always show your client that you are listening carefully by maintaining eye contact and nodding – not all clients will pause for breath, so you will need to listen very carefully.
- Use positive body language – keep your arms open and look interested.
- Always try to respond to clients in a positive helpful manner.
- If you need to encourage a client to end a conversation, use closed questions, keep to the subject matter and the purpose of the discussion and summarise any agreed points.

ACTIVITY

Think of an occasion where you were trying to make an appointment and you got an unprofessional response. Write down what you felt was bad about the person you were dealing with. How did it make you feel? Did you go back again?

ACTIVITY

What would you do and say if a client enquired about a therapist who had recently left your salon?

ATTENDING TO CLIENTS AND ENQUIRIES

For all salon enquiries it is important that you clearly identify the purpose of the enquiry. As a receptionist you might deal with the following types of enquiry:

- telephone enquiries
- face-to-face enquiries
- electronic enquiries by email or text message.

It is important to be able to answer and deal with these enquiries professionally and to give accurate information to any visitor to the salon. You might need to deal with:

- appointment enquiries – to make, alter or cancel an appointment
- enquiries about the salon's opening and closing times
- enquiries about the prices of services and products
- enquiries from product representatives or area sales managers selling or promoting their stock
- wholesale deliveries from suppliers to the salon – for example general stock, such as wax, cotton wool or specific branded goods
- cold sales calls – people trying to contact the salon manager without prior arrangement or trying to introduce the salon to new services and products that they have not requested.

INDUSTRY TIP

You must, where possible, make sure you know the prices for all services and treatments that your salon offers and for retail products that you stock. Make sure you have a retail price list to hand so you can refer to this if you are unsure as it is important to make sure you give the correct information.

INDUSTRY TIP

Check whether product representatives have an appointment and whether the appointment is in the diary. Make the person they are coming to see aware that the representative has arrived at the salon.

INDUSTRY TIP

Any deliveries should be left in a safe location, ideally in the unpacking area. The goods will need to be signed for to confirm that they have arrived at the salon.

INDUSTRY TIP

Most salons will get cold calls both over the phone and in person and you need to make sure you follow the salon's procedure for dealing with them. Some of the callers can be quite time-consuming and cause delays for the salon.

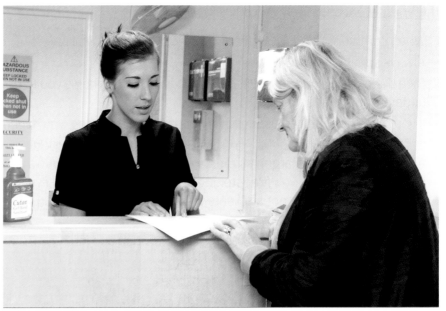

Offer assistance if the client has any queries

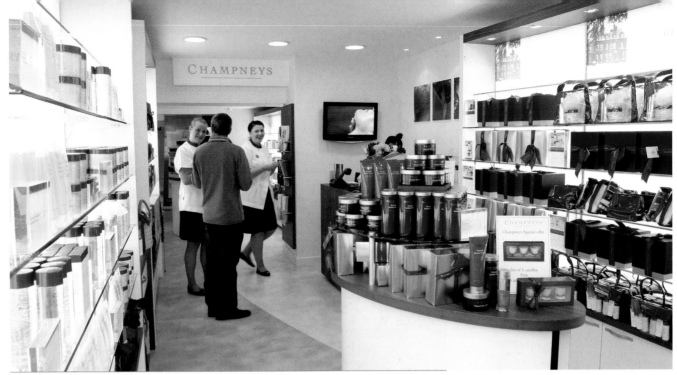

Therapists attending to a customer in a retail area

Always make sure that you deal with enquiries within the limits of your own authority. This means that you should only deal with something if you have permission to do so or it is part of your job description. If you have not been told you have approval to do something then it is not within the limits of your authority and you should refer enquiries to the relevant person.

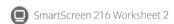
SmartScreen 216 Worksheet 2

ACTIVITY

Discuss who you would refer enquiries to if they are outside the limits of your authority.

Telephone enquiries

When the telephone rings, try to answer the phone promptly – ideally within three rings, using a pleasant and friendly tone of voice and speaking clearly. You should use your salon's correct greeting. Smile while you talk on the phone and you will have a happier sounding voice. When you answer, state the salon's name (as per your salon's policy) and say something along the lines of: 'Good morning/afternoon, Head to toe salon, Hannah speaking. How might I help you?'

INDUSTRY TIP

One reason for saying 'Good morning' or 'Good afternoon' before the salon's name is because on the phone clients do not always hear the first thing you say properly. By the time you say the salon's name, they are listening fully.

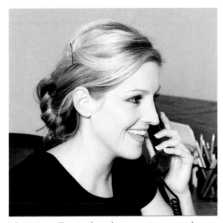

Face-to-face enquiry

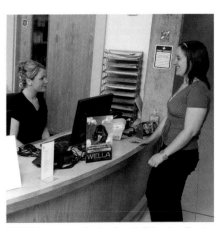

Always smile on the phone – you sound happier

Maintain eye contact when talking to clients

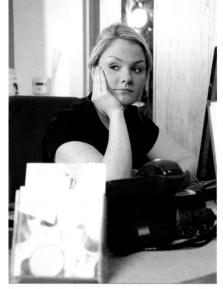

Receptionist with poor posture and lack of interest

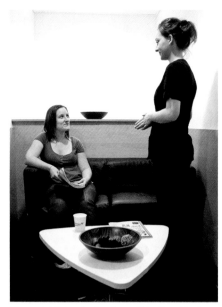

Therapist introducing herself to the client

Face-to-face enquiries

Greet your client as soon as they walk into the salon if you are in the reception area. If you are doing something else, such as dealing with another client, or you are on the phone, it is important just to smile, nod and make eye contact. You should always greet your clients promptly and warmly.

As clients arrive, always confirm their name and appointment details to make sure the booking is correct. It will also allow you to confirm any service changes that the client might request and make the necessary adaptations. You should then tell the therapist promptly of their client's arrival.

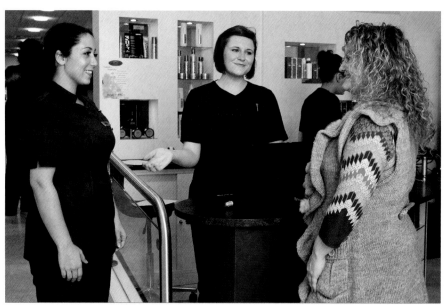

Receptionist taking the client to the therapist

Offer the client a seat in the reception area or take them to the waiting area if it is away from the reception. Offer to take and hang up their coat or look after any other items, such as umbrellas or shopping bags. Ask them whether they would like a magazine to read while they are waiting. You must maintain a friendly yet professional approach at all times.

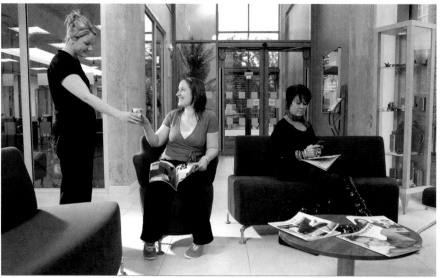

If a client has to wait, offer them a drink

ACTIVITY

Write down the different types of questions you can use. Now write down when you think you would need to use the different types of question. You can refer to Chapter 205/213 Promote products and services/display stock to help if you need to.

Electronic enquiries

Some salons receive booking enquiries by email or text message. This can be through direct contact with the salon or through the salon's website. You must always send a reply to the client confirming the details in the same way you would face to face or on the telephone. If the client's request cannot be met then a further few emails or text messages might be required to offer alternative times and confirm the appointment. You might need to contact them by telephone to clarify any complications.

Some larger businesses have electronic appointments systems that clients can access through the salon's website and book their appointments themselves. They will then receive an automated email reply confirming the appointment.

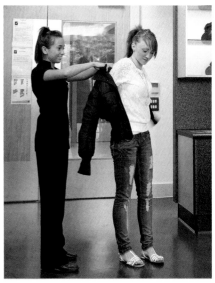
Helping a client with her coat

ACTIVITY

Write a response to the following appointment request that a client has sent by email.

ONLINE BOOKING SYSTEM

Hello

I would like to book with Aoife at 3.30 pm on Wednesday 22nd October for a facial. Please can you let me know if you can do this.

Bryony

Unfortunately you are unable to offer the time or therapist she is requesting.

Ask your tutor to check your reply and give you feedback.

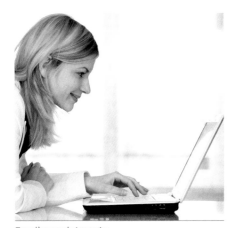
Email appointments

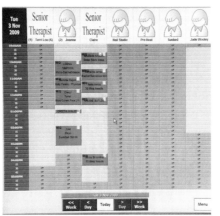
Computer screen view of appointment booking system

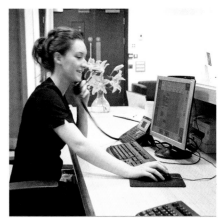
Telephone booking

ACTIVITY

Can you think of some open questions that might be asked at reception?

ACTIVITY

Can you think of some closed questions that might be asked at reception?

COPING DURING BUSY PERIODS

The reception area can be very busy at times and you will have to balance the needs of different people. Clients visiting the salon in person can see how busy you are but people calling the salon cannot, so try not to let the telephone ring more than three times before you answer it. You can always excuse yourself from the person in the salon to pick up and answer the phone and then ask the client on the phone to wait a few moments. You will need to identify who needs your attention first and avoid upsetting those who are still waiting to be seen.

When you are rushed off your feet, apologise to clients for keeping them waiting, suggest they take a seat, offer them a drink, keep them informed about the situation and tell them that you will not keep them waiting for longer than necessary. If you are really busy, ask for help from a colleague.

MANAGING CLIENTS' NEEDS AND EXPECTATIONS

As a therapist or a receptionist, you will meet a variety of people with different needs and expectations. You might encounter:

- An unexpected client who thinks they have booked an appointment: apologise and explain to the client that you do not have the appointment recorded in the appointment book. See if you can find the appointment elsewhere. See if you can fit the client in – for example, it might be possible to offer them an appointment with another therapist instead.
- Double-booked appointments: usually down to human error, eg if the receptionist was distracted and wrote the appointment in the wrong place (but more often it is the client's error).
- Late arrivals: be tactful as you do not want to upset the client even though they are late. There are a number of reasons why clients are late and many do not do it deliberately. If there is not enough time to complete the service, explain to the client or alternatively make the client aware that you will not be able to offer a full treatment and offer them the option of having part of the treatment or a reduced treatment or the option of rebooking for another time.
- A client who wishes to change their appointment service: ask the client when they would like to change their appointment to and look for an alternative.
- A client who is not sure of what service to book and when to book it: be patient and find out as much information as you can. Give the client some suggestions and be helpful.
- Clients from different cultures or those whose first language is not English: be friendly and if you need to, write information down. Use

simple language. Do not be frightened to say that you do not understand something or to ask the client to repeat what they have said.

- A client with **mobility** needs or disabilities: sometimes it is easiest to just ask the client what will help them. Someone with a mobility problem might have to use a downstairs treatment room if this is an option and have a foot stool or access to an adjustable couch. A client who is hard of hearing might need you to talk to them face to face and you will need to remember to do this or write information down for them. If the client has a guide dog you will need to make sure there is room for the dog to lie down.
- A client who wants to complain: apologise and listen to the complaint. If you can deal with the complaint then do so, otherwise refer it to the manager.
- An angry client: see Chapter 203 on pages 184–185 for guidance on dealing with an angry client.

INDUSTRY TIP

If you have clients who are always late or who forget on a regular basis, send them a text or get the receptionist to give them a quick call a few hours before their appointment to remind them. The cost of a text or call is less than a missed appointment.

INDUSTRY TIP

Remember if a client needs to bring in a guide dog that it is a working dog and not a pet, you should acknowledge the dog but do not make a fuss of it and distract it from its work.

Mobility

The ability to move.

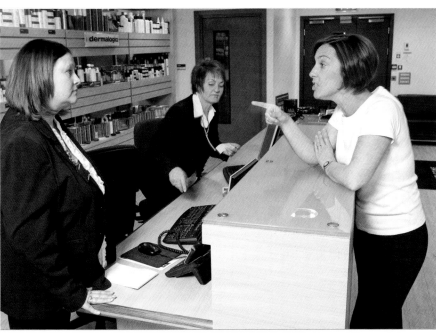

An angry client

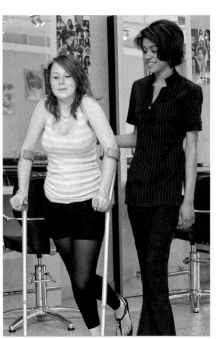

A client with mobility needs

WHY DON'T YOU...
discuss with a colleague how you would handle each of the above situations professionally. Make a list of things that you would need to consider in each situation and the issues you might need to overcome.

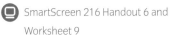 SmartScreen 216 Handout 6 and Worksheet 9

TAKING MESSAGES CORRECTLY

The receptionist will need to deal with any messages that have been left on an answer machine. This might include cancelling appointments, calling clients back to make appointments and passing messages onto members of the team so that they are aware of any changes to the appointment book.

The receptionist must also take a message if a person is not available to deal with a telephone call or speak to the person or client personally.

You must make sure that all the details are recorded clearly and that you pass them on when that person is free.

When taking a message for someone, make sure you write clearly. Make sure you cover all the information needed:

■ who the message is for
■ the date and time the message was left
■ a brief but accurate description of the message
■ who the message is from
■ the contact details of the caller/visitor, such as their email address or telephone number – be sure to write the contact number down accurately
■ the action to be taken (eg to return their call and the best time to call)
■ whether the message is urgent or a general enquiry
■ the name of the person who has taken the message (ie you).

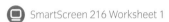 SmartScreen 216 Worksheet 1

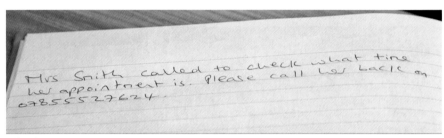
A brief, accurate message requiring action

INDUSTRY TIP

If you are unsure, always ask twice. If you cannot spell a name or if you are not sure you have heard correctly, ask the client to spell it.

When taking messages, make sure you follow the salon's procedures for recording the message details and when to pass them onto the correct person. If you take down information, such as a contact number, incorrectly, the message becomes useless or if you fail to pass on the message, the person expecting the return call could be annoyed. If this is a client, you could lose the appointment, costing the salon business and revenue and the salon could get a poor reputation for being unreliable.

BOOK APPOINTMENTS

In order to make sure that a salon runs smoothly, it is important that appointments are booked carefully and correctly.

In this part of the chapter you will learn about:
■ making, recording and confirming appointment bookings
■ confidentiality
■ legislation.

MAKING, RECORDING AND CONFIRMING APPOINTMENT BOOKINGS

When you make appointments for the salon's clients, you need to make sure they are booked carefully, to fit in with the services offered and staff availability, as well as the client's request. Your role will involve dealing with clients' requests and identifying their requirements accurately.

ACTIVITY

With a friend or colleague, try out a role play booking an appointment in a busy reception area.

What was difficult for you as the client and as the therapist/receptionist?

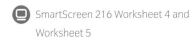 SmartScreen 216 Worksheet 4 and Worksheet 5

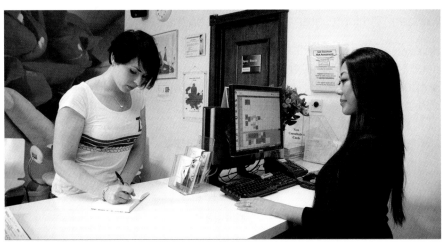

As a receptionist, you will deal with clients' needs and requests

SCHEDULING APPOINTMENTS

When you have confirmed with the client the type of service or treatment required, the preferred time and date and the therapist that they have requested, you must record the appointment either in the appointment book or on an electronic booking system.

There are many electronic booking systems on the market and you must be trained by your salon manager before using such a system. Written appointment systems tend to follow a set format in most salons. The book will have columns with times along the side. At the top of each column will be the therapists' names and the bookings for each therapist will be in the column under their name. The times that the therapist works (and does not work) should be clearly marked in the appointment book.

As a guide, the abbreviations that salons tend to use in written appointment books are shown in the table below.

Service/treatment	Abbreviation	Service/treatment	Abbreviation
Half leg wax	½ LW	Eyelash tint	Elt
Full leg wax	FLW	Eyelash extensions	Elx
Bikini line wax	BL	Threading	Th
Under arm wax	UA	Make-up	M-Up
Facial	Fac	Full body massage	FBM
Manicure	Man or m/c	Back massage	BM
Deluxe manicure	Del. Man or D m/c	Reapplication of polish	Re – V (T for toes, F for fingers)
Pedicure	Ped or p/c	Lip wax	Lip
Deluxe pedicure	Del. Ped or D p/c	Chin wax	Chin
Eyebrow shape	Ebs	Lip and chin wax	L & CW
Eyebrow tint	Ebt		

Appointment times

Most salons will have slightly different appointment times and scheduling procedures. When you first start, you must always check your salon's policy before booking in any clients. You might be given a list to help you. However, most appointment systems have booking spaces based on 15-minute intervals, such as 10 am, 10.15 am, 10.30 am, and so on. Some work on 10-minute intervals depending on the service required.

Below is a guide for a variety of service and treatment times. You might need to adapt and vary these times according to the clients and the products you are using. Many salons will allow additional time for a consultation.

Service/treatment	Time allocated
Half leg wax	20–30 minutes
Full leg wax	45 minutes
Bikini line wax	15 minutes
Under arm wax	15 minutes
Lip wax	10 minutes
Chin wax	10 minutes
Lip and chin wax	10 minutes
Facial	60–75 minutes
Manicure	45 minutes
Deluxe manicure	60 minutes
Pedicure	60 minutes
Deluxe pedicure	75 minutes
Eyebrow shape	10 minutes
Eyebrow tint	10 minutes
Eyelash tint	20 minutes
Make-up	30–60 minutes depending on the make-up application being carried out
Reapplication of polish	15–20 minutes

WHY DON'T YOU...
find out if the abbreviations above differ from your salon's system.

Paper-based appointment booking system

ACTIVITY

Mock up an appointments page. See how many treatments you could book in one day for two therapists.

Booking services accurately

It is extremely important that you book in services correctly, as incorrect bookings can mean that:

- services or treatments do not run to time
- clients might be kept waiting
- the therapist's time is wasted
- therapists have to rush treatments
- clients are double booked
- clients do not turn up as expected because the wrong time has been put into the appointment book.

Confirming appointments

When you have booked an appointment, make sure you have entered the information correctly and have taken a contact number. Repeat back to the client the booking information, confirming the treatment, time, date and the therapist's name.

CONFIDENTIALITY

As the receptionist, you will need to take clients' contact details when making appointments or recording messages. Clients' contact details are confidential and need to be kept safe and secure. Never leave them lying around for unauthorised people to see.

When you are taking down clients' person details or you are having a personal conversation with a client, think carefully as to who is around and can overhear conversation. Not all clients want the general public to know their personal business. If possible find somewhere private away from the reception to confirm intimate treatments.

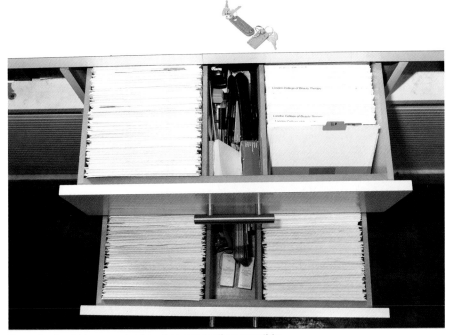

Records should be organised so they are easily accessible

When completing client record cards and consultation records, any verbal discussion should be completed away from the reception area – again to maintain confidentiality.

As part of your role you might be accessing client records and preparing record cards for the therapists and it is important therefore that you comply with the Data Protection Act (DPA). If any information about staff or clients is kept on a computer, your salon manager must register the salon with the Data Protection Register.

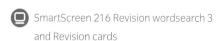
SmartScreen 216 Revision wordsearch 3 and Revision cards

ACTIVITY

Write a list of the requirements you are expected to comply with under the Data Protection Act. See what you can remember and then refer to the Legislation chapter to see if you have covered everything.

Following the Data Protection Act and your salon's policy for client confidentiality maintains professionalism, enhances the salon image and avoids a bad reputation and unnecessary loss of clients. Clients have the right to take legal action against the salon if their personal information is not kept confidential and in line with the Data Protection Act.

LEGISLATION

In addition to being aware of the requirements of the Data Protection Act in ensuring that client confidentiality is maintained, you also need to be familiar with the following legislation when working on reception:

- The Sale of Goods Act – goods must be as described in any promotional material, meet the British safety standards and be of satisfactory quality.
- The Consumer Protection Act – goods must comply with certain safety standards; clients can sue for damages if they do not.
- The Prices Act – the prices of products must be displayed and clients must be given accurate information.
- The Trade Descriptions Act – the description of any goods must be accurate and not misleading.

HANDY HINTS

You can find more information on all the legislation that you need to be familiar with when working on the reception in the Legislation chapter.

ACTIVITY

Take each of the above pieces of legislation and write a list of what you must do as an employee to meet the requirements of each Act when you are working in the salon.

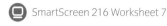
SmartScreen 216 Worksheet 7

DEAL WITH PAYMENTS

At the end of every treatment or retail sale, there is a payment **transaction**. Payment might be in the form of cash, a card or a cash equivalent, such as gift vouchers. It is important that you are able to process the payment correctly without errors. You must also be aware of security when processing payments.

Transaction

A business deal where something is bought or sold.

In this part of the chapter you will learn about:

- handling payments
- payment discrepancies and **disputes**
- end-of-the-day totals
- keeping payments safe and secure.

HANDLING PAYMENTS

It is very important that the receptionist is **competent** at working out the correct total of the bill and the change at the end of the client's treatment or service. Incorrect bills can lead to embarrassment for everyone and the business will suffer loss of income.

CALCULATING COSTS

You must be knowledgeable about the pricing structure for the services and treatments offered by your salon and the prices of the retail products that are available in your salon.

To calculate a client's bill you could use:

- a calculator
- a till
- an electronic point of sale (EPOS) device or scanner
- a pen and paper.

ACTIVITY

Research the cost of your salon's retail products and services and compare them with those of a competitor or a salon on the Internet. Is there much variation in the prices? If yes, why do you think this is?

ACTIVITY

Using the price list below, which includes VAT, calculate the total amount from treatments/services and retail products that each of the therapists has brought in the salon.

Which therapist has brought in the most revenue? Do you think there is a reason for this? How have retail sales made a difference to the totals? Do you think this is important? If so, write down why. Discuss these answers with your tutor.

Therapist – Andie		Therapist – Hannah	
Treatments and retail products sold		Treatments and retail products sold	
Facial	£48	Man (manicure)	£28
Eyelash tint	£12	Make-up	£35
Eye make-up remover	£15.30	Lipstick	£14
Pedicure	£33	Nail polish	£9.50
Cleanser	£21.50	Half leg wax	£14
Moisturiser	£42.50	Eyebrow shape	£8
Total		Total	

Disputes

An arguement or disagreement.

Competent

Having the ability, skill or knowledge to do a task.

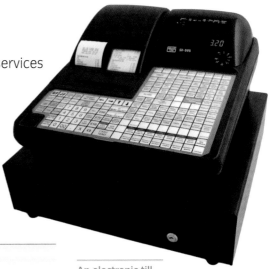

An electronic till

SmartScreen 216 Worksheet 6

INDUSTRY TIP

Treatments, services and retail products are usually subject to value added tax (VAT) and prices should therefore be displayed inclusive of VAT. VAT is currently charged at 20 per cent – in addition to the basic cost. If the government changes the rate of VAT, the salon needs to revise its prices to reflect this so you need to be up to date with these changes.

Although it is good practice to work through these tasks and calculate the bills with a calculator, it is likely that your salon will have an electronic point of sale system where the computer works out the cost for you. These have touch screen buttons for each service and might also have a barcode scanner for retail products. You still need to be careful that you are entering the correct amounts and pressing the correct buttons.

ACTIVITY

Using your salon's prices for each of the treatments and retail products, repeat the previous activity. How do the totals compare?

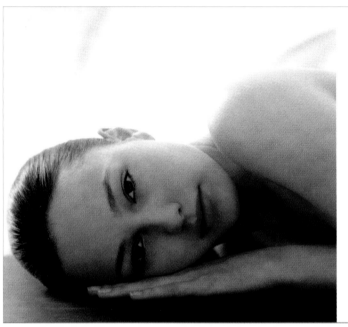

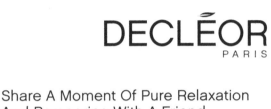

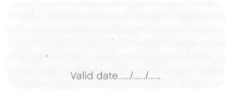

Share A Moment Of Pure Relaxation And Pampering With A Friend

Take delight in the relaxing benefits of a Decléor Aromatherapy Face or Body Treatment and it will be our pleasure to offer you and one friend £10 off from both your treatments.

Valid date....../....../......

Restriction may apply. Please mention this offer when booking your appointment. Offer only available on treatments over £50, only one offer per client.

An example of a promotional discount voucher

Informing clients of the costs

When you are confirming the total bill with your client, you should do so politely. Start by explaining the cost of the treatment, then the cost of any retail products and, finally, give them the overall cost. This will give your client the opportunity to decline the retail products if the costs are higher than expected. However, this should not happen and there should not be any surprises with the bill if the retail product prices are clearly displayed and if you have previously informed the client about the price of the treatment.

TYPES OF PAYMENT

When you have calculated the cost of the treatment and any retail goods to be purchased, you will need to find out how the client is going to pay and record the sales correctly, following your salon's policy.

Payment by cash

If your client chooses to pay with cash, check all notes and coins to make sure they are not forged or damaged in any way.

If you are happy that the cash is genuine, take your client's money and count it but do not place it in the till until your client has received their change. Leave it in the sight of both you and the client. Cash payment issues are easier to resolve if the money has not been placed in the till and you can confirm exactly how much money the client gave you.

When you have calculated the required change, count this out as you hand it to your client.

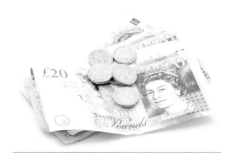
English notes and coins

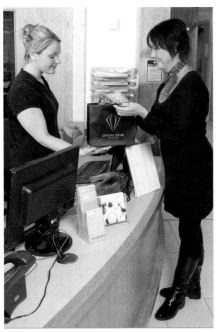
Count money carefully

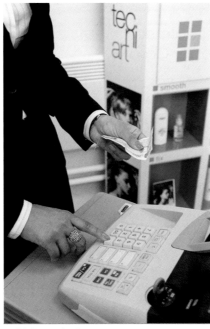
Hold the cash given to you

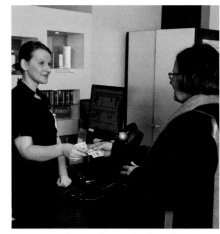
Count the client's change back to them

Forgeries

If you think you have been given a forged note, check the note with your salon manager and inform the client. Politely ask them for an alternative method of payment. Always follow your salon's policy and make sure you know what to do if you encounter cash that is not genuine or non-legal tender.

Payment with cash equivalents

Your client might want to pay with a cash equivalent, such as:

- gift vouchers
- discount vouchers from introductory offers or promotional offers
- loyalty card points
- traveller's cheques.

Cash equivalents are used instead of cash payments but work in the same way. Some salons might give vouchers, instead of cash, as change if the total bill does not come to the total value of the voucher. However, you must check this against your salon's policy.

When taking vouchers, you must record the value of the voucher being used and the total of the bill and check that the voucher is in date and valid. Vouchers are often numbered so that each voucher has a unique number reference. This helps to prevent forgeries being used. The number can then be tracked on a computer or simple tracking sheet to show how much the voucher was for, when it was sold and when it was **redeemed**.

INDUSTRY TIP

Make sure you monitor the amount of change in the till so that there is always enough change to give clients when needed.

INDUSTRY TIP

Check your salon's policy for accepting £50 notes and confirming that the notes are genuine.

WHY DON'T YOU...
visit http://www.bankofengland.co.uk/banknotes/current for more information about banknotes.

INDUSTRY TIP

It is a criminal offence to pass on a banknote that you know to be counterfeit. If you have a note that you believe is counterfeit, you must take it to the bank as soon as you can. The bank can then send the note for analysis and notify the police.

Redeem

To exchange for payment of goods or services.

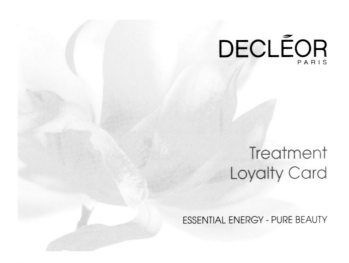

ESSENTIAL ENERGY - PURE BEAUTY

A loyalty card

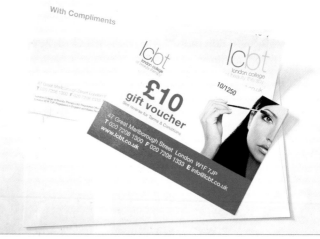

A valid gift voucher is a method of payment

INDUSTRY TIP

Whichever method of payment is used, it will cost the salon money to process it into the bank. Cheques can cost a business about 70p to bank, debit card payments around 21p to process and credit cards about 1.5–2 per cent of the total payment to process. Banks also charge money to process cash.

INDUSTRY TIP

If a cheque is written for more than the amount on the cheque guarantee card, the business will not accept it as the money is not guaranteed.

INDUSTRY TIP

A takings' sheet is a sheet of paper used by salons to record the revenue they have taken over the course of the day. The sheet will contain a record of every treatment given and all retail sales the salon has made by the therapists. This allows the therapists to see whether they are meeting their targets and allows the business to see which therapists are the most productive. These sheets are particularly important if the salon does not have an electronic computer system and if the therapists are working on a **commission** basis for the sales of treatments and products.

Commission

A percentage of the value of the sales that a therapist creates.

Payments by cheque

Cheque payments are still an acceptable method of payment but are becoming less popular with many salons no longer accepting them as a method of payment. Cheques need to be guaranteed with a cheque guarantee card which means that the banks will honour the payment to the retailer up to a set amount.

Processing cheques correctly

If your salon still accepts cheques, you must complete several checks to make sure that they are completed correctly.

When you inform the client of the total bill, your client will need to complete the cheque in front of you with the following information:

- the salon's name
- the amount in words
- the amount in figures
- the date
- their signature.

The client will need to provide you with a cheque guarantee card. You must then write on the back of the cheque the limit of the cheque guarantee card, the card number and the expiry date.

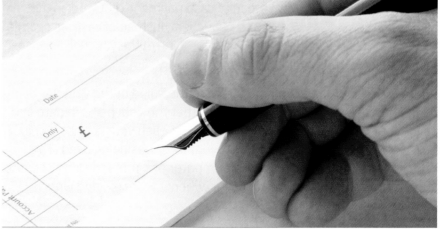

A cheque must be signed in front of you

Payment by card

Debit cards and credit cards have become a very popular and easy payment method. However, because of the fees that businesses have to pay to the credit card companies, these are costly and not all salons will accept them as a form of payment.

If your salon takes card payments and this is your client's chosen payment method, then you need to find out whether your client is using a debit or credit card.

With debit cards the payment is taken immediately from the client's bank account. Credit card companies request payment from the client on a monthly basis.

The procedure for paying with a debit or credit card is the same and you will use a chip and PIN (personal identification number) machine (called a merchant machine), a card reader or a chip and PIN terminal. Your salon will give you training on how to process card payments as the process varies slightly from one machine to another.

INDUSTRY TIP

Always check that the payments are made correctly. If authorisation for a payment is declined, inform the client tactfully. This can often be something as simple as an interruption to the connection but it could also mean that there are not enough funds in the client's account.

INDUSTRY TIP

Chip and PIN cards are designed to prevent fraud. Only the cardholder should know the PIN and they are the only person who needs to touch the card, unless there is a query. Discreetly look away as the client enters their PIN (personal identification number).

WHY DON'T YOU...
check with you salon manager what your salon's card limits are.

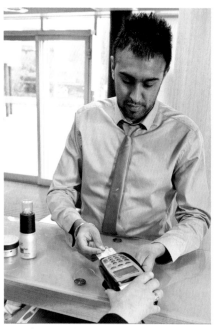

A card transaction

 SmartScreen 216 Handout 10

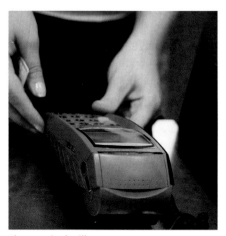

The terminal will prompt you

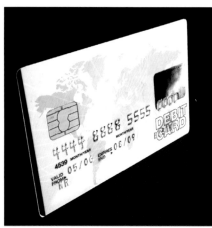

A debit card

PAYMENT DISCREPANCIES AND DISPUTES

As the receptionist, it might be part of your role to identify and resolve payment discrepancies or disputes and you must make sure that you do so within the limits of your own authority. Any payment discrepancies or disputes that are outside of your authority must be referred to the relevant person – this might be a manager or a more senior therapist. Payment disputes could be disagreements over the total bill, overcharging or undercharging, insufficient funds in the client's accounts, suspect tender or invalid payments.

INVALID CURRENCY

Invalid currency includes banknotes that have expired, notes with incorrect markings or even foreign currency. Some large salons in the UK accept Euros – particularly those in tourist areas. Check your salon's policy about receiving payment in Euros.

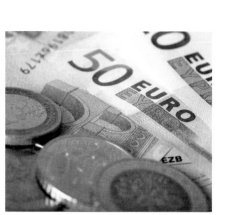

Euros

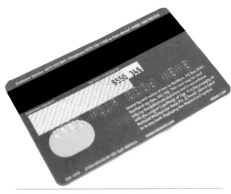

An unsigned card is an invalid card

INVALID CARDS

Invalid cards might be ones that:

- are unsigned
- are out of date
- look or feel counterfeit
- have an unclear hologram.

A card might also be invalid if the cardholder's name does not match the client's name or if a warning appears on your card machine.

INCORRECT COMPLETION OF CHEQUES

Cheques that have been incorrectly completed might have the incorrect amount in figures or words, an incorrect date or a counterfeit signature.

SUSPECTED FRAUD

If a card is declined by the merchant terminal, the card cannot be authorised or the card company suspects fraudulent spending on the card, it does not necessarily mean that the client has committed fraud and you must not accuse the client. If, however, you do suspect that fraud is taking place, excuse yourself from your client taking the card with you and inform your salon manager.

If the merchant terminal informs you that the card is stolen or counterfeit, you must follow the step-by-step instructions on the merchant terminal. The merchant provider might need to be contacted and the salon should have this number somewhere that is easily accessible. You might be told you must retain the card and in some cases, call the police. Always make sure you manager is aware of the situation before you act.

In all of the above situations, you would need to inform the client tactfully that their payment has been declined or cannot be accepted and ask for an alternative payment method. If the client does not have an alternative payment method, then ask your salon manager what you should do.

INDUSTRY TIP

Always try to resolve payment discrepancies or disputes as discreetly as possible to avoid embarrassment to both clients and staff, to avoid unhappy customers and therefore loss of profit and so that the till balances at the end of the day.

END-OF-THE-DAY TOTALS

At the end of the day, the receptionist or salon manager needs to check the days' takings. For security reasons, this should be done when the salon is closed. This procedure checks that the money in the till matches the amount that the salon has expected to take. Most tills will give a print-out to show how much has been received for each different method of payment – cash, card, voucher and cheque. The amount taken in card payments should match the print-out from the card terminal. Some till systems will also show how much has been taken by each therapist and how many retail products have been sold. These figures are all kept and form part of the salon's accounts.

KEEPING PAYMENTS SAFE AND SECURE

Every salon will have its own policy for maintaining security of payments.

To prevent **breaches** in security you must follow your salon's policy for the reception area.

Breaches

To fail to follow security procedures.

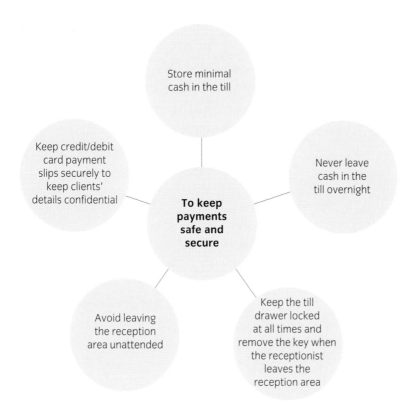

Store minimal cash in the till

Keep credit/debit card payment slips securely to keep clients' details confidential

To keep payments safe and secure

Never leave cash in the till overnight

Avoid leaving the reception area unattended

Keep the till drawer locked at all times and remove the key when the receptionist leaves the reception area

You must also make sure that client records are kept in a lockable cabinet.

> **INDUSTRY TIP**
>
> In many salons the reception is not manned permanently. It is a good idea to have a door with a buzzer or chimes that sound as the door is opened so that you know someone has come into the salon. Another alternative is a pressure-sensitive buzzer or bell that is located under a door mat that sounds when someone stands on the mat.

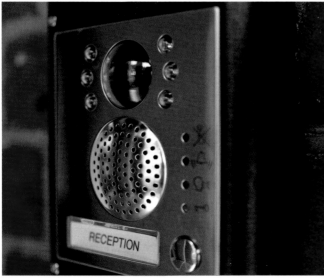

An intercom/buzzer entry device

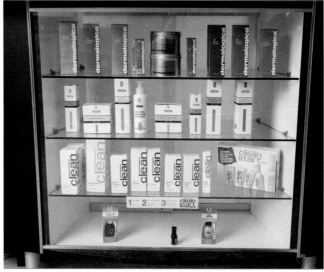

A lockable cabinet

TEST YOUR KNOWLEDGE

Use the questions below to test your knowledge of Chapter 216 to see how much information you have retained. These questions will help you revise what you have learnt in this chapter.

Turn to page 601 for the answers.

1. Why is it important that a treatment is booked for the correct time?
   a) To keep the therapist ahead of their appointments
   b) To make the salon look busy
   c) To avoid the client being charged for extra time
   d) To manage therapists' time cost effectively

2. Which **one** of the following is the first step in the booking process when dealing with a new client?
   a) Take the client's name
   b) Ask their preferred time
   c) Take the client's contact details
   d) Ask which therapist they require

3. When answering the telephone, the receptionist should ideally pick the call up before:
   a) it has rung three times
   b) it has rung five times
   c) it has rung seven times
   d) it has rung nine times.

4. Which **one** of the following is a method of verbal communication?
   a) Talking
   b) Smiling
   c) Eye contact
   d) Nodding

5. Why should a message be passed on as soon as possible?
   a) To be considerate to the caller
   b) The message might be urgent
   c) The message might be personal
   d) It might be a sales call

6. Which **one** of the following is the main reason that confidentiality must be maintained?
   a) The client will be unhappy
   b) The salon will get a poor reputation
   c) The client might take legal advice
   d) Clients might pass on information

7. Why is it important to book appointments correctly?
   a) To avoid clients having insufficient time
   b) To avoid the client turning up at the wrong time
   c) To make sure that the therapist is not working all day
   d) To make sure you have enough time for retail opportunities

8. Security should be maintained by:
   a) keeping the door locked if the reception is empty
   b) taking the keys out of the treatment room door when you have opened it
   c) keeping the till shut when it is not in use
   d) putting the appointment book under the desk.

9. When booking an appointment, which of the following is not required?
   a) The client's name
   b) Any contra-indications to treatment that the client might have
   c) The client's contact number
   d) Whether the client is new to the salon

10. When a client walks into the salon, what is the first thing that the receptionist should do?
    a) Look at the client and say 'Can I help you?'
    b) Acknowledge the client with a smile
    c) Refer to the client by their full name
    d) Look up what the client has booked in for

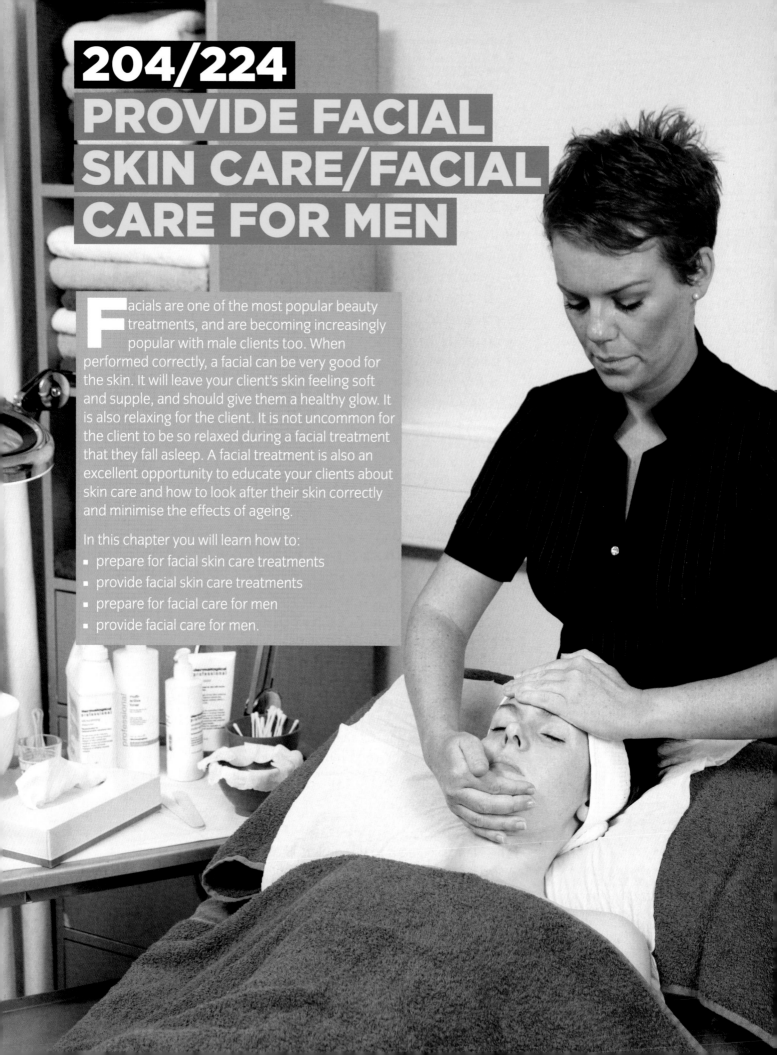

PROVIDE FACIAL SKIN CARE/FACIAL CARE FOR MEN

Facials are one of the most popular beauty treatments, and are becoming increasingly popular with male clients too. When performed correctly, a facial can be very good for the skin. It will leave your client's skin feeling soft and supple, and should give them a healthy glow. It is also relaxing for the client. It is not uncommon for the client to be so relaxed during a facial treatment that they fall asleep. A facial treatment is also an excellent opportunity to educate your clients about skin care and how to look after their skin correctly and minimise the effects of ageing.

In this chapter you will learn how to:

- prepare for facial skin care treatments
- provide facial skin care treatments
- prepare for facial care for men
- provide facial care for men.

PREPARE FOR FACIAL SKIN CARE TREATMENTS AND FACIAL CARE FOR MEN

Before you can carry out facials, it is important you are prepared. Health and safety requirements should be carried out for every service, but knowing how to set up your service area, which products and tools you should use and how to carry out an effective consultation are also essential for facial treatments.

In this part of the chapter you will learn about:

- health and safety
- the treatment environment
- skin care products
- consultation
- preparing the client
- skin analysis
- skin types and conditions
- contra-indications.

HEALTH AND SAFETY

The treatment area should be fully prepared before the client arrives. This will make sure that your client can fully relax. You should make sure that all work surfaces have been cleaned. Any equipment that needs to be sterilised, such as sponges and mask brushes, should be ready before you begin. Make sure that any equipment or products that you need are ready and easily accessible before you start so that you do not have to interrupt your treatment to go and get anything.

You should then excuse yourself and let the client know you are going to wash your hands. Refer to Chapter 202 Follow health and safety practice in the salon for a hand-washing guide.

POSITIONING YOURSELF

For health and safety you need to decide how best to position yourself. If you are going to stand you should make sure you are not leaning or overstretching as this will cause muscular aches, strains and fatigue. Ideally you should sit when you are carrying out a facial so that you can keep your back straight and your feet flat on the floor to maintain your posture.

TREATMENT ENVIRONMENT

The client also needs to be comfortable during their treatment. It is especially important for facial treatments to have a calm, pleasant and relaxing atmosphere. You can find information on how to prepare the treatment environment in Chapter 203 Client care and communication in beauty-related industries.

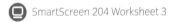 SmartScreen 204 Worksheet 3

HANDY HINTS

Look back at Chapter 202 Follow health and safety practice in the salon for advice on how to follow safe and hygienic working practices.

TREATMENT COUCH

The treatment couch should be covered and there are several different ways to prepare the treatment couch. Each tutor/college will show you a way. Also there are several different ways to prepare the client on the couch.

Whatever method you are shown for setting up your couch, make sure the couch is protected, neat, tidy and ready for the client.

ENVIRONMENTAL CONDITIONS

The following should all be checked and adjusted if necessary so that the client can relax during their treatment:

- subtle lighting – make sure there will not be any lights shining into your client's eyes
- soft, gentle, relaxing music – although some clients might actually prefer to have their treatment in silence
- warm, cosy room temperature
- good ventilation – to keep the air fresh and to prevent any draughts
- pleasing aroma – the room should have a pleasant smell
- client privacy – make sure the client feels that the treatment is private
- no unnecessary noise during the facial – avoid sounds that might disturb the client, such as stirring masks vigorously, opening packaging or moving around on a wheeled stool during the treatment
- hazard free – you should make a quick check of your working area for hazards and remove these to reduce any risks.

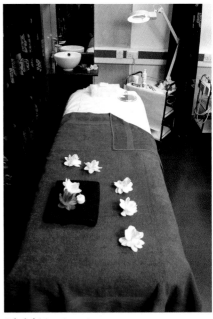

A bright treatment space

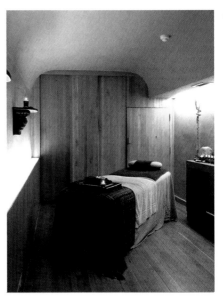

A rustic treatment room

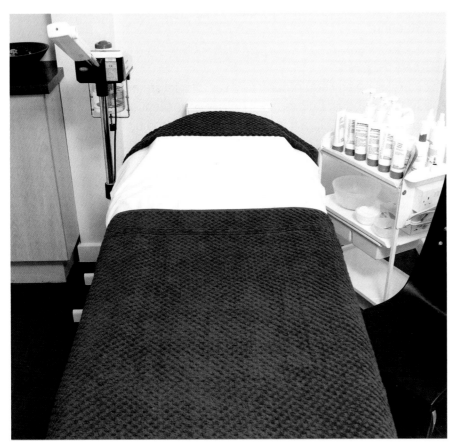

A college treatment space

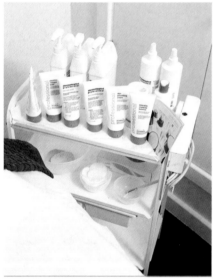

Consumables

Items that need to be replaced.

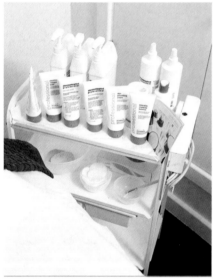

Your trolley should be organised

FACIAL TROLLEY

The trolley should be clean and set up in an organised way. There are lots of different ways to set up the trolley – your tutor/employer will show you how they want you to set up your trolley and you should follow this. Consider having the following **consumables** and equipment easily accessible. Your tutor might have taught you differently but these are some items that you might consider:

- cotton wool – some dry and some damp
- tissues – neatly laid out
- plastic or disposable spatulas for removing products from jars
- mask brush
- facial complexion/manual cleansing brush
- sponges/facial mittens or cleansing cloth
- a range of skin care products – these should be positioned so that they are in a logical order for use. Products should include:
  - eye make-up remover
  - cleanser
  - toner
  - exfoliant
  - massage cream or oil
  - masks
  - moisturisers, including eye and lip moisturisers
- two bowls/containers for damp and dry cotton wool
- cotton buds
- bowl for mixing the mask
- headband.

EQUIPMENT

If you are using any equipment, such as a facial steamer or hot towel caddy, these should be prepared before your client arrives. Check all the equipment to make sure it is safe to use; you should check for any damage, frayed flexes or broken plugs. Plug in electrical equipment and turn on the main switch. Make sure there are no trailing wires. Check the water level of the steamer and top up if necessary with the correct water. Turn on the hot towel caddy and place damp facial towels inside. Make sure that the magnifying lamp is clean, close at hand and that you can see through the magnifying lens clearly.

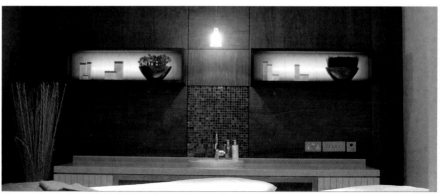

The treatment room should be calm and tranquil

SKIN CARE PRODUCTS

There are a variety of different skin care products for different skin types and conditions. In this chapter you will be given some general product guidance. It is very important that you have a good knowledge of the products you are using. You should be able to describe the texture and feel of the product. You also should know what each product contains, the skin type or condition it is suitable for and the benefits and features of using it. Each product company will have their own products and you will be given training on these.

CONSULTATION

You can find more detailed information on the consultation process and communication techniques in Chapter 203 Client care and communication in beauty-related industries.

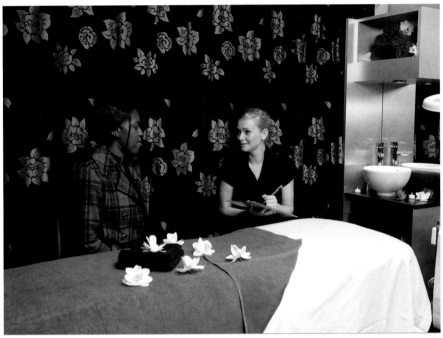

Use open body language during the consultation

The aim of a consultation is to find out what results the client is expecting from their treatment. Treatment objectives for facials usually fall into two categories:

- skin imporvement
- relaxation.

With regards to the client's expectations concerning changes to their skin, you need to be tactful and provide the client with a treatment plan that will aim to meet their expectations. You might need to recommend regular facials, perhaps supported with a skin care routine at home for maximum results.

It is now a good idea to **summarise** exactly what your facial treatment will include and what you are going to do to meet your client's treatment objectives and priorities. It is important that your client understands the treatment process.

Summarise

To give a short account of the main points.

COMMUNICATION AND BEHAVIOUR

At all times in the salon it is important that you behave in a professional manner. Professional behaviour is covered in Chapter 201 Working in beauty-related industries and can be reviewed on pages 130–134. Make sure you always follow salon requirements and work cooperatively with others to maintain a safe and pleasant working environment.

When you communicate with your client, you should follow the communication guidance given in Chapter 203 Client care and communication in beauty-related industries.

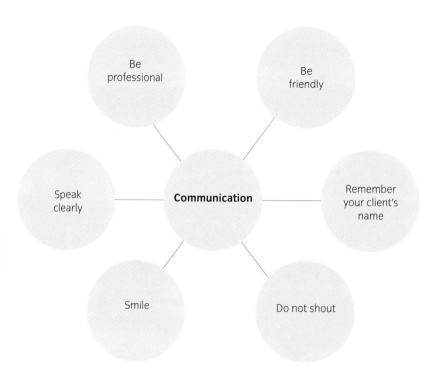

INDUSTRY TIP

Where possible you should leave the client to get undressed in private.

INDUSTRY TIP

All jewellery should be placed in the client's handbag or a secure pocket so that it is safe, secure and there is no risk of the client leaving it behind.

INDUSTRY TIP

When clients make an appointment for a facial, you might find it useful to enquire whether they wear contact lenses or not. If they do, then suggest that they either remove them before they come into the salon or bring their contact lens solution and the barrel with them so that they can remove their lenses and keep them safe during the treatment.

INDUSTRY TIP

If your client needs assistance getting on the couch, make sure you offer this. You might need to provide a step if the couch cannot be adjusted and offer them an arm to lean on as you help them onto the couch.

Modesty

Needs to be protected to avoid embarrassment.

PREPARING THE CLIENT

A good way to start your facial is to make sure your client is comfortable. The client might be nervous – give clear instructions as to how you want them to get prepared.

- If the client is wearing contact lenses, ask them to remove them. This is for comfort and is also a good idea because if any product gets in the eyes, it will attract to the lenses and make vision cloudy.
- Ask the client to remove their jewellery, including earrings and facial piercings (also watch, bracelets and rings if the facial includes an arm and hand massage).
- Ask the client to remove their shoes.
- Ask the client to remove their top. Ladies can leave their bra on but should lift their arms out of the straps. A male client will need to have the upper chest uncovered.

If possible, you should leave the client while they are getting prepared to protect their **modesty**. Instruct the client to lie face upwards on the couch when ready and cover themselves with the cover.

CLIENT COMFORT

When the client is on the couch, you can then make them comfortable. Make sure they are warm enough. Place a cushion under the client's knees for comfort. This helps to tilt the pelvis so that the back is more comfortable. Ask the client if they want their arms tucked under the cover or out.

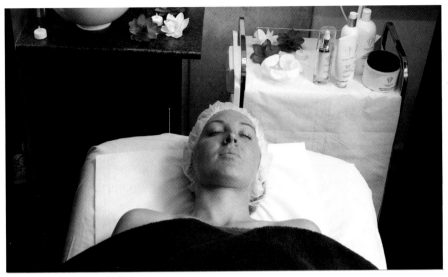

Client prepared for a facial

Cover the client with a towel, blanket or duvet leaving the **décolleté** area uncovered. In the winter the client will need something warmer so they do not get cold during the treatment and in the summer something lighter, possibly even just a towel across the chest if it is very warm. Apply a headband to protect the client's hair and make sure all stray hairs are tucked under the band.

SKIN ANALYSIS

Before reading through the next section, you should make sure you have read the section on the skin in the Anatomy and Physiology chapter. You should be familiar with all the skin characteristics discussed in this chapter. This will give you a greater understanding of why a skin analysis should always be carried out before every facial, even on a regular client.

Our skin is changing all the time and there are lots of factors, such as ill health, that can cause changes in our skin. The skin should be analysed after a **superficial** cleanse with a light, gentle cleanser. While you are doing this, you can assess the skin to find out which cleanser to use for the second deeper cleanse. The skin should be viewed using a magnifying lamp so that you can see it up close and in detail.

A skin analysis is carried out to:

- check for contra-indications
- identify specific areas for treatment
- make sure that a suitable treatment plan is provided
- make sure the client is treated with products suitable for their skin type and condition
- build a **rapport** with the client and gain their confidence
- check progress following a previous treatment.

INDUSTRY TIP

It is unnatural to lie completely flat so for comfort the natural curves of the body should be supported (neck, back and behind the knees). Try to achieve this for your client by supporting the neck with a small cushion or folded towel and by placing a cushion behind the knees.

Décolleté

Lower neckline – in beauty therapy this includes the neck and upper chest down to where the bust line starts.

INDUSTRY TIP

Some clients get very hot – you should always check with the client what amount of cover is comfortable for them.

Superficial

On the surface; not deep or penetrating.

Rapport

An easy understanding of feelings and attitudes between two people.

Pigmentation

The colouration of tissues by pigment.

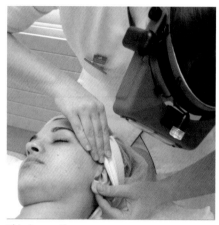

Skin inspection

INDUSTRY TIP

Avoid stating a specific skin type when you first look at your client's skin. In reality, the majority of people have a combination skin type. However, not all combination skin is the same. Analyse the skin first and make your assessment based on the skin's condition, characteristics and your observations. Make a note of these on your record card before naming a skin type. Remember, initial impressions can be misleading and if you decide on a skin type before you have carried out a thorough analysis, your client's skin will not get the maximum benefit from the treatment. Some clients might be more concerned about treating a skin condition, eg sensitivity or ageing, rather than their skin type, so there are lots of factors you must consider.

INDUSTRY TIP

To determine whether the client's skin is dehydrated, lightly pinch the skin around the facial contours and eye area. Does the skin show good elasticity and spring back into shape quickly? Or does it show signs of dehydration and look parched between the fingertips?

SKIN ANALYSIS CONSIDERATIONS

When inspecting the skin you should consider the following factors:

- The skin's age and how it is being affected by the ageing process. Are there changes to elasticity and muscle tone?
- Is the **pigmentation** on the face even or patchy?
- The pH balance of the skin. This is the acidity of the skin, which will affect whether it is obviously oily or dry.
- What is the texture of the skin – how does it feel to the touch? Is it smooth or coarse, showing signs of dryness or poor exfoliation? A tacky feel will indicate high oil content.
- The skin's temperature. Is it warm or cool? A dry skin tends to feel warm and a very oily skin can feel cool.
- Does the client have good bone structure? This helps to minimise some signs of ageing.
- Are there any skin imperfections or skin abnormalities, such as comedones, thread veins, papules, scar tissue, moles or superfluous hair?
- With male clients, look at the growth pattern of facial hair, how much there is and its texture.

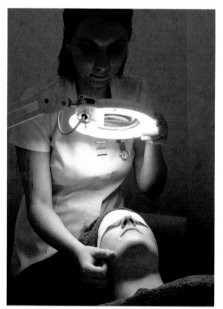

Skin analysis using a magnifier and lamp

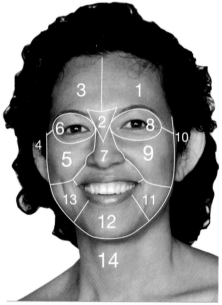

Face mapping

INDUSTRY TIP

If you have access to a woods lamp, these are really useful. This is a special lamp which uses ultraviolet light in the dark to highlight the skin's imperfections. It helps to show the client the condition of their skin to support your analysis.

Look at each of the main areas of the face rather than at the face as a whole. Check the neck, chin, each cheek, nose, bridge of the nose and the forehead.

Make a note of anything you can see or feel. When you have done all of this you can then decide on your client's skin type and condition.

Several factors can affect the condition of a client's skin and should be considered in your skin analysis, treatment plan and recommendations. These include:

Skin condition

Skin condition (central node) connects to:

Occupation – if the client works outside or in extremes of temperature this will have an adverse effect on the skin. It can make the skin dry, dehydrated and increase **photo-ageing**.

Smoking – cigarettes contain lots if unhealthy toxins. Smoking affects the quality of oxygen absorbed in the lungs. It destroys vitamin C, which is important for healthy skin and affects the production of collagen, causing premature ageing.

Drinking too much alcohol on a regular basis or binge drinking can increase the risk of liver damage. This is an important organ which helps to process nutrients and remove toxins from the body.

Lack of home care and use of incorrect products – this will mean that the skin might be neglected, unprotected and there is a higher risk of aging more rapidly.

Social habits

It is important to get enough sleep as a lack of sleep can make the skin look dull. When we are asleep, the body spends a lot of time repairing itself.

A lack of activity or exercise can make both the body and skin sluggish. This can be seen as dull skin that might be prone to congestion due to poor circulation.

History of the skin – where does the client come from? A client could have spent some years living abroad in very different climates. A client who has lived in a hot country will be more prone to photo-aging. If the skin is exposed daily to high levels of ultraviolet light it will be become damaged and the effects of aging will be more obvious at a younger age.

Stress – this damages the body in many ways. When we are stressed, the body is too busy preparing to defend itself and does not work well. When we are very stressed, the immune system suffers and we are more likely to become ill.

Diet and fluid intake – if the client has a poor or unhealthy diet (this can include too little food as well as too much) it will mean that the body does not have the essential nutrients it needs to repair and keep the body in a healthy state. It is important to take in enough fluids to prevent dehydration. Water is best as in its pure state it does not contain any chemicals that the body will need to work hard to remove.

Some medication can alter the skin's texture, eg steroids can cause the skin to become thinner and more fragile.

General state of health – if this is poor it is quite likely that the skin will reflect this and look dull. If the client is healthy the skin will usually be healthy too.

Photo-ageing
Damage to the skin caused by exposure to UV light.

ACTIVITY

Carry out a skin analysis on a colleague and make a note of everything you see, but do not write down a skin type. If you can, carry out a skin analysis on someone older than yourself and on a young child (if they will stay still for long enough!). Compare and discuss your results in your class.

SKIN TYPES AND CONDITIONS

We treat skin according to its skin type and characteristics. The skin type is based around the level of natural oil and moisture the skin has. The condition of the skin is in addition to the skin type and tends to be affected by internal and external factors. It is important to consider this in your choice of skin care and the techniques you will use during a treatment. Further information can be found in the Anatomy and Physiology chapter on pages 2–30.

INDUSTRY TIP

It is important that you understand how lifestyle has an impact on the anatomy and physiology of the body. There is further information on how internal and external factors affect the body in the Anatomy and Physiology chapter.

INDUSTRY TIP

Recommend that clients drink water rather than tea, coffee, fizzy drinks and alcohol as these can all make the body dehydrated.

INDUSTRY TIP

Recommend that clients get a good 8 hours sleep regularly if they can (and you should too!) This is the recommended amount to keep the body working well.

Skin type or condition	What does it feel like?	What does it look like?	What are the characteristics?	Cause of skin type or condition	How skin ages
Dry	Fine texture or slightly coarse if very dry and neglected	Paler tone, pinkish or rosy due to dilated capillaries	▪ matte or crepey appearance ▪ dehydrated, causing skin cells to lift slightly; might lead to flaky patches and more leathery look to skin ▪ skin might appear more transparent and be highly vascular so that it is red, with capillaries visible through the skin's surface ▪ no prominent pores ▪ warm to touch	▪ photo-ageing ▪ hormonal changes, such as during and following the menopause ▪ lack of skin care ▪ exposure to air conditioning ▪ smoking ▪ crash diets, lack of proper nutrition ▪ illness	Skin prone to early signs of ageing
Oily	Medium texture; might be coarser around the nose and cheeks; might be moist to the touch	Sallow, grey appearance and skin tone	▪ shiny ▪ open, relaxed pores ▪ comedones ▪ flaky patches due to poor desquamation	▪ hormonal changes, eg puberty ▪ ethnic origin, eg Afro-Caribbeans might have a more oily skin	Tends to show signs of ageing at a slower rate
Balanced (normal)	Medium to fine texture	Healthy, vibrant glow	▪ even distribution of secretions; no blemishes	▪ most of us start off with a balanced skin. As we grow our environment and changes in our body alter its appearance	Ageing will be at a normal rate and will depend on other influencing factors, such as lifestyle and diet

Skin type or condition	What does it feel like?	What does it look like?	What are the characteristics?	Cause of skin type or condition	How skin ages
Combination	Variable in different parts of the face; the skin will have a combination of the different characteristics depending on skin type	Oily or dry characteristic depending on skin type	▪ typical characteristics of a dry/balanced/oily skin; commonly oily T-zone and dry cheeks and neck	▪ see skin types above as applicable	The different areas of skin will age according to the characteristics of each type – see the information above
Sensitive	Might have coarse texture or be delicate and fine	Prone to blemishes, has a rosy appearance and is warm to the touch	▪ flushes easily ▪ burns easily in the sun ▪ rapid change in colour when exposed to temperature change ▪ skin might be reactive to touch and colour easily ▪ might be sensitive to product ingredients and susceptible to allergic reactions	▪ dry and dehydrated skin types ▪ use of incorrect products ▪ allergies	Prone to premature ageing
Dehydrated	Feel of the skin will depend on skin type; if the skin is squeezed very gently between the fingers, fine lines will be visible	There might be no obvious change to the skin's appearance	▪ very fine lines around the eye area and jaw ▪ skin absorbs creams rapidly	▪ lack of hydration ▪ use of incorrect, harsh products ▪ illness	Prone to premature ageing
Mature	The skin has a more padded appearance caused by the slowing of new skin cell production; lines and wrinkles can easily be felt	Dull; lifeless; lack of colour	▪ lines ▪ crepey appearance ▪ papery appearance ▪ fine lines around jaw ▪ loss of elasticity and tone ▪ pigmentation changes ▪ lentigines or age spots	▪ collagen is not replaced very quickly so the activity of the skin and replacement of new skin cells slows down	Ageing has already begun

SmartScreen 204 Worksheet 5

CONTRA-INDICATIONS

A contra-indication is a reason why a treatment might be restricted or prevented. It might be an absolute contra-indication, which means the client cannot be treated at all, or one which might require the treatment to be restricted and/or modified. If you think that the client should seek medical advice then suggest this but, remember, you are not a medical practitioner and you should not make any form of diagnosis.

In some cases the contra-indication will just restrict the treatment. Examples are a bruise or an area of open skin, eg eczema. You will need to work around these areas. In other cases the treatment will need to be modified. For example, if the client has a product allergy you might be restricted in the products and the treatment you can offer.

You should always explain the situation to the client if you are going to have to avoid an area or modify a treatment. The client must agree to this before you start.

ACTIVITY

Make a list of contra-indications that would prevent you from carrying out a facial. For each one, state whether you could offer an alternative treatment and what this treatment would be.

ACTIVITY

Make a list of 10 contra-indications that would restrict a facial treatment. Next to each one, write down how you would modify the treatment.

Contra-indications are covered in the Anatomy and Physiology chapter. Make sure you are familiar with the contra-indications listed below, especially those relating to the skin.

- **Prevent treatment:** fungal infection, bacterial infection, viral infection, infestations, severe eczema, severe psoriasis, severe skin conditions, eye infections, during chemotherapy, during radiotherapy.
- **Restrict treatment:** broken bones, recent scar tissue, hyper-keratosis, skin allergies, cuts and abrasions, epilepsy, diabetes, high and low blood pressure, skin disorders, undiagnosed lumps and swellings, product allergies.

 SmartScreen 204 Worksheet 6

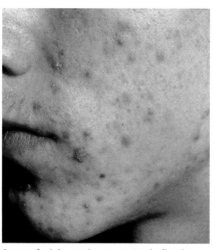

Severe facial acne is one contra-indication that can prevent a facial treatment

PROVIDE FACIAL SKIN CARE TREATMENTS AND FACIAL CARE FOR MEN

Before you start your facial, you must have a good understanding of the products you will be using and their ingredients. Different products will vary and it will be impossible to cover every ingredient here. You must make sure that you know the manufacturer's instructions on how to use the products. You should know the key ingredients and the benefits of each product. You should be given the important ingredients of the skin-care range you are using in a training manual. Most skin care products have the ingredients listed on the box or the product container.

In this part of the chapter you will learn about:

- emulsions
- exfoliants and facial scrubs
- warming devices
- facial massage
- face masks
- moisturisers
- completing the facial
- home care and aftercare advice
- contra-actions
- completing records
- good practice
- men's grooming.

EMULSIONS

In **cosmetic science**, creams and lotions are grouped together and generally referred to as emulsions. An **emulsion** consists of two liquids mixed together. One liquid is often purified water (aqua). The other liquid is usually oil. An emulsifier is added to make sure that these two liquids remain evenly mixed and do not separate.

There are two main types of emulsion:

- A water-in-oil emulsion is where the water is dispersed in the oil. These are rich, heavy creams, such as night creams.
- An oil-in-water emulsion is usually lighter than a cream. General moisturisers, lotions and milks fall into this category. Gels are transparent oil-in-water emulsions and usually contain a cellulose thickener.

COMMON COSMETIC INGREDIENTS

Products must by law have their ingredients listed. This is important so that you know what they contain and can avoid certain ingredients if you need to. For example, if a client has a nut allergy you could check the label to make sure the product is nut free. The ingredients are always listed in order of amount, so the top ingredient would be in the largest quantity and the items at the bottom of the list in the smallest amounts.

Cosmetic science
The research and development of skin care and cosmetic products.

Emulsion
Creams and lotions made up of two liquids mixed together.

Every product will be slightly different as each manufacturer will want unique features for their product to make it different from another manufacturer's product. Some common ingredients are described in the table. When you become familiar with these ingredients, you will be able to link them easily to features and benefits.

INDUSTRY TIP

Essential oils and vegetable oils used in products are usually listed by their Latin names, which is why you will not always recognise them.

Ingredient	Purpose	Examples
Preservative	substance added to keep a product balanced and safe, and to prevent it from decaying; prolongs its **shelf life**	vitamin C, isopropyl alcohol
Emollient	an action or substance that softens the skin	wheat-germ oil, linoleic acid, allantoin, sweet almond oil, shea butter, beeswax
Humectant	substance that holds water and prevents the product from drying out	glycerol, sorbitol, lactic acid, urea, hyaluronic acid, salicylic acid
Buffer	controls the **pH** of the product and prevents changes in the acidity or alkalinity; a pH that is too high or too low can irritate the skin	glycolic acid, potassium hydroxide, malic acid magnesium carbonate, lactic acid
Antioxidant	holds harmful molecules together and minimises their destructive power; prevents the chemical deterioration of the product (antioxidants also assist in the repair of damaged cells)	grapeseed extract, ascorbic acid, benzoic acid
Emulsifier	stabilises the ingredients and keeps the ingredients evenly **distributed** so they do not separate	glycerol stearate, **acetyl alcohol**

Shelf life

The length of time a product can stay stable or usable before opening; after this period of time the product might not be usable and will start to go off.

Humectant

An ingredient that draws water to it.

pH

An abbreviation of the 'potential of **Hydrogen**' – a measure of the hydrogen ion concentration of a substance.

Hydrogen

A gas that has no colour or smell.

Distributed

Spread over an area.

Acetyl alcohol

An example of an emulsifier.

Ingredient	Purpose	Examples
Solvent	the liquid in which other molecules are dissolved	purified water (aqua), isopropyl alcohol
Thickener	increases the **viscosity** of a product	cellulose, beeswax, xanthan gum
Essential oil	a delicate oil made up of tiny organic molecules produced from plants and trees; commonly extracted by the **distillation** of leaves, flowers (petals), seeds, stalks, bark and roots; added to products to provide various therapeutic effects	rose, cedar wood, cinnamon
Perfume	added to give a product a pleasing smell and to mask the smell of some of the raw ingredients	essential oils

Viscosity

How runny or thick a product is; a viscous product is one that is very thick.

Distillation

Purifying or separating a mixture by using evaporation or boiling.

ACTIVITY

Look at three products you have in your salon and see if you recognise any of the ingredients. What is the largest ingredient in each product?

pH LEVELS

Different products will have different pH levels. A product that is used daily should ideally have a pH level that is similar to that of the skin, ie pH 4.5–6. If a product is very alkaline, eg a bar of soap (face soap can have a pH of 7; soap for the body can be as high as pH 9) it will be very drying on the skin, stripping the natural oil content from the surface. This is what makes the skin feel tight following its use. If a product is more acidic (below pH 4.5) it will cause irritation to the skin. Some salon treatments use products with different pH levels to achieve a specific effect, eg glycolic acid peels, and must be used by carefully trained professionals and the skin carefully rebalanced following treatment to prevent any skin irritation.

CLEANSERS

A cleanser should be easy to use, have a pleasant feel on the skin and be economical. Cleansers are used for the following reasons:

- to remove make-up
- to remove surface debris, including dead skin cells and pollution
- to allow the skin's acid mantle to function better.

We describe cleansers by how viscous (runny or thick) they are.

Cleansing waters

These have a very light texture and a more liquid-like consistency. Some are very light gels. Cleansing waters are designed for quick, easy use and do not usually need to be used in conjunction with a toner. They are a good product to recommend to clients who only need a light cleanse and who are not wearing make-up.

Wash-off cleansers

These are light cleansers that can be applied and worked into the skin before washing off. They are created for clients who like the feel of water on the skin as part of the cleansing process. Many products for oily or problem skin fall into this category. Some wash-off cleansers produce a foam. The product is gently made into a foam by rubbing it into the fingers before applying it to the skin. This makes application easier and it can be easily rinsed off.

Gel cleansers

These cleaners have a light, non-greasy feel to them and a transparent appearance. They are usually applied to the skin, followed by a little water and the cleanser is then worked into a foam. Many cleansers for men are gel-based cleansers. Shaving gels work in a similar way. Gels are usually recommended for oily or combination skin.

Cleansing milks

These have a light, more liquid texture and can be poured easily. If they are very liquid (like milk) they will need to be applied to a cotton pad before application to the skin.

- They are generally good for young or oily skin as they have a light, non-oily (water-in-oil) texture.
- They are great for sensitive skin as they are light and easily worked into the skin.
- Some milks are made for dry skin with an oil-in-water formula and a richer feel.

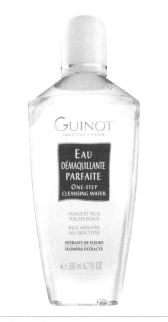

Cleansing water

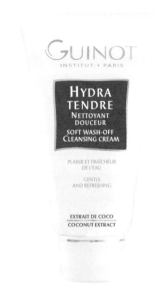

Wash-off cleanser

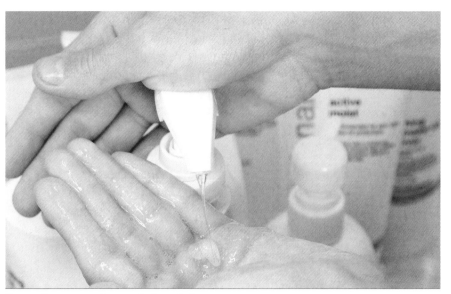

Pumps dipsense a set amount of product

Cleansing lotions

These are the most popular type of cleanser. They can be applied directly to the skin and massaged gently in, before removing with damp cotton wool. Their texture is usually light and they are easy to pour and use.

Cleansing creams

These are richer and have a creamy texture. Some are almost solid and need to be warmed before use to make the product liquefy (become runny). Creams are good for removing heavy make-up and are used on drier skin.

Cleansing bars and soaps

These were originally designed for clients who liked the feel of soap and water. They still tend to be more alkaline and therefore have a drying effect on the skin, making the skin feel tight. They are not a popular choice now as most people are aware that they are not a good product to use as part of a good skin care routine.

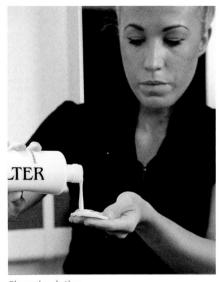

Cleansing lotion

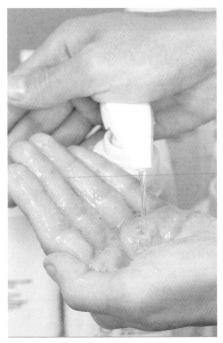

Pump action gel cleaners

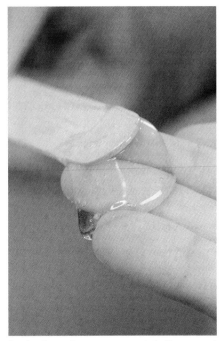

For hygiene always use a spatula if you need to remove products from a pot or jar

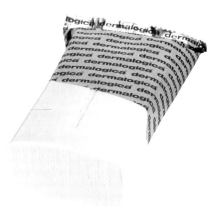

Cleansing bar

Eye make-up remover

This is a product specially designed for removing make-up from the delicate eye area. It is more gentle than a normal cleanser to avoid any stinging sensations should the product get into the eyes.

> **INDUSTRY TIP**
>
> Cleansing wipes are wipes which are soaked in a cleanser. They are popular as they are easy to use. They are effective cleansers as they usually have a high mineral content. However, they should not be used all the time as they can clog the skin as the cleanser leaves a surface residue. Products that do this are described as **comedogenic**. They are quite expensive to use when you compare them to the number of applications obtainable from a cleanser and the fact that one wipe is often not enough to remove make-up thoroughly.

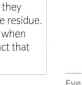

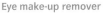

Eye make-up remover

Comedogenic

An ingredient or product that blocks the skin and causes comedones.

ACTIVITY

Make a chart listing all the different skin types and skin conditions. Next to each skin type, write the name of the cleanser that you have in your salon that is suitable to use for that skin type and condition.

You could add to this the features and benefits of each of the cleansers you have chosen. Think about feel, smell, packaging, etc.

How to use a cleanser

Cleansers can be used in different ways. The table below offers guidance as to how each product is best applied and removed.

Cleanser	Application	Removal
Cleansing water	Apply the product to damp cotton wool and wipe over the area to be cleansed. Repeat the process until the skin is clean.	As the product is applied using cotton wool there is no separate removal technique required.
Cleansing milks	If the product is very liquid, apply to damp cotton wool and wipe over the area to be cleansed. Repeat the process until the skin is clean. If the milk is slightly thicker, place a small amount of product onto the fingertips. Apply directly to the skin using the fingers. Gently massage into the skin using circular movements.	If the product is applied using cotton wool there is no separate removal technique required. If the product is applied using the fingertips, remove from the skin using damp cotton wool.
Cleansing lotions	Apply a small amount to the fingertips and warm by rubbing the fingertips together. Apply directly to the skin from the hands. Gently massage into the skin's surface to loosen make-up or surface debris.	Remove from the skin using damp cotton wool.
Cleansing creams	Apply a small amount to the fingertips and warm by rubbing the fingertips together. Apply directly to the skin from the hands. Gently massage into the skin's surface to loosen make-up or surface debris.	Remove from the skin using damp cotton wool.
Cleansing gels or foaming cleansers	Place a small amount of product onto the fingers and add a little water to liquefy the product or create a foam. Apply directly to the skin using the fingertips. Gently massage into the skin using circular movements.	Rinse well with lukewarm water until all the cleanser is removed.
Cleansing bars	Work the bar into the hands with a little water to loosen the surface of the cleansing bar. Work the product into the skin using gentle circular movements.	Rinse well with lukewarm water until all the cleanser is removed.

SALON CLEANSE

The cleansing routine shown in these step-by-steps is just one way of doing it; your salon or training establishment might show you a different cleansing routine that they will want you to use.

Make sure the client's hair is secured in a headband and that all loose, stray hairs are tucked up into the headband out of the way.

Cleansing the eyes and mouth

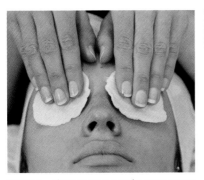

STEP 1 – Place some eye make-up remover onto two round pads of damp cotton wool. Ask your client to close their eyes. Place the pads onto your client's eyes and press gently downwards, working the cleanser onto the lashes. Leave the pads in place to loosen the eye make-up.

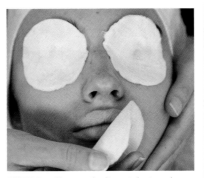

STEP 2 – Cleanse the lips – take two damp pads of cotton wool and place a little cleanser onto one pad. Press the two pads together so that the cleanser is now on both pads. Support the side of the mouth with one hand and wipe across the mouth with the pad in the other hand. Alternate the pads. If the client is wearing lipstick this should be repeated until you have removed the lipstick.

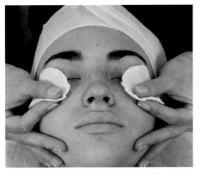

STEP 3 – Return to the eyes. Gently remove the pad from one eye, wiping gently across the eye area from the outer eye to the inner eye.

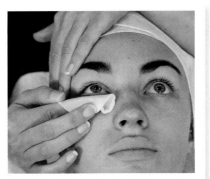

STEP 4 – Ask your client to look up and clean under each of the eyes with the pad from that eye until the area is clean. Repeat with the other eye.

> **INDUSTRY TIP**
>
> You do not want to chat all the way through a facial but you will want to let the client know what you are doing. You can do this by placing a hand on the client's shoulder before applying a product. Always let your client know when you are about to apply hot towels or cold cotton wool pads so that they are prepared and will not be shocked by the change in temperature.

> **INDUSTRY TIP**
>
> The skin around the eye is very delicate and one of the thinnest areas of skin on the body. It is one of the first areas to show the signs of ageing. It should be treated gently and always gently supported. As it is different from other areas of the face, it is a good idea to recommend that the client uses specific eye products, eg eye make-up removers and eye creams, to hydrate the skin. Using incorrect products or products that are too rich can make the tissue around the eye area puffy.

> **INDUSTRY TIP**
>
> When you work around the eye to cleanse the area, you should always place the hand you are not cleansing with on the skin to support it. The skin around the eye is very delicate; you should avoid stretching or pulling the skin.

> **INDUSTRY TIP**
>
> If the client is wearing lots of eye make-up, especially mascara, you might need to work the cleanser more thoroughly onto the eyelashes using a cotton bud or the tip of your ring finger.

> **INDUSTRY TIP**
>
> Always use different pads to cleanse each eye; never use the same pad. This is necessary to avoid any possible cross-infection.

Cleansing the face

The first cleanse is a superficial light cleanse that covers the décolleté, neck and face. This gently cleanses the face and removes any surface residue or make-up so that you can decide more accurately which products are best suited to the skin. For the superficial cleanse you should use a light lotion cleanser suitable for all skin types.

When you have carried out a skin analysis on clean skin, you can then carry out a deep cleanse. You do not need to cleanse the eyes and lips again – just the face. This cleanse follows the same routine as the superficial cleanse but is carried out more slowly, with smaller, deeper circular movements, making sure that the whole facial area has been thoroughly cleansed.

Female facial cleansing

Before you start, put some cleanser onto your fingertips. Rub the fingertips together away from your client's head and face to warm the product.

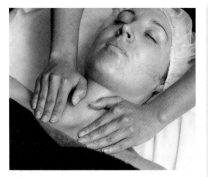

STEP 1 – Starting with the fingertips on the sternum, apply the cleanser to the décolleté.

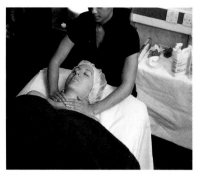

STEP 2 – Work the cleanser into the skin with the fingers, using large circular movements and working across the décolleté.

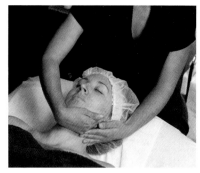

STEP 3 – Moving up onto the neck, make upward sweeping movements using the whole hand to mould to the shape of the neck. Keep movements light and avoid any pressure over the throat as this can be unpleasant for your client.

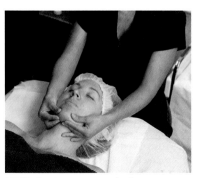

STEP 4 – Continue onto the face. Start on the chin using quick circular movements with the thumbs and then work upwards and outwards with the fingertips, using small circular movements.

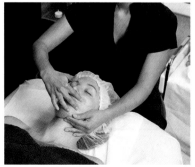

STEP 5 – Using the thumbs or fingertips, work around the nose, taking care not to close the nostrils and prevent breathing.

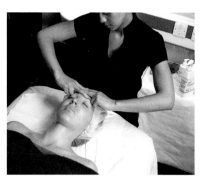

STEP 6 – Slide the hands up the bridge of the nose and cleanse over the forehead using quick circular movements. Finish with the fingertips of one hand on each temple.

Male facial cleansing

For male clients, apply the cleanser in reverse to work with the facial hair growth.

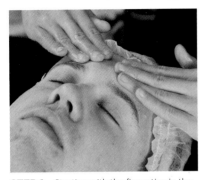

STEP 1 – Starting with the fingertips in the centre of the forehead, cleanse the forehead using circular movements.

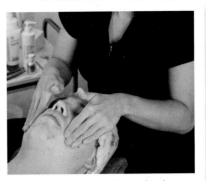

STEP 2 – With one hand on each side, work down the face using circular movements of the fingertips, working in towards the nose.

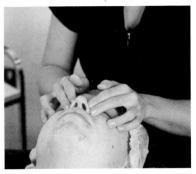

STEP 3 – Work around the nose using the thumbs or fingertips.

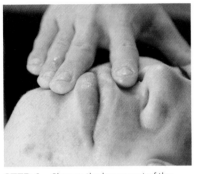

STEP 4 – Cleanse the lower part of the face, sliding two fingers around the lips.

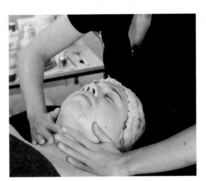

STEP 5 – Sweep the hands down the neck, following the direction of hair growth.

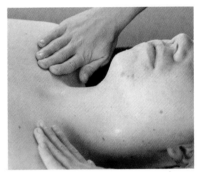

STEP 6 – Massage across the décolleté using the fingertips. Slide the hands around to the back of the shoulders and neck. To finish, bring the fingers over and onto the face and finish with the fingers on the temples.

Removing the cleanser

For female clients: remove the cleansing product from the skin with damp cotton wool, sponges or cleansing mittens, working from the décolleté up the neck and from the centre of the face outwards, up to the forehead.

For male clients: place sponges or cleansing mittens onto the forehead and using both hands, remove the cleanser by working outwards across the forehead, passing gently under the eyes. Then work gently down the face to work in line with the direction of hair growth. Avoid using cotton wool as it will snag on the hair stubble.

Blot the skin dry. Perform a skin analysis and change the products if necessary.

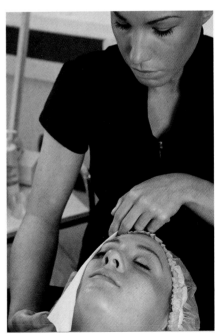

Blot the skin dry after removing the cleanser

Desquamation

Shedding or removal of the outermost layer of the skin.

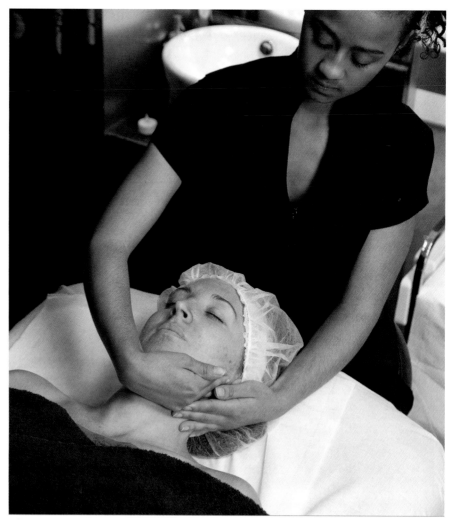

When working cleanser into the neck, avoid applying pressure to the throat

Manual cleansing brush

Deep cleansing can be carried out using a small manual cleansing or complexion brush. These have soft, synthetic bristles so that they do not drag or scratch the skin. They are used to work a cleanser deeper into the skin's tissues to aid **desquamation** and remove impurities.

Method for using a cleansing brush

Before you begin, make sure the cleansing brush you are using has been disinfected. Ask your client to close their eyes and then apply damp cotton pads to protect their eyes and prevent any product splashing into them.

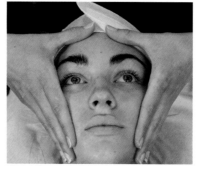

STEP 1 – Apply cleanser to your client's skin with the hands.

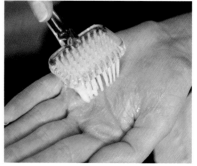

STEP 2 – Dampen the cleansing brush in warm water.

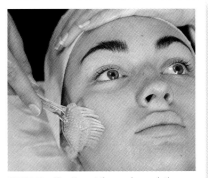

STEP 3 – Starting at the neck, work the brush gently into the skin using small circular movements. Press the bristles slightly into the skin as you circle the brush. Do not scrub the skin. Work over the entire face.

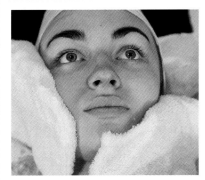

STEP 4 – Remove the cleanser with either a hot towel or damp cotton wool. Tone the skin (see below).

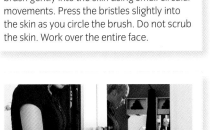

STEP 5 – Clean the brush with an antibacterial soap. Spray with an antibacterial spray. Allow to dry and then store in a UV caddy.

TONERS

Toners have the following benefits:

- They remove any remaining cleanser (an additional cleanse). This helps to prevent any unwanted product sitting on the skin and causing blocked pores or skin **congestion**.
- They restore the acid mantle. We need to balance this so that the skin does not have to overwork trying to rebalance itself.
- They refine the pores.
- They refresh the skin.
- They balance the pH levels following cleansing.

Toners can be used with any skin type depending on the **formulation** and ingredients, so it is important to check the manufacturer's recommendation before use. Different names are given to different strengths of toning products.

Astringents

The strongest toners are astringents and these are used on very oily skin. They contain alcohol, which is very good for **degreasing** the skin's surface but is quite strong. It makes the skin work hard to rebalance and restore its pH following application. On other skin types alcohol can be very dehydrating.

Rosacea

This condition is a chronic long-term skin disorder causing redness and swelling of the face. It is caused by congestion and enlargement of the superficial blood capillaries on the face. It leaves the skin prone to flushing. More information on this condition can be found in the Anatomy and Physiology chapter.

Congestion

Blocking or obstruction of an area; in this context it refers to blocking or obstruction of the skin.

Formulation

How something is created.

Degreasing

Removing grease.

Tonics

These are toners that are used on dry or more delicate skin. They have no alcohol content and are gentle on the skin.

Fresheners

These are very mild toners for dry or delicate skin. They can also be used as a 'pick-me-up' in hot weather to freshen the skin. Many are made from floral waters. This is the fragrant water that is left after extracting essential oils from flowers, eg rose, or orange flower water.

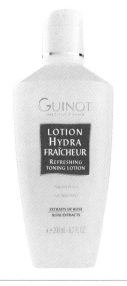

A freshener toning lotion

How to use a toner

A toner can be applied in three ways:

- The most common way to apply a toner is by placing it onto damp cotton wool pads. The pad is then gently wiped over the skin's surface until the whole face has been covered. This will complement and complete a cleanse.

- A spritzer is a toner applied using a fine spray that gently drops onto the skin in a fine mist. It is applied from behind the head, first making sure the client has their eyes and mouth closed. Usually two or three quick pumps of the spray is adequate. This is a great way of freshening the skin.

- A further method is used in more specialised treatments. A piece of gauze, large enough to cover the face, is soaked in toner and then gently laid over the facial area.

204/224 PROVIDE FACIAL SKIN CARE/FACIAL CARE FOR MEN

INDUSTRY TIP

Alcohol in products will degrease and dehydrate the skin.

INDUSTRY TIP

Encourage clients to use the same brand of cleanser and toner as these are designed to work together to give the best results. Some cleansers and toners are incompatible (will not work together) so the skin might not be cleansed properly.

INDUSTRY TIP

Always use a toner unless the directions on a cleanser state that one is not required. If you do not use a toner when one is required, it can take the skin 8 hours to repair and rebalance its acid mantle following cleansing.

INDUSTRY TIP

It is more hygienic and cost-effective, both in the salon and at home, to use products, eg toners and cleansers, that have a pump dispenser rather than a pouring bottle.

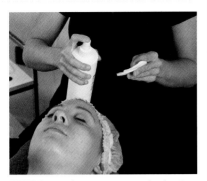

STEP 1 – Apply toner to two pads of cotton wool pressed together. Open the pads.

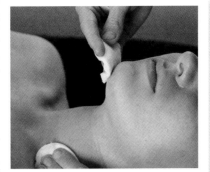

STEP 2 – Tone the face starting at the décolleté. Slowly place the pads onto the skin (the toner will be cold).

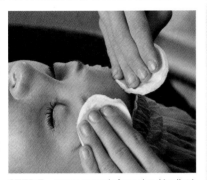

STEP 3 – Wipe upwards from the décolleté to the neck, lower face, cheeks and finally across the forehead.

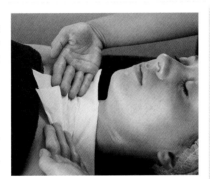

STEP 4 – Open a tissue and place it across the lower part of the face/neck. Press down to blot the skin dry, remove and place on the upper part of the face; press down and remove. When you do this, make sure you do not cover your client's nose. Check with the fingertips that the skin is dry.

INDUSTRY TIP

Warn the client what to expect – that the sprizter might feel cold as the mist drops onto the skin. Ask the client to breathe in, then spray over the face from the head downwards as the client breathes out.

INDUSTRY TIP

Some brands of toner use a spritzer-type spray. This is a toner in a natural spray dispenser. To apply a spray toner, ask the client to first close their eyes and mouth.

INDUSTRY TIP

When you cleanse, tone, exfoliate and massage, check that your movements are gentle around the nose and that you are not closing the client's nasal passages. This will be unpleasant for the client and might make them feel **claustrophobic**.

Claustrophobia

Fear of enclosed or confined spaces.

Dermabrasion

Very deep skin exfoliation using electrical equipment with either crystals or a diamond head attachment.

EXFOLIANTS AND FACIAL SCRUBS

To exfoliate means to peel off the scales. The function of an exfoliant is to:

- give a deeper cleanse
- remove the build-up of dead skin cells
- remove impurities
- improve the appearance and texture of the skin.

Exfoliation can be carried out manually using a product, which is what we will be looking at here, or using chemical or mechanical equipment, such as **dermabrasion**.

TYPES OF EXFOLIANT

Different types of exfoliant are available depending on the skin type, skin condition and the depth of exfoliation required. All types of skin benefit from regular exfoliating; most clients would benefit from a weekly exfoliation treatment. An exfoliant can also be known as a scrub. The texture of an exfoliant can vary from a rich cream to a thick paste.

Exfoliant	Benefit	Application	Active ingredients	Skin condition	Precautions
Gritty exfoliants/ scrubs	Exfoliants often contain tiny **beads** (mechanical exfoliation) that, when massaged into the skin, lift off the dead skin and clean away any unwanted surface debris. **Enzyme** A protein that speeds up a chemical process where one substance is changed into something different.	Applied to the skin and gently massaged into the surface. The product is removed with warm water and facial mittens or sponges. **Bead** Tiny circular ball.	The beads can be made from polyethylene balls that are a smooth, synthetic exfoliant. Alternatively the exfoliant can be derived from fruit or nut kernels. These tend to be harsher than beads and scratch away at the skin to exfoliate.	Both types are good on coarse skin with lots of dead skin cells that need to be removed to improve the skin texture. They are good for: ■ oily skin, to stimulate the skin and remove some of the surface congestion ■ skin that has poor circulation ■ skin that needs revitalising and brightening ■ evening out the skin's texture, eg a fading tan.	They should not be used on sensitive or delicate skin as they might irritate the skin. Be aware of clients with nut allergies and always check the ingredients before use.
Exfoliants with enzymes	The **enzymes** in these exfoliants gently break down the dead skin on the surface. They loosen the cement that holds the skin cells together so that the dead skin can be easily removed.	The product is applied to the skin either using a mask brush or by placing a small amount of product on the fingertips and distributing this over the facial areas, leaving a fine film on the skin's surface. The product is left for a very short time to dry. There are three different methods of removal depending on the product brand and skin condition. Rinse off, leaving a soft, smooth skin. Rub off using the ring and middle finger while carefully supporting the surrounding skin. As the product is rubbed away it forms granules that help to exfoliate the skin. Remove with damp cotton wool or warm mittens.	Contain enzymes (chemical exfoliation).	A good option for more delicate or sensitive skin as they do not overstimulate the skin's surface if removed with damp cotton wool or warm mittens.	Be aware of your client's skin sensitivity and amend use as required.

Exfoliant	Benefit	Application	Active ingredients	Skin condition	Precautions
Exfoliants with alpha hydroxyl acids (AHAs)	Alpha hydroxyl acids (AHAs) are another common exfoliating ingredient and are usually derived from fruit acids. Like enzymes, they penetrate around the dead skin cells and weaken the bonds that hold the cells together.	Different products have different percentages of AHAs and this will affect the way the product is applied and the length of time it is left on the skin. Lower percentage AHAs are applied to the skin and left for a short period of time to work. They are then thoroughly rinsed off, leaving a soft, smooth skin.	Alpha hydroxyl acids – the amount of AHAs varies depending on the fruit acids used.	Suitable for most skin types. Many types can be used on sensitive skin.	All traces of the product should be removed, as some AHAs continue to work if left on the skin and might cause sensitivity.
Exfoliants with beta hydroxyl acids (BHAs)	These are a more specialist product and additional training is usually provided by the company that supplies it.	Follow the manufacturer's instructions.	Beta hydroxyl acids (BHAs).	Suitable for most skin types. Many types can be used on sensitive skin.	Follow the manufacturer's instructions.

EXFOLIATION IN THE SALON

When the skin has been thoroughly cleansed, you can move onto exfoliation. It is important that you follow your product brand's instructions on how to use their exfoliant as these products differ in their application. It is also important that you **educate** clients about exfoliating their skin so that they can get the maximum benefits from their products. It is equally important that the clients are told how often to exfoliate; if they overexfoliate their skin they can make it sensitive. You must make sure you know the product you are using so that you can give the clients accurate advice for using the products according to their particular skin type and condition.

As a general guide, most clients will benefit from exfoliating weekly but should not exfoliate more than twice a week.

APPLYING AN ENZYME-BASED EXFOLIANT

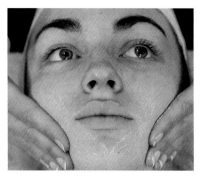

STEP 1 – Make sure the skin is dry. Place a small amount of the product onto the fingertips of one hand; press the fingertips of both hands together to distribute the product.

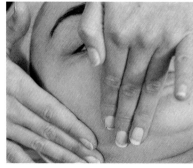

STEP 2 – Press the product gently onto your client's face and neck. Leave for a minute to dry slightly – but not fully.

STEP 3 – Use one hand to support the skin and with the other hand gently rub the skin to remove the product.

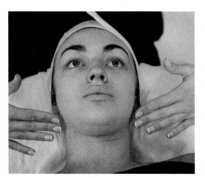

STEP 4 – Brush off any excess product.

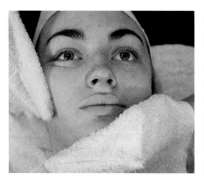

STEP 5 – Wipe the skin with warm mittens, sponges or damp cotton wool to remove any excess product.

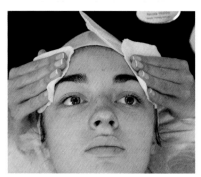

STEP 6 – Tone the skin.

APPLYING A SCRUB-BASED EXFOLIANT

Male clients tend to prefer a scrub exfoliant rather than a cream as it feels more beneficial to their skin. You can use scrub-based exfoliants with a steamer to keep the product moist while you work it into the skin. This prevents the product from dragging or causing excess friction.

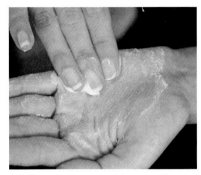

STEP 1 – Place some exfoliant into the hands and add a little warm water.

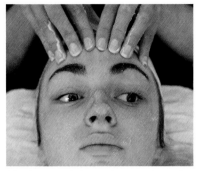

STEP 2 – Work the product over the neck and up onto the face using small circular movements.

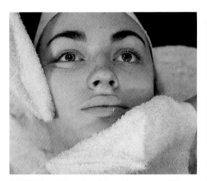

STEP 3 – Wipe the skin with warm mittens, sponges or damp cotton wool to remove any excess product.

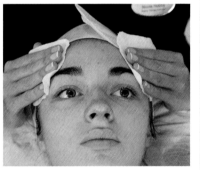

STEP 4 – Tone the skin.

INDUSTRY TIP

Recommend that male clients use a scrub for 2 minutes in the shower (no longer otherwise it will make the skin sensitive) if they suffer with ingrown hairs and/or razor rash.

ACTIVITY

Get some different types of exfoliant (eg smooth beaded, nut kernel, enzyme and AHA). Use each on a different area of skin and compare and contrast the texture, feel and result of each.

WARMING DEVICES

Warming is used during a facial treatment mainly to help deep cleanse the skin. This is particularly beneficial where there are **comedones** and blocked pores as the process will help to soften the skin and aid **extraction**. Warming the skin also helps the products to **penetrate** the skin more easily. In addition, it prepares the facial muscles and helps them to relax. You can find out more information about the skin and facial muscles in the muscles section of the Anatomy and Physiology chapter. The type of warming device you use will depend on what you have access to. Both methods (steamer or hot towels) achieve similar results.

HANDY HINTS

Look back at the Anatomy and Physiology chapter for information on the position and action of the muscles of the head, neck and shoulders; the bones of the head, neck and shoulders; and the structure and function of the blood and lymphatic system for the head, neck and shoulders.

Comedones
Blackheads.

Extraction
Removal or taking out.

Penetrate
When something, eg a substance, enters into another thing.

HANDY HINTS

Look back at the Anatomy and Physiology chapter for more information on the layers of the epidermis.

SmartScreen 204 Worksheet 7

Asthmatic

A person who suffers from a chronic condition that causes difficulty in breathing.

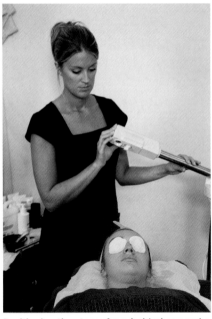

Positioning the steam from behind can make it easier for the client to breathe during treatment

Menopause

The time when a woman's body begins to change – it signals the end of a woman's reproductive years. Hormone levels change and periods stop.

EFFECTS OF WARMING THE SKIN

- The stratum corneum or horny layer is softened.
- Superficial circulation increases, helping to remove waste products.
- The pores relax and open so that perspiration can flow out more easily.
- Warming has a soothing effect on the sensory nerve endings.

STEAMERS

Facials steamers can be a free-standing unit or a small hand-held device. Both have a small water tank and a heating element to heat the water.

Steamers have the following effects when used during a facial treatment:

- They deep cleanse the skin and aid in extraction of comedones and blocked pores.
- They hydrate the skin.
- They stimulate the circulation in pale, dull and lifeless skin.

You should avoid using steaming treatments on **asthmatics**, as they might find it difficult to breathe easily through the steam if you use a facial steamer.

You should avoid using both steaming and warming treatments on the following:

- Claustrophobic clients – as they might react adversely to the steaming mist; it can make them feel anxious.
- Excessively greasy skin – as the steamer might be too stimulating on the sebaceous glands.
- Excessive broken capillaries on the cheeks – as the heat will aggravate them and increase the high colour of the skin.
- Rosacea – as above.
- Reduced skin sensitivity – as the client will be unable to tell you if the skin is getting too warm, resulting in possible heat damage to the skin's surface.
- **Menopausal** women – the heat might bring on a hot flush, causing the client discomfort.

INDUSTRY TIP

If you have a client who is claustrophobic do not wrap them up too tightly. It is a good idea to leave their arms out of the blanket or cover. Avoid setting masks, warming devices that cover the face fully and steaming as this can make them feel confined. Check whether they want eye pads or not as they might find this makes them feel anxious.

INDUSTRY TIP

Some exfoliants are more effective when applied with steam as the heat activates the product, giving better results.

Using a facial steamer (mechanical warming)

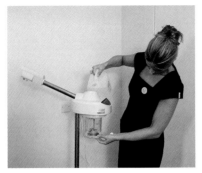

STEP 1 – Check the machine before your client arrives. Fill the tank with distilled water, making sure it is not filled past the safety mark. Check that the steamer head is at a safe angle and that the neck and head are not too low, which might cause the vapour to dribble or spit.

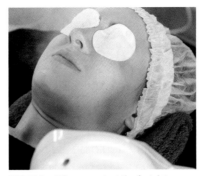

STEP 2 – When you start the facial, turn the unit on. The average time to heat up is 9 minutes for a free-standing steamer. When you are ready to apply the steam, cover your client's eyes with damp cotton wool and protect any sensitive areas with petroleum jelly and damp cotton wool.

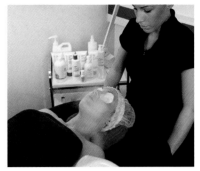

STEP 3 – Warn the client what to expect, and position the steaming unit correctly.

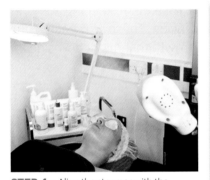

STEP 4 – Align the steamer with the highest point of your client's face (this is usually their nose). The steamer can be positioned to the side of your client. They should be raised slightly and their face turned towards the steamer. The steamer can also be placed behind the couch so that the steam passes down the face. This is a good position as it prevents too much steam falling directly on the nose, making it hard to breathe. Steaming can be applied for 3–10 minutes, but this depends on the type of skin, client preferences and the desired results.

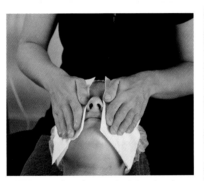

STEP 5 – When the required time has been completed, blot your client's skin dry.

INDUSTRY TIP

Dry skin (providing there is no sensitivity) might benefit from a longer steam as it will hydrate and stimulate the sweat and sebaceous activity in the skin. Steam for between 5 and 10 minutes at a distance of 37–45 cm (15–18 inches).

The reverse might apply to oily skin – too much heat can be overstimulating but gentle steaming will help to soften the skin and open the pores for extraction. Place at a distance of 25 cm (10 inches) for approximately 5–7 minutes.

For combination skin, 5–7 minutes at a distance of 30–37 cm (12–15 inches) is ideal.

INDUSTRY TIP

For health and safety reasons, make sure there are no trailing cables.

INDUSTRY TIP

Most units will have a cut-off mechanism so that if the water level falls too low the unit will turn off automatically.

ACTIVITY

Produce a quick chart for steaming. List the different skin types, how far the steamer should be away from the skin, how long each skin type should have and why. Check your answers with your colleagues.

HOT TOWELS (MANUAL WARMING)

Facial towels can be simply rolled and placed in a bowl of hand-hot water. Alternatively, the towels can be placed in a hot towel caddy or warmer. These are small cabinets that heat the towels or mittens inside by means of gentle steam. The caddies are useful as they will keep the towels hot and damp until you are ready to use them, keeping the treatment flowing. Some have UVC bulbs inside. These are special light bulbs that help slow down any bacterial growth that might be inside the caddy.

Using a hot towel caddy

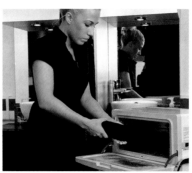

STEP 1 – Take clean cleansing mitts or towels and dampen with hot water. Place inside the caddy and turn on the unit. Leave the towels for about 15 minutes before using. Remove from the caddy.

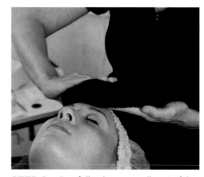

STEP 2 – Carefully place a small part of the towel onto your client's skin and check that the temperature is comfortable.

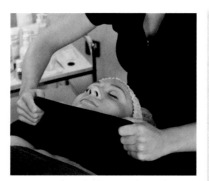

STEP 3 – Place the first towel onto the neck and gently roll the towel open and up the face.

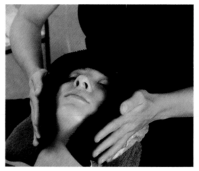

STEP 4 – Apply a second towel to the forehead and gently open and roll the towel down.

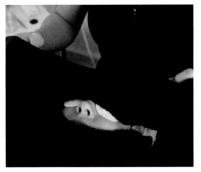

STEP 5 – Wrap the towels securely around the face and onto the neck. Make sure that the nose is fully exposed so that the client is comfortable and can breathe easily. Leave for a couple of minutes but do not let the towels fully cool.

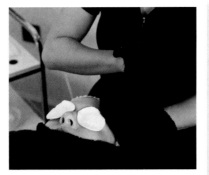

STEP 6 – Lift the towels off slowly as it will feel quite cold to the client as the skin is exposed.

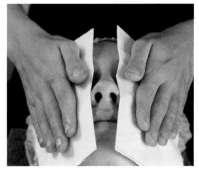

STEP 7 – Blot any excess moisture with a tissue.

EXTRACTION

The aim of extraction is to remove any visible comedones or blocked pores. It is really important that you carry out the process correctly to avoid any risk of skin damage. Warming the skin prior to extraction helps to make extracting easy as the skin is softened and the pores are relaxed. Many facials do not include extractions any more as the process is not very relaxing.

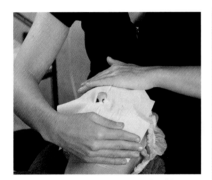

STEP 1 – Make sure the skin is dry; blot with a tissue if necessary.

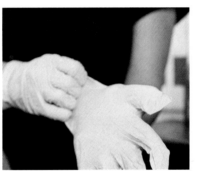

STEP 2 – Put on disposable gloves. The gloves will help prevent the hands slipping on the skin and minimise any risk of cross-infection.

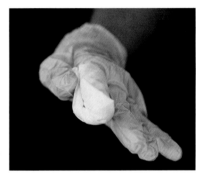

STEP 3 – Fold two tissues and cover the index fingers of both hands.

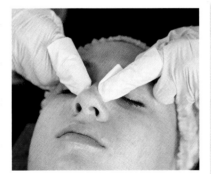

STEP 4 – Place the fingers around the comedone or blocked pore. Using the pads at the side of the index fingers, lift the skin under the comedone or blocked pore and gently roll the skin in a back and forth action to extract the contents. Do not use your nails as this will mark the client's skin. (This is one important reason why your nails should be short.)

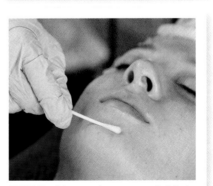

STEP 5 – When you have removed all that you are intending to, wipe the area with a mild liquid antiseptic to reduce any risk of cross-infection.

FACIAL MASSAGE

This is one of the most enjoyable parts of a facial. It is deeply relaxing. The massage should take approximately 20 minutes of an hour-long facial but the timing might need to be adapted to suit the client's skin type and condition.

PHYSIOLOGICAL EFFECTS OF A MASSAGE

- Improves the texture of the skin by desquamation and the application of a suitable **massage medium** which has a skin-smoothing effect.
- Increases the circulation to the skin and muscles. The improved circulation gives the skin a healthy glow.
- Increases the supply of oxygen and **nutrients** to the **intercellular** tissues. Stimulates the removal of waste products from the intercellular tissues.
- Stimulates sweat and sebaceous activity, making the skin more supple.
- Increases the activity of the cells (metabolism).
- Relaxes the muscle fibres and relieves tension.
- Promotes relaxation. Releases **endorphins**, giving the client an increased sense of wellbeing.

ACTIVITY

Do you know the difference between physiological and psychological? Make a list of what you think both words mean in the context of the treatments we give. Compare your answers with your colleagues. What psychological effects do you think a facial will have?

Massage medium
Product applied to the skin during a massage.

Nutrients
Substances that help us grow.

Intercellular
Found between cells.

Endorphins
Chemicals released by the pituitary endocrine gland that affect the transmission of electrical signals within the nervous system. When endorphin levels are high in the body we feel less pain and fewer negative effects of stress.

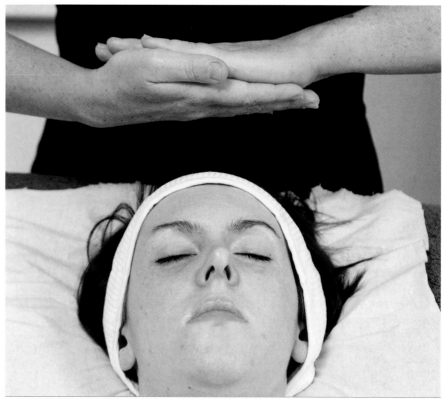

About to begin a facial

MASSAGE MEDIA

A massage medium is used during a massage to give the hands something to glide on. This makes the massage more comfortable and prevents dragging and excessive friction on the skin. The medium also leaves the skin feeling soft and supple. Oils and creams can be used on any skin type, depending on the manufacturer's instructions. It is important to be aware of which product you can use on each skin type and condition. If you use a product designed for dry skin on oily skin it will be too rich for the skin and will leave your client's skin feeling very oily.

There are two main types of massage media:
- Oil – traditionally used more for dry and sensitive skin as clients with oily skin will not like the idea of having more oil added to the skin's surface.
- Cream – traditionally used for oily skin types.

INGREDIENTS

Oils can be natural oils, eg grapeseed, sweet almond or macadamia nut. They might have essential oils blended into these base oils to give them a pleasant smell and a therapeutic effect, such as relaxation. An oil medium might also be made from a mineral oil base. Some companies produce products that look and feel very similar to oils but are actually oil free.

Creams can be produced to suit any skin type. Some are rich and creamy and others are light emulsions. Massage creams should be warmed in the hands before applying; this warms the cream for the client's comfort but also makes the product spread more easily.

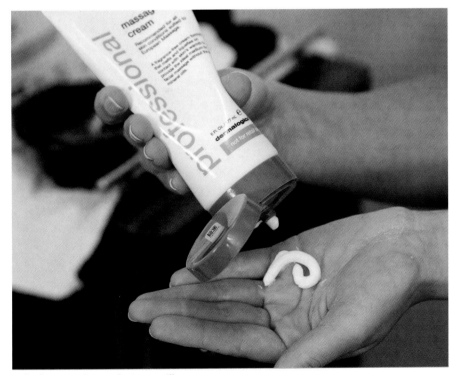

Only dispense the product you will use

There is a huge variation in product brands. Make a list of the products you have in your establishment that you can use for a massage. Next to each product, write down which skin type and condition it is suitable for and then discuss your list with your colleagues.

MASSAGE TECHNIQUES

Effleurage

A massage routine always starts and finishes with effleurage. It is the movement used to apply the massage medium. Effleurage movements are light, stroking movements and can be applied with the palms of the hands, fingertips or thumbs. Effleurage can be applied **superficially** or deeply, quickly or slowly. Effleurage is used to link other movements and keeps the massage flowing at a continuous pace.

The effects of effleurage are:

- an increase in circulation, bringing oxygen and nutrients to the skin's tissues and removing waste products
- relaxation of the muscles and skin tissues
- removal of dead skin cells (desquamation) as the hands glide over the skin.

Petrissage

Many of the movements used during a facial massage will be a variation of petrissage. These are **kneading** movements and involve applying pressure, rolling or lifting the tissues up or over the **underlying** muscles and organs. Petrissage movements can involve the whole of the surface of the palm of the hand, the pads of the thumb, fingers or knuckles. These movements are deeper and more stimulating than effleurage movements.

Superficially

Lightly on the surface.

Kneading

Massage technique that involves compression of the tissues.

Underlying

Found under something.

INDUSTRY TIP

To help improve flexibility and to help your understanding of petrissage movements, take some play doh or a stress ball and work it between your fingers and hands.

Petrissage along the mandible

The effects of petrissage are:

- an increase in circulation, bringing oxygen and nutrients to the skin's tissues and removing waste products. A visible erythema will be seen on the skin's surface
- relaxation of the skin's tissues
- desquamation
- a temporary improvement in the tone of the muscle fibres
- stimulation of cell renewal
- relaxation of the muscles and removal of the lactic acid that builds up during muscle activity, reducing muscular aches
- assistance of the lymphatic system. You can find out more about the lymphatic system of the face in the Anatomy and Physiology chapter on page 84.

Frictions

Frictions are a type of petrissage movement but have a very different purpose. They are quick movements, applied using the finger or thumbs in either a rubbing or circular action to stimulate the skin and create friction.

The effects of friction are:

- vasodilation and rapid increase in circulation seen as an erythema on the skin's surface
- loosening of tightness in the skin, such as scar tissue, by stretching the collagen in the skin's tissues
- loosening of glueyness in the muscle fibres, which can be felt as either tightness or uneven muscle tissue. This helps to relieve muscular tension
- desquamation
- stimulation of the circulation and a temporary plumping effect when applied along fine lines and wrinkles, eg the forehead.

Tapotement

Tapotement is also known as percussion movements. Tapotements are stimulating movements that are light and brisk. Examples of tapotement on the face are light tapping and slapping movements using the fingertips.

The effects of tapotement are:

- a rapid increase in circulation, bringing oxygen and nutrients to the skin's tissues and removing waste products. A visible erythema will be seen on the skin's surface
- relaxation of the skin's tissues
- stimulation of cell renewal
- relaxation of the muscles and removal of the lactic acid that builds up during muscle activity, reducing muscular aches
- stimulation of the superficial nerve endings, causing a temporary toning and tightening of the skin
- assistance in removal of static lymph from the tissues.

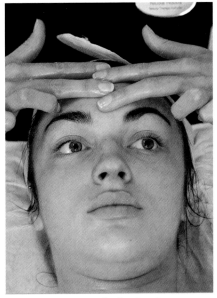

Scissor friction over the forehead

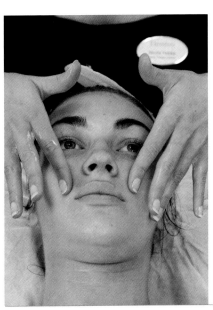

Raindrop tapotement over the cheeks

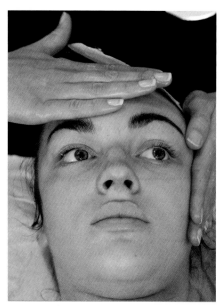
Running vibrations over the forehead

Sedation
Calming.

Vibrations

The muscles of the therapist's lower arm and hands are held taut to produce a mild trembling through the fingers or thumbs. This is then applied to the client's skin. The aim is for the vibrations to travel through the skin to the nerve endings, with minimal surface stimulation. These movements are applied sparingly.

The effects of the vibrations are:

- gentle stimulation of the deeper skin layers
- stimulation of the nervous system
- relaxation and **sedation**
- very effective assistance in the removal of static lymph from the tissues.

ACTIVITY

Explain why you think it is important to use effleurage to link different massage movements. How will this benefit your client's massage?

ADAPTING MASSAGE TECHNIQUES

Massage movements should be adapted to suit the clients' skin type and treatment objectives. Some examples are below.

- A client with greasy skin will require a calming and soothing massage to reduce sebaceous activity.
- A client with dry skin will require more stimulating movements to stimulate cellular renewal.
- A client with sensitive skin will need to have calm, slow techniques to avoid overstimulating the skin and causing irritation.
- Massage on a male client will need to be adapted to make sure all the movements work across or down the face. Avoid movements against the natural hair growth as this can be uncomfortable on the fingers – especially if there is stubble.

ACTIVITY

Sandra is a mature client in her 50s. She is concerned about the fine lines around her mouth and eyes. Her skin is a combination skin type and its condition is dehydrated. What massage techniques would be appropriate to use and what should you avoid? How will you adapt your facial massage to meet the client's objectives?

INDUSTRY TIP

It is a good idea to do regular hand exercises to help improve the suppleness of your hands and fingers. Try the following:

- Put your hands together. Keeping the fingers together, draw the palms apart.
- Place the hands on a flat surface and try and lift each finger one at a time.
- Pretend you are playing a piano on a soft surface.
- Lock your hands together and rotate your hands at the wrist, going clockwise and anticlockwise.
- Make tight fists with your hands, then open your hands and stretch your fingers as much as you can.

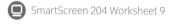
SmartScreen 204 Worksheet 9

MASSAGE ROUTINE

A good massage will be flowing, rhythmic and continuous, using a range of techniques. Maintain contact with the skin at all times, using effleurage to link your movements where necessary.

Below is a suggested routine to give you an idea of a facial massage using a variety of massage techniques. Your college, salon or the product brand you are using will have a massage **sequence** that you will be taught.

First select a massage medium suitable for your client's skin type and condition. Apply to the hands and warm gently by rubbing the hands together away from your client's head and face. Apply the medium to the skin with light effleurage movements, starting across the décolleté and moving up the neck and face.

INDUSTRY TIP

Make sure your hands are warm – this will be more comfortable for the client. In addition, warm muscles and tendons are more flexible so this will help protect your hands from strains. A simple way to achieve this is to place your hands in warm water before the massage.

Sequence

A particular order that you follow.

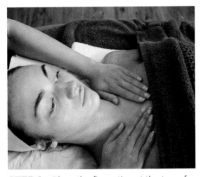

STEP 1 – Place the fingertips at the top of the sternum. Divide the hands and effleurage across the décolleté, around the shoulders and up the back of the neck. While maintaining contact, return the hands over the shoulders and back to the sternum. Repeat four times.

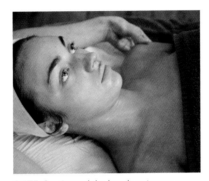

STEP 2 – Spread the hands out across either side of the chest and thumb-knead the front of the deltoid muscle. Knead around the deltoid to the back and then, turning the hands, thumb-knead across the top of the trapezius up to the occipital bone. Repeat step 1.

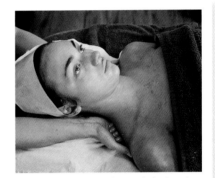

STEP 3 – Make loose fists with the hands and use the knuckles to knead across the chest. Slide around the deltoids and knuckle-knead across the upper trapezius.

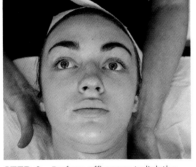

STEP 4 – Perform effleurage to link the movements. Using both hands and alternating strokes, massage the back of the neck. Repeat four times. Support the base of the skull and 'ease' the spine with a gentle stretch.

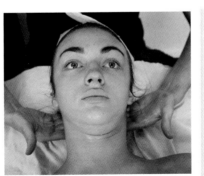

STEP 5 – Place the fingertips at the base of the skull into the occipital hollow; apply static vibration.

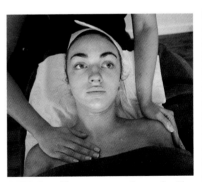

STEP 6 – Effleurage across the neck with your right hand, starting at the left shoulder and moving across the pectorals, around the deltoid and up the right side of the neck until the fingers reach the occipital bone. The left hand supports the left shoulder to keep the area stable. Repeat effleurage with the left hand, working from the right deltoid across the pectorals and around the deltoid up the left side of the neck, supporting the right shoulder with the right hand. Repeat four times.

INDUSTRY TIP

Do not stretch the neck on a client who has suffered a neck or **whiplash** injury.

Whiplash

An injury to the muscles and joints of the neck caused by a sudden jolt, resulting in a violent movement of the neck beyond its normal range of movement. The head is usually thrown forwards and then backwards, as in a car accident.

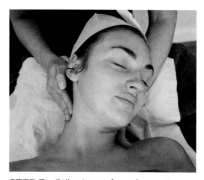

STEP 7 – Following on from the previous effleurage movement, gently turn your client's head to the left as you come up the right side of the neck. Finger-knead along the sternocleidomastoid, behind the ear and upper trapezius on the right side of the neck. Perform effleurage to turn the head back to the centre and a second effleurage to turn the head to the right. Repeat the finger-knead on the left side.

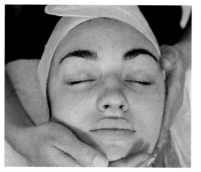

STEP 8 – Effleurage the mandible left to right, using one hand to effleurage and the other to support. Swap hands to perform an alternate movement. Repeat twice.

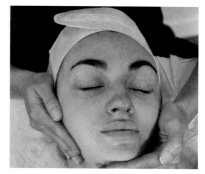

STEP 9 – Perform running vibrations across the mandible from left to right, using one hand to apply the running vibration and the other to support. Swap hands to perform an alternate movement. Repeat twice.

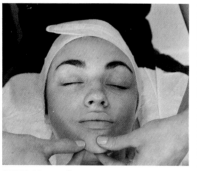

STEP 10 – Perform tapotement using the fingertips in a pincer movement to the mandible – the fingers gently pinch the skin and flick off.

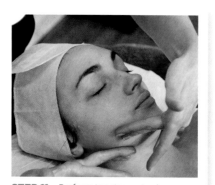

STEP 11 – Perform tapotement using gentle fingertip slapping below the mandible and lower cheeks to flick and lift the tissue.

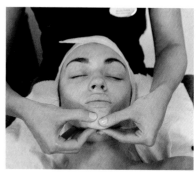

STEP 12 – Carry out a thumb-knead to the mentalis.

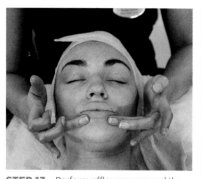

STEP 13 – Perform effleurage around the mouth using the ring fingers; working around the orbicularis oris muscle, starting at the top of the lip and circling around to the bottom.

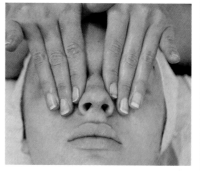

STEP 14 – Using the fingers, start on the mentalis and draw the fingers up the sides of the nose to the bridge; divide the hands and sweep down under the eyes, across the cheeks to the temple and circle. Repeat twice.

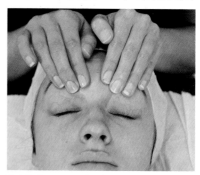

STEP 15 – Using the fingertips, start on the mentalis and draw the fingers up the sides of the nose to the bridge. Use the fingers to lift the eyebrows then slide the hands to the temples and circle. Repeat twice.

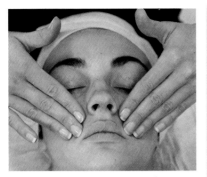

STEP 16 – Link the movements with effleurage. Draw small circles up the face from the chin, following the mouth-to-nose line (like a corkscrew) up the sides of the nose. Gently massage over the nose using the fingertips, then slide up the bridge of the nose onto the frontalis. Divide the hands over the frontalis and slide the fingers back down the cheeks to the mentalis. Repeat twice.

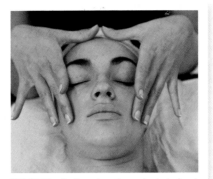

STEP 17 – Perform tapotement – 'raindrop' tapping across and over the face using light fingertip tapping.

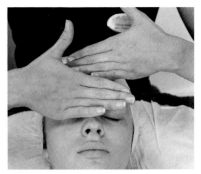

STEP 18 – Perform effleurage from the tip of the nose up to the frontalis in a continuous stroking movement, alternating the hands. Repeat four times.

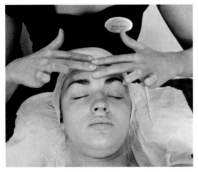

STEP 19 – Perform scissor frictions across the frontalis. This involves working the middle finger of one hand into a V shape made by the index and middle fingers of the opposite hand, working the frictions into any visible lines.

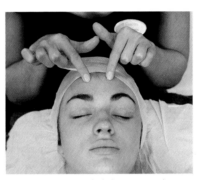

STEP 20 – Draw petal shapes over the frontalis with the tips of the index fingers, working from the centre to the left and back across the frontalis to the right.

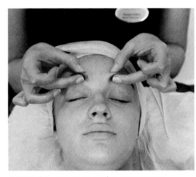

STEP 21 – Starting at the corrugator muscle, work out over the eyebrows, gently pinching them.

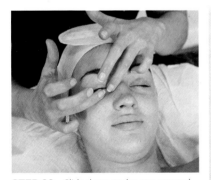

STEP 22 – Slide down under one eye and, using alternating ring fingers, apply a drainage effleurage under the eye from the inner eye to the outer eye.

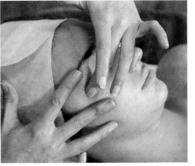

STEP 23 – Support the outer edge of one eye with one hand and apply gentle frictions to any visible lines on the outer eye area. Make sure you support the skin adequately. Repeat steps 22 and 23 with the other eye.

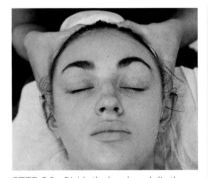

STEP 24 – Divide the hands and slip them over the ears so that the ear is between the index and middle fingers. Slide the fingers down and gently knead the skin around the ear. Repeat four times.

ACTIVITY

When you are happy with your massage routine, think about how you will need to adapt it for a male client.

- Make a list of all the things you will need to consider.
- Practise your routine on a male client.

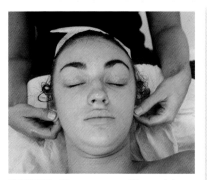

STEP 25 – Massage around the ear lobes and ear with the thumb and fingers. Repeat four times.

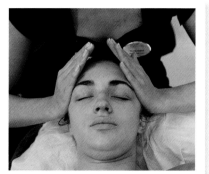

STEP 26 – Place the palms onto the temples and gently massage with circular movements.

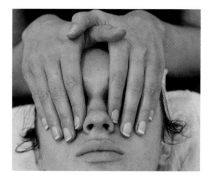

STEP 27 – Place the fingers over the eyes and rest for a few moments to finish.

ACTIVITY

Using your college's massage routine, list each movement and write down what technique each massage movement is.

ACTIVITY

Explain why you think that a massage routine always starts with effleurage.

FACE MASKS

A face mask is any substance that is spread over the face, neck and upper décolleté area and left for a period of time to have an effect on the skin. Depending on the ingredients and application of the mask, you will find one to achieve almost any objective. There are occasions when you might want to apply more than one mask to suit different skin types and conditions. This will also help to maximise the results.

USE AND EFFECTS OF DIFFERENT MASKS

- **Cleansing** – these masks often have a clay base that absorbs surface impurities and excess oils. They also desquamate.
- **Stimulating** – some masks have a thermal ingredient, which makes the mask warm up when it is applied to the skin. This stimulates blood circulation and increases sweat and sebaceous activity.
- **Hydrating** – these masks leave a film of moisture or oil on the skin's surface to nourish it. Some of these masks can be left on and the residue massaged into the skin or, when the client uses them at home, they can be left on overnight.
- **Peeling** – these are plastic-based masks that set after application and then peel off, lifting off dead skin cells and impurities.
- **Soothing** – these masks have soothing and cooling ingredients, causing **vasoconstriction**.
- **Brightening** – these masks literally brighten the appearance of dull or tired-looking skin.

INDUSTRY TIP

When the body is relaxed the body temperature drops slightly. Keep this in mind and check that your client is still warm enough. If the client is cold they will lose their deep state of relaxation. Feel the skin and check for goose bumps. Offer the client another blanket if they are cold. It is a good idea when the mask is on to pull the covers up and over the client's shoulders to keep them cosy. To protect the duvet or blanket, place a small tissue over the edge at the base of the neck where the mask finishes.

Vasoconstriction

Tightening of a blood vessel making it narrower.

Masks can be divided into two main categories:

- **Setting** – this type of mask will set on the skin's surface after application, changing from a liquid or mobile form to a solid, firm or dry texture. Setting masks include peeling masks, modelling masks, thermal masks, clay-based masks and paraffin masks.
- **Non-setting** – these masks do not change in structure while they are on the skin. They include warm oil masks and biological or natural masks.

Think carefully about your choice of mask and its suitability for both the client's skin type and skin condition. Take care when you are applying masks to very nervous or claustrophobic clients. Claustrophobic clients might prefer to keep their eyes uncovered. Avoid using a setting type of mask with such clients.

Wax-based masks

These masks are applied in a liquid form and harden as they dry or cool on the skin's surface. They form a waterproof layer on the skin, making it sweat. This process encourages deep cleansing of the skin's pores. Some of these masks are applied over a piece of gauze to make it easier to remove from the skin. A small hole is cut out so the nose can be left uncovered. The gauze is smoothed over the face and the mask applied over the top. The gauze can be used as a guide for application, making sure the gauze is fully covered with the mask.

Rubber/latex-based masks

These have to be mixed and applied quickly. They form an elastic, waterproof layer over the skin. They retain the skin's heat, leading to an increase in the skin's temperature and circulation. The mask dries and is lifted or peeled off the skin. As the mask is removed, it lifts off trapped surface debris and exfoliates the skin.

Do not use these masks on clients with a latex allergy or if they are claustrophobic.

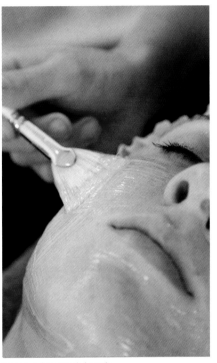
Using a fan mask brush

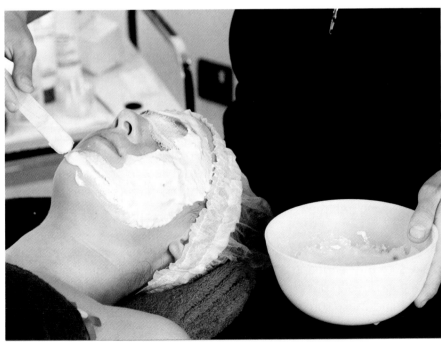
Using a spatula to apply a mask

Humectant

Something that is able to absorb water.

Hydrocolloidal gels

These are gel masks with a high water content. As the water evaporates from the skin it causes a tightening sensation. **Humectants** are added to prevent the mask from drying out by absorbing water from the air.

Earth-based mask

These have a natural earth ingredient, such as clay. The clay dries and contracts on the skin. They are very good cleansers as they absorb excess grease, oil and surface debris. Examples of earth ingredients are kaolin, white clay, aluminium silicate and bentonite. These masks usually have other ingredients added to counter the drying effects of the clay, including vegetable oils and floral waters.

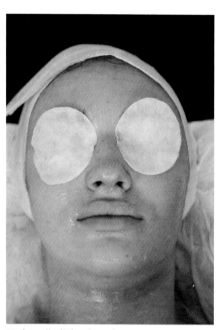

Hydrocollodial gel mask

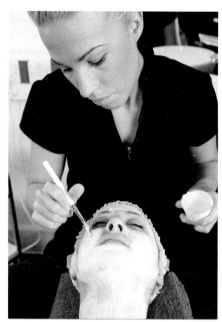

Earth/clay-based mask

ACTIVITY

Make a table of the masks you have in your salon using the following headings:

Type of mask, active ingredient, benefit, skin type suitable for, skin condition suitable for, precautions needed.

APPLYING AND REMOVING A MASK

In a professional facial, a face mask is always applied to cleansed skin following a facial massage unless specified otherwise by the brand manufacturer. Some cleansing masks are applied before massage so that the nourishing or active ingredients of the massage are left on the skin following treatment.

PREPARING FOR MASK APPLICATION

Make sure the headband is protected with tissue. Even with male clients it is a good idea to put on a headband to avoid any product getting into the hairline. Make sure stray hairs are tucked securely into the headband.

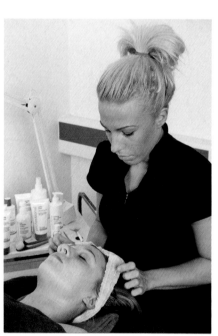

All traces of mask must be removed

THE CITY & GUILDS TEXTBOOK

You will need the following:

- mask
- mask brush or spatula
- bowl of warm water
- sponges or hot towels
- toner
- additional tissues
- mask (mixing) bowl.

In addition, some masks require gauze for the mask to sit on.

APPLYING A MASK

If the mask is to be applied using a mask brush, use long, sweeping movements to apply the product. Avoid dabbing the mask on as this will disturb the client. Using a brush will give an even application of the product on the skin. Some rubber masks need to be applied using a spatula.

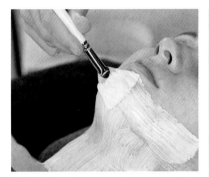

STEP 1 – When you are using a mask brush to apply the mask product, start at the base of the neck. In some cases you might apply a mask to the décolleté area.

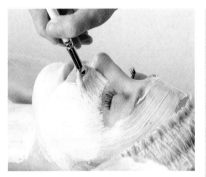

STEP 2 – Apply the mask evenly, avoiding the hairline and taking care around the eyes.

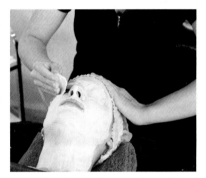

STEP 3 – When you have evenly applied the mask, add eye pads to your client's eyes.

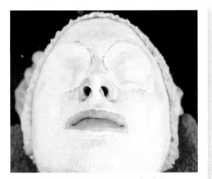

STEP 4 – When you have applied the mask, make sure your client is warm and comfortable.

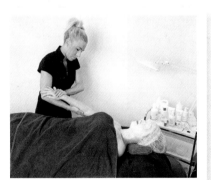

STEP 5 – You might want to offer your client a complementary hand and arm massage.

INDUSTRY TIP

Always refer to the manufacturer's instructions when you are applying a mask.

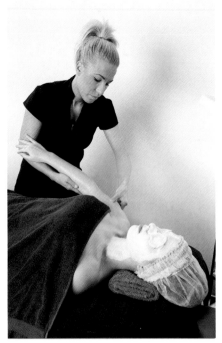

Arm massage while mask is active

Applying a rubber-based mask

Rubber masks can be tricky to control when you apply them. Follow the step-by-step instructions below, but see the previous mask application photos for guidance.

STEP 1 – Apply eye pads first.

STEP 2 – Mix up the mask in a bowl with a spatula. Usually these masks are mixed with warm water but an additional liquid might be supplied that you mix together with the powder base. Do not use a brush as the product will be very difficult to remove from the bristles and will not help application.

STEP 3 – Apply the mask, starting from the centre of the face on the nose. Work outwards across the cheeks and over the face. Applying the mask this way means that if it runs you can collect and smooth the runs as you go. It also helps to get a good even application on the face.

STEP 4 – Apply the remaining mask to the neck.

STEP 5 – Make sure you do not take these masks too near the hairline and always make sure you apply a sufficient amount around the edge as this will make the mask easier to remove.

While the mask is having its desired effect on the skin, you might choose to give the client a scalp massage or a hand and arm massage. This is a relaxing addition to the treatment and reassures the client that they are not left alone. Make sure that your client is aware that you will be including this in their facial treatment when you carry out your consultation.

Removing clay-based masks

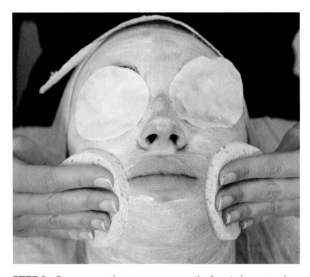

STEP 1 – Press warm, damp sponges over the face to loosen and soften the mask. Gently wipe the sponges over the face, rinsing them in warm water, until you have removed all traces of the mask.

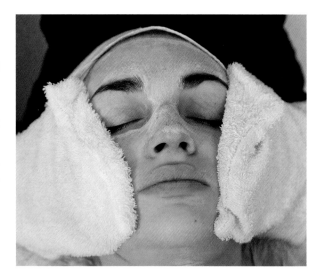

STEP 2 – Alternatively, you can use mittens from a hot caddy. Press the warm mittens over the face to loosen and soften the mask, gently removing the residue.

Removing setting masks

The removal routine below shows the removal of just one type of setting mask. Always refer to the manufacturer's instructions as this might vary.

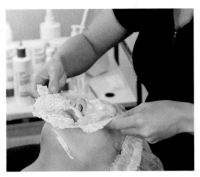

STEP 1 – Gently lift the edges of the mask to make sure the mask is ready to be removed.

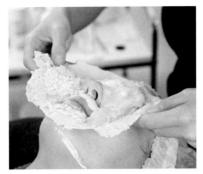

STEP 2 – Take care when you are removing the mask away from your client's face.

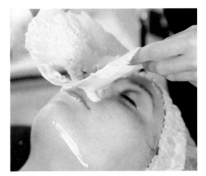

STEP 3 – Check that the entire mask has been removed, especially around the hairline, nostrils and under the chin. Make sure you remove any mask residue that is left on the skin.

Next step of facial procedure

Tone the skin and blot the skin with tissue to make sure it is dry.

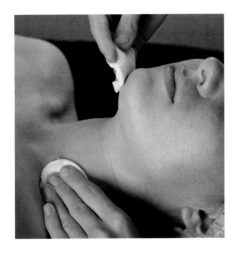

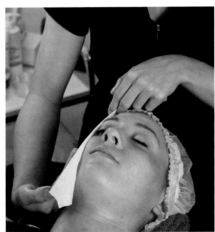

MOISTURISERS

To complete the facial you need to make sure that your client's skin is protected and nourished. Apply a day moisturiser, or a night cream if the facial is being carried out in the evening. Apply eye and lip care.

There is a huge selection of moisturisers, many of which promise to provide the user with fantastic results. The basic functions of a moisturiser are to:

- protect the skin and act as a barrier against the elements
- replace, hold and attract moisture to the skin (humectant)
- smooth the skin texture
- provide a smooth base for make-up, acting as a barrier between the make-up and the skin underneath.

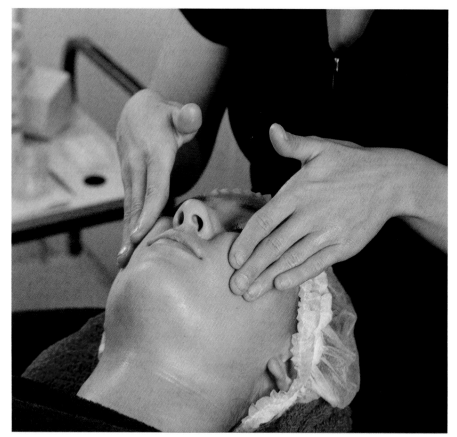

Completing the facial by applying moisturiser

MOISTURISERS FOR THE DAYTIME

When you are selecting a moisturiser for a client, it is important to ask the client about the type of product they like the feel of, as this will encourage them to use one daily. There are so many to choose from it is usually possible to find something that will meet your client's needs. A product to be used on younger skin will have different ingredients from one that is marketed for more mature skin. This is because different age groups will be looking for different benefits from their product. The skin will have a different structure as it ages and the product will be aiming to minimise the signs of ageing.

The texture of the moisturiser will vary according to the skin type and condition it is intended for. Creams tend to be heavier and richer and are more suitable for dry or more mature skin as they have a higher oil content. Clients who like a light product will prefer a lotion with a lighter texture or a gel. Gels are water-based products so have a light, non-greasy feel to them and are good on oily or young skin. You need to make sure you understand how the structure and function of the skin changes as we age as this will affect the advice you give. You can find further detail on the skin and ageing in the Anatomy and Physiology chapter on pages 13–14.

INDUSTRY TIP

Encourage clients to be economical with their products. It is better to apply a small amount and add more if needed than to put too much on in one go and waste it. If your client's skin is really dehydrated you can recommend another application of moisturiser at midday if they are not wearing any make-up. Some companies produce a hydrating spray that can be applied over make-up during the day.

Moisturising product	Features	Benefits	Skin type and condition suitable for	Examples of ingredients	Home use
Moisturising lotions	A light product that is easily absorbed into the skin. Lotions can come in a container with a pourable lid or in a pump dispenser.	▪ protect the skin and act as a barrier against the elements and pollution ▪ replace, hold and attract moisture to the skin (humectant) ▪ smooth the skin's texture	This will depend on the product manufacturer as these can be made for all skin types. A product for younger skin will be lighter than one for more mature skin, which will have a richer feel.	Humectants and hydrators; hyaluronic acid; **ceramides and lipids** (mineral and vegetable oils); glycerol. **Ceramide** A fatty acid (lipid). **Lipids** A broad group of chemicals, including waxes, fats and fat-soluble vitamins.	Apply a small amount to the skin every day, morning and night.
Matifying lotions	A daily moisturiser with a matt-effect finish. Usually supplied in a pump dispenser.	▪ hydrate and protect the skin without leaving the skin feeling greasy or looking shiny as these products have a matte finish	Oily and combination skin.	Humectants and hydrators; hyaluronic acid.	Apply to the skin in the morning.
Moisturising creams	More concentrated and richer than a lotion. Creams usually come in a pot or tub and need to be removed using a small spatula.	▪ protect the skin and act as a barrier against the elements and pollution ▪ hydrate the skin by replacing, holding and attracting moisture to the skin ▪ smooth and refine the skin's texture ▪ soften the skin	Dry, dehydrated skin. Young dehydrated skin will require a cream that is rich but easily absorbed whereas mature, dry or dehydrated skin might need a rich nourishing, heavier textured cream.	Hyaluronic acid; vitamins A and E; humectants and hydrators; antioxidants; ceramides and lipids (mineral oils and vegetable oils); myristic acid (**isopropyl myristate**). **Isopropyl myristate** An non-oily liquid that reduces the oiliness of a product.	Apply to the skin every day, morning and night.

204/224 PROVIDE FACIAL SKIN CARE/FACIAL CARE FOR MEN

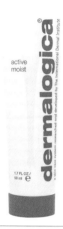

Balm

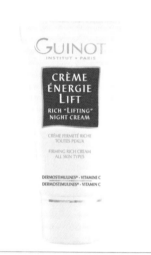

Night cream

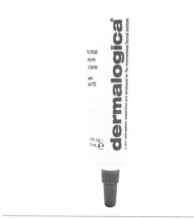

Eye cream

OTHER MOISTURISING PRODUCTS

Balms

Balms are often marketed to be unisex, ie aimed at both the male and female market. Men find the term 'balm' less feminine and are more likely to purchase it than if the product is called a moisturiser. Balms are often very light, matte moisturisers with a high water content but this is not always the case. Some are quite solid and only a small amount is required because when the product is warmed it becomes quite liquid and easy to apply.

Balms are supplied in a variety of containers depending on the consistency of the product. Balms have the same benefits as other moisturisers:

- They protect the skin and act as a barrier against the elements and pollution.
- They hydrate the skin.
- They refine and smooth the skin's texture.

Application will depend on the product brand and ingredients as balms can be made for all skin types and conditions. They might contain beeswax, essential oils, carnauba wax and oils, such as avocado, jojoba and almond. They should be applied to the skin every morning and/or evening as per the manufacturer's instructions.

Night creams/products

Night creams are a rich, creamy oil-in-water emulsion, usually supplied in a tub or pot. Applying a separate cream at night is not a gimmick. The skin works very differently at night under different influences from that experienced during the day. The body, and in particular the skin, goes through a period of repair at night. A night-time cream will slowly feed the skin while it repairs and regenerates to prevent and reduce the signs of ageing.

Night creams are available for all skin types and conditions. They might contain shea butter; oils, such as wheatgerm, almond and essential oils; hyaluronic acid; vitamins A and E; humectants and hydrators; antioxidants; ceramides and lipids (mineral oils and vegetable oils); and acetyl alcohol.

A thin layer of cream is applied at night onto cleansed skin. Night creams should be included in the skin care routine soon after age 25 if the client is willing to invest in additional skin care products.

Eye creams

As the skin around the eyes is very thin it will absorb products quickly. Eye creams might come in a tub or tube dispenser. They are richer than eye gels and regenerate and plump up the tissue around the eye, minimising the appearance of fine lines and wrinkles.

Eye creams are particularly effective on dry or mature skin. The tissue around the eye area is much thinner than anywhere else on the body so it is important to use a product that is designed with this in mind.

Eye creams might contain floral water, cornflower, hyaluronic acid, green tea and vitamins C and E. They should be applied to the skin every day, morning and/or night as per the manufacturer's instructions.

Eye gels

Eye gels are a lighter product than a cream. They tend to be water-in-oil emulsions so that they penetrate easily without leaving any surface residue. They are supplied in a tube or pump.

Eye gels calm and soothe the eye contour area. They reduce signs of tiredness, puffiness and dark circles. They are suitable for younger skin, dehydrated, combination and oily skin and can contain floral waters, witch hazel, tea and cornflower.

They should be applied to the skin every day, morning and/or night as per the manufacturer's instructions.

SPECIALIST PRODUCTS

Many specialist products can be used in the salon and/or as part of the home care routine. When you go through your training you will cover these products. They include serums, ampoules, lip and neck creams.

Neck creams

In addition to the face, the neck also needs hydration and protection. Neck creams are rich, intense products that help to minimise the appearance of ageing of the neckline and décolleté. The neck is one of the first areas to show signs of ageing. Neck creams work to restore the different needs of the skin of the neck and to minimise these signs. Neck creams:

- hydrate and smooth wrinkles along the neckline
- nourish the skin, leaving it smooth and revitalised.

Some neck creams have lifting effects and work on reducing age spots.

Neck creams are suitable for mature skin, especially clients over 40. They might contain proteins; vitamins A, C and E; shea butter; vegetable oils, such as wheatgerm, almond and essential oils; hyaluronic acid; humectants and hydrators; antioxidants; and acetyl alcohol.

Many clients neglect to include the neck and just treat their face, yet it is still exposed to the same elements. Recommend this product to mature clients (40 plus). It should be applied morning and evening along the neckline and décolleté.

> **INDUSTRY TIP**
>
> Eye products should only be applied by dotting them gently around the socket bone of the eye, not directly into the eye area. Too much product can make the eye area puffy. Measure out your product so that you have an amount the size of a grain of rice. This will be enough for both eyes.

> **INDUSTRY TIP**
>
> Ageing starts as early as age 25; the body's ability to renew itself starts to slow and the sebaceous activity starts to drop. Additional skin care, such as eye creams and night creams, should be encouraged from this age to support the skin and to prevent the signs of ageing.

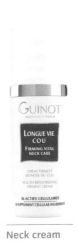

Neck cream

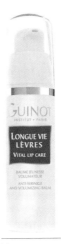

Lip cream

Lip products

Clients are now much more aware about protecting and nourishing their lips. In the past this has been an often neglected area. Some long-lasting lipsticks can be dehydrating and the lips need extra protection in the sun and when it is very cold.

Lip treatment products can come in an easy to apply lipstick, or a pot or tube. They:

- hydrate and moisturise the lips, leaving them soft and smooth
- soften fine lines and wrinkles around the lip
- protect the lips.

Some products leave a natural shine on the lips.

Lip products are suitable for all skin types and conditions. They might contain shea butter; sunflower, coconut or grapeseed oil; aloe vera; vitamin E; rice; and essential oils.

Recommend lip products to all your clients to use as required, to leave the lips feeling smooth and to give a natural gloss finish to the lips.

Serums

Serums are light-textured products that almost have a liquid feel. They are absorbed quickly and easily into the skin. Some products marketed for everyday use are now described as serums but here we will describe the more specialist products that you can find within a branded product range.

Serums can come in a pump dispenser or ampoule. They are designed to have an intensive or boosting effect on the skin, enhancing the results of the facial treatment. They can be used on all skin types and conditions as per the manufacturer's instructions.

Serums can contain humectants and hydrators; ceramides and lipids (mineral and vegetable oils); glycerol; essential oils; and vitamins.

Some serums are salon-exclusive products and are not for retail. Others can be retailed to the client to enhance their normal skin care routine and might be used for a short period, eg 7 days, or for a longer period, such as a month. They are normally applied before or instead of a moisturiser or night cream.

Serum

Ampoules

These are small glass or occasionally plastic bottles that contain a small amount of liquid with active ingredients. They are used to boost or intensify the results of a facial treatment or skin care routine at home.

Ampoules can be used in different ways depending on the manufacturer's instructions and the nature of the special ingredients they contain. They are formulated for a very specific treatment and might contain very fragile ingredients, eg essential oils. When the bottle has been opened they need to be used straight away or within a few days, otherwise the ingredients' lose their effect.

They can be mixed with massage media or used with specialist masks or before moisturising, to enhance the effects of the treatment.

Sun protection products with SPF

SPF stands for sun protection factor. The number next to the SPF tells you how much protection the product will give – but this will depend on the client's skin type and how easily they tan. If a client can stay in the sun for 15 minutes without getting sunburnt, a product with an SPF of 15 will give them 15 times that protection so they would be able to stay in the sun for 3¾ hours. However, the effectiveness of the product also depends on how well it has been applied and how strong the sun is.

Sunscreens work by absorbing some of the damaging UVB rays, preventing skin damage and premature ageing. They are suitable for all skin types and conditions. Their use is especially important after treatment with AHAs and BHAs, dermabrasion and glycolic peels.

Sunscreens might contain zinc oxide, vitamin E, wheat, soya oils and natural filters. The product should be applied to the skin at least 20 minutes *before* exposure to the sun so that it can settle into the skin and form a protective layer. A generous application is advisable, making sure the area (face or body) is fully covered.

INDUSTRY TIP

When you retail a product to a client with SPF to protect their skin, make sure you stress that they reapply it if they have been in water – even if the sunscreen is water-resistant, just to be safe. Dermatologists recommend that you use at least a factor 15, even if you tan easily, to keep the skin protected.

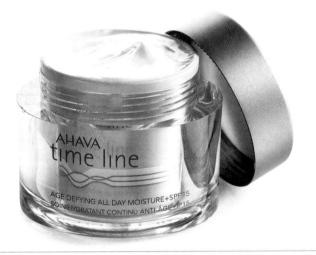

Moisturiser with SPF

INDUSTRY TIP

Many moisturisers contain sunscreens (SPF). However, these can limit the other skin care qualities of the product.

ACTIVITY

Make a chart and compare the moisturisers you have in your salon. Apply each product to the back of your hand and use the following headings to record the differences between them:

What is the texture like? How well has it absorbed? What does it smell off? How does the skin feel after use?

ACTIVITY

Investigate the moisturising products you have in your salon. Try to find a lotion, a cream and a gel. Look at the ingredients on each of the products.

- How different are they?
- Are many of the ingredients the same?
- Do the ingredients occur in a different order, showing different quantities in the formula?

INDUSTRY TIP

Using something new on a client will encourage them to think about and experience the benefits of the product to them and increase the chance of a retail sale.

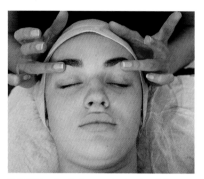

STEP 1 – Apply the product using little tapping movements on your client's skin, following the orbicularis oculi muscles.

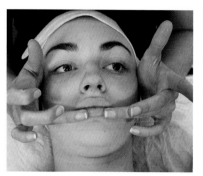

STEP 2 – Apply to your client's lips using the ring fingers, making sure the lips are fully covered.

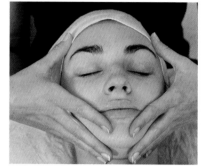

STEP 3 – Select a suitable moisturiser for your client's skin type. You will need no more than a five pence piece sized amount to cover the face and neck.

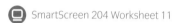

SmartScreen 204 Worksheet 11

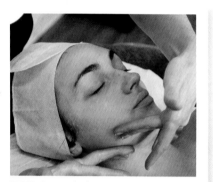

STEP 4 – Apply the moisturiser over the chin and lower face, across the cheeks, up the nose and across the forehead, using light effleurage movements.

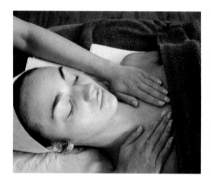

STEP 5 – You might choose a neck cream for the décolleté and neck area on a more mature client. Warm the neck cream with your fingertips and smooth across the décolleté and neck area using light effleurage movements.

INDUSTRY TIP

Let your client know when the treatment is complete. Recommend that your client sits up slowly as they might feel lightheaded, and offer them a glass of water. You can now give your client the aftercare advice they need.

INDUSTRY TIP

When you are using eye products, use them sparingly. A grain of rice sized amount is all you need.

INDUSTRY TIP

When you are using lip products, use them sparingly. A pea sized amount is all you need.

INDUSTRY TIP

When you are working around the lip and eye areas, always remember to use your ring fingers as these use the least pressure.

HOME CARE AND AFTERCARE ADVICE

Following a facial you should give your client suitable aftercare advice to follow. This consists of recommendations that your client should follow to maximise the short-term benefits from their facial treatment.

Home care advice consists of recommendations that your client should follow to maximise the long-term benefits of the treatment. These will include a suitable skin care routine, products and possibly lifestyle changes.

Leave the skin
free of make-up
until the next day

Follow a home care
routine to maintain
treatment results
and objectives

Avoid touching
the skin

**Home care
and aftercare
advice**

Relax and avoid
any strenuous activity

Avoid UV lamps and
sunbathing as the skin
will be more sensitive due
to stimulation during a
facial and the
products applied

Avoid any further
treatments to the
area, such as
depilation, for
24 hours

Depilation
Hair removal.

INDUSTRY TIP
If the client has had the facial in the morning,
recommend a light cleanse, tone and
moisturise before going to bed. If the facial
has been given later in the day, advise the
client that they will not need to do anything
else to their skin that day.

Recommend the client
follows a home skin care
routine to maintain the
treatment results
and objectives

Advise the
client what to do if
they have any
reactions or
contra-actions to
the treatment

Recommend suitable
professional products
for your client to use
so that they can
maximise the
long-term benefits

**Home care –
long-term
advice**

If
the client
needs to improve a
skin condition, advise
them to have a course of
facials, eg weekly for 6
weeks, to help improve the
skin condition. This can
be offered at a special
incentive price

Advise the clients
to have regular facials to
maximise the results and slow
down the signs of aging on the
skin. For more mature skin, once a
month is ideal if the client can
afford to do so. If the client has
concerns about their skin a
treatment programme should
be devised and discussed
with the client

INDUSTRY TIP

Look back at the Anatomy and Physiology chapter for further information on how natural ageing, lifestyle and environmental factors affect the condition of the skin and muscle tone.

Where appropriate, discuss any lifestyle changes that your client could make to improve their skin. Be tactful and discuss only issues that have been raised to avoid offending the client. The client will need to be told the benefits of the suggestions you make.

Increase physical activity to improve circulation, the skin's cell renewal and appearance

Eat a healthy diet – diet does have an impact on the skin. If you are not consuming enough essential vitamins and minerals this will have a negative impact on the skin. The skin needs certain minerals and vitamins and a balanced diet to renew and repair

Reduce caffeine and alcohol intake. Both of these dehydrate the body and the skin

Recommended lifestyle changes

Reduce the amount you smoke or give up smoking altogether. Smoking destroys vitamin C, which is essential for the skin. It also affects oxygen uptake and its circulation. Without oxygen the skin cannot renew and repair effectively

Find time to relax and de-stress. Stress affects the immune system and slows down the body's ability to repair

ACTIVITY

Review the lifestyle changes that you might discuss with the client – make a list of the benefits that the client might gain from following the advice you give.

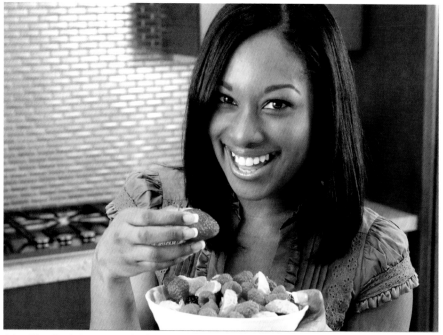

A healthy diet is important for healthy skin

CONTRA-ACTIONS

A contra-action is an adverse reaction that can happen during or after a treatment. The table lists some contra-actions that might occur and the actions to take if they do.

Contra-action	What to be aware of	Action to follow
Severe erythema	This might be due to overstimulation of the skin or it could be a sign that the skin is reacting adversely to a product.	Review what you are doing. If you are applying a massage, are you using appropriate techniques?
Overheating	If the skin is feeling very warm you should consider that the client might be having an adverse reaction.	Remove the product you are using with lukewarm water. Apply cold compresses to the skin to reduce the circulation.
Allergic reaction to a product	The skin will feel hot and the client will experience tingling or itching; the skin will feel irritated.	Remove the product completely with lukewarm water. Apply a cold compress. Stop the treatment. Refer the client to a medical practitioner if the irritation does not subside. Sometimes this reaction can be delayed and it might occur when the client has returned home. In this case advise the client to remove all traces of the product with warm water and apply a cold compress.
Swelling	This might occur in conjunction with an allergic reaction – see advice above.	As above.
Tissue damage resulting in blood loss	This can only happen as a result of poor practice. It can be as a result of scratching the client with long or poorly manicured nails, or damage caused by jewellery. It can be due to using products or tools in an inappropriate way causing damage to the skin, eg using a comedone extractor and scraping the skin too firmly, causing skin grazes.	Put on a pair of disposable gloves before treating the area to avoid any direct contact with the blood. Cleanse the area with an antiseptic first-aid wipe taken from a sealed package for hygiene. Tell the client that the skin has been broken and advise caution.

INDUSTRY TIP

For skin irritation it is often best to suggest that the client speaks to a pharmacist rather than a GP. It will be quicker and the pharmacist will usually have something that can be purchased over the counter without the need for a prescription, such as antihistamine.

INDUSTRY TIP

Always use lukewarm water on the skin as this is close to body heat. Very hot or very cold water should be avoided if there is any irritation as extremes of temperature make the skin react adversely, causing vasodilation or vasoconstriction. If a client has broken capillaries this can also aggravate the condition.

COMPLETING RECORDS

Now that your treatment is complete, you should make a note of what you have done during your facial, recording details of any products you have used, recommended or given a sample of to your client. It is useful to make a note of anything that the client specifically requested, eg an extra headrest or no eye pads (if they were claustrophobic). Note any reactions the client had, particularly if they were adverse ones. When your information is complete, file the card away. Maintain confidentiality and privacy – do not leave it lying around in the salon for other clients to see.

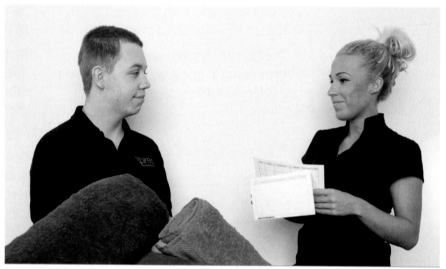

After completing the record card, remember to file it away

GOOD PRACTICE

Tidy your work area and leave it ready for the next treatment. Make sure you place lids securely back on any pots. Dispose of rubbish carefully in the bin. Clean and disinfect your sponges, complexion and mask brushes. Wash your mask bowl and put towels into the laundry area ready to be washed. Make sure the room is clean, tidy and ready for the next service.

MEN'S GROOMING

In this section we will be looking at shaving. Facial treatments have been covered in the facial section above and guidance has been given on how to adapt these for male clients. You can find information about improving the appearance of brows to enhance facial features for male clients in Chapter 210/218/225.

SHAVING

For many men, shaving is a daily routine. Shaving removes hair growth, cutting it close to the skin's surface. It also has an exfoliating effect as the blades scrape off the dead skin cells.

Shaving can be carried out using an electric shaver. This is a quick, dry method but tends not to give a very close finish. Wet shaving is more effective and involves using a shaving product and a razor. There are three different types of razor:

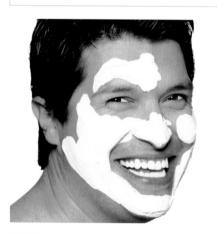

- cut-throat – a single long blade with a protective cover
- double-faced – double blade
- disposable – these come in different designs with different numbers of blades (up to 5) and swivel heads.

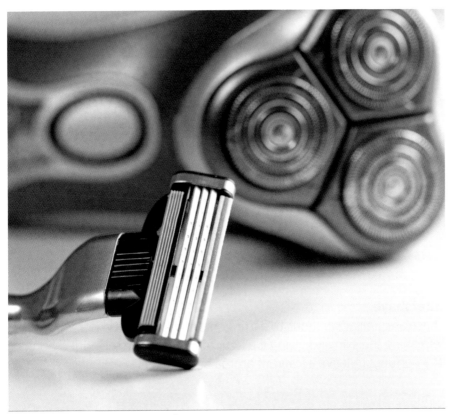

A disposable razor and an electric shaver

INDUSTRY TIP

Men should be advised to change their blades or dispose of their razor (if disposable) after approximately 10 shaves.

INDUSTRY TIP

Be careful of the terms you use with male clients. Use masculine phrases when talking to your client, eg balms not moisturisers, washes rather than cleansers, scrubs instead of exfoliants, grooming rather than pampering.

INDUSTRY TIP

Do not use blunt blades as these will drag the skin and increase the risk of shaving rashes and ingrown hairs.

MENS' GROOMING PRODUCTS

Shaving gels, creams and foams

These are applied to help lift the hairs. They also provide a slippery surface for the razor, making the shaving process easier and minimising the risk of shaving rashes. Use a clear gel if you are not shaving a complete beard area and if there are areas that are to be left, such as sideburns. The clear product will allow you to see clearly where you are shaving.

INDUSTRY TIP

The average male has over 15,000 hairs distributed over a third of his face.

Shaving serums and oils

These lubricate the skin and provide a perfect base for a close shave. They will also help to minimise the risk of a shaving rash. These are an alternative product to shaving gels or foams for clients with drier skin.

Aftershave balms

The application of balms following shaving will help to cool and calm the skin, and reduce any redness and razor-burn stinging (see page 321).

Moisturisers, fluids and emulsions

Men should be encouraged to use a moisturiser to help replace the oils that have been lost following shaving in addition to all the same benefits we have described for female clients (see pages 307–314). Like all moisturisers, these will help to keep the skin hydrated, supple and youthful. A huge range of moisturisers are now formulated and marketed to male clients.

INDUSTRY TIP

A good product to recommend to male clients is a 2-in-1 face wash and exfoliator. A combined product will encourage them to see the benefits of the skin care without it taking up too much time. Male clients do not like routines that seem feminine so this is a good alternative.

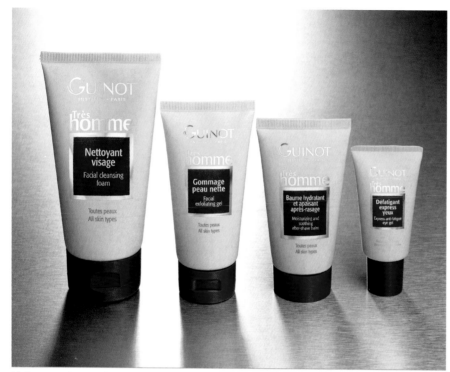

Male grooming products

Aftershave moisturiser

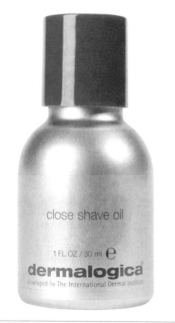

Shaving oil

Aftershave

These are similar solutions to astringents. They refine the pores, refreshing the skin and giving it a tight feel. They have the added bonus of a perfume to leave a fragrant aroma on the client's skin.

SHAVING THE SKIN

It is important that you understand the shaving process so that you can advise clients in the procedure and promote the best products to benefit the clients. With male skin care ranges expanding in the choice of products, this is an area where you can easily lose a sale through lack of knowledge. The shaving procedure described below will help you to understand the shaving process in more detail. You will not be expected to do this in the salon.

Procedure for a shaving service

1 Cleanse the skin using a light, water-soluble cleanser to make sure there is no oily residue on the skin. It also makes sure that the skin is clean before beginning. Rinse well with lukewarm water.

2 Place some shaving product in a bowl and dampen slightly with water. Work into a lather or foam using a shaving brush.

3 Work the shaving foam into the skin using small circles. This will help to lift the stubble and hairs.

4 Begin the shaving process. Rinse the blade regularly under running water to remove hair and clean the blade. This also helps to minimise cross-infection.

5   Begin at the sides of the face over the masseter muscle. Start at the top of the muscle and work down. Hold the skin taut with the opposite hand to minimise any discomfort. Use slow, deliberate strokes against the direction of hair growth. Repeat on the other side.

6   Shave down the cheek area to the mandible.

7   Work underneath the mandible and down the neck.

8   Work into the centre of the face, including the upper lip. Ask the client to pull their upper lip down over their upper teeth to keep the skin stretched. Move to the lower lip and chin. Ask the client to pull the lip over the lower teeth to keep the skin stretched.

9   Rinse the skin well with cool water to constrict and close the pores.

10 Apply an aftershave skin balm.

11 Apply a moisturiser, eye product and lip balm.

Following shaving, the client should be advised always to rinse their razor well under running water. They should rinse the shaving brush out well and squeeze or flick it to remove any excess water. The brush should be placed in a stand so that the water drips away from the handle.

Contra-actions to shaving

There are three contra-actions to shaving that a client might experience:

- **Shaving rash** can be caused by several factors. The most common is using a blunt blade, causing irritation on the skin's surface. Another common cause is failing to keep the blade clean during and following shaving. Lack of sufficient shaving product can also cause razor rash and irritation.

- **Cuts** are usually caused by a lack of skin support during shaving or an incorrect procedure. Clients should be advised to take extra care when they are using a new blade.

- **Ingrown hairs** – the most common cause of ingrown hairs is incorrect shaving, in particular shaving against the hair growth. Regular use of an exfoliant and a moisturiser will help to minimise ingrown hairs. Special products can also be recommended that are designed to help reduce ingrown hairs.

Aftercare advice following shaving

Advise the client to avoid the following immediately after shaving as the skin will be more sensitive and more likely to react to exposure:

- sunbathing and sunbeds (natural and artificial UV)
- excessive heat, such as saunas or steam baths
- perfumed products – this includes aftershave. Clients should be advised to use a suitable aftershave balm to calm and soothe the skin instead.

Additional grooming for eyebrow shaping can be found in Chapter 210, page 584, which applies to both men and women.

HANDY HINTS

If you are unsure of any of the muscles or bones mentioned in this sequence, review the information on the muscles and bones of the face in the Anatomy and Physiology chapter.

INDUSTRY TIP

Clients who like to use a shaving brush should be advised to always dry brushes so that the water runs away from the handle. This prevents rotting and the bristles becoming smelly.

Use the questions below to test your knowledge of Chapter 204/224 to see how much information you have retained. These questions will help you to revise what you have learnt in this chapter.

Turn to page 601 for the answers.

1. Which light is the best type to use for observing the skin during analysis?
   a) Magnifying lamp
   b) Fluorescent lighting
   c) Spot lights
   d) Flexible lamp

2. Which **one** of the following is the best advice to give a male client prior to coming in for a facial treatment?
   a) Use a low alcohol aftershave
   b) Have a close shave
   c) Use their normal shaving cream
   d) Do not shave for at least 48 hours prior to facial treatment

3. What can be tested during the manual examination of the skin by lightly pinching the skin in the main facial area?
   a) Elasticity
   b) Circulation
   c) Skin type
   d) Sebum production

4. A shiny nose on a client will indicate which **one** of the following skin types?
   a) Combination
   b) Dehydrated
   c) Dry
   d) Sensitive

5. Exfoliation would be beneficial to young skin to:
   a) remove stale make-up from the skin's surface
   b) deep cleanse the skin in preparation for massage
   c) rejuvenate the skin and give it a healthy glow
   d) remove dead skin cells, excess surface oils and surface debris.

6. Why is a water-soluble cleanser more suitable for oily skin?
   a) Has a light liquid texture
   b) Leaves minimal reside of oil on the skin
   c) Quicker to apply to the skin
   d) Can be rinsed off with water

7. Which **one** of the following is the main reason why distilled water can be used in a facial steamer?
   a) To generate pure steam
   b) To prevent the build-up of limescale
   c) To reduce the cost of servicing
   d) To increase vapour production

8. Which **one** of the following best identifies how a hot towel should be positioned on the client's face?
   a) Fold around the face leaving the nose and mouth exposed
   b) Fold in half and lay across the face
   c) Wrap around the head and face
   d) Fold in four and press onto the client's skin

9. Which **one** of the following is a function of a moisturiser?
   a) Removes traces of toner prior to make-up
   b) Provides a smooth base for make-up
   c) Makes blending of make-up products easier
   d) Prevents make-up from seeping into pores

10. Why should further facial treatments be recommended to a client?
    a) To maximise the benefits and effects of the treatment
    b) Relaxation and enjoyment of the treatment
    c) Therapists will gain more experience
    d) Increased profits for the salon

11. Which **one** of the following could show client satisfaction with the facial treatment they have received?
    a) Completing the treatment within the set time
    b) Offering the client a refreshment
    c) Giving the client a treatment discount
    d) The client books another treatment

12. Which **one** of the following might be an indication of dry skin in a client?
    a) Formation of fine lines around the eyes
    b) Prominent thread veins on the neck
    c) Small comedones around the nose
    d) Good bone structure and facial contours

13. Which **one** of the following is an essential part of the therapist's preparation?
    a) File and clean the nails
    b) Make sure a refreshment is available for the client
    c) Display aftercare products
    d) Make sure that all equipment is ready

14. How should a facial massage be adapted for a client with oily skin with pustules?
    a) Increase massage around the neck and shoulders, avoid pustules, keep movements slow and light
    b) Follow the normal facial massage routine but increase the time of the massage
    c) Increase effleurage and deep petrissage movements but avoid tapotement
    d) Avoid areas where pustules are present and apply a lot of circular frictions using a massage oil

15. Which **one** of the following descriptions will usually identify a sensitive skin condition?
    a) Shiny nose and sallow complexion
    b) Tendency to redness; skin warm to the touch
    c) Presence of thread veins and milia
    d) Fine lines around the eyes and flaky skin

Starting out with a qualification in beauty therapy I decided very early on that I wanted to run my own skin care business. Having never really connected with the 'beauty' side of the industry I knew my destiny was rather to help people achieve the best possible skin health.

I gained valuable experience in salon management and consultancy before setting up on my own. My greatest life changing moment was finding Dermalogica; a unisex line who share my vision for achieving skin health without luxury, gimmicks or 'miracle' cures.

As the Education Manager for Dermalogica I have a team of over 70 people in the education department to motivate and inspire. Believing passionately that education sets you apart from others, I thoroughly enjoy delivering educational presentations globally and contributing to trade and consumer publications alongside writing curriculum.

Our industry has changed dramatically in recent years and is set to continue to evolve. In order to keep up with those changes and meet the needs of today's customer, attending on-going training is vital.

Every day I am privileged to meet incredible therapists who through education, passion and sheer hard work have made themselves successful and financially independent in the skin care industry.

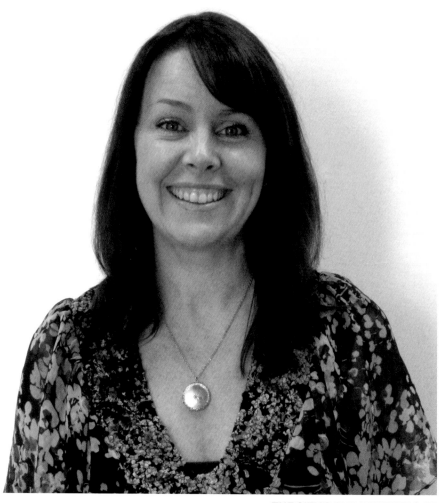

REMOVE HAIR USING WAXING/THREADING TECHNIQUES

The removal of body hair is not a recent fashion – the ancient Egyptians were removing body hair in 300BC! Today, waxing is one of the most common treatments carried out in the salon, from a quick eyebrow shape to larger areas, such as the legs, leaving the area smooth and hair free. Waxing is a skill that requires practice so that you are quick and efficient in carrying out the treatment.

Threading has become much more widespread in western salons in recent years. It has been used in Arabic and Asian countries for centuries. A twisted loop of cotton thread is used and rotated rapidly over the skin to trap and remove unwanted hairs from their roots. When the therapist is experienced in carrying out threading, it is a fast, neat and inexpensive method of hair removal.

In this chapter you will learn how to:

- prepare for waxing treatments and threading services
- provide waxing treatments
- provide threading services
- aftercare and home care advice.

PREPARE FOR WAXING TREATMENTS AND THREADING SERVICES

Before you carry out hair removal treatments, it is important to be prepared. Health and safety requirements should be followed for every service and knowing how to set up your service area, which products and tools you should use and how to carry out an effective consultation are essential for waxing treatments and threading services.

In this part of the chapter you will learn about:

- health and safety
- the treatment/service environment
- consultation
- sensitivity testing
- contra-indications to waxing treatments and threading services
- equipment and tools for waxing treatments and threading services
- products for waxing treatments and threading services
- treatment timings
- preparing your work area
- preparing the client.

INDUSTRY TIP

Habia has produced a booklet called *The Code of Practice for Waxing*. This booklet gives recommendations to beauty therapists. It has been approved by environmental health practitioners across the UK and is endorsed by several high-profile manufacturers and suppliers. It is a voluntary code, but it is recommended that all professional beauty therapists follow it. It states the minimum level of performance and practice expected in health and safety enforcement related to waxing. The booklet includes guidance on waxing systems, hygiene, operational procedures and salon safety.

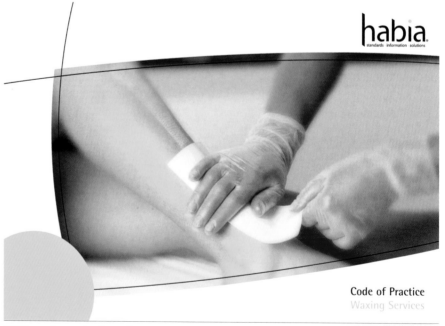

habia
standards · information · solutions

Code of Practice
Waxing Services

Habia waxing code of practice

HEALTH AND SAFETY

One of the most important health and safety requirements for waxing is PPE. Wear disposal gloves to maintain personal hygiene and reduce any risk of cross-infection. For threading, you can wear gloves if you want. However, they can affect the threading process and restrict the roll of the thread as it can catch on the gloves. Put gloves on clean, dry hands. Gloves should be made from nitrile or PVC and should also be powder free. (Powder is applied to the inside of the gloves to make their application easier, but it actually dries to skin out). Avoid latex gloves due to latex allergies. Remove gloves by turning the outer surface inside out to avoid the contaminated surface of the gloves being exposed in the waste bin.

Some therapists also like to wear a waxing apron. This might be a personal choice or one of the salon's policies.

DISPOSING OF WASTE

You should have a waste bin that is lined with a dustbin liner. For hygiene purposes, the bin should have a lid that can be opened and closed easily, ideally with a foot pedal. To make sure you are being **hygienic**, dispose of your waste as you work and do not let it collect on a trolley or work surface. Place bin liners with waxing strips inside another bin liner before placing in an external bin.

> **HANDY HINTS**
>
> Refer back to Chapter 202 for information on other health and safety requirements related to waxing treatments and threading services.

TREATMENT/SERVICE ENVIRONMENT

The salon environment is very important in making the client feel relaxed and comfortable during their treatment. Before carrying out the treatment, you should carry out a quick check of your working area for hazards and remove these to reduce any risks.

> **HANDY HINTS**
>
> You should be familiar with the health and safety legislation. Review the Legislation chapter (pages 91–113) before working through this chapter as it has an effect on your working practices. You need to make sure you are working safely and legally.

 SmartScreen 206 Worksheet 3

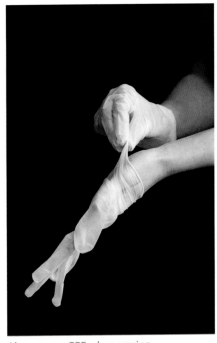

Always wear PPE when waxing

Hygienic
Clean.

 SmartScreen 202 Worksheet 8

> **HANDY HINTS**
>
> Review Chapter 202 for removing gloves to make sure you are following the procedure correctly.

> **HANDY HINTS**
>
> Additional information on waste disposal can be found in Chapter 202 on page 156–157.

> **HANDY HINTS**
>
> Further information on risk assessment can be found in Chapter 202 Follow health and safety practice in the salon.

 SmartScreen 206 Worksheet 2

Prior to carrying out the treatment, the factors in the table below should all be checked and adjusted if necessary.

Environmental factor	Why it is important
Lighting	▪ Good bright overhead lighting is essential so that the area to be treated can be seen clearly during the treatment. If you can see well, you will be able to see clearly the hair that needs to be removed. ▪ Lighting should not cause any shadows as these will create areas of poor visibility and strain your eyes.
Temperature	▪ A warm room temperature is essential. ▪ For some waxing treatments the client will be undressing and if the client gets cold this will affect the waxing process. ▪ It is always better if the client is warm as the hairs will be removed more easily both during waxing and threading.
Ventilation	▪ The room needs to smell fresh and be well ventilated. ▪ A stale or stuffy room will be unpleasant and uncomfortable. ▪ Good ventilation will make sure the air is circulating to keep you alert and reduce cross-infection from stale air.
Aroma	▪ There should be a pleasant aroma in the room so that it smells fresh and inviting.
Privacy	▪ The client will feel more comfortable and relaxed if they feel the treatment is private. They will not want to feel they are being exposed unnecessarily. ▪ Keep treatment room doors or curtains closed. ▪ Make sure windows are covered so that there is no view from outside into the room. ▪ Leave the room if the client needs to undress for the waxing treatment they are having (eg full leg wax). ▪ Cover areas you are not working on with a towel where possible so that you protect the client's modesty.

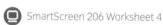 SmartScreen 206 Worksheet 4

HANDY HINTS

Consultation techniques are covered in more detail in Chapter 203 on pages 166–176. You will find information here on verbal and non-verbal communication techniques, the use of visual aids and the importance of completing client record cards. Look back at this chapter to remind yourself about consultation techniques before you continue.

CONSULTATION

Before you carry out a waxing treatment or threading service, you will need to have a consultation with your client to find out what results the client is hoping to see from their treatment; you will then know what your treatment objectives are. To make sure your client leaves satisfied, it is important to listen to them carefully and match the treatment objectives to their needs. This is also a good opportunity to think about any retail products that the client might benefit from so that you can incorporate this advice into your treatment.

Waxing is a very personal treatment and although it is important with all treatments to make the client feel comfortable and at ease, it is especially important if the client is going to have to undress and expose parts of their body to you. You must always behave professionally and make them feel that their modesty, privacy and comfort is important.

SENSITIVITY TESTING

There are some tests that should be carried out prior to all waxing treatments.

PATCH TEST

Any client who has not had waxing treatments before should have a patch test 24 hours before their first waxing treatment. This is important for clients who have a history of allergies or skin sensitivity. This might also be a wise procedure to carry out if there is any concern about a client's health (eg if the client has started to take new **systemic** medication or if they become pregnant).

The patch test involves applying a small amount of wax to an area, such as the ankle or wrist. Cleanse the area, apply the wax and remove in the normal way. Apply aftercare lotion or cream to complete the patch test. Record the patch test and date the client record card.

HEAT SENSITIVITY OR THERMAL TESTING

This test involves two parts:

1 The first part is to check the temperature of the wax before applying it to the client. Apply a small amount of wax to the inner part of your wrist to check the temperature of the wax. Remove it using a small eyebrow strip. Do not use the same strip on the client for hygiene reasons.

2 The second part is the application of a small amount of wax to the client's skin to check that the temperature is suitable for their skin. Remove with a strip as normal. If the temperature needs adjusting, this should be done and checked again before starting.

TACTILE TESTING

This test checks that the client's skin is not damaged by testing their senses. The test involves applying a sharp/blunt or rough/smooth item randomly, but with care, to the area to be treated while the client is not looking. The client is asked to state what sensation they can feel.

Systemic

Affecting one of more of the systems of the body.

INDUSTRY TIP

If you change the brand of product you use or start using a new wax, always make sure you carry out new patch tests on any clients who need them.

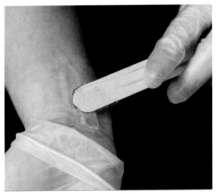

Check temperature on wrist

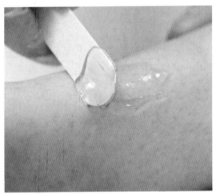

Checking temperature on the client

HANDY HINTS

At all times in the salon it is important that you behave in a professional manner. Look back at the section on Professional behaviour in Chapter 201 (pages 130–134).

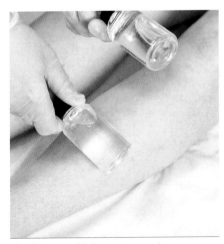

Checking sensitivity to temperature

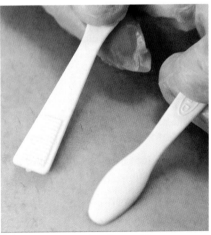

Tactile testing on the client's skin

WHY DON'T YOU...
with a colleague carryout a patch test, tactile test and heat sensitivity test.

INDUSTRY TIP

Many clients are more sensitive when they are pre-menstrual. If your client is more sensitive during this period, it might be a good idea to advise them to avoid booking an appointment at this time.

INDUSTRY TIP

Clients who have an allergy to wax or have very sensitive skin often cope well with threading as an alternative.

INDUSTRY TIP

Be very cautious with clients who are using skin care products containing retinol, glycolic acid or AHAs when you are carrying out facial waxing as the skin might be more sensitive. If the client has been having professional glycolic treatments or peels, waxing should not be carried out until the skin has had a suitable time to recover.

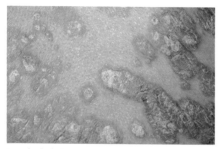

Psoriasis is just one contra-indication that can prevent waxing

Hyper-keratosis

Thickening of the skin caused by an excessive amount of keratin.

Phlebitis

This is inflammation of a vein. This is a painful condition that can affect one or more of the veins of the leg. The skin is visibly red and inflamed around the area of the affected vein and can feel quite warm to the touch. Do not treat the affected area.

CONTRA-INDICATIONS TO WAXING TREATMENTS AND THREADING SERVICES

A contra-indication is a reason why a treatment cannot be carried out. It might a general contra-indication that means the client cannot be treated at all or one that might require the treatment to be restricted. If there is a reason why you cannot carry out the treatment you should tactfully explain why to the client. If you think that the client should seek medical advice then suggest this but remember you are not a medical practitioner and you should not make any form of diagnosis.

In some cases contra-indications will just restrict the treatment. For example, a skin tag or mole can be covered with some petroleum jelly to stop the wax sticking and pulling on the skin. It might be that the treatment will need to be adapted. For example, if the client has a prominent varicose vein, you will have to work around the area to avoid any possible damage to the skin and the underlying vein as the wax is pulled off. When you need to avoid an area or adapt a treatment, you should always explain why to the client.

Contra-indications that *prevent* waxing include:

- fungal infections
- bacterial infections
- viral infections
- infestations
- severe eczema
- severe psoriasis
- severe skin conditions
- deep-vein thrombosis
- chemotherapy
- radiotherapy
- urinary infections/diseases.

Contra-indications to waxing that *restrict* treatment include:

- broken bones
- recent scar tissue
- **hyper-keratosis**
- skin allergies
- cuts and abrasions
- epilepsy
- diabetes
- skin disorders
- recent fractures and sprains
- undiagnosed lumps and swellings (oedema)
- product allergies
- circulatory conditions and **phlebitis**
- hyper-sensitive skin
- recent cosmetic surgery and tattoos
- recent laser treatment
- recent mircro-dermabrasion treatment.

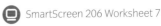

ACTIVITY

Make a list of the contra-indications that restrict treatment. Explain how they restrict the waxing treatment and how you might have to adapt the treatment.

EQUIPMENT AND TOOLS FOR WAXING TREATMENTS AND THREADING SERVICES

It is important to make sure that all your equipment is prepared before your client arrives. Check all the equipment to make sure it is safe to use. You should check for any damage to the equipment, frayed flexes or broken plugs. Make sure there are no trailing wires. Plug in the wax heater and magnifying lamp, if you are going to use one, and switch them on at the mains. Check that the wax heater is on a stable surface.

EQUIPMENT

Equipment	Preparation and use	Additional information
Wax heater 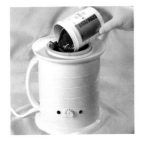	▪ Plug in the wax heater and switch it on at the mains. ▪ Turn on the wax heater and allow enough time for the wax to heat up fully prior to the waxing treatment – this usually takes about 10–20 minutes depending on the wax. Hot wax might take a bit longer to heat if you are using a larger (1 kg plus) heater. ▪ For hot wax, the heater should be turned up to high until the edge of the wax begins to melt and then turned down to the normal working temperature. ▪ Adjust the temperature if necessary.	▪ Wax should be melted in a specially designed heater. The heater should have a **thermostatic** control. This is to make sure that the temperature of the wax can be maintained at suitable working temperatures. ▪ Always make sure you are familiar with the manufacturer's instructions for the heater you are using. ▪ Roller and flat-head applicator cartridges must be heated in heaters that are specially designed to fit the cartridges. **Thermostat** A device that controls temperature or that turns on when a temperature reaches a certain point.
Magnifying lamp 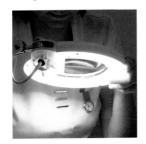	▪ Plug in the magnifying lamp if you are going to use one and switch it on at the mains. ▪ Make sure that the magnifying lamp is clean and that you can see through the magnifying lens clearly.	▪ A magnifying lamp is useful for checking that you have removed all stray hairs.

Tools	Preparation and use	Additional information
Wax strips 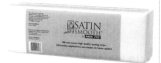	<ul><li>There are *two* main types of wax strip – muslin and paper – that can be used in conjunction with warm wax to remove the wax from the skin.</li><li>Make sure you have plenty of strips on your trolley for your treatment.</li><li>Make sure you have cut up some smaller strips and have these ready on your trolley for using on small areas, such as the face.</li></ul>	<ul><li>Your choice of wax strip will be your personal preference as they both achieve the same end result:<ul><li>**muslin strips** – these are light and very flexible, but they absorb some wax residue</li><li>**paper strips** – these are stiffer than muslin. The wax adheres to the surface and is not absorbed into the material.</li></ul></li></ul>
Spatulas 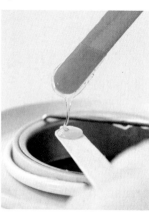	<ul><li>You should have several spatulas on your trolley. You should have large and small spatulas for different areas of the body.</li><li>Your selection of spatulas should be disposable and are usually made of wood.</li><li>Practise spatula methods – the Habia code of practice recommends *two* methods for using a spatula:<ul><li>*One-dip method* – a spatula is dipped into the wax and used once and then thrown away.</li><li>*Drizzle method* – this uses one spatula to place into the pot and a second spatula to apply the wax. The wax pot spatula is used to collect the wax and then it is drizzled onto the working spatula to avoid any contamination of the wax. This method will add time to the waxing process even when you are proficient.</li></ul></li></ul>	<ul><li>Smaller spatulas should be used for small areas on the face – these are the size of a lolly stick.</li><li>Some spatulas have slanted ends to help give a more precise application.</li></ul>
Cotton thread 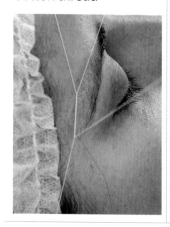	<ul><li>This is used to create the threading loop.</li><li>The thread should be prepared just before you start the treatment by pulling off the desired length of thread in front of the client for use with the preferred technique (mouth, hand, neck) ready to start.</li></ul>	<ul><li>Make sure the thread is 100 per cent cotton.</li><li>The thread should be made from good quality cotton that does not break easily.</li><li>Never use a synthetic thread.</li></ul>

Tools	Preparation and use	Additional information
Tweezers 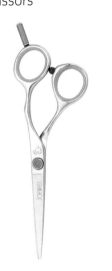	<ul><li>Tweezers should be sterilised in an autoclave and placed in a chemical disinfecting solution in a jar on the trolley for easy access during the treatment.</li><li>Tweezers are used for removing strays hairs following waxing and threading.</li><li>They might also be used following an eyebrow wax to shape the eyebrows to give further definition.</li></ul>	<ul><li>Make sure you are using stainless steel tweezers so that they can be put into an autoclave for sterilisation.</li><li>When you have finished using the tweezers, make sure that they are wiped over with a disinfectant solution to remove any stray hairs and grease before they are sterilised again.</li></ul>
Scissors	<ul><li>Scissors should be sterilised in an autoclave and placed in a chemical disinfecting solution in a jar on the trolley for easy access during the treatment.</li><li>Scissors are used for cutting very long hairs to make it easier to wax without pulling unwanted hair (eg along a bikini line).</li><li>They might also be used for a scissor-over-comb technique to cut long, unwanted eyebrow hairs. An eyebrow comb or disposable mascara brush is used to hold the long hair up away from the eyebrows so that you can trim the long hair.</li><li>Scissors that are used for cutting cotton should only be used for that purpose and should still be stored in a chemical solution for hygiene in between treatments.</li></ul>	<ul><li>Make sure you are using stainless steel scissors so that they can be put into an autoclave for sterilisation.</li><li>When you have finished using the scissors, make sure that they are wiped over with a disinfectant solution to remove any stray hairs and grease before they are sterilised again.</li></ul>
Mirror 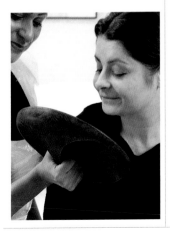	<ul><li>You should have a clean mirror handy to give to the client during consultation if they are having any facial threading or waxing. They can show you exactly how much hair they would like removed.</li><li>You should also give the client the mirror on completion of the treatment to make sure they are happy with what you removed.</li></ul>	<ul><li>Always make sure the mirror is kept clean and free from fingerprints.</li></ul> **INDUSTRY TIP** Clean the magnifying lens and hand-held mirror with a mirror cleaning cloth rather than a window cleaning product as these tend to leave smears.

Tools	Preparation and use	Additional information
Eyebrow brush and comb	▪ These should be washed in hot soapy water and stood in a chemical disinfectant solution. ▪ They are used to brush the unwanted hairs up out of the way before threading or waxing. ▪ They might also be used to comb through the eyebrow hair and lift the hairs up so that very long hairs can be trimmed with scissors.	▪ It is better to use disposable mascara brushes to maintain hygiene.
Disposable gloves	▪ These are used to protect the therapist and client from cross-infection. ▪ They protect the therapist's hands from exposure to chemicals.	▪ Use powder-free, nitrile, vinyl or PVC gloves.

INDUSTRY TIP

Try to avoid heating up warm wax by turning the wax heaters onto full. If you forget to turn the heater down in time the wax will get too hot for you to use. The excessive heat can also affect the properties of the wax. It is better to know how long it will take for the wax to melt at a lower temperature and allow it to melt gently.

ACTIVITY

Practise with both types of wax strip and write down how they compare. Which do you prefer and why? Do you prefer to use one or the other on a particular area?

CONSUMABLES

Remember, a consumable is something that you can only use once during the treatment. Here is a list of the consumables you will need for providing waxing and threading treatments.

Consumable	Use	Additional information
Cotton wool	▪ Cotton wool discs are used for applying cleanser and lotions.	▪ Cotton wool is used following treatment to avoid direct contact with the skin and prevent cross-infection.

Facial tissues	▪ Facial tissues are used to:
	  ▪ protect clothes (eg pants) from wax
	  ▪ blot moisture from the skin.	

Orange wood stick	▪ Orange wood sticks are used to measure eyebrow length during eyebrow shaping.	
Couch roll	▪ Couch roll is used for hygiene reasons to cover the couch. ▪ A sheet might also be placed on the floor for the client to stand on. ▪ It is also used to clean equipment.	▪ If you use couch roll on the floor, check that the paper will not slip.

Make sure you are being economical and cost-effective with your wax strips. As a rough guide you will need:

3–4 strips for a half leg

7–8 strips for a full leg (without bikini line).

Put wax heaters onto a timer plug so that they start to heat up 15 minutes before the salon opens. This will make sure your wax is ready for the first appointment.

For further detail on how to use orange wood sticks to mark out eyebrows during eyebrow shaping, refer to Chapter 210/218/225 on pages 560–600.

PRODUCTS FOR WAXING TREATMENTS AND THREADING SERVICES

Listed below are all the products you will need to carry out waxing treatments and threading services.

Products	Preparation and use	Additional information
Disinfecting chemical solution	▪ Place diluted disinfectant (eg Barbicide or Sterilsafe) into a glass jar to keep metal tools clean and hygienic during the treatment.	▪ Make sure that the solution is diluted and disposed of according to the manufacturer's instructions.
Petroleum jelly	▪ This is a barrier cream that can be used to cover small skin imperfections, such as a mole or a skin tag. ▪ It prevents the wax from sticking to the contra-indication and causing any damage to the area.	▪ Only use a tiny amount – enough to just cover the area.
Cleanser	▪ If the client has make-up on their face, it is a good idea to cleanse the skin first to remove the make-up before applying a disinfection cleanser.	▪ It is suggested you use a light lotion suitable for all skin types – even sensitive skin.
Pre-wax lotions or sprays	▪ This is a solution that is applied to the skin to remove any surface oils and debris and to make sure the wax adheres well to the hair and skin. ▪ They can also be used to cleanse the skin before threading.	▪ Pre-wax solutions might be lotions or sprays. Any products, such as body lotion, left on the skin will reduce the grip or bond of the wax.

Products	Preparation and use	Additional information
Pre-threading cleanser	■ This is a light disinfectant product, such as Steritane, that is used to cleanse the skin before threading. ■ It is applied to the skin to remove any surface oils and debris and during threading to make sure the cotton rolls easily over the skin.	■ The skin should still be prepared and cleansed prior to threading like any other treatment.
Powder	■ Powder is used to make sure the skin's surface is dry especially in intimate areas and under the arms. ■ The powder is used to absorb excess moisture helping to keep the skin dry. ■ When used in conjunction with hot wax it forms a surface on the skin preventing the wax from sticking and pulling the skin so it must only be used in small quantities. ■ It can be used to the same effect with warm waxes but again must only be used in small quantities as too powder much will prevent the wax from sticking.	■ Purified talc is still commonly used but these days there is a move towards using talc-free powders, such as corn starch. There are many hazardous chemicals in talc and it can be quite harmful if inhaled continually. ■ Powder should be applied carefully and ideally from a powder applicator to minimise the amount of powder in the air. ■ When you are applying powder, keep the product close to the skin and avoid shaking the container vigorously.

Soothing lotions	■ Soothing lotions are applied after waxing or threading because they:
	  ■ soothe the skin
	  ■ have an antiseptic effect to minimise any contra-actions
	  ■ remove any wax residue from the skin's surface following waxing.
		■ Depending on the salon's preference, this product could be a cream, lotion or an oil-based product.

Wax equipment cleaner 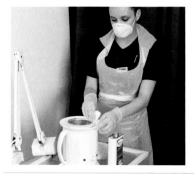	■ Pour the cleaner onto a tissue to remove wax from equipment and floors. ■ If the product has a spray, spray it onto the surface to be cleansed and leave for a few moments before wiping away with a piece of tissue or couch roll.	■ It is recommended that you use gloves when you are working with this product. ■ If you are cleaning the wax heater, make sure it is turned off, but still warm, so that you can remove the wax easily.

TYPES OF WAX

There are a number of different types of wax to choose from when you are carrying out a waxing treatment. It is therefore important that you know about the different types of wax available, how to prepare them and the ingredients within them.

Waxing product	Preparation and application	Ingredients
Warm wax (also known as honey wax or cream wax) 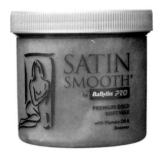	■ This is a semi-solid wax which, when heated, becomes liquid. The working **consistency** should be quite runny but not so runny that it is difficult to collect on a spatula and apply. ■ There are many different types of warm wax so it is important that you are familiar with the manufacturer's instructions for the wax you are using. ■ The working temperature of warm waxes varies between manufacturers but an average working temperature is 40–45°C but can be as low as 35°C. ■ Warm wax can come in a variety of colours from a clear, honey colour to opaque waxes which are cream, pink or pale green in colour.	■ Warm wax is made of refined gum resins, gum rosin and hydrocarbon tackifiers that give the wax its adhesive qualities. ■ Additional additives, such as chamomile or lavender, might be included to give a soothing effect or tea tree oil to give an antiseptic effect. **Consistency** The thickness or smoothness of a substance.
Sugar paste 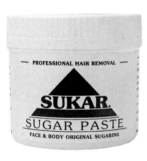	■ Sugar paste is a special type of wax. It comes from traditional methods of waxing which are still used in the Mediterranean and Arab countries. ■ The formula for sugar paste has changed little during its history and is made from a lemon and sugar base or a sticky emulsion of oil and honey. ■ The paste is worked with the hands to apply it and remove it.	■ It contains a high quantity of sugar (sucrose) or honey. ■ Today, sugar paste, like other waxing products, also contains oils and additional additives, such as olive oil or aloe vera extract, to reduce discomfort. ■ Real sugar paste will always be water soluble.
Sugar wax 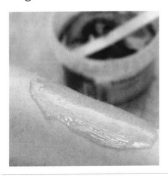	■ This is a wax that has some of the qualities of sugar paste but is warmed, applied and removed using the same methods as warm wax.	■ Sugar wax is a marketing move to introduce a new product but many do not see it as a true sugaring product.

Waxing product	Preparation and application	Ingredients
Hot wax – film, hard or peelable waxes 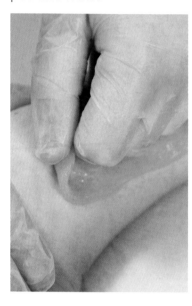	<ul><li>Hot waxes include film, hard or peelable wax. The wax can come as blocks of wax, chunks or pellets.</li><li>Whichever form the wax comes in, it is important to make sure it is fully melted before use.</li><li>Hot wax always has a hotter working temperature, hence the name hot wax, than warm wax. However, today this is not always the case and it is important to be familiar with the individual manufacturer's specifications.</li><li>A typical beeswax hot wax has a working temperature of 60–62°C. Film, hard and peelable waxes all have lower working temperatures which is why they have increased in popularity.</li><li>Always check the manufacturer's instructions for the brand of product you are using to be sure.</li></ul>	<ul><li>Hot wax has come a long way from its original beeswax formula. It used to also be known as beeswax due to its main ingredient.</li><li>Film wax and peelable waxes are other names given to this method but the application is the same.</li><li>All hot waxes are made from flexible resins. Additional additives, such as azulene and lavender, might be included to have a soothing effect.</li></ul>

INDUSTRY TIP

Wax temperatures vary as do the thermostats on wax heaters. Wax is made to be compatible with specific brands of wax heaters so it is important you check the manufacturer's instructions and always monitor the temperature of wax in a universal (non-specific) heater.

INDUSTRY TIP

Always use the correct size spatula for the area you are waxing.

TREATMENT TIMINGS

The table below states the industry accepted timings for different waxing treatments and threading services. Treatments will vary from client to client and might need to be modified and adapted depending on the client's skin type, hair growth and their expectations of their treatment, so these treatment times are just a guide.

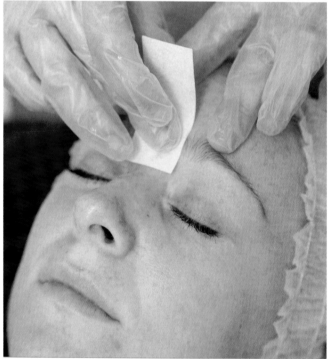

Waxing between the eyebrows

Treatment area	Treatment/service times
Half leg wax (ankle to the knee or just above the knee)	Up to 30 minutes
Full leg wax (ankle to the bikini line)	Up to 45 minutes
Underarm wax	Up to 15 minutes
Bikini line wax	Up to 15 minutes
Eyebrow wax	Up to 10 minutes
Lip and chin wax	Up to 10 minutes
Face threading	Approximately 30 minutes (depending on size of area)

<table>
<tr><td>INDUSTRY TIP</td></tr>
<tr><td>These times can be flexible.</td></tr>
</table>

INDUSTRY TIP	
These times can be flexible.	

Please note at Level 2 you are not expected to undertake Brazilian waxing. The technique is included in intimate waxing at Level 3.

ACTIVITY

Find out the timings of waxing treatments in your local salons.

PREPARING YOUR WORK AREA

The treatment area should be fully prepared before the client arrives. Make sure that all work surfaces have been cleaned and that any equipment or products that you need are ready and in easy reach before you start.

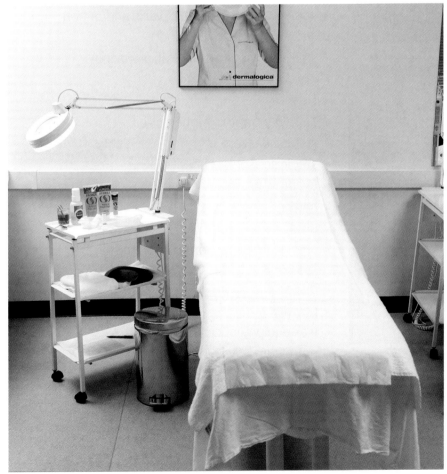

Prepared treatment area for waxing

TREATMENT COUCH

The couch should be neat, tidy and ready for the client. For leg and bikini waxing the treatment couch should be covered with a protective cover – this might be a plastic cover or couch roll.

For threading, the couch just needs to be protected with a piece of couch roll. If the client is sat on a semi-reclining chair rather than a couch, this should be protected in the same way.

INDUSTRY TIP

Plastic covers can get very hot and sticky so make sure they are covered with a small washable cotton sheet and/or couch roll.

PREPARING YOUR TROLLEY

The trolley should be clean and set up in an organised way. You should have the following consumables and equipment easily accessible:

Waxing trolley

If you are carrying out a waxing treatment, your trolley should contain:

- dry cotton wool discs or squares
- facial tissues
- disposable spatulas – large and small
- wax heater(s) – securely positioned on a stable trolley
- adequate supply of wax (warm and/or hot)
- wax strips (muslin or paper)
- small cut wax strips (for facial waxing)
- pre-wax lotion
- cleanser
- after-wax/soothing lotion or oil
- sterile tweezers
- sterile scissors
- eyebrow brush and comb
- mirror
- orange wood sticks
- chemical disinfection solution to stand tweezers and scissors in (eg Barbicide)
- disposable gloves
- powder
- wax equipment cleaner
- petroleum jelly.

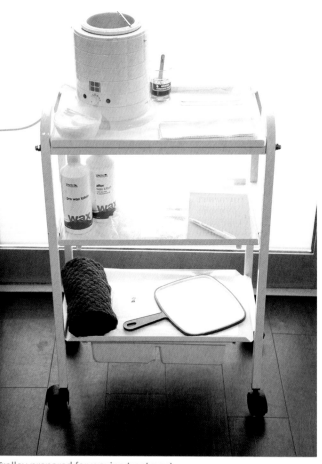

Trolley prepared for waxing treatment

Threading trolley

If you are carrying out a threading service, your trolley should contain:

- cotton thread
- dry cotton wool discs or squares
- facial tissues
- pre-wax lotion/antiseptic lotion
- cleanser
- after-wax soothing lotion or oil
- sterile tweezers
- sterile scissors
- eyebrow brush and comb
- mirror
- chemical disinfection solution to stand tweezers and scissors in (eg Barbicide)
- disposable gloves.

PREPARING THE CLIENT FOR WAXING

Always check whether the client has had previous waxing treatments. If the client has not had waxing before you need to advise the client that the hair growth must be long enough for you to wax. As a guideline, the hair on the body needs to be about 1 cm long or about 2-weeks' growth following shaving. Advise the client to wear lose clothing if they are having a leg or a bikini wax. This is to allow the air to circulate following treatment and to prevent any restrictive clothing rubbing on sensitive areas following the treatment.

SKIN AND HAIR ANALYSIS

When your client is settled and comfortable on the couch, you should carry out a skin and hair analysis. You should do this before starting any waxing or threading treatment, regardless of the area. This should be done as you prepare the area to be treated by wiping it over with a pre-wax solution or cleansing product.

The purpose of your analysis is to:

- look at the hair growth and hair growth patterns
- check for contra-indications
- check the skin type and condition.

 SmartScreen 206 Worksheet 5

Skin types and conditions

We tend to think of skin types and conditions only in relation to the face but the body can also have different skin types. The skin can be dry, dehydrated, mature, oily or normal and different areas of the body can have different skin types. There is detailed information about different skin types in the Anatomy and Physiology chapter on pages 16–17. You should make sure you are able to recognise different skin types and conditions before beginning any waxing treatment since they can impact on the waxing process. If the skin is oily, it might be necessary to use more powder to absorb any excess oil and help the wax stick better.

Achilles tendon

The tendon that attaches the **gastrocnemius** (see page 73) to the calcaneus (heel bone).

Gastrocnemius

Muscle forming the calf.

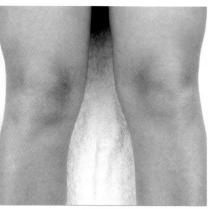

Dry skin on knees

If the skin is very dry, the wax will help to remove some of the scaly dead skin leaving healthy skin underneath. This is a good time to advise the client of the benefits of exfoliating and moisturising. Dry skin can hold onto the wax and draw the wax into the dry skin. This can cause problems with removal in areas where the skin is particularly dry (eg over the knees and along the **Achilles tendon**). When the wax is removed, it can take away more of the dry skin cells than wanted making the skin sore.

> **INDUSTRY TIP**
>
> If you have an area of wax that will not come off, do not keep trying to remove it as the skin will become sore and even bruised. Apply another patch of wax that covers the affected area and the troublesome patch of wax to make a slightly larger patch and then remove as normal.

> **HANDY HINTS**
>
> Make sure are familiar with the information on skin types and characteristics in the Anatomy and Physiology chapter on pages 2–30.

ACTIVITY

Work with three colleagues and compare the skin on your legs. Is there a difference? For each of your three colleagues, write down three reasons why the skin is different on each of them. Now ask each colleague a few questions to see if you can find out why. For example, do they moisturise?

Very sensitive skin can appear to react adversely following a treatment. It is only when the client has had a couple of treatments that they will know that this is a normal reaction for their skin and how long it will take for their skin to settle down. Mature skin will need to be supported and stretched well to compensate for loss of elasticity in the skin.

PROVIDE WAXING TREATMENTS

In this part of the chapter you will learn about:

- advantages and disadvantages of waxing
- wax application techniques
- body waxing
- facial waxing
- completing a waxing treatment.

> **INDUSTRY TIP**
>
> Always get the client to remove their shoes before they get onto the treatment couch. When you want to relax, you kick off your shoes – it has the same effect during the treatment and helps the client to relax.

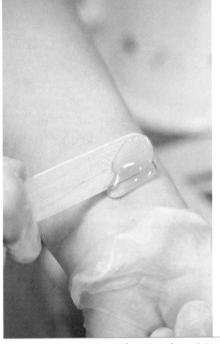
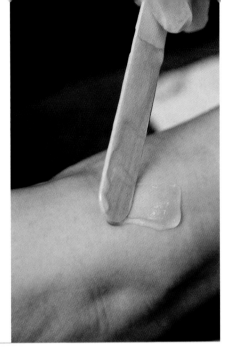

Testing the temperature of wax on the wrists

SmartScreen 206 Worksheet 1

ADVANTAGES AND DISADVANTAGES OF WAXING

Advantages	Disadvantages
A large area can be treated at one time.	It is more expensive than shaving, tweezing or threading.
Regrowth will have fine ends rather than blunt ends (as you get with shaving) as it will grow from the root.	There might be a tendency for ingrown hairs.
The effects last longer than many other methods of **depilation** – around 3–6 weeks depending on the area.	Clients need to wait for the hair to grow so that it is long enough as there needs to be enough hair growth for the wax to stick to.
Instant results.	Can be uncomfortable and for some people quite painful.
	As the hair is removed from the roots there will be a shadow created by the blunt hair that is visible in the hair follicle.

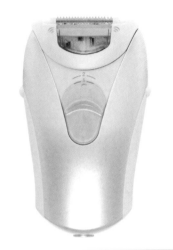

An electrical depilator

Depilation
To remove hair from the body.

WAX APPLICATION TECHNIQUES

WARM WAX TECHNIQUES

Warm wax is suitable for use on all types of hair growth. It can be used for waxing small or large areas.

Spatula method

Warm waxes are applied to the skin in a thin layer in the direction of hair growth using a spatula. If the wax is too thick it will drag on the skin and be uncomfortable. The code of practice recommends *two* methods for applying the wax to a spatula:

INDUSTRY TIP

Before you begin the treatment, wash your hands with an antibacterial hand wash. Make sure you are wearing disposable gloves to minimise cross-infection and before applying wax to any area always make sure you test the wax on both yourself (on your wrist) and your client to make sure the temperature is suitable.

1 **one-dip method** – a spatula is dipped into the wax and used once and then thrown away
2 **drizzle method** – this uses one spatula to place into the pot and a second spatula to apply the wax. The spatula in the wax pot is used to collect the wax and then it is drizzled onto the working spatula to avoid any contamination of the wax. This method will add time to the waxing process even when you are proficient.

Application

When you have the wax on the spatula, hold the spatula at a maximum angle of 45°. Place the spatula on the skin and allow the wax to drop onto the skin.

Apply the wax with a long sweeping action (like spreading honey on bread). Do not drag the spatula or try to spread the wax further as this can be uncomfortable. This should be a quick sweeping action.

Apply a muslin/fabric or paper wax strip over the top of the wax and rub once or twice to stick the strip to the wax.

Lift the edge of the wax strip to get a grip and then remove it by pulling against the direction of hair growth. Pull the strip back on itself, rather than directly upwards as this is uncomfortable and can break the hairs.

Used wax strips should be disposed of as clinical waste.

WHY DON'T YOU...
practise drizzling the wax from one spatula to the other (ie from the spatula in the wax pot to the working spatula). Remember you must not let the spatulas touch. You need to make sure you are not drizzling the wax anywhere but onto the second spatula.

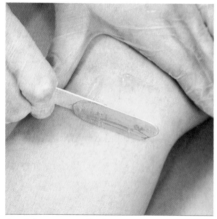
Applying wax to the leg

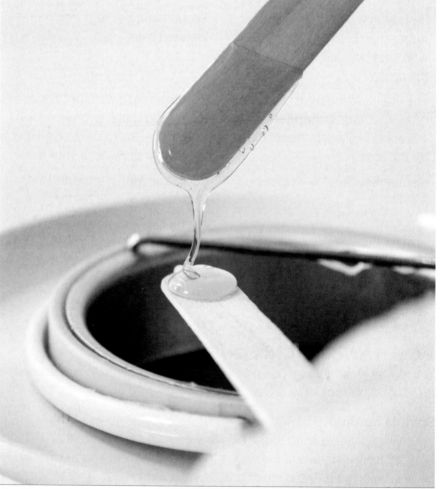
The drizzle method

Roller application

The roller application is a really quick method of applying wax without any mess. The wax comes in a special cartridge that fits into the wax heater. Attached to the top of the cartridge is a roller.

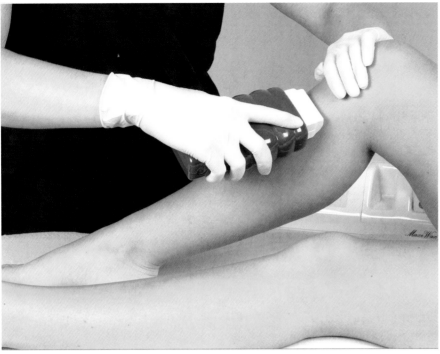

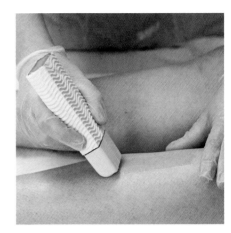

Roller application

The wax must be at a good working temperature so that it flows well and does not drag on the client's skin as this can be uncomfortable. Insulated sleeves that can be pushed onto the roller are used to protect the therapist's hands from the heat of the wax cartridge.

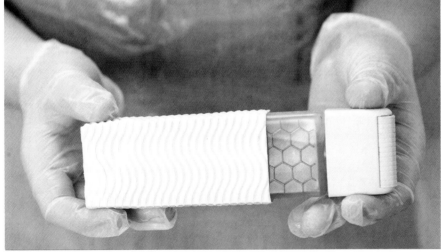

Protective heat sleeve

Ideally, each client should have their own roller head which should be sterilised in between uses. Alternatively, roller heads can be disposed of after a single use. There are different sized roller heads and cartridges for treating different parts of the body.

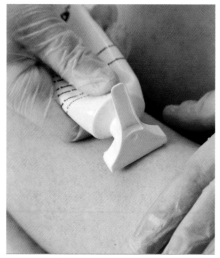

Waxing with a flat-head applicator

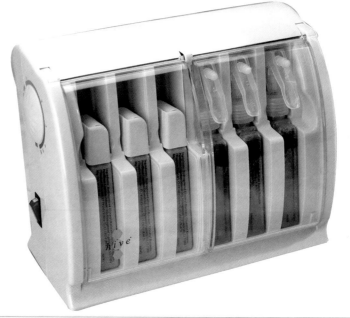

Cartridge heater

After applying the wax using the roller method, remove it and dispose of it in the same way as for the spatula technique above.

Flat-head applicators

These are like the roller in that they attach to a tube of wax. The wax is very gently squeezed in the tube to force the wax onto the flat-head applicator and from the applicator onto the skin. The applicator is then drawn over the area where the wax is to be applied.

The flat-head applicator is disposed of after each client to maintain hygiene. There are different sized applicator heads for treating different parts of the body.

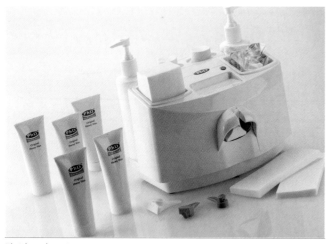

Flat-head system

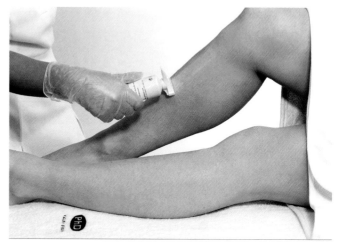

Application of flat-head waxing system

ACTIVITY

Make sure you have a go at using different methods of wax application as it is valuable experience. You should make sure you use at least two methods of warm wax application (including spatula) and hot wax application. You need to perfect quick efficient techniques in more than one type of wax application.

SUGAR PASTE APPLICATION

Sugar paste is applied in the same way as warm wax, using a spatula, and removed with wax strips. It has a lower working temperature than warm wax. Traditional sugar paste has a very unique application:

- Warm the sugar paste so that it is soft and can be shaped into a ball.
- Apply the ball of sugar paste to the skin and work it into the hair growth.
- Using controlled movements, lift and pull the sugar paste from the skin against the hair growth to remove the hair.

HOT WAX TECHNIQUE

Hot wax works better on stronger, coarse, **terminal hair**, such as that under the arms and around the bikini line.

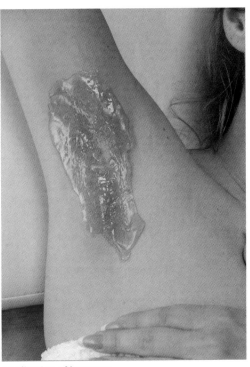

Application of beeswax

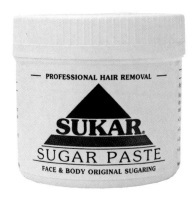

Sugar paste

Terminal hair

Terminal hair is thick and coarse in texture, is deep rooted with a rich blood supply and contains a lot of pigment. It has much more nerve supply than vellus hair so removal of terminal hair tends to feel more uncomfortable for the client.

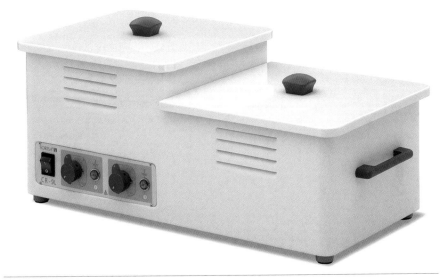

Large dual hot wax heater

INDUSTRY TIP

Hot wax is used for intimate waxing as it gives better results.

Application

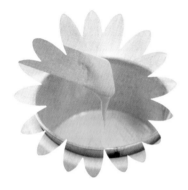

Hot wax blocks

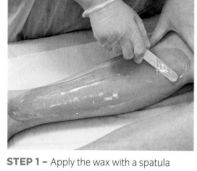

STEP 1 – Apply the wax with a spatula against the direction of hair growth, lifting the hairs into the wax.

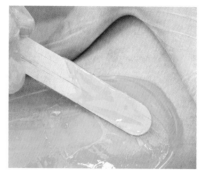

STEP 2 – Hold the spatula flat to the skin and use it in a clockwise and anticlockwise direction to apply the wax and trap the hairs.

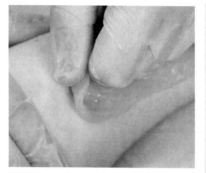

STEP 3 – Make sure the patch of wax has good thick edges to make it easier to remove. Give the wax a few seconds to harden and then flick up a corner of the patch with your thumb to loosen it.

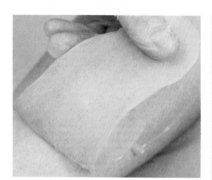

STEP 4 – When there is an area or wax to grip hold of, pull the patch quickly against the direction of hair growth.

WHY DON'T YOU...

practise your hot wax technique on a large area, such as a leg. This will help you to master the art of application, spatula control and getting really good edges to your wax.

> **INDUSTRY TIP**
>
> Do <u>NOT</u> use your nails to 'flick' as this can cause bruising.

> **INDUSTRY TIP**
>
> Hot wax is more expensive to use than other types of wax and it is for this reason that it is kept for smaller areas since it is not cost-effective to use it on larger areas.

> **INDUSTRY TIP**
>
> Beeswax (used for hot wax applications) used to be recycled. It is now unacceptable for hygiene reasons to recycle the wax.

> **INDUSTRY TIP**
>
> If you are planning to go on and do intimate waxing at Level 3 you need to perfect your technique for hot wax.

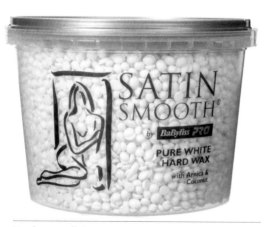

Hard wax pellets

ACTIVITY

The analysis of used hot wax is great for studying the hair growth cycle. Wax an underarm or eyebrow and then turn the wax over and examine the hair that you have removed. Can you define clearly the different stages of the hair growth cycle? Also, note the different length of the hairs that were growing in the skin.

INDUSTRY TIP

It is better to use hot wax on the face than warm wax as it tends to produce less erythema and does not leave a sticky residue.

INDUSTRY TIP

If there are little bits of hot wax residue left on the client's skin, take a patch of freshly removed wax that is still a little **tacky**, turn it over and press the unused tacky side onto the wax to lift it off.

Tacky

Glue like and sticky.

INDUSTRY TIP

If you are using beeswax, remember to remove it while it is still a little tacky. If it sets hard, it will become brittle, crack and become difficult to remove without picking off the pieces. This will be uncomfortable for the client.

WAXING

FULL AND HALF LEG WAX

Before starting the treatment, ask your client to remove their lower clothing, leaving their underwear on. They do not need to remove any upper clothing.

When the client is on the couch, cover them with a towel to maintain their modesty and to keep them warm. If the client is having a full leg wax, offer them a tissue to tuck into their underwear to protect them.

INDUSTRY TIP

Encourage clients to remove trousers, leggings and skirts even if they are only having a lower leg wax as there is a risk that the wax might get on their clothes. Rolling trouser legs and leggings up will also affect their circulation.

INDUSTRY TIP

This is not the only sequence you can use for waxing legs. Refer to your tutor or trainer for guidance.

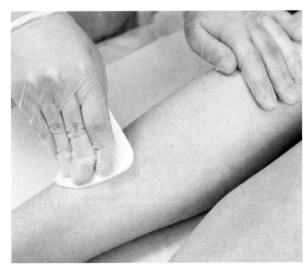

STEP 1 – Wipe the area to be waxed with a pre-wax lotion to remove dead skin and any local **pathogens**.

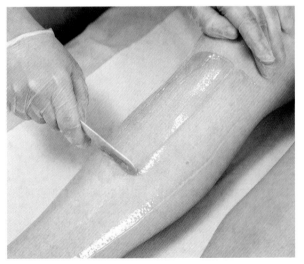

STEP 2 – Begin by applying the wax to the front of the first lower leg, from the knee to the ankle.

Pathogens

Bacteria, viruses or other micro-organisms that can cause disease.

INDUSTRY TIP

When you are cleaning the area, it is important that you assess your client's hair growth direction as every client is different.

INDUSTRY TIP

Make sure your client is in a semi-reclined position so that you can work on the front of their legs.

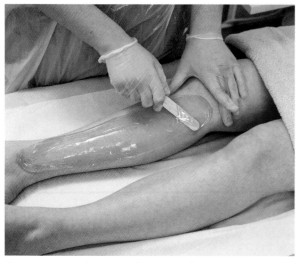

STEP 3 – When you have applied the wax to the lower leg, remove it – starting at the ankles and working up the leg to the knee.

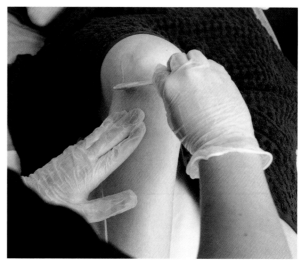

STEP 4 – Ask your client to bend their knee upwards while you apply the wax over the knee area. This will keep the skin stretched. Work in small patches to avoid bruising.

INDUSTRY TIP

If you are applying the wax using a roller, make sure the wax is flowing well. You can use a wax strip to get the roller moving by rolling the head onto the wax strip and then applying the wax to the skin. Use long sweeping applications to cover the area.

INDUSTRY TIP

NEVER apply wax to the back of the knee as there are lymph nodes here and the skin is significantly thinner, making it more prone to bruising.

INDUSTRY TIP

It is important to be economical when you are working with wax in order to maximise profits and keep waste to a minimum. For a half leg wax, you should be aiming to use 2–4 wax strips. For a full leg wax (excluding the bikini line) you should use 4–6 wax strips.

Waxing the toes

Ask the client if they want you to include the top of the foot and toes. If they do, remove the wax from the toes using a small wax strip.

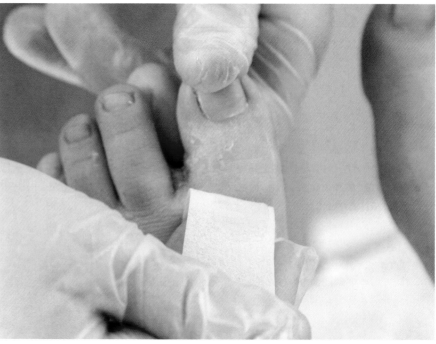

Full leg wax

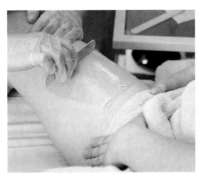

STEP 1 – If your client is having a full leg wax you now need to move on to the upper leg.

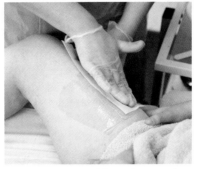

STEP 2 – There are different hair growth patterns on the upper leg and you should apply the wax separately to each pattern so that you know which direction to remove the wax strips in.

For step 3 repeat the full and half leg wax steps you have learnt so far on the other leg.

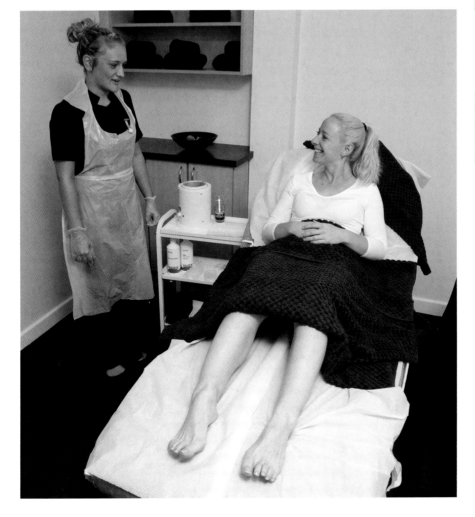

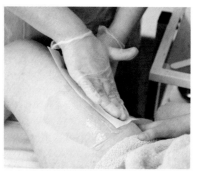

STEP 4 – Remove the wax from the upper leg, getting the client to help keep the skin stretched. When you are removing the wax from the inner thigh, ask your client to turn their knee outwards slightly.

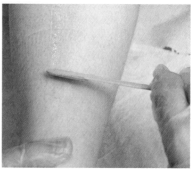

STEP 5 – When you have completed waxing the front of the legs, ask your client if they would like their toes waxed. If they do, follow the procedure on page 350. Ask your client to sit forward while you lower the couch. Lift the towel and ask your client to turn over so that you can work on the backs of the legs. Start at the bottom of the leg furthest away from you and work up the leg repeating on the other leg. Stop at the knee if you are only carrying out a half leg wax.

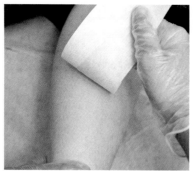

STEP 6 – Remove the wax from the lower leg.

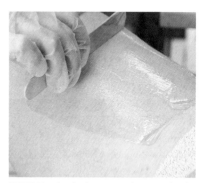

STEP 7 – Apply the wax to the upper back of the leg.

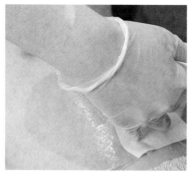

STEP 8 – Remove the wax from the upper back of the leg.

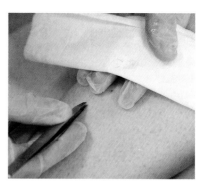

STEP 9 – Remove any stray hairs with tweezers and a piece of tissue.

BIKINI LINE WAXING

Before you begin, ask your client to remove their lower clothing leaving their underwear on. Offer the client a pair of disposable pants if they want to wear them.

Application of warm wax to the bikini line

The diagram illustrates the typical hair growth direction – but every client is different and it is important you assess each client carefully.

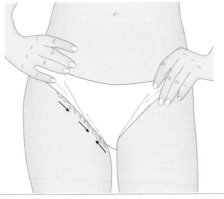

Direction of hair growth

INDUSTRY TIP

Advise the client when they book that they should wear some old underwear, ideally a pair of knickers that matches the bikini line they are being waxed to. Your salon might have the option to provide the client with disposable pants to wear should they client choose to.

INDUSTRY TIP

If the client has very long hair this should be trimmed with sterile scissors to prevent the long hairs catching and pulling as this is quite uncomfortable.

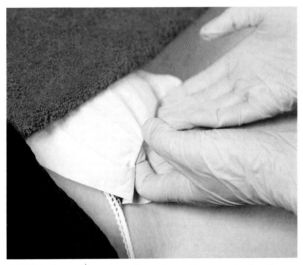

STEP 1 – Offer the client two tissues to tuck into their underwear if they are wearing their own.

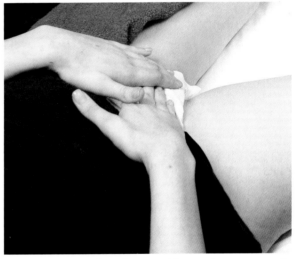

STEP 2 – Get the client to lift one knee up and drop the knee outwards to stretch the skin in the area and to improve accessibility. Ask the client to show you the hair they would like waxed.

INDUSTRY TIP

Some bikini areas might need a lot more hair removal. You need to adapt your treatment depending on the person you are waxing.

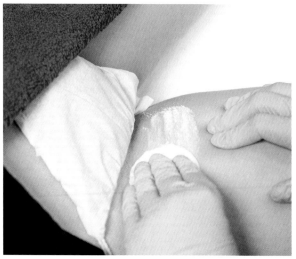

STEP 3 – Apply pre-wax lotion to the area using cotton wool. Observe the hair growth as you do this. Dry the skin with a tissue.

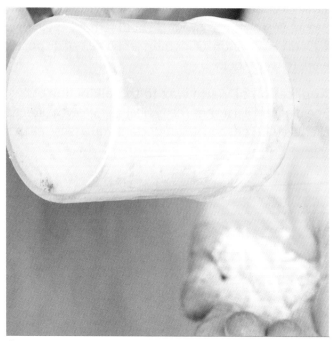

If you are using hot wax, a dusting of talc can help

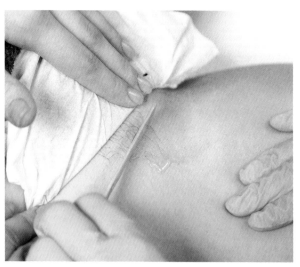

STEP 4 – Apply the wax to one side of the bikini area.

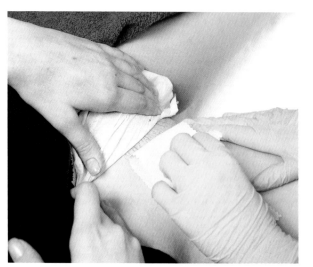

STEP 5 – Ask the client to help stretch the skin and then remove the wax by applying a strip over the top and pulling against the direction of hair growth. Repeat on the other side. Some clients might require additional hair to be removed from the upper thigh. Complete the treatment (see pages 361–362).

INDUSTRY TIP

A couple of firm rubs over the wax strip is enough to make them stick. If you keep rubbing the strips, it does not make the wax stick any better but instead it stimulates the circulation and increases sensitivity.

INDUSTRY TIP

Some bikini areas might need a lot more removal. You need to adapt your treatment depending on the person you are waxing.

Application of hot wax to the bikini line
Working on both sides at the same time

Follow the steps above on pages 341–342 for the preparation of your client.

Follow the steps above on pages 341–342 for the preparation of your client.

INDUSTRY TIP

Keep applying wax to the areas where the hair is growing to complete the bikini wax sequence.

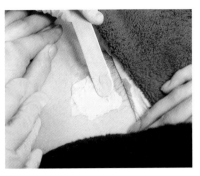

STEP 1 – Apply hot wax against the direction of hair growth in an even application, making sure the edges are thick.

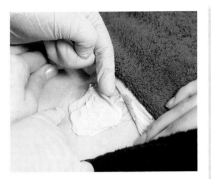

STEP 2 – Remove the patch by flicking up a small lip of wax to provide an area to grip. Pull the wax patch firmly in the direction opposite to hair growth to remove it. Repeat on the other side.

UNDERARM WAXING

Follow the steps above on pages 341–342 for the preparation of your client.

Follow the steps above on pages 341–342 for the preparation of your client.

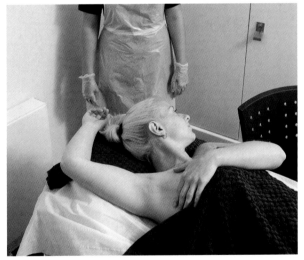

STEP 1 – Ask the client to remove their upper clothing. They can leave their bra on if they want to.

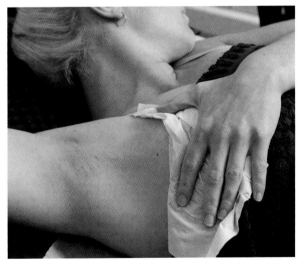

STEP 2 – Make sure tissues are in place to protect your client's underwear and towels.

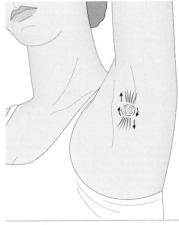

Circular hair growth

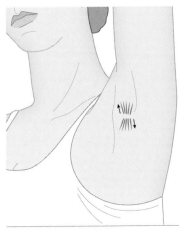

Two-way hair growth

INDUSTRY TIP

If there are bits of hot wax left on the client's skin it is most likely that this is because the wax has not been applied thickly or evenly enough. To remove these bits of wax, you can either apply a new patch of wax over the top and use it to remove the bits of wax or turn a freshly removed patch upside down and press the tacky surface onto the remaining bits of wax and lift them off.

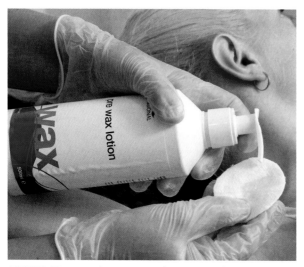

STEP 3 – Apply pre-wax lotion to the area with cotton wool.

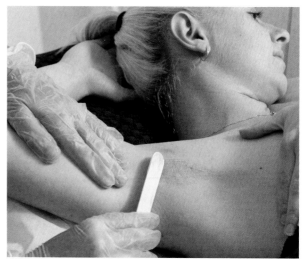

STEP 4 – Apply the wax according to the direction of hair growth and the method you are using.

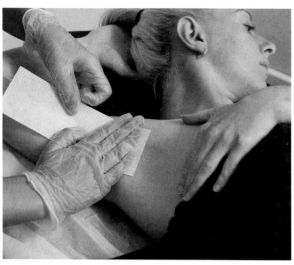

STEP 5 – Apply a wax strip over the wax and rub a couple of times to stick the strip to the wax.

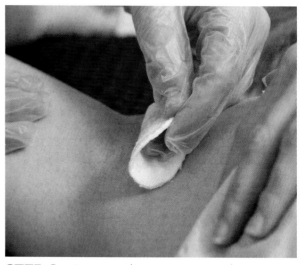

STEP 6 – Remove the strip against the direction of hair growth. Apply aftercare lotion to the waxed area.

WHY DON'T YOU...

ask one of your colleagues to wax your underarms. Do one side with hot wax and the other with warm wax. What difference did you notice? Did you prefer one type of wax over the other? Did the hairs grow back differently? Did one method last longer than the other? Discuss your findings with your tutor.

Application of hot wax to the underarm areas

When you are using hot wax, make sure you remember the following tips:

- Always apply the hot wax against the direction of hair growth.
- Make sure wax patches are not too big on the underarm area.
- Make sure you create a thick lip around the wax to get hold of.
- Remove the wax patch against the direction of hair growth quickly and effectively to avoid discomfort.
- Refer to the image on page 355 for reference.

FACIAL WAXING

EYEBROW WAXING

During the consultation offer the client a hand mirror and ask them what they are looking for from their eyebrow wax. What shape are they trying to achieve? Repeat back to the client what they have asked you to do so that you are both clear about the objectives of the treatment.

> **INDUSTRY TIP**
>
> Avoid going over any area more than twice when waxing as this will cause skin sensitivity and you could end up removing skin as well as hair growth.

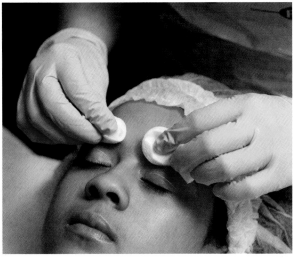

STEP 1 – Ask your client to lie on the couch. If your client is wearing make-up, wipe over the eyebrow area with a cleanser. Then wipe the area with a pre-wax lotion.

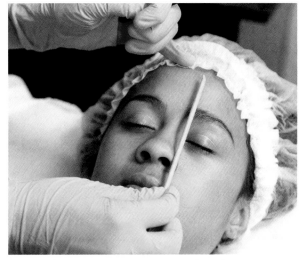

STEP 2 – Use an orange wood stick to measure out correctly the eyebrow shape you are working to.

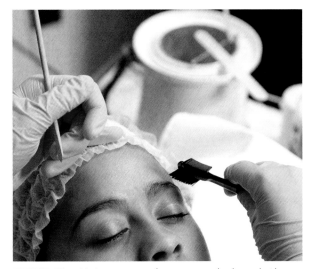

STEP 3 – Using an eyebrow comb, brush the eyebrow hairs that are not going to be waxed out of the way.

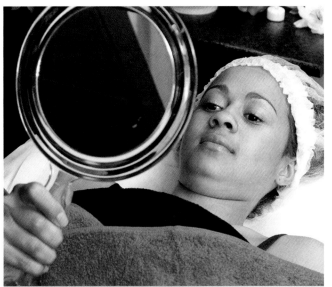

Always make sure your client checks they are happy with the result

Application of warm wax to the eyebrows

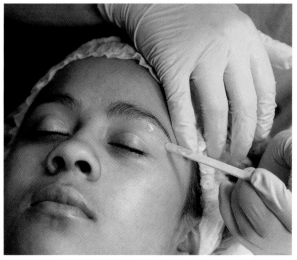

STEP 1 – Apply the warm wax in the direction of hair growth, being careful not to catch any hairs you do not want to remove.

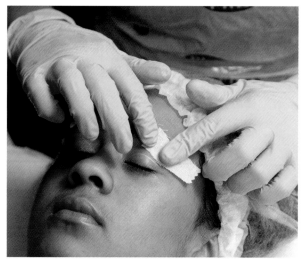

STEP 2 – Place a small wax strip over the top of the wax.

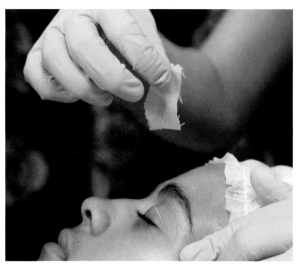

STEP 3 – Support the skin on the temple at the side of the face with one hand and stretch the skin gently. Remove the strip against the direction of hair growth. Repeat on the other eyebrow.

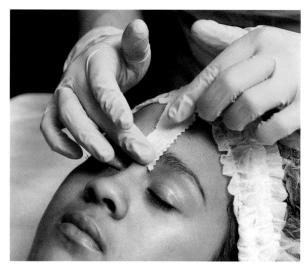

STEP 4 – Wax in between the eyebrows if required.

INDUSTRY TIP

Wooden stirring sticks make excellent waxing spatulas for small areas.

INDUSTRY TIP

Dispose of the strip, never use the wax strip twice as the wax can catch on parts of the eyebrow and remove hairs that you do not want to remove.

INDUSTRY TIP

When you first start eyebrow waxing and are nervous about accidentally removing hairs, apply a very light application of petroleum jelly to the hairs you do not want to remove. This will prevent the wax from sticking to the hairs.

INDUSTRY TIP

When you are treating the face area do not be tempted to use large spatulas and split them as they can leave splinters which are a health and safety hazard.

Application of hot wax to the eyebrows

Follow the same preparation for the previous waxing step-by-steps.

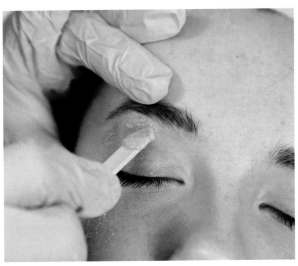

STEP 1 – Apply the wax against the direction of hair growth and in between the eyebrows if required.

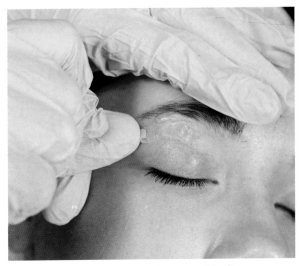

STEP 2 – Support the skin. Quickly flip up a corner of wax to give you something to grip.

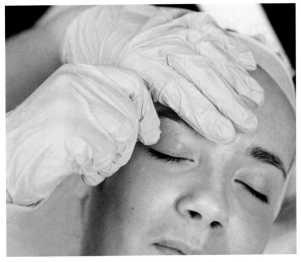

STEP 3 – Remove the wax by pulling firmly against the direction of hair growth. Using the same procedure, remove the wax from the other eyebrow and in between the eyebrows if required.

Complete the eyebrow wax by following the steps on pages 361–362.

INDUSTRY TIP

Remove any stray hairs with tweezers to refine the eyebrow shape.

INDUSTRY TIP

Remember, it is advisable not to remove hair from above the eyebrow line when you are waxing as this causes the eyebrow to lose its softness. Hair should only be removed from below the eyebrow line.

INDUSTRY TIP

To increase your speed with hot waxes, you will need to learn to work with more than one patch at a time and work in a **systematic** pattern.

Systematic
Working in a particular order.

WHY DON'T YOU...
ask one of your colleagues to wax your eyebrows. Do one eyebrow with hot wax and the other with warm wax. What difference did you notice? Did you prefer one wax to the other? Did the hairs grow back differently? Did one method last longer than the other? Discuss your findings with your tutor.

LIP AND CHIN WAX

Follow the same preparation for the previous waxing step-by-steps.

Application of warm wax to the upper lip

Cleanse the area to be waxed

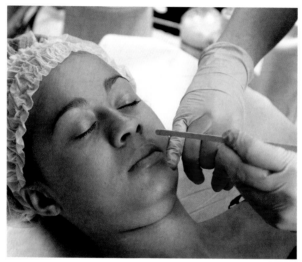

STEP 1 – Apply the warm wax in the direction of hair growth on one side of the lip.

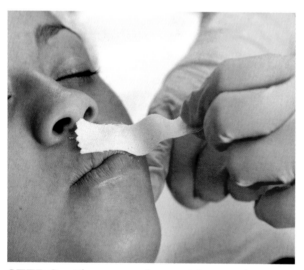

STEP 2 – Place a small wax strip over the top of the wax and rub it with one finger tip.

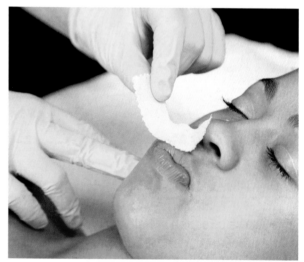

STEP 3 – Pull the strip against the direction of hair growth to remove the hair. Repeat on the other side.

Complete the lip wax by following the steps on page 361–362.

Application of warm wax to the chin

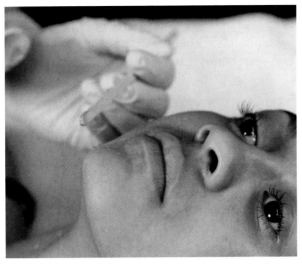

STEP 1 – Apply the wax down the chin in the direction of hair growth, making sure you cover the whole area that is to be waxed.

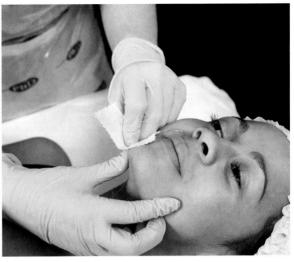

STEP 2 – Remove the wax by placing a small strip on the area to be waxed and pulling each strip against the direction of hair growth to remove the hair.

Application and removal of hot wax to the upper lip and chin

- Divide the upper lip area into two. Apply the wax to one side of the upper lip against the direction of hair growth.
- Support the side of your client's cheek and lift the skin very gently to stretch it. Flick up the wax and remove it by pulling against the direction of hair growth.
- Repeat on the other side.
- Complete the chin wax by following the steps below.

COMPLETING A WAXING TREATMENT

- Check the area you have waxed for any stray hairs and remove these with tweezers.

INDUSTRY TIP

If the client has been using products containing Retin-A or Accutane, do not wax over the areas of skin the products have been used on. Products containing these ingredients thin the skin and are therefore contra-indications to waxing.

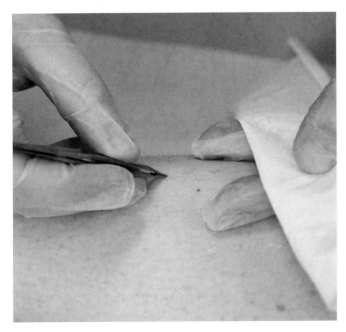

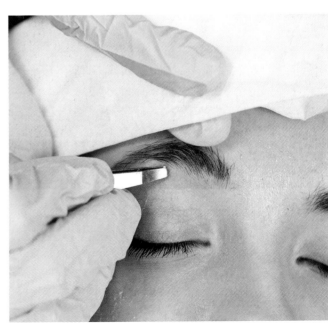

- Ask the client to check whether they are happy with the finish.
- To complete the treatment, apply an after-wax or soothing product. For all areas other than the legs, you can use a cotton wool pad to apply after-wax lotion or oil. For larger areas (ie the legs), apply after-wax lotion or oil with your hands. Either wear disposable gloves or, when you have washed your hands, use a cotton wool pad.

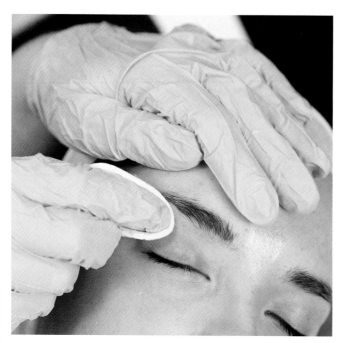
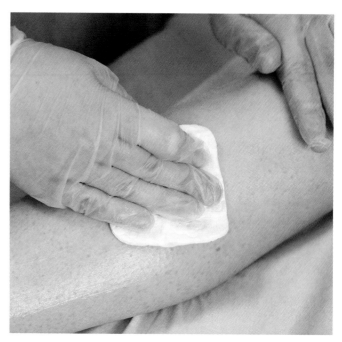

You can now remove your gloves and wash your hands.

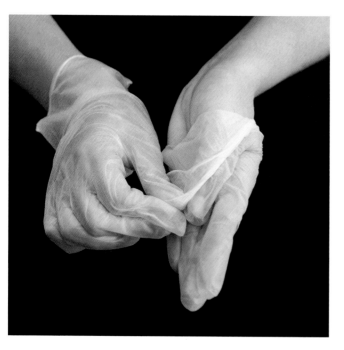
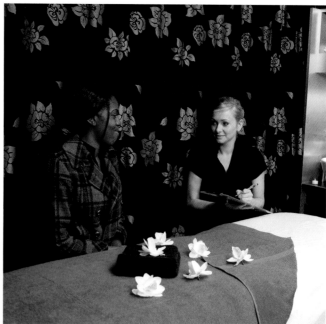

Giving aftercare advice for waxing

Give your client aftercare and home care advice.

PROVIDE THREADING SERVICES

In this part of the chapter you will learn about:
- advantages and disadvantages of threading
- preparing for threading
- threading techniques
- carrying out threading services
- completing a threading service.

ADVANTAGES AND DISADVANTAGES OF THREADING

The following table shows the advantages and disadvantages of threading compared to other methods of hair removal.

Advantages	Disadvantages
A cost-effective method of hair removal – only a few items are required and thread is very cheap.	Only a small area can be treated at one time.
Regrowth will have fine ends rather than blunt ends (as you get with shaving) as it will grow from the root.	Can be uncomfortable and for some people quite painful.
The effects lasts longer than many other methods of depilation; around 3–6 weeks depending on the area.	Clients need to wait for the hair to grow so that it is long enough. There has to be enough hair growth for the cotton to pull out.
Instant results.	
Skilled therapists can provide a very fine and precise finish.	

PREPARING FOR THREADING
- Carry out a consultation and find out the client's treatment objective.
- Ask the client to remove their shoes and sit on the couch in a semi-reclined position.
- Wash your hands. You can wear disposable gloves if you prefer but these can catch on the thread and restrict your technique.
- If the client is wearing make-up, first use a little cleanser to remove the make-up from the area to be threaded and apply a pre-threading cleanser (eg Steritane) to the area to make sure the skin's surface is clean.
- You will now need to prepare your thread to the desired length and twist the thread.

THREADING TECHNIQUES
There are different techniques used to prepare and twist the thread but all threading techniques use a good quality cotton thread. Avoid synthetic threads as they can damage the skin.

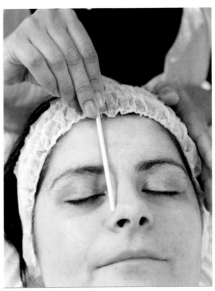

Use an orange wood stick to measure where hairs need to be removed

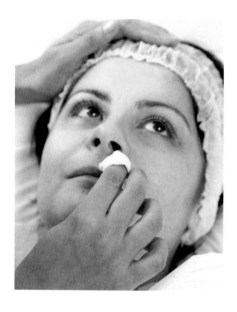

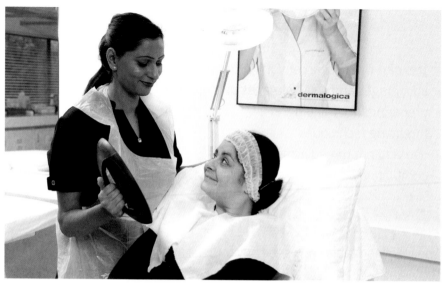

ACTIVITY

See if you can find some different types of threads (eg sewing thread) and compare them with the cotton used for threading. Write down how the threads differ? Which breaks more easily? Does one thread have more stretch than the other? When you wrap the thread around your fingers is there a difference in how it feels? Discuss these findings with your tutor.

TECHNIQUE 1: USING THE MOUTH AND NECK

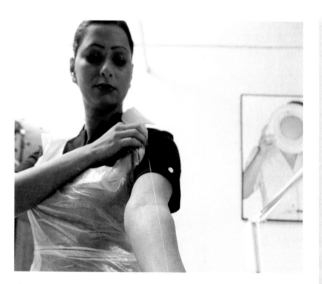

STEP 1 – Take a piece of thread that is approximately 60 cm long. This is roughly the length of your arm.

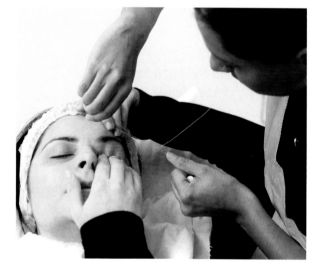

STEP 2 – Place one end in your mouth and grip it with your teeth and lips. Place one hand halfway along the length and draw the other end across the middle.

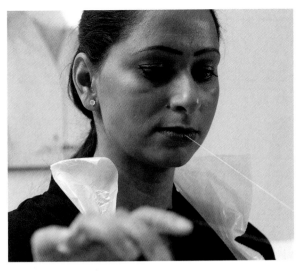

STEP 3 – Twist the middle four times to create a loop.

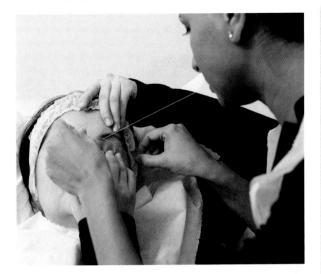

STEP 4 – Move the loop using your index and middle finger of your dominant hand to enlarge the loop and rotate the twisted cotton. With the other hand hold the other end of the thread to maintain stability. Hold the thread in your mouth **taut**, to maintain even pressure, as you draw the loop carefully over the skin's surface to remove the hair. Your head is moved to maintain the **traction** in the thread.

Taut
Stretched or pulled tight.

Traction
Grip.

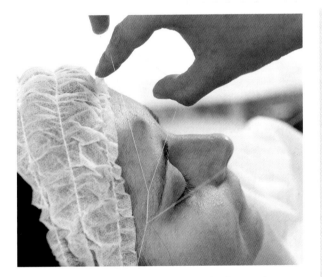

STEP 5 – Open the thread to pluck out the hairs from the root by widening the finger and thumbs of one hand.

Another version of this technique involves tying the thread to a second piece of thread that is loosely tied around your neck rather than being gripped in your mouth.

ACTIVITY

There are other techniques using hand threading. In a group research what they are and how they differ.

TECHNIQUE 2: USING THE HANDS

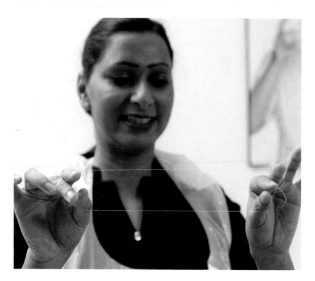

STEP 1 – Wrap the ends of the thread around the thumb and index finger of one hand.

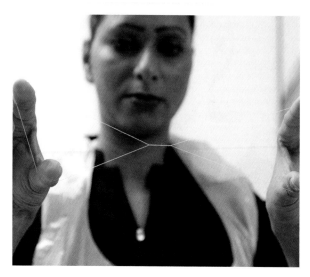

STEP 2 – Use your free hand to twist the loop to create the twisted thread.

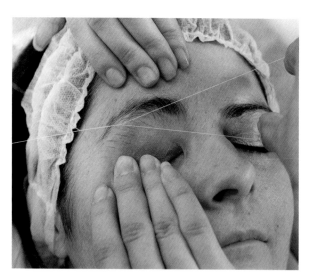

STEP 3 – Work with both hands to move the thread and hold it taut. The hand within the loop mainly holds the loop taught while the thumb and finger draw the twisted thread back and forth. Open the thread to pluck out the hairs from the root by widening the finger and thumbs of one hand.

WHY DON'T YOU...
practise threading on a large area, such as a leg, to help you perfect your technique.

ACTIVITY

Practise each different technique to see which technique you are most comfortable with. Write down two differences that you noticed between the techniques you used.

CARRYING OUT THREADING SERVICES

GENERAL GUIDELINES FOR THREADING SERVICES

- Place the thread onto the skin in the area you are going to treat. Work in an organised way so that you cover the area to be threaded fully.
- You must make sure that the skin is fully stretched wherever you are carrying out threading.
- You should be skimming over the surface of the skin rather than applying pressure to the skin. Applying too much pressure on the skin can result in damage to the skin caused by the thread.
- Work with your fingers to open and close the circle of thread so that the twist in the thread moves over the hairs to be removed, catches them in the thread and pulls them out from the root.

EYEBROW THREADING

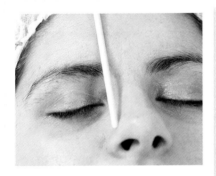

STEP 1 – Use an orange wood stick to measure out correctly the eyebrow shape you will be working to.

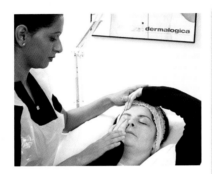

STEP 2 – Ask the client to close their eyes and assist you by placing their fingers onto their eyelid and stretching their eyelid.

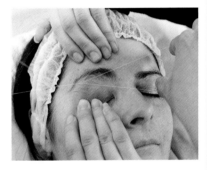

STEP 3 – Using your preferred threading technique, work from the outer eye in towards the bridge of the nose.

INDUSTRY TIP

Some cultures require more definition and sometimes remove hair from above the eyebrow.

UPPER LIP THREADING

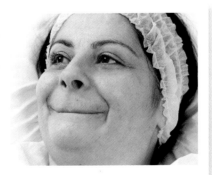

STEP 1 – Ask the client to pull their lip over their teeth to make sure their skin is firmly stretched.

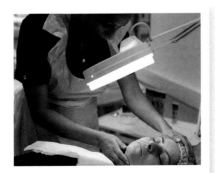

STEP 2 – Turn your client's face slightly to one side to check the direction of hair growth.

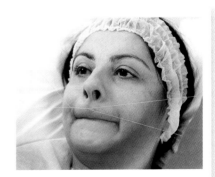

STEP 3 – Using your preferred threading technique, work from one side of the lip into the centre.

CHIN THREADING

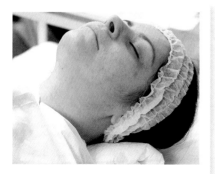

STEP 1 – To stretch the skin, place a bolster or a small rolled-up towel under your client's neck.

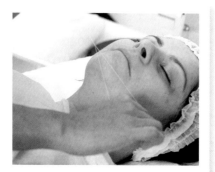

STEP 2 – Remove all unwanted hair by widening one hand and pushing the wound section of cotton towards the other hand, pulling the individual hairs from the root.

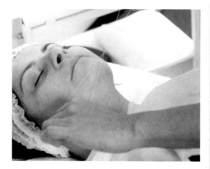

STEP 3 – Turn the face the other way and then repeat to the other side.

FACIAL THREADING

Other areas of the face might need to be threaded. You must discuss the treatment objective with your client and choose your preferred method before carrying out the treatment.

ACTIVITY

Working with a colleague, make a table of the advantages and disadvantages of hot wax, warm wax and threading as methods of hair removal.

COMPLETING A THREADING SERVICE

- Check that your client is satisfied with the service. Ask them to look at the area you have threaded to make sure they are happy with the result. This gives them the opportunity to let you know if you have missed any hairs. They are looking at the area from a different angle and might be able to see any stray hairs.

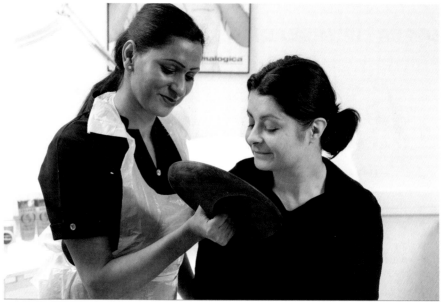

Show your client the finished result

- When you have removed all the hairs from the area, you can dispose of your thread.
- Apply a soothing aftercare solution using a cotton wool pad. While you are applying this, you can give your client aftercare and home care advice.
- When you have finished the service, wash your hands using an antibacterial hand wash and dry well.

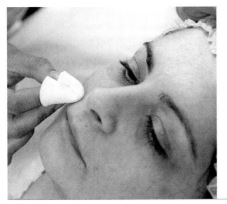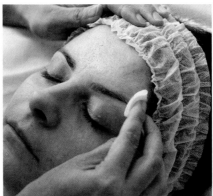

Apply the aftercare solution

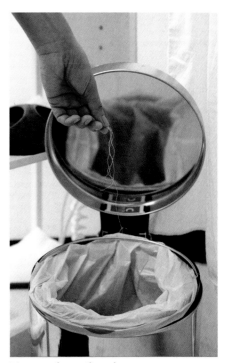

Dispose of your thread

AFTERCARE AND HOME CARE ADVICE

Following a waxing treatment or threading service, you should give your client suitable advice to maximise the benefits of their treatment and maintain the treatment. Aftercare advice will be the same for every client and will be advice on how to reduce the risk of infection following treatment. Home care advice will be more specific advice tailored to each client's needs and will include product recommendations and skin care advice.

In this part of the chapter you will learn about:
- aftercare advice
- home care advice
- contra-actions to waxing treatments and threading services
- completing the client record card
- tidying your work area
- alternative methods of hair removal.

AFTERCARE ADVICE
Advise your client to follow the aftercare advice for 12 hours (or until the next day) after waxing or threading as the skin will be sensitive and the hair follicles will be open. They need to give the skin the opportunity to heal and repair from any temporary surface damage.

Following waxing treatments and threading services, the client should avoid:
- touching the skin
- wearing make-up following a face wax

- ultraviolet (UV) light and sunbathing as the skin will be more sensitive and more likely to burn
- exposure to excessive heat, such as saunas or steam baths
- swimming pools, hydro pools and jacuzzis as the skin might be more sensitive to the chemicals in the water and more susceptible to cross-infection from the communal water
- wearing tight-fitting clothing around the waxed area to prevent any irritation of the skin
- perfumed products, such as perfumes, body lotions and body treatments as the pores of the skin are open and the skin will be more sensitive
- self-tanning products as these will be attracted to the skin's open pores leaving a spotty, pigmented appearance.

You should also:

- recommend to your client when they should return for their next waxing treatment or threading service to maintain the results
- recommend products to your client to maintain their treatment at home
- advise your client what to do if they have any contra-actions.

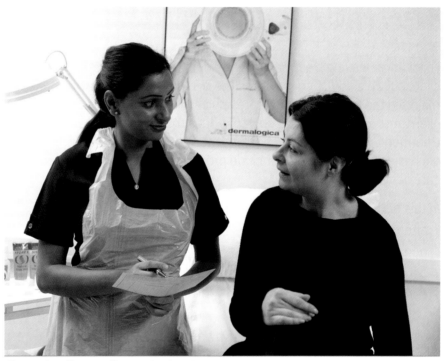

Always give aftercare after any treatment

INDUSTRY TIP

Recommend products throughout the treatment, as the opportunity arises, rather than give them a hard sell on completion of the treatment. For example, if the client has dry scaly skin, you could recommend an exfoliant or body lotion.

HOME CARE ADVICE

The following spider diagram shows the home care advice you should provide your clients following a waxing treatment or threading service.

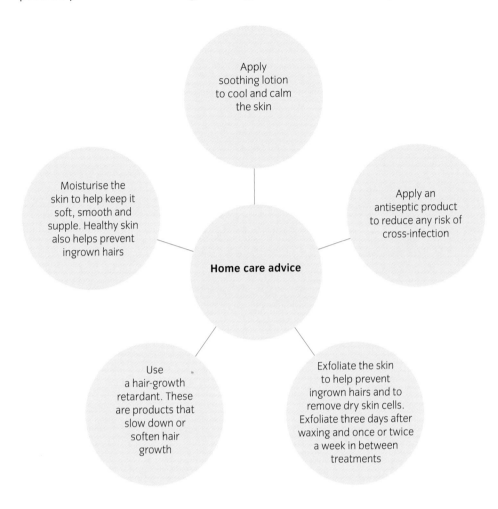

Apply soothing lotion to cool and calm the skin

Moisturise the skin to help keep it soft, smooth and supple. Healthy skin also helps prevent ingrown hairs

Home care advice

Apply an antiseptic product to reduce any risk of cross-infection

Use a hair-growth retardant. These are products that slow down or soften hair growth

Exfoliate the skin to help prevent ingrown hairs and to remove dry skin cells. Exfoliate three days after waxing and once or twice a week in between treatments

CONTRA-ACTIONS

A contra-action is an **adverse** reaction to a treatment suffered by a client. It can happen during or after treatments. If a contra-action occurs during the treatment or service, you need to stop straight away and remove the product that is causing the reaction. If it happens after the treatment, you should advise your client to seek medical attention by contacting their GP.

It is important to be able to recognise the signs of contra-actions that might occur and know what action to take if they do occur.

Adverse

Unpleasant, difficult or harmful.

Contra-action	Is it a normal or adverse reaction?	Cause/reaction	Treatment
Erythema	Normal reaction.	▪ Erythema is caused by trauma to the skin from the adhesive properties of the wax. ▪ The heat of the wax causes **vasodilation** of the surface capillaries. The pulling of the hairs from the hair follicles has the same effect during both threading and waxing. This increase in the circulation can be seen as reddening of the skin. ▪ A normal erythema can take anything from an hour to several hours to return to normal depending on the skin's sensitivity and colour.	▪ Apply a soothing aftercare lotion, keep the area cool and avoid tight clothing. **Vasodilation** Dilation of the blood vessels.
Swelling	Some swelling is normal but it should only be mild. Excessive swelling is an adverse response.	▪ Following waxing, the circulation is increased in response to the trauma to both the skin and hair follicles and histamine is released into the skin from the dermis to repair and minimise any risk of infection. ▪ This reaction gives the skin the appearance of a 'plucked' chicken as there is a tiny amount of swelling around each hair follicle. ▪ This contra-action is most common around the bikini line and under the arms where the hair growth is strong.	▪ It is important to apply a soothing, antiseptic lotion to calm the skin. ▪ Keep the area cool and free from tight clothing

Contra-action	Is it a normal or adverse reaction?	Cause/reaction	Treatment
Allergic reaction to a product	Adverse reaction.	▪ If there is a possibility that a client has an allergy, you should carry out a patch test of the product prior to application (see page 329). ▪ A client might also react to an aftercare product applied to skin that is sensitive following waxing or threading. ▪ The skin will feel hot and the client will feel irritation, tingling or itching.	▪ Remove the product completely with lukewarm water. Apply a cold compress. ▪ Refer the client to a medical practitioner if the irritation does not subside. ▪ Sometimes this reaction can be delayed and it might occur when the client has returned home. ▪ In this case, advise the client to bathe the skin with lukewarm water and apply a cold compress. ▪ They should seek advice from a medical practitioner.
Bruising	Adverse reaction.	▪ Bruising usually occurs as a result of a poor waxing technique. ▪ It is unlikely that bruising will occur during a threading process. ▪ Bruising can occur on clients with very fragile skin. ▪ There are some blood disorders (eg anaemia) that might make a client more susceptible to bruising.	▪ If bruising occurs, it is important to review your waxing technique. ▪ Failure to stretch the skin during waxing will increase the risk of the skin lifting and the tiny skin capillaries being torn which will appear as a bruise. ▪ Applying warm wax too thickly can increase the risk of bruising when the wax is removed.

Contra-action	Is it a normal or adverse reaction?	Cause/reaction	Treatment
Removal of skin	Adverse reaction to waxing.	▪ This is quite literally the removal of the upper layers of the epidermis rather than just the removal of the dead skin cells. ▪ If the wax is too hot, it can take off the outer layers of the skin. ▪ This leaves the skin sore and red. The area where skin has been removed can usually be seen as a more shiny patch of skin and there might be superficial peeling around the edges of the area. ▪ Removal of skin can also occur following prolonged exposure to the sun. Clients are unaware that their skin has been burnt as there are no signs of erythema on the skin's surface. It can take up to 8 hours for the effects of the sun on the skin to be visible.	▪ If peeling of the skin occurs, you need to review your techniques. ▪ Make sure that the area is well-stretched when you are removing the wax. ▪ Make sure that the skin is dry – if necessary apply a very light dusting of powder. ▪ Avoid going over an area twice as this will cause additional exfoliation of the skin and increase the risk of skin removal. ▪ Make sure the wax is applied thinly.. ▪ When you are carrying out a bikini line wax, avoid waxing directly over the top of the inguinal ligament.
Bleeding **Virgin hair** This is hair that has not been waxed before.	Adverse reaction. This is quite common when you are waxing **virgin hair** that is strong and coarse on the bikini line and under the arms.	▪ When the hairs are pulled from the hair follicles a tiny haemorrhage occurs as the blood vessels nourishing the hair bulb are broken and bleed into the hair follicle. ▪ Bleeding is visible as a tiny red spot within the empty hair follicle. ▪ With very strong terminal hair this bleeding might be greater and can visibly flow onto the skin's surface.	▪ Never touch the area directly without wearing gloves. ▪ Apply an antiseptic/soothing lotion with a cotton wool pad.
	Adverse contra-action with threading.	▪ With threading, this can occur if the therapist is heavy handed and applies too much pressure to the thread causing it to cut into the skin. ▪ This is one reason why cotton thread is used rather than synthetic thread.	▪ If this occurs, review your threading technique as it is likely that you are holding the cotton too tightly to the skin.

Contra-action	Is it a normal or adverse reaction?	Cause/reaction	Treatment
Ingrown hairs	An adverse contra-action.	▪ A common cause of ingrown hairs is incorrect waxing and threading (eg removing hair in the wrong direction). ▪ There are two types of ingrown hairs. The first type can be seen just below growing along just below the surface of the skin. The second type are ingrown hairs that are coiled within the hair follicle and grow downwards – these are more likely to becoming infected. ▪ Some clients are more prone to ingrown hairs. Clients with curly hair might find ingrown hairs more common but generally ingrown hairs are a result of fine, soft regrowth that struggles to push through the hair follicle and above the skin. Dry and suntanned skin can make it difficult for hairs to grow through the skin easily as the skin is thicker and coarser.	▪ Regular use of an exfoliant and a moisturiser will help to minimise ingrown hairs. There are also products that are manufactured specifically to inhibit hair growth and reduce ingrown hairs.

ACTIVITY

Work with three colleagues and compare the skin on your legs. Is there a difference? Write down three reasons why your skin might be different. Now ask each of your colleagues a few questions to see if you can find out why (eg do they moisturise?). For each of your colleagues, write down three pieces of aftercare advice or recommendations you can give them to improve their skin.

COMPLETING THE CLIENT RECORD CARD

Now that you have completed the waxing treatment or threading service, make notes about the treatment or service that you have carried out. In your notes include details of the area treated and, if it was a waxing treatment, the type of wax used. Be sure to include any details that might help with future treatments.Note any contra-actions the client has had, particularly if they were adverse. When your information is complete, file the card away. Always maintain confidentiality and privacy. Do not leave client record cards or treatment plans lying around in the salon for other clients to see.

TIDYING YOUR WORK AREA

Tidy your work area and leave the area ready for the next client. Make sure rubbish is disposed of carefully in the bin. Clean your tweezers and scissors with surgical spirit or a disinfectant solution to remove any hairs or grease from the surface before placing them in an autoclave or sterilising solution. Wipe the plastic couch cover with an antiseptic spray. Clean around the wax heater with wax cleaner. Place towels into the laundry area ready to be washed.

 SmartScreen 206 Worksheet 6

ALTERNATIVE METHODS OF HAIR REMOVAL

There are many methods that are available for removing hair – both temporary methods and permanent methods. The various methods available are not always suitable for every client or every area of the body. You should be aware of the different methods of hair removal that are available so that you can advise your client on which method is best for them.

Method	Temporary or permanent	How the treatment works	Advantages	Disadvantages
Electrolysis A specialist technique that is taught at Level 3 within the general beauty therapy route	A permanent method of hair removal for removing hair from a small area.	A tiny stainless steel or gold-plated probe is inserted into the individual hair follicles and used to **cauterise** or destroy the cells that produce the hair. When the hair cells have been cauterised, the hair can be removed easily from the skin. It can be carried out almost anywhere on the body but it is a fairly uncomfortable treatment. It is important to master the technique correctly to avoid any risk of damaging the skin and scarring.	▪ Removes the hair permanently. ▪ Treats specific problem hairs. **Cauterise** To burn the skin with a heated instrument.	▪ Can be uncomfortable. ▪ Takes a long time to see the results as the hair-producing cells might need to be treated several times before they are fully removed so that new hairs no longer grow. ▪ A risk of skin damage if the therapist carrying out the electrolysis is not careful or properly trained.
Laser hair removal and Intense Pulsed Light (IPL):	Popular methods of permanent hair reduction.	Laser hair removal involves a precisely controlled laser passing through the skin in the areas of hair growth. The laser is attracted to and heats the darker areas of the skin (ie the melanin) in the hair follicles without affecting the skin around them. The laser is limited in terms of its depth of penetration and what it can treat. IPL is the use of a series of synchronised light pulses rather than a laser. Each pulse of light causes the temperature within the hair shaft to increase which destroys the keratin in the hair. It also causes damage to the **germinating** cells in the **dermal papilla** so that the hair cannot reproduce. There is short-term discomfort during the treatment and erythema can last approximately 24 hours.	▪ Treats larger areas of hair growth to reduce hair permanently. ▪ IPL allows a larger area to be treated at once. **Germinating** To begin to grow after being **dormant**. **Dormant** Something that is temporarily inactive or not in use. **Dermal papilla** The base of the follicle is attached to the blood supply and provides oxygen and nutrients, stimulating hair growth throughout the anagen phase.	▪ Different laser equipment works on different wavelengths which can result in varying results. ▪ Treatment is very uncomfortable. ▪ The cost per treatment is expensive (however, this needs to be weighed up against the cost of other types of hair removal treatments over a long period of time). ▪ Not all types of hair and skin colour can be treated with good results – laser and IPL cannot successfully treat blonde or white hair. ▪ With IPL, several treatments will be required to treat larger areas which can make this quite an expensive method of hair removal.

Method	Temporary or permanent	How the treatment works	Advantages	Disadvantages
Ultrasonic treatment	Long-term, temporary hair removal.	A new introduction to the long-term, temporary hair removal market, this treatment uses ultrasonic sound waves. The ultrasonic sound waves are passed down the hair follicle and transform into **thermal** energy. This causes a rapid rise in the temperature of the hair follicle which **inhibits** hair growth. **Thermal** Heat. **Inhibits** Prevents.	■ A virtually pain-free method of hair removal. ■ Can be used to treat specific hairs. ■ Ultrasonic waves can be used on any skin or hair colour, even white, unlike light waves, as they do not need melanin to be present for them to work.	■ Treatment is still new. ■ Process can be quite slow. ■ Some regrowth. ■ More expensive than other methods of hair removal.
Depilatory creams	Temporary hair removal from the surface of the skin.	When applied to the skin, the creams seep into the opening at the top of the hair follicle. The alkaline product (often containing calcium thioglycolate) causes the hair to swell and absorb the product further. The ingredients cause the sulphur bonds in the keratin protein in the hair to break and the hair dissolves. The dissolved hair is then washed from the skin's surface. It is advisable to carry out a patch test before using these types of products to check for skin sensitivity.	■ Quick and easy to use. ■ A cheap method of hair removal. ■ The client can use these products at home. ■ Can be used on small or large areas. ■ Added ingredients have a softening effect on the skin. ■ The results last for about a week.	■ Patch testing should be carried out before use as allergies are quite common. ■ Can be messy when treating large areas. ■ Some products can have quite a strong off-putting smell. ■ Can cause skin sensitisation and the skin can remain sensitive for up to 24 hours after application.

Method	Temporary or permanent	How the treatment works	Advantages	Disadvantages
Shaving	Temporary hair removal.	Shaving can be done using electrical or disposable razors. Disposable razors come in a variety of styles and include one or more blades for a closer finish. Flexible heads give good skin contact while shaving. Disposable razors can be used with a shaving product, such as a cream or foam, to help maintain contact with the skin and improve the process. Further information of shaving can be found in Chapter 204.	▪ Quick and easy to use. ▪ Clients can use this method at home. ▪ Can be used on small or large areas. ▪ Shaving products contain additives to leave the legs feeling soft and silky. **Folliculitis** An inflammation of the hair follicles.	▪ If used on dry skin (which is not recommended), razors can catch and snag the skin, causing damage. ▪ The use of unclean blades can result in razor rash (skin sensitisation) and **folliculitis**. ▪ Razors produce a blunt cut which leaves the hair coarse when it regrows. ▪ If razors are not used carefully, there is the possibility of cutting the skin causing bleeding, infection and skin scarring. ▪ Results are very temporary and only last a few days and the area can still have dark stubbly appearance in the hair follicles. ▪ Regrowth has coarse ends which initially makes the hair appear darker as it grows back.

Method	Temporary or permanent	How the treatment works	Advantages	Disadvantages
Electrical depilators	Temporary hair removal.	There are a variety of different machines available. All of them are hand-held electrical devices that have a small rotating coil. The device is moved over the skin and hairs and the coil traps the hairs plucking them from their roots.	▪ The client can use this method at home. ▪ Requires a good technique but it is quick to use when this is mastered. ▪ A cheap method as there is only the initial cost of the epilator.	▪ Can be uncomfortable to use as the hairs are plucked. ▪ Can cause ingrown hairs. ▪ Only suitable for large areas of hair growth. ▪ As the method can be applied to the skin randomly, it can lead to distorted hair growth. ▪ It still requires the hair to be a certain length so that the coil can catch hold of the hairs.

INDUSTRY TIP

Abrasive mitts are often marketed as helping minimise hair growth but they tend to be quite ineffective and if used too roughly can make the skin sore. They are, however, excellent for discouraging and lifting ingrown hairs from the skin.

TEST YOUR KNOWLEDGE

Use the questions below to test your knowledge of Chapter 206/219 to see how much information you have retained. These questions will help you to revise what you have learnt in this chapter.

Turn to page 601 for the answers.

1. In which **one** of the following areas of the body might blood spots appear as a normal contra-action to waxing?
   a) Under the arm
   b) The lower leg
   c) The eyebrows
   d) The upper lip

2. Which **one** of the following alternative methods of hair removal will produce coarse regrowth?
   a) Shaving
   b) Threading
   c) Depilatory creams
   d) Tweezing

3. Which **one** of the following adverse contra-actions could occur during threading if too much pressure is applied with the thread?
   a) Bruising
   b) Swelling
   c) Bleeding
   d) Erythema

4. Which **one** of the following contra-indications would restrict waxing?
   a) Recent scar tissue
   b) Chemotherapy
   c) Radiotherapy
   d) Herpes zoster

5. Which **one** of the following contra-indications would require referral to a medical practitioner?
   a) Chloasma
   b) Vitiligo
   c) Impetigo
   d) Eczema

6. Normal erythema during waxing is caused by:
   a) an allergic reaction to a product
   b) the client being too warm
   c) poor application technique
   d) increased blood supply to the skin.

7. Which **one** of the following alternative methods of depilation would be the most suitable for a client who has severe varicose veins – a contra-indication that prevents leg waxing?
   a) Shaving
   b) Plucking
   c) Threading
   d) Depilatory cream

8. Which **one** of the following can be applied to protect a small blemish when carrying out waxing?
   a) Moisturiser
   b) Petroleum jelly
   c) Aftercare lotion
   d) Pre-wax lotion

9. A client should be advised to avoid exposure to ultraviolet (UV) rays after waxing to prevent:
   a) urticaria
   b) tanning
   c) burning
   d) pigmentation.

10. How should you apply aftercare lotion following an underarm wax?
    a) With your hand
    b) With cotton wool
    c) With a tissue
    d) By using the client's hand

11. Why should you examine hair growth prior to waxing?
    a) To check the direction of growth for the correct application of wax
    b) So that you know what type of hair growth you are removing
    c) To be able to advise the client which aftercare products to use at home
    d) To check the area for contra-indications

12. How long should you allow for an underarm wax?
    a) 15 minutes
    b) 10 minutes
    c) 20 minutes
    d) 25 minutes

13. Which **one** of the following products should be applied to the skin after cleansing prior to applying hot wax?
    a) Petroleum jelly
    b) Pre-wax spray
    c) Moisturiser
    d) Powder

14. When would you need to use a pair of scissors to cut the client's hair?
    a) Prior to a bikini wax if the hair is very long
    b) To remove hair that the client does not want waxed
    c) When there is a contra-indication to waxing
    d) To create a tidy area to wax around

15. Aftercare advice should be given to a client:
    a) if a contra-action occurs
    b) after the first treatment only
    c) after every treatment
    d) from time to time to remind the client what to do at home.

CASE STUDY: JANICE BROWN

My father was horrified the day I told him I was not going to university but had successfully enrolled on the City & Guilds Beauty Therapy course at Chesterfield College. I had a pretty tough time from him, but stuck to my guns. What a great decision!

The professional beauty industry is innovative, challenging, frustrating and always great fun to be involved in. During my career journey I have experienced most aspects of the industry: providing treatments, managing salons, working in sales, teaching, training, giving demonstrations, helping set standards, writing (I am the co-author of the *Encyclopedia of Hair Removal*) and research and development. I currently own and run Hof Beauty Ltd along with my husband Robert.

I can honestly say that I have loved every single role. The industry provides an endless supply of learning opportunities where no two days are ever the same.

My father did eventually admit that I had made the right choice!

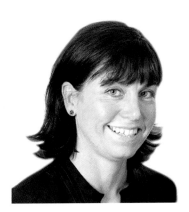

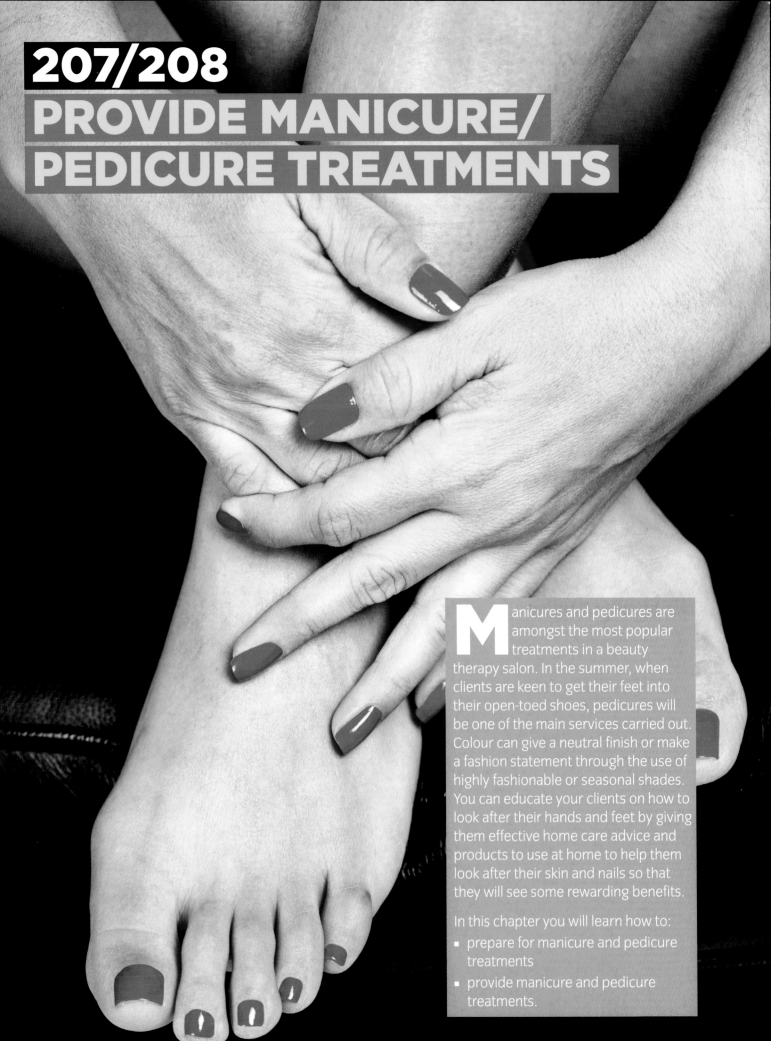

207/208
PROVIDE MANICURE/ PEDICURE TREATMENTS

Manicures and pedicures are amongst the most popular treatments in a beauty therapy salon. In the summer, when clients are keen to get their feet into their open-toed shoes, pedicures will be one of the main services carried out. Colour can give a neutral finish or make a fashion statement through the use of highly fashionable or seasonal shades. You can educate your clients on how to look after their hands and feet by giving them effective home care advice and products to use at home to help them look after their skin and nails so that they will see some rewarding benefits.

In this chapter you will learn how to:

- prepare for manicure and pedicure treatments
- provide manicure and pedicure treatments.

PREPARE FOR MANICURE AND PEDICURE TREATMENTS

Before you carry out manicure and pedicure treatments, it is important to be prepared. You must follow health and safety requirements for every treatment. Knowing how to set up your treatment area, which products and tools you should use and how to carry out an effective consultation are essential for manicure and pedicure treatments.

In this part of the chapter you will learn about:

- health and safety
- preparing for manicure and pedicure treatments
- consultation for manicure and pedicure treatments
- nail care products
- preparing the client and yourself for manicure and pedicure treatments.

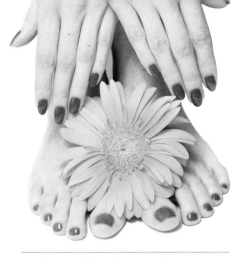

Matching polish on fingers and toes

HEALTH AND SAFETY

It is very import to follow all health and safety regulations when you are carrying out manicure and pedicure treatments.

METHODS OF STERILISATION

Prior to carrying out a treatment, you must make sure your tools are properly sterilised before your client arrives.

Manicure tools

For a manicure, make sure that the following tools are prepared and have been sterilised.

HANDY HINTS

You need to make sure you are familiar with the legislation that is relevant to carrying out manicure and pedicure treatments – especially health and safety legislation. You can find all the information you need in the Legislation chapter on pages 91–113. It is recommended that you answer the 'Test your knowledge' questions in the Legislation chapter successfully before working through this chapter.

Tool/equipment	Image	Sterilisation method
Metal tools (including cuticle nippers, clippers and cuticle knives)	**BARBICIDE** + GERMICIDE + FUNGICIDE & VIRUCIDE	<ul><li>Wipe metal tools with a disinfectant, such as surgical spirit or isopropyl alcohol, to remove any grease or debris and sterilise them in an **autoclave**.</li><li>Alternatively, place these smaller tools into a chemical sterilising solution (eg Sterilsafe). Immerse the tools fully to sterilise all parts of the tools and place them in a jar containing a disinfectant solution.</li></ul>

Autoclave

A machine that uses high-pressured steam to kill all micro-organisms. It is used to sterilise small metal tools.

Tool/equipment	Image	Sterilisation method
Other items (eg wooden hoof sticks and buffers)		• Wipe these over with a sanitising product to remove any grease and debris.
Emery boards		• Ideally, you should only use these once, but this is not always practical and so you must spray them with a sanitising spray before and after every use and allow to dry before use. • It is recommended that you do this in view of the client so that they can see you are maintaining high standards of hygiene.
Nail brush		• Wash nail brushes in hot soapy water. • Spray with a disinfectant spray.
Nail care attachments (eg cuticle pusher and hard skin remover)		• Wash in hot soapy water. • Spray with a disinfectant spray or, if possible, soak in a chemical sterilising solution.

Pedicure tools

In addition to the tools and equipment listed above, you will also need to prepare and sterilise the following tools for pedicure treatments.

Tool/equipment	Image	Sterilisation method
Foot rasps		▪ Scrub the rasp clean with hot, soapy water using a nail brush (kept specifically for this purpose) to remove dead skin tissue. Allow to dry. ▪ Depending on the type of rasp, spray it with a disinfectant spray or place in a chemical sterilising solution.
Toe separators		▪ Soak in a chemical sterilising solution, such as Milton Sterilising Fluid, or give them to the client.
Foot/spa bath		▪ Wash with hot water and antibacterial cleaner. ▪ Spray with disinfectant spray. ▪ Regularly clean with a sterilising liquid (eg Milton Sterilising Fluid) or tablet. ▪ Place the liquid or tablet into the foot spa and dilute with water as per the manufacturer's instructions. ▪ Turn on the foot spa and allow the liquid to work its way through the equipment for a few moments. ▪ Many spa baths now have disposable liners that can be used during treatment and then thrown away.

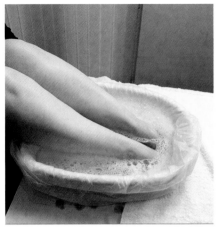

A pedicure bowl with disposable liner

Accessible

Easy to access.

INDUSTRY TIP

Some salons still use toe separators but they are not recommended for hygiene reasons. If you do use them, you should follow the instructions above for sterilisation.

INDUSTRY TIP

Remember the basic rules of COSHH:

Follow the manufacturer's instructions – exactly as written.

Dilute products exactly as per the manufacturer's instructions – do not guess.

Never mix products (eg cleaning products) unless the manufacturer states that it is safe to do so.

Check containers that are not in use are sealed properly.

Rotate stock to avoid products deteriorating.

Do not store products near heat.

Only store products in designated containers.

Keep products away from heat or naked flames – particularly aerosols.

Avoid prolonged and frequent exposure to or use of hazardous products.

Wear personal protective equipment (PPE) as appropriate.

Make sure unused products and empty containers are disposed of properly.

HANDY HINTS

You will find further information on how to prepare your general treatment environment in Chapter 203.

HANDY HINTS

You will find more information on health and safety and risks and hazards in Chapter 202 on pages 144–146.

EQUIPMENT SAFETY CHECKS

If you are using any equipment, such as thermal mitts, thermal booties, paraffin wax, a nail care machine or an overhead lamp to give you extra lighting, check that it is ready and safe to use before your client arrives. Check for any damage to the equipment, such as frayed flexes or broken plugs. Plug in the electrical equipment and turn on the main switch to make sure that it is working correctly. Make sure that there are no trailing wires.

DISPOSAL OF WASTE

You should have a bin that is easily **accessible** during the treatment. The bin should be lined with a dustbin liner and it should have a lid that can be opened and closed without causing you to interrupt the treatment. To make sure you are being hygienic, dispose of your waste as you work and do not let it collect on a trolley or treatment surface. Do not let the bin become so full that the lid cannot close. Empty the bin at regular intervals if not after every treatment.

TREATMENT ENVIRONMENT

The client needs to be comfortable during their treatment. Prior to treatment, check the following and make adjustments so that the client can relax during their treatment.

Lighting

There should be good, bright overhead lighting with no shadows in your working area. You need to be able to see the client's hands and feet clearly so that the treatment can be carried out safely and effectively. If you cannot see clearly, it will affect the finish of your treatment and might leave the client dissatisfied.

Heating

There should be a warm and cosy room temperature so that the client is comfortable and can relax.

Ventilation

You need good ventilation to avoid the build-up of odours and fumes. Stale air will make you feel tired. Preventing a build-up of fumes is especially important when you are working with nail enhancements and nail polish products as these have very strong odours and can be hazardous for your health. Make sure that there are no draughts as this will be uncomfortable for both you and your client.

Music

Play soft, gentle background music that is not too noisy or too loud as this will affect your ability to listen to your client's needs and treatment objectives.

Health and safety

Hazards and risks could cause injuries. Make a quick check of your working area for hazards and either remove these, or reduce any risks that might cause hazards. Make sure you monitor health and safety constantly.

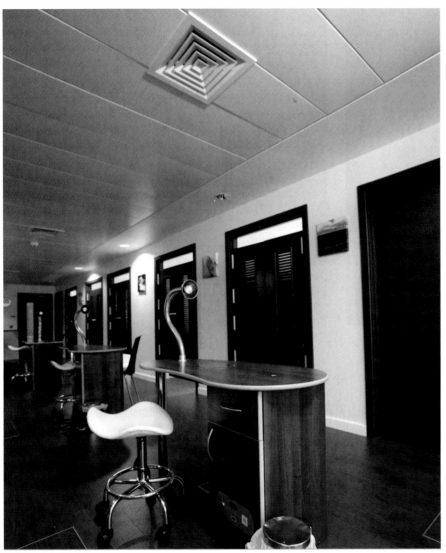
An example of a nail station with ventilation and extraction

INDUSTRY TIP

Choose your music and your radio station carefully, especially if you are playing the radio. You do not want to play music that might put clients off coming into the salon or studio or have radio discussions that might offend clients.

PREPARING FOR MANICURE AND PEDICURE TREATMENTS

Prepare the treatment area before the client arrives. Make sure that all work surfaces are clean and that any equipment or products are ready before you start. Check that any equipment that needs to be sterilised is sterilised before the client arrives so it is ready before you begin.

ACTIVITY

Check how your working environment compares with that of a real working salon. Make a list of any changes you would make.

PREPARING THE MANICURE TREATMENT AREA

Protect and cover the treatment area, whether this is a couch or manicure table. Either fold a small towel to create a wrist rest or use a small manicure cushion and cover this with a hand towel and a small piece of couch roll.

INDUSTRY TIP

Check your tools regularly for wear and tear. If your tools are not working well they will affect your work. You can get special oil to use on the hinges of small tools (eg cuticle nippers) to keep them working smoothly. They should be oiled occasionally by putting a single drop of oil on the hinge and working the tool to get the oil into the hinge. Metal tools will be affected by sterilisation over time and these should be replaced when they start to show any signs of wear and tear, such as rust.

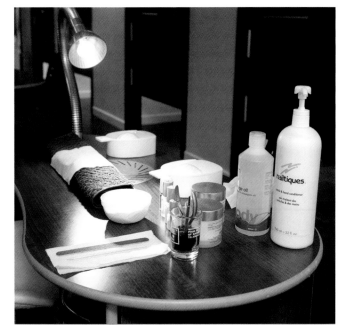

Manicure table set up

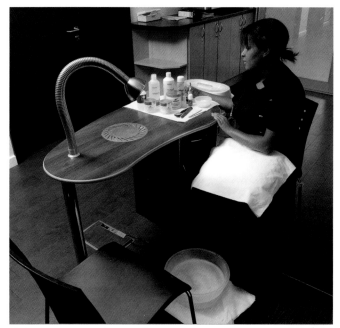

Therapist preparing for a pedicure

PREPARING THE PEDICURE TREATMENT AREA

For pedicures, if the client is sitting on a couch, protect it with a couch cover and a towel and place a piece of couch roll across the foot of the couch. If the client is sitting in a chair, protect the floor area with a towel or bath mat covered with a piece of couch roll.

PREPARING YOUR TROLLEY

The trolley should be clean and set up in an organised way. You should have the following consumables and equipment easily accessible:

- cotton wool pads or lint-free nail wipes/pads
- tissues
- plastic or disposable spatulas for removing products from pots
- nail care products – these should be positioned so that they are in a logical order for use. This order might vary depending on the product brand you are using. Products should include:
  - sanitising spray
  - nail enamel remover
  - cuticle cream
  - hand soak/wash
  - cuticle remover
  - hand mask
  - massage cream
  - base coat
  - a selection of nail varnishes
  - top coat
  - quick-dry spray
  - a bowl for the client's jewellery (if required)
  - emery boards (soft and normal)
  - hoof stick
  - orange wood sticks

- jar containing a chemical sterilising solution (eg Barbicide or Sterilsafe) to stand your metal tools in to keep them sterilised during the treatment
- nail brush
- couch roll – for covering the towel when you are painting the nails.

For a pedicure you will not need the hand soak/wash or hand mask but you will also need:

- foot rasp
- exfoliant
- foot mask
- toenail cutters/nippers
- foot spray
- foot bath.

ACTIVITY

From memory, set up a trolley for a manicure and pedicure treatment. Get your tutor to check that you have included all the tools and products you will need.

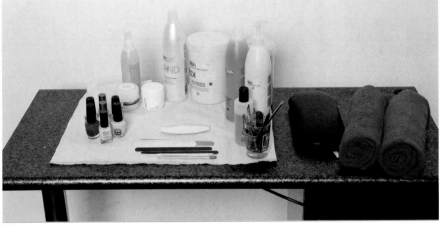

Selection of manicure products

CONSULTATION FOR MANICURE AND PEDICURE TREATMENTS

At all times in the salon, and especially during the consultation, it is important that you behave in a professional manner. You should always work cooperatively with others and follow the salon's requirements.

When you communicate, you must make sure that you follow the communication guidance given in Chapter 203. Use an appropriate friendly tone and speak clearly. Make sure you talk directly to the client when you can and use the client's name so that they know you are talking to them and to make them feel reassured and at ease. Check that the client understands what you are saying and give them the opportunity to ask questions.

INDUSTRY TIP

Placing a small piece of lint in the bottom of the sterilising jar will help to protect the tips of metal tools.

WHY DON'T YOU...
from memory, make a list of the things that you need for a pedicure.

HANDY HINTS

Professional behaviour is covered in Chapter 201. Look back at pages 130–134 if you need to remind yourself.

INDUSTRY TIP

Remember, being professional means being polite, using appropriate language (both verbal and non-verbal), listening carefully and being approachable at all times.

Up-sell

To offer or promote a more deluxe product or treatment.

CARRYING OUT YOUR CONSULTATION

Carry out your professional consultation to identify the treatment objective. The consultation is your opportunity to **up-sell** the treatment you are giving if this is possible or desired by the client. For example, if the client is having a standard manicure or pedicure you could offer them a deluxe treatment.

To make sure your client leaves satisfied, it is important to listen to them carefully and match the treatment objectives to their expressed needs. The client might have several treatment objectives including:

- to reduce and/or even out the length of the nails
- to smooth out any irregularities on the nail plate
- to improve the condition and appearance of the cuticle
- to condition, rehydrate and nourish the nail and skin
- to exfoliate the skin
- to provide an attractive and/or a protective covering to the nail plate.

INDUSTRY TIP

Not all clients want a colour polish applied. They might just want a conditioning treatment applied to the nails. Male clients will have a buffed, polish-free finish and some female clients might also prefer this option.

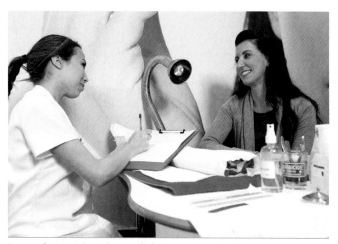
Remember to 'plant the seed' during a consultation!

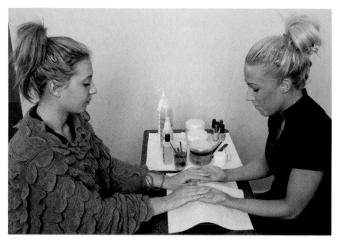
Analysing a client's nails

When you have agreed the treatment objectives, it is a good idea to summarise exactly what the manicure or pedicure treatment will include. When you have agreed the treatment plan with your client, you should ask them to sign and date it to agree and consent to the treatment.

THE SKIN AND NAIL ANALYSIS

You should always carry out a skin and nail analysis before every manicure and pedicure, even on regular client. Our skin is changing all the time and there are lots of factors, such as ill health, that can make our skin and nail structure change.

Give the skin and nails a quick spray with a skin sanitiser. Analyse the skin and nails before starting the treatment to:

- check for contra-indications
- identify specific areas for treatment
- make sure that a suitable treatment plan is provided
- make sure the client is treated with suitable products (as many nail companies now offer a range of treatment programmes)
- build a rapport and gain the client's confidence
- check progress if the client has had previous treatments.

INDUSTRY TIP

Clients might only spend one hour in the salon having a treatment which is one hour of professional care. If they have one treatment a month, that equates to 12 hours of care in a year. Twelve hours is plenty of time to advise them about good practice and educate them on how to achieve their desired aims.

HANDY HINTS

For more information on consultation techniques, look back at Chapter 203 (pages 166–176).

Look at each nail plate in turn. Make a note of anything you can see or feel. When you have done this you can then decide on your client's skin and nail type and condition. During the skin and nail analysis, you should also be checking for any contra-indications to treatment, such as nail disorders and diseases.

HANDY HINTS

Refer to the Anatomy and Physiology chapter to make sure you are familiar with common nail disorders and diseases so that you are able to recognise them.

HANDY HINTS

You will find further information on the structure of the skin and nail in the Anatomy and Physiology chapter (pages 1–90). You need to make sure you review these sections and are familiar with this information to help you understand about the skin and nail analysis.

Factors affecting the condition of the nails and skin

When you are carrying out the skin and nail analysis, there are a number of day-to-day and lifestyle factors that can affect the condition of a client's skin that you should take into consideration. These will affect your treatment plan and recommendations.

Factor	Effect on the nails and skin
Occupation	If the client works outside or in extremes of temperature, this will have an adverse effect on their skin and nails. Varying temperatures can cause dryness, dehydration and increase photo-ageing. If the client comes into contact with chemicals within their job and their hands are not properly protected, their skin could be dry or they might even have contact dermatitis.
Time to commit to treatment	If the client leads a busy lifestyle – a busy job and/or has lots of other responsibilities – how much time do they have to spend on improving or maintaining the condition of their hands and/or feet?
Daily lifestyle and habits	Smoking affects the repair and condition of the skin. Cigarettes contain unhealthy **toxins**. Smoking affects the quality of oxygen absorbed in the lungs. Nicotine can stain the skin and nails on the fingers that hold the cigarette.
	A lack of sleep will slow down the skin's ability to repair itself. It is while we are sleeping that the body repairs itself.
	People who drink too much alcohol (either regularly or through binge drinking) are at a high risk of damaging their liver. The liver is an important organ that helps to process nutrients and remove toxins from the body.
A lack of home care and the use of incorrect products	If there is a lack of home care, the skin and nails might be neglected. For example, a lack of care to the feet can lead to the build-up of hard skin on the heels.
	The use of products that do not benefit the client will result in a lack of incentive to keep up a skin/nail care routine as the client will not see positive results.
Medication	Some medication can alter the skin and nails (eg steroids can thin the skin).
General state of health	If the client's general health is poor, it is quite likely that their skin and nails will reflect this and they might look dull or dehydrated. If the client is healthy, it is likely that their skin will be too. White marks that are even across the nail can be an indication that the client has had an illness when the nail was being produced. Ill health can take its time to show in the nails because of the amount of time it takes the nails to grow. Consistent ridges that are evenly placed across the nails at the same position on the nail bed can also be an indication of poor health.

Toxin
A poison.

HANDY HINTS

There are many factors that can affect the way the nail grows and you should review these in the Anatomy and Physiology chapter on pages 37–49.

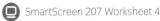 SmartScreen 207 Worksheet 4

When carrying out your inspection of the skin and nails, you should consider the following factors and adapt your treatment as necessary.

Factor influencing treatment	Consideration or cause	Adaptation of the treatment
■ Loss of elasticity in the skin. ■ Ridges and dryness in one or more of the nail plates.	■ The age of the skin and nails. ■ How are the nails and skin being affected by the ageing process?	■ Use an extra hydrating massage cream or hydrating anti-ageing mask. ■ You might also have access to anti-ageing serums that can be used to add extra luxury to the nail service. ■ Recommend that the client uses hydrating products at home, such as hand cream, foot cream and cuticle oils.
■ The texture of the skin and nails – do they feel dry?	■ Dry skin, hands and cuticles might be a sign of neglect or exposure to harsh products and chemicals.	■ Use hydrating, conditioning products. ■ Recommend that the client uses both conditioning and **hydrating** products at home or that they use protective gloves.
■ How warm or cool the skin's temperature is.	■ This will give you an indication as to what the client's circulation is like. ■ Poor circulation (cold hands and feet) will affect the condition of the skin and nails.	■ Poor circulation will benefit from massage to increase the circulation. ■ Buffing the finger nails will also help to stimulate the circulation to the nails to improve nail growth.

■ Skin or nail imperfections or abnormalities, such as:
  ■ **corns**
  ■ **calluses**
  ■ **bunions**
  ■ thickened toes nails
  ■ **thread veins** (feet)
  ■ discoloured nails
  ■ scar tissue
  ■ damage to the nail plate.
	■ The cause will vary depending on the imperfection found.	■ Treatment might need to be adapted and the area avoided to prevent any harm or further tissue damage.

■ The client's natural nail shape.	■ Which shape will best complement the client's natural nail shape?	■ Shape the nail according to the natural shape for the best result. ■ You should also consider the client's wishes and advise the client if their request is not achievable.

Corns

Corns are smaller than calluses and can be found on the top or between the toe joints. Some people also have corns on the first joint of their middle finger as a result of the pressure from holding a pen (writer's lump).

Callus

An area of hard skin produced by the body to protect a particular area. Calluses are formed as a result of pressure or friction (eg from poorly-fitting shoes). Calluses are commonly found on pressure points under the ball of the foot or at the back of the heel where shoes often rub.

Bunion (hallus valgus)

A painful condition where the metatarsophalangeal joint of the big toe becomes enlarged and moves out of place. The big toe bends in towards the other toes creating a lump on the side of the foot.

Thread veins

Small capillaries visible through the skin's surface.

Hydrating

To increase moisture.

INDUSTRY TIP

Most clients will have an idea as to what shape they would like their finished nails to be. If they are unsure you can use the shape of their natural nails, by using the cuticle at the base of the nails as a guide, to indicate the best shape.

HANDY HINTS

Refer back to the chapter on Anatomy and Physiology to recap on skin and nail imperfections or abnormalities.

Nail types and nail conditions

During the consultation, it is important to establish the client's nail type and any nail conditions that might be contra-indications to treatment.

Nail or cuticle condition	Characteristics	Cause
Healthy nails/cuticles (normal)	■ An even pink colour. ■ The nail plate is smooth and free from any irregularities or imperfections. ■ The nail plate is flexible and strong.	■ Good circulation and a healthy diet. ■ No major medical problems.
Dry nails/cuticles	■ A dull and powdery appearance. ■ They lack any sheen to the surface. When you stroke across the nail plate you will feel a slight drag.	■ There is a lack of natural moisture in the nail plate. ■ An unbalanced diet. ■ Frequent hand washing. ■ Contact with drying external agents (such as cleaning chemicals).
Damaged nails/weak soft nails	■ The nail plate will be extremely soft, thin and very weak. ■ The free edge will disintegrate when filed. ■ They might also be prone to peeling or flaking.	■ This might occur for a variety of reasons. ■ They commonly occur after nail enhancements. ■ Poor diet. ■ Lack of natural hydration in the nail. ■ Certain medical conditions. ■ Frequent contact with harsh chemicals.
Peeling nails *(lamellar dystrophy)*	■ An opaque appearance to the nail plate.	■ Peeling is caused by a separation of the layers of the nail plate causing the nail to peel along the free edge. ■ Peeling might also be caused by an unbalanced diet.

Nail or cuticle condition	Characteristics	Cause
Brittle nails (onychorrhexis) (*on-i-ko-rek-sis*) (*fragilitas unguium*)	■ Hard and inflexible. ■ They do not bend easily if at all. ■ The nail will crack, break or shatter easily, often breaking below the free edge line.	■ A lack of natural hydration in the nail. ■ An unbalanced diet. ■ Poor circulation in the elderly. ■ Certain medical conditions. ■ Frequent contact with harsh chemicals. ■ Too many manicures and too frequently.
Excessive/overgrown cuticles (pterygium) (*terr-e-gee-um*)	■ Excessive growth of the cuticle that grows up and along the nail plate. ■ The extended growth might be slight but in some cases it can extend over a large portion of the nail plate. ■ As the nail grows, the cuticle can become torn and hangnails occur.	■ Excessive growth of the cuticle. ■ It can be the result of damage to the nail matrix.
Bitten nails (onychopaghy) (*ony-co-fagy*)	■ The individual might bite the nail some way below the normal free edge and some people might also bite the surrounding skin and cuticles as well. ■ The skin can become quite sore, inflamed and tender. ■ The nail tip can look **bulbous**. **Bulbous** Swollen and rounded.	■ This is a nervous habit.
Hangnails	■ The cuticle splits and tears at the sides of the nail plate, as the nail plate grows and moves upwards.	■ Uneven growth ■ Dry cuticles. ■ Incorrect cutting of the cuticles causing the cuticle to split and tear.

Nail or cuticle condition	Characteristics	Cause
Horizontal and longitudinal ridges 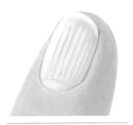 *Longitudinal ridges*	■ Horizontal ridges in the nail plate that run across the nail from side wall to side wall. ■ These ridges can be so pronounced that they cause a weakness in the nail structure and the nail can break. ■ They can be seen clearly and felt as changes to the texture of the nail plate. ■ Longitudinal ridges run from the cuticle to the free edge. ■ They can be seen clearly and felt as changes to the texture of the nail plate. **Rheumatism (also referred to as arthritis)** A medical condition that causes inflammation of the joints, pain and loss of movement.	■ Trauma to the nail, matrix or nail bed. ■ Illness. ■ Poor circulation and conditions, such as chilblains. ■ They become more common as we age. ■ Damage to the nail matrix. ■ In some cases, the damage affects the whole nail plate and, as it reaches the free edge, the nail splits. ■ **Rheumatism**. ■ Poor circulation and fine ridges are common in old age.

HANDY HINTS

You will also need to be aware of the different skin types and conditions. Information about skin types and conditions can be found in the Anatomy and Physiology chapter on pages 1–30. Make sure you are familiar with this information as you will need to be confident when you are providing treatments and offering aftercare advice.

WHY DON'T YOU...

carry out a skin and nail analysis on a colleague and make a note of everything you see on their hands and nails. (You can do their feet if you prefer.) If you can, also carry out a skin and nail analysis on someone older than yourself and on a young child (if they will stay still for long enough). Compare and discuss your results in your class.

Contra-indications

A contra-indication is a reason why a treatment cannot be carried out or why a treatment might have to be modified. A contra-indication might *prevent* the treatment so that the client cannot have the treatment at all or just *restrict* it so the treatment will need to be modified. If you think that the client should seek medical advice, recommend this but remember you are not a medical practitioner and you should not make any form of diagnosis.

As part of your consultation, you will need to look for contra-indications that will either prevent or restrict treatment. You should always explain to the client that you going to have to avoid an area or adapt a treatment.

Contra-indications that prevent nail treatments

INDUSTRY TIP

A normal nail has about 18 per cent moisture content. If this drops below 16 per cent, the nail becomes brittle and if it becomes more than 25 per cent, the nail becomes soft.

Contra-indication	Description and cause
Onychia (*oh-nik-ee-uh*)	■ A bacterial infection of the nail fold causing the skin around the base of the nail to become red and inflamed. ■ There might also be pus visible.

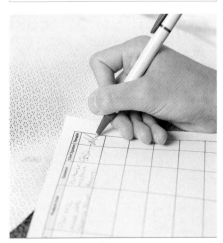

Completing a record

INDUSTRY TIP

There are lots of thing that can alter the colour of the nail plate. Hair colour or dyes can temporarily change the colour of the nail plate. People who smoke are likely to have stained nails and skin on the hand used to hold the cigarettes as a result of the nicotine in the cigarettes. Most staining is only temporary and will either fade or grow out with the nail.

Atrophy

To waste way, weaken and shrivel.

INDUSTRY TIP

If you have clients who wear nail enhancements, look out for mould. It is quite rare but occurs when enhancements are not maintained properly and where nail enhancements have lifted – providing an ideal moist warm environment in which mould can grow. It looks like a green ink stain on the nail plate.

INDUSTRY TIP

Onyx is the Greek medical term for nail.

Onych… means 'of the nail' and appears as a prefix in most nail-related words (eg onycholysis).

Contra-indication	Description and cause
Onychatrophia (**atrophy**) (*on-ee-chat-tro-fi-ah*) 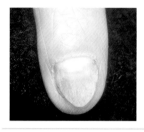	▪ Wasting of the nail plate. ▪ The nail plate looks dull and cloudy and might even completely come away from the nail bed. ▪ It is caused by injury, use of strong chemicals and by some diseases.
Onychoptosis (*on-ee-chop-toe-sis*) 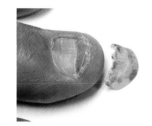	▪ Shedding of the nail plate. ▪ Caused by ill health, disease or trauma to the nail plate.
Fungal infections, eg tinea pedis (athlete's foot) 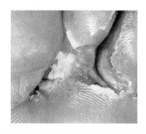	Symptoms include irritation and sometimes a distinct odour. The fungus lives on keratin and likes a moist warm environment. White spongy looking skin might crack, split and peel. Commonly found between the toes but can also affect larger areas of the foot. These prevent you from carrying out nail services because of the risk of cross-infection.
Bacterial Infections, eg furuncles (boils) and carbuncles, or impetigo 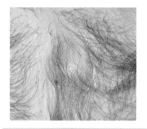	See page 28 for descriptions and causes of these infections. Some bacterial infections are very contagious and you should not feel under pressure to treat any infected area. These prevent you from carrying out nail services because of the risk of the bacteria growing underneath the nail.
Viral infections, eg verrucae (plantar warts) 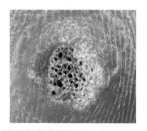	Verrucae occur on the soles of the feet. The weight of the body makes the wart grow inwards. Particularly contagious in damp warm moist conditions. These prevent you from carrying out nail services because of the risk of cross-infection.

Contra-indication	Description and cause
Infestations, eg pediculosis corporis (body lice) 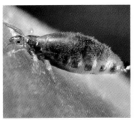 Body lice	Body lice are caused by tiny parasitic insects that lays their eggs on clothing and feed on the skin. Symptoms include intense itching at the site of the infestation, usually in the skin's creases (eg the elbows). More information on infestations is avilable on page 30. These prevent you from carrying out nail services because they are contagious.
Onycholysis (severe nail separation) (*on-ee-KOL-e-sis*) 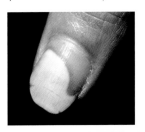	Severe separation of the nail from the nail bed. Nail plate looks white not pink. If you tap the surface of the nail you will hear a hollow sound. This prevents you from carrying out nail services because the condition of the nail plate is too poor to be worked on.
Severe eczema 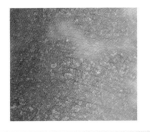	Areas of extreme dryness. The irritated skin is itchy. Can be caused by an internal irritant (eg a food intolerance) or by contact with an external allergen (eg animal hair or a product). Can prevent you carrying out nail services because the service might cause the condition to worsen or result in a reaction.
Severe psoriasis 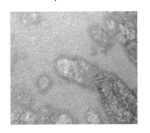	Skin cells are produced very quickly and build up on the skin's surface leaving very itchy scaly patches with a white pearly surface. Skin can crack and bleed. The exact cause is unknown. It is linked to stress and is often hereditary. The nail service you carry out might cause the condition to worsen or result in a reaction.
Severe skin conditions 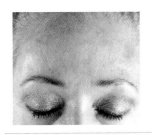	These are severe cases of sensitive, dehydrated or mature skin. See page 280 for more information on each of these conditions.

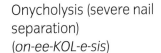

INDUSTRY TIP

We often say that the nail is the window to our health and tells us what is going on inside us. When you have surgery, surgeons use the nail plates to tell how much oxygen there is in the body. Nails appear pink as a result of the blood present in the nail bed showing through the transparent nail plate. Blue nails are the result of poor circulation.

Contra-indication	Description and cause	How the treatment can be modified
Onychogryphosis (*on-e-koh-gri-foh-sis*)	■ Crooked, curved, thickened nails. ■ The nail plate becomes enlarged and misshapen. The nail can become claw like or curve forwards or sideways. ■ It usually only affects the toenails. ■ It is usually caused by poor circulation. ■ It is not infectious.	■ The nails might be very difficult to cut so might need to be referred to a chiropodist or podiatrist.
Onychauxis (hypertrophy) (*on-e-corx-is*)	■ Thickened nails. ■ This condition is common on the toenails and might affect one or more of the nail plates.	■ Thickened toenails can be very difficult to cut and are best cut before soaking. ■ They should be cut with toenail clippers and the nail clipped in little pieces to get the desired length. ■ Trying to cut the nail in one go can be uncomfortable for the client. ■ If the nails are very thick it might be advisable to refer the client to a chiropodist.
Onychomalacia (eggshell nails) (*on-ee-chom-al-a-c-ah*)	■ Thin, weak, soft nails. ■ They are often more cloudy in appearance. ■ The condition can be caused by illness, a dietary **deficiency** or stress. **Deficiency** Something lacking.	■ Take extra care when you are working on these fragile nails.
Broken or fractured bones	Broken bones in the area being treated (hand or foot) can either prevent or restrict the service but it will depend on the severity of the break. See page 59 for more information on different types of breaks and fractures.	If it is only a small break then you should be able to work around the area. Larger breaks might prevent you from carrying out the treatment.
Recent sprains	When a ligament is overstretched or torn. A common area for sprains is around the ankle joint. A sprain can occur as the result of a fall when the full force of the body's weight is placed onto a joint.	The area will be very tender so be careful when you are working around it.

Contra-indication	Description and cause	How the treatment can be modified
Recent scar tissue	When the skin is broken, blood cells move into the wound and the blood clotting process starts. This is the body's way of healing tissue damage, but scar tissue sometimes remains.	The skin will be very tender to touch so be careful when you are working around the area and explain to your client why you are avoiding the area.
Hyper-keratosis	Thickening of the skin caused by an excessive amount of keratin. This thickening is often produced to protect the underlying tissue from rubbing, pressure and irritation. Commonly affects elbows, knees and the soles and heels of the feet.	Do not treat the affected area.
Skin allergies	When an allergic reaction occurs, the immune system produces antibodies in response to allergens that most other people would not find harmful. Common allergic conditions include urticaria, erythema, dermatitis and eczema.	Do not treat the affected area.
Cuts and abrasions	When a cut or abrasion is present, you need to avoid the area and work around it. A cut or abrasion will heal within a short space of time.	The skin will be very tender and you could risk cross-infection, so either apply a plaster to the affected area or be very careful when you are working around it.
Varicose veins	Bulging surface veins that look blue/green and bulbous. They are caused by the valves in the veins breaking down, which results in a stagnation of blood and causes obstruction, making the veins bulge.	Do not treat the affected area as it might be very painful to touch.
Epilepsy	Uncontrolled electrical activity in the brain. Seizures range from the sufferer having a blank expression and not responding, to a grand mal seizure which is when the individual becomes partially unconscious and suffers uncontrollable movements. Often has no known cause but can be triggered by a brain injury or a chemical imbalance. Photo sensitive epilepsy is caused by flashing lights.	If the client's condition is controlled and they know what triggers their seizures (and can avoid the trigger) there is no reason why they should not have safe treatments, eg a manicure or pedicure.

Contra-indication	Description and cause	How the treatment can be modified
Diabetes	There are two types, type 1 and type 2. Refer to page 86 for more information on both types.	If your client has diabetes, be very careful not to cut the cuticle and to keep the nail enhancements short. This is to reduce the risk of infection – diabetes can slow down the body's ability to fight off infections.
Phlebitis	This is inflammation of a vein. This is a painful condition that can affect one or more of the veins of the leg. The skin is visibly red and inflamed around the area of the affected vein and can feel quite warm to the touch.	Do not treat the affected area.
Product allergies	The client might suffer an allergic reaction to a product that has been applied to the skin. The skin will feel hot and the client will feel irritation, tingling or itching.	Check throughout the service that the products you are using are not causing any kind of allergic reaction.
Undiagnosed lumps and swellings	Any swelling that suddenly becomes noticeable to you should be looked at by a doctor. Most swellings are usually innocent and not malignant, but it is foolish to ignore any lump or bump that was not there before.	Avoid the area, as you are not certain of the cause, and advise the client to see their GP.

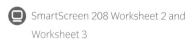

SmartScreen 208 Worksheet 2 and Worksheet 3

SmartScreen 206 Worksheet 1

ACTIVITY

From memory, write a list of the all the nail diseases and conditions that you can think of that would prevent a nail treatment. Now write a second list of all the nail diseases and conditions you can think of that might restrict a manicure or pedicure. Next to each condition, explain how you would modify your treatment. Check your answers with your tutor.

NAIL SHAPES

During the consultation you must also consider the nail shape that the client wants and whether it is suitable for their nail type.

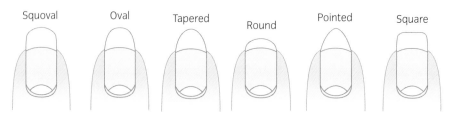

Squoval   Oval   Tapered   Round   Pointed   Square

NAIL CARE PRODUCTS

There are lots of nail care products available for different nail and skin types. Before looking at specific products, it must be stressed that all products are different and that you should make sure you are familiar with the manufacturer's information for the brands that your salon uses. Different products will vary a lot and the information given in this chapter is only basic guidance. You must make sure that you know the manufacturer's instructions for the products you are using. You should know the key ingredients and be able to:

- describe the benefits of each product that you work with
- know the skin type or condition each product is suitable for
- describe the texture and feel of each product.

The table below shows some of the ingredients that are commonly found in manicure and pedicure products:

HANDY HINTS
Look back at the Anatomy and Physiology chapter for further information on nail shapes (page 41).

WHY DON'T YOU...
make a prompt card for the products you use in your salon. Using a table format, write the name of the product, its benefits, its main ingredients and its retail price. Laminate the card and keep it somewhere close by so that you can refer to it.

Ingredient	Example	What it does	Which products contain this ingredient
Preservatives	■ Vitamin C ■ Isopropyl alcohol	■ Preservatives are added to a product to keep it stable, safe and prevent it from decaying. ■ They also prolong the products shelf life.	■ All products contain preservatives
Emollients	■ Wheat germ oil ■ Sweet almond oil ■ Shea butter ■ Beeswax	■ An emollient softens the skin.	■ Massage cream ■ Cuticle cream ■ Cuticle oil
Emulsifiers	■ Glycerol stearate ■ Cetyl alcohol	■ Emulsifiers stabilise the ingredients and keep ingredients evenly distributed so they do not separate.	■ Massage cream ■ Cuticle cream
Thickeners	■ Cellulose ■ Beeswax ■ Xanthan gum	■ Thickeners increase the **viscosity** of a product. **Viscosity** Thickness.	■ Massage cream ■ Cuticle cream ■ Cuticle removers
Clarifying agents	■ Butyl alcohol	■ Clarifying agents are used to prevent the product from becoming cloudy.	■ Nail polishes
Solvents	■ Butyl alcohol	■ Solvents keep the ingredients dissolved. ■ They also prevent the ingredients from setting or going hard.	■ Nail polishes
Perfumes (synthetic and man-made)	■ Lemon oil ■ Rose oil	■ Perfumes are added to give a product a pleasing smell. ■ They also mask the smell of some of the raw ingredients.	■ Hand cream mask ■ Foot spray
Kaolin	■ China clay (hydrate aluminium silicate)	■ Kaolin is a white or cream-coloured powder that absorbs moisture.	■ Foot masks

Ingredient	Example	What it does	Which products contain this ingredient
Silica	■ Sand	■ A white powder derived from nature; 12 per cent of rocks are formed from silica. It has excellent oil absorbing qualities.	■ Hand masks ■ Foot masks
Polyethylene balls	■ A polymer (substance formed from combining lots of small molecules (monomers) of ethylene) ■ It is produced from petroleum gas or dehydration of alcohol	■ Added to products to give tiny smooth balls that gently exfoliate the skin when massaged over the surface.	■ Foot scrub
Mineral oils	■ Mineral oil	■ Used in products as a lubricant, protective agent and a binding agent.	■ Massage oil ■ Massage cream
Ethyl alcohol	■ Ethyl alcohol	■ Used as an antibacterial agent.	■ Fragrances ■ Alcohol-based lotions ■ Nail preparation products
Isopropyl alcohol	■ Isopropyl alcohol	■ Used as an antibacterial agent and solvent.	■ Antibacterial sprays, eg hand or foot preparation sprays ■ Equipment sanitising sprays or wipes
Potassium hydroxide	■ Potassium hydroxide	■ Used to emulsify products.	■ Cuticle remover
Benzalkonium chloride	■ Benzalkonium chloride	■ Used as an antibacterial agent.	■ Surface disinfectants
Beeswax	■ Beeswax	■ A waxy emulsifier.	■ Moisturisers, hand or foot creams
Acetone	■ Acetone	■ Used as a solvent.	■ Nail enamel remover ■ Acrylic nail solvent

You need to know and understand the benefits of the products that you are using when carrying out nail care treatments and how to use them. The table below outlines the main products used in carrying out nail care treatments, the main ingredients within the products, the benefits of each product and how to use them.

Product	Benefit	Use	Main ingredients
Sterilising fluid, eg Sterilsafe and Barbicide	■ Sanitises small metal or plastic tools (such as cuticle nippers) and keeps them sanitised in between treatments.	■ The sterilising fluid is placed into a storage jar or container used for holding tools. ■ It is essential that the fluid is diluted exactly according to the manufacturer's guidelines, using specific measures, so that the chemicals work properly. ■ Another type of sterilising fluid is used to clean pedicure spas or foot baths which is corrosive and therefore not suitable for sterilising tools.	■ Glutaraldehyde ■ Quats (quarternary ammonium compounds) ■ Alcohol (eg ethyl alcohol) ■ Hypochlorite (a form of chlorine used in Milton Sterilising Fluid)
Skin sanitiser and sanitising sprays	■ Antibacterial products that kill bacteria to limit the spread of germs and infections.	■ Spray over the client's hands or feet before beginning a treatment. It should be applied as part of the skin analysis check.	■ Ethyl alcohol ■ Benzalkonium chloride
Nail polish remover	■ Contains chemicals that break down and dissolve nail polish so that it can be removed easily.	■ For best results, apply to the nail using a cotton lint-free pad and hold in place for several seconds. ■ This will give the product time to penetrate into the polish so that it can be wiped easily from the nail plate without excessive rubbing.	■ Acetone (ideally this should be avoided as it is very dehydrating) ■ Ethyl acetate ■ Butyl acetate ■ Glycerine (or a similar ingredient to counter the drying effect of acetone)
Hand and foot soak	■ Used to cleanse and soften the skin. They usefully have an antibacterial ingredient to restrict bacterial growth in the water while the treatment takes place. ■ Foot soaks often have a deodoriser to freshen the feet and make them smell pleasant.	■ Place a small amount of product (a single pump for a manicure or two or three pumps for a pedicure) into a manicure bowl or a foot spa. ■ Soak the client's fingertips or feet. ■ This product can also be used on a nail brush for deep nail cleansing or to clean the nails and remove any excess grease before applying polish to the nail plate.	■ Panthenol ■ Triclosan

INDUSTRY TIP

It is advisable not to allow the hands or feet to soak for too long as the nail plate is **porous** and will absorb a certain amount of water making the nail plate expand. This is why nails are filed before they are soaked. If the nails are allowed to soak for a long period of time, the amount of time that the nail polish lasts will be affected.

Porous

Containing minute holes through which water and air can pass.

Product	Benefit	Use	Main ingredients
Buffing paste	■ Buffing paste has an abrasive (exfoliant) action for the nail plate and smoothes out irregularities in the nail.	■ Apply a tiny amount, about the size of a grain of rice, to the nail plate and then buff with a chamois buffer.	■ Stannic oxide ■ Kaolin ■ Silica
Exfoliants	■ Exfoliants contain special ingredients that have a gritty texture and help to: 　■ give a deeper cleanse 　■ remove dead skin cells 　■ brighten the skin 　■ improve the appearance and texture of the skin. ■ Exfoliants can also contain **enzymes** or alpha hydroxy acids (AHAs) that gently break down the dead skin on the surface. ■ They loosen or weaken the **intracellular bonds** that hold the skin cells together so that they can be easily removed.	■ Massage into the area (hands, lower arm, lower leg and feet) using firm circular movements until most of the product has been absorbed into the skin. ■ Brush off any exfoliating grains that are left and then place the hand/foot into water to soak. ■ Brush over the area with your fingertips to remove any leftover exfoliant. ■ Remove the foot or hand and dry with a towel. **Enzymes** Proteins that speed up chemical reactions. **Intercellular bonds** Proteins that hold cells together and prevent them from falling apart.	■ Polyethylene balls ■ Nut kernels ■ Salt ■ Oatmeal ■ Seeds ■ Plant fibres ■ Alpha hydroxy acids (AHAs) ■ Acids (fruit)
Cuticle cream	■ Used to soften and nourish the cuticle.	■ Apply a tiny amount, usually about the size of a grain of rice, to the cuticle and massage it in. ■ It might be combined with a thermal treatment to enhance the benefits.	■ Water ■ Soft paraffin ■ Mineral oil ■ Beeswax

Product	Benefit	Use	Main ingredients
Cuticle remover	▪ Lifts and dissolves the cuticle. ▪ Helps to remove any loose or stubborn (eponychium) skin.	▪ Apply to the cuticle area using the tip of an orange wood stick. ▪ Using gentle circles, push back the cuticle. ▪ Cuticle remover should not be applied to living tissue or left on the skin for long periods as it can cause irritation.	▪ Potassium hydroxide ▪ Trisodium phosphate **INDUSTRY TIP** Potassium hydroxide in cuticle remover can be quite effective at removing stains, such as discolouration resulting from the use of dark nail polishes.

Nail conditioners	▪ There are a variety of nail conditioners available to treat particular nail conditions, such as peeling nails, brittle nails or weak nails, following the application of nail enhancements.	▪ These can be applied in the form of a treatment cream or oil and a small amount massaged into the nail plate.
		▪ More commonly they are designed to be applied like a clear polish that is applied over the nail plate and the free edge to seal it.
			▪ Ingredients will vary depending on the nature of the conditioner and can include:
			  ▪ vitamins
			  ▪ calcium
			  ▪ complex strengtheners
			  ▪ proteins
			  ▪ natural vegetable oils, such as wheat, jojoba or almond oil

Nail strengtheners	▪ Provides strength to the nail plate. These products often have a flexible plastic base.	▪ There are different strengtheners available – some are a liquid formula that is just applied to the free edge area and others are applied to the whole nail plate like a clear nail polish. ▪ Do not get these products on the nail wall or cuticle as they can be drying and can cause irritation.	▪ Aluminium sulphate ▪ Plazitsers (these change the structure of a product to make it hard, like plastic) ▪ Acrylic
Paraffin wax	▪ The product, in its warm state, makes the blood vessels **dilate** thereby increasing the circulation. ▪ The warmth is also very soothing and relaxing for the client. ▪ It also causes the skin to sweat and the pores to open.	▪ Apply paraffin wax in its liquid state by brushing it carefully onto the skin to form an even layer over the skin. ▪ Wrap the skin in plastic film and keep it warm for about 10–15 minutes. ▪ The wax can then be removed like taking off a glove. The remaining residue is a film of paraffin oil that can be massaged into the skin.	▪ Mineral oil **Dilate** To become wider or larger.

Product	Benefit	Use	Main ingredients
Cuticle oil	■ An oily product that softens and nourishes the skin and the nails – especially the cuticle.	■ Massage a single drop into the cuticles and nail plate.	■ Naturally occurring oils (eg almond oil)
Base coat	■ The base coat (the first product applied to the nail in the nail painting sequence) has several benefits: ■ It prevents discolouration of the nail plate when using coloured nail polish. ■ It provides a smooth surface for applying the nail polish to. ■ It helps the nail polish last longer. ■ It acts as an adhesive agent between the nail plate and the nail polish. ■ It can also contain ingredients to help correct and balance the condition of the nail plate.	■ Apply in a smooth, even layer covering the nail plate. **INDUSTRY TIP** Nail polish might chip because: ■ the nail plate is flaking or peeling ■ there is grease on the nail plate ■ no base coat was applied ■ there is too much solvent in the nail polish making it thin in consistency ■ the quick-dry product set the polish too quickly. **INDUSTRY TIP** Nail polish might flake or peel because: ■ the polish has been applied too thickly ■ no top coat was applied ■ there was grease on the nail plate ■ the layers of polish were not allowed to dry before adding additional layers.	■ Nitrocellulose ■ Butyl acetate ■ Ethyl acetate ■ Isopropyl alcohol
Cream nail polish	■ Forms a strong, coloured coating to enhance the appearance of the nail plate.	■ Apply in a smooth, even layer covering the nail plate. **INDUSTRY TIP** To prevent nail polish from thickening around the top of the bottle, use a tissue (not cotton wool as this will leave fibres) to wipe around the top of the bottle after use with nail polish remover and make sure the lid is replaced securely and tightly. Keep nail polishes away from direct sunlight or heat – but do not store them in a fridge as the cold can affect them as much as the heat.	■ Nitrocellulose ■ Resins ■ Butyl acetate ■ Ethyl acetate ■ Isopropyl alcohol ■ Pigments

Product	Benefit	Use	Main ingredients
Crystalline-coloured nail polish	■ Gives a crystalline or frosted appearance. ■ Forms a strong, coloured coating to enhance the appearance of the nail plate.	■ Apply in a smooth, even layer covering the nail plate.	■ Nitrocellulose ■ Resins ■ Butyl acetate ■ Ethyl acetate ■ Isopropyl alcohol ■ Pigments ■ Bismuth oxychloride
Top coat GLOSSER	■ It provides a protective layer to the polish. ■ Some top coats give a high-gloss finish to the nail polish. ■ It gives a sheen to the nail polish. ■ It seals and protects the nail polish.	■ Apply a top coat at the end of the nail painting sequence after the application of nail polish. ■ Apply in a smooth, even layer covering the nail plate when the nail polish is dry to the touch. **INDUSTRY TIP** If you apply top coat before the nail polish is dry enough, it will pick up the colour pigments from the polish and discolour the clear top coat.	■ Basic ingredients are the same as for base coats: ■ Nitrocellulose ■ Butyl acetate ■ Ethyl acetate ■ Isopropyl alcohol ■ Also has a high-gloss finish
Quick-dry nail products	■ These products contain an ingredient (usually an alcohol) that evaporates quickly, cooling the nail polish and helping it to set more quickly. **INDUSTRY TIP** Always wait a good couple of minutes before applying a quick-dry nail product otherwise the nail polish will ripple and the polish will be ruined.	■ If you are using a product in droplet form, place one drop of the product onto each nail and rotate the nail from left to right to spread the product over the nail plate. ■ If you are using a product with a brush applicator, use the brush to apply the product to the whole nail plate.	■ Methyl ethyl ketone ■ Cyclomethicone ■ Dimethicone **INDUSTRY TIP** Avoid quick-dry nail products that are aerosol sprays as these can be problematic for asthmatic clients.
Massage creams	■ Massage creams have a higher oil content than lotions and nourish the skin leaving it soft and silky. ■ The product is richer than a lotion and more suitable for a dryer skin type, or ageing or sun-exposed skin.	■ Apply the massage cream to your hands and warm it between your hands before applying it to the client. ■ For the hands, one pump from a bottle should be enough to cover each hand and, for the feet, two pumps from the bottle should be enough for both feet. ■ Massage the cream into the area, using a range of relaxing movements, until it is fully absorbed.	■ Purified water ■ Mineral oil ■ Vegetable oils ■ Beeswax ■ Shea butter

Product	Benefit	Use	Main ingredients
Massage lotions	<ul><li>A lotion has a lighter texture compared to a cream and is absorbed into the skin more easily than a cream.</li><li>They condition and soften the skin without leaving any surface residue.</li></ul>	<ul><li>Apply the massage lotion to your hands and warm it between your hands before applying it to the client.</li><li>For the hands, one pump from a bottle should be enough to cover each hand and, for the feet, two pumps from the bottle should be enough for both feet.</li><li>Massage the lotion into the area, using a range of relaxing movements, until it is fully absorbed.</li></ul>	<ul><li>Purified water</li><li>Mineral oil</li><li>Vegetable oils</li></ul>
Hand creams	<ul><li>Hand cream or lotion is quick and easy to apply.</li><li>It is light in texture and should be absorbed easily by the skin leaving it feeling smooth and nourished. Hand creams usually have a pleasing fragrance.</li><li>Hand creams containing mineral oils that sit on the surface of the epidermis and provide a protective barrier – they give a soft, smooth feeling.</li><li>Natural vegetable oils (eg sweet almond oil) penetrate more readily into the upper epidermis and are better for nourishing the skin.</li></ul>	<ul><li>Apply as required to the hands.</li><li>Make sure that you have enough product to cover the hands leaving them feeling nourished and hydrated.</li></ul>	<ul><li>Glycerol</li><li>Water</li><li>Colour</li><li>Perfume</li><li>Isopropyl myristate</li><li>Methyl cellulose</li><li>Triethanolamine</li></ul>

ACTIVITY

Are there any particular nail polish application techniques that you are required to use in your salon (eg do you need to use a top coat with all colours)? Discuss these with your tutor.

PREPARING THE CLIENT AND YOURSELF FOR MANICURE AND PEDICURE TREATMENTS

PREPARING THE CLIENT FOR A MANICURE TREATMENT

Ask your client to remove their jewellery and place it in a small bowl on the treatment table so that they can see it. This will also help you to remember to get your client to put their jewellery back on before you begin applying the nail polish.

PREPARING THE CLIENT FOR A PEDICURE TREATMENT

Ask your client to:

- remove their shoes and socks or tights
- remove tight trousers (if they prefer) to avoid getting any products on them.

POSITIONING YOURSELF FOR MANICURE AND PEDICURE TREATMENTS

For health and safety reasons, you also need to decide how best to position yourself. Make sure you are not leaning or overstretching as this will cause muscular aches and strains. Ideally, you should sit so that you can keep your back as straight as possible and your feet flat on the floor to maintain your posture. Poor posture will lead to muscular fatigue and, in some cases, strain or injury.

> **INDUSTRY TIP**
>
> When the client calls to make an appointment for a pedicure, make sure you advise them to bring some open-toed sandals or flip flops to wear after their treatment. This will help to avoid smudging their nail polish. It is amazing how many clients think all polish dries instantly and that they can put socks and enclosed shoes back on without it affecting their polish. It is a good idea to keep a supply of disposable flip flops that can be sold to clients who forget.

> **INDUSTRY TIP**
>
> The guidance given in this chapter is general guidance and might need to be adapted according to the products you are using. Some nail products have very set methods of application and so you need to make sure you are familiar with the particular techniques that are appropriate for the products you are using.

PROVIDE MANICURE AND PEDICURE TREATMENTS

Now that you know the products you will need and have carried out your consultation, you are ready to carry out manicure and pedicure treatments.

In this part of the chapter you will learn about:

- nail tools and techniques
- manicure and pedicure treatments and techniques
- completing the manicure and pedicure treatment
- aftercare and home care advice.

> **WHY DON'T YOU...**
>
> from memory, make a list of all the special conditioning products that are available in your salon that you can use on your clients' hands or feet. Include treatment base coats. Discuss your answers with your tutor.

 SmartScreen 208 Worksheet 8

> **INDUSTRY TIP**
>
> You need to remember to get the client to put their trousers back on before you begin applying the nail polish.

> **HANDY HINTS**
>
> Look back at Chapter 202 (page 148) to remind yourself of how to wash your hands effectively.

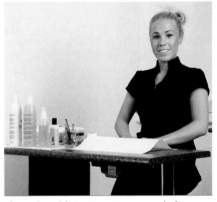

Therapist with treatment area ready for a client

WHY DON'T YOU...
see if you can find range of different emery boards in your salon and compare them. (If you have access to emery boards used for nail enhancements then include these too.) Write a short list comparing the different grit and thickness of each emery board. Next to each emery board, write down what the emery board would be used for and check your answers with your tutor.

NAIL TOOLS AND TECHNIQUES

There are a lot of tools that you will need to carry out a manicure or pedicure treatment. Using tools incorrectly can cause damage and even injury to the client. Refer to the spider diagram below for one way of carrying out a manicure or pedicure service. This will help you to know when you should use each tool discussed in the table.

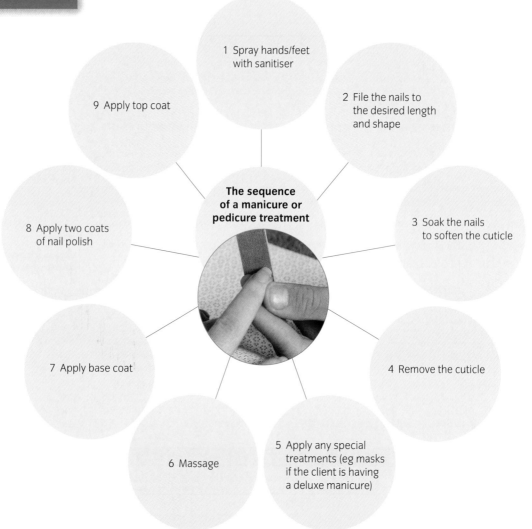

1 Spray hands/feet with sanitiser

2 File the nails to the desired length and shape

3 Soak the nails to soften the cuticle

4 Remove the cuticle

5 Apply any special treatments (eg masks if the client is having a deluxe manicure)

6 Massage

7 Apply base coat

8 Apply two coats of nail polish

9 Apply top coat

The sequence of a manicure or pedicure treatment

Good nail painting techniques can take time to perfect as you will need to develop your technique across a range of products. Only constant practice will make sure you master these.

INDUSTRY TIP

While service times are important, when you are learning it is best to take your time and get what you are doing right before worrying about timings. When you can do something well then you can set yourself time targets.

Tool	Use	Technique	Additional information
Emery boards 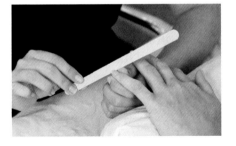	Used to file the nail into shape or to smooth away rough edges.	<ul><li>The correct way to hold an emery board is to hold the end of the board between the thumb, index and middle finger.</li><li>Hold the file at a 45° angle to the nail edge. At this angle the emery board will file the fibres of the nail down so that they can be removed easily.</li><li>The filing technique should be a long, light and sweeping movement.</li><li>File from one edge of the nail to the centre, repeat to the other side, alternating with a few strokes to each side.</li><li>When you have reached the desired length and shape of the free edge, **bevel** the free edge by taking the nail file down the free edge to remove any fluffy nail fibres.</li></ul> **Bevel** To smooth and round off.	<ul><li>For a manicure, the emery board should be softer – around 240–400 grit.</li><li>For a pedicure, the emery board should be around 180–240 grit.</li></ul> **INDUSTRY TIP** It is important to use good quality emery boards as cheap emery boards can have unfinished edges that are sharp and can cut the skin. **INDUSTRY TIP** Never use a sawing motion (ie working the file backwards and forwards) when you are using an emery board to file the nails. This action will create friction and heat in the nail plate and can cause the nail layers to separate. **INDUSTRY TIP** Emery boards come in varying degrees of coarseness (grit) – commonly between 80 and 400 grit. The higher the number, the softer the file. If the emery boards are cushioned this reduces the pressure and softens the effect.

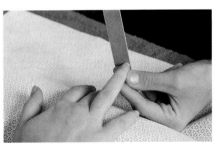

INDUSTRY TIP

To make sure you are filing the nail into a **symmetrical** shape, hold the emery board on its thin side down the centre of the nail and look to make sure that the nail is filed evenly on both sides.

Symmetrical

Two halves that are exactly the same – one being a mirror image of the other.

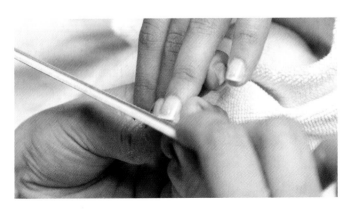

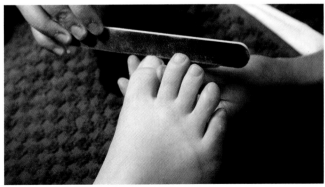

ACTIVITY

Look under the free edge of your nail. Describe what you can see. What part of the nail structure do you think this is?

Tool	Use	Technique	Additional information
Cuticle knife	A metal tool that is used to lift the cuticle gently from the nail plate.	▪ Dip the knife into water before use and then with the blade flat to the nail plate, use tiny circles to lift the cuticle off the nail plate. **INDUSTRY TIP** Make sure that metal tools (such as cuticle knives) are made from stainless steel as these are more robust and less likely to rust when in contact with water over a period of time. **INDUSTRY TIP** Make sure you sterilise all your metal tools in an autoclave before use.	▪ Incorrect use can cause damage to the matrix and damage to the skin. ▪ It can also cause damage to the nail plate and scratch it if it is used dry.
Hoof stick	A small wooden or plastic stick, with a rubber hoof-shaped attachment at the end.	▪ Dampen the hoof stick before use and apply it to the nail plate near the cuticle using little circles to gently lift and push back the cuticle.	▪ Hoof sticks might be plastic or wooden. **INDUSTRY TIP** Plastic hoofs sticks are more practical as they can be disinfected more easily. Wooden hoof sticks tend to bend when they get wet.
Cuticle nippers	A metal tool that is used to remove any loose dead cuticle.	▪ Carefully hold the cuticle nippers and trim away any loose skin. ▪ For hygiene reasons, any skin that is removed should be wiped from the cuticle nippers with a cotton pad or tissue and not onto the manicure towel.	▪ Do not trim away healthy skin. ▪ If cuticle nippers are used incorrectly and you cut away too much skin, you can leave the area sore and open to infection.
Nail scissors	If the toenails are curved, nail scissors might be required to make them easier to cut. They might also be used to cut down the length of the free edge on fingernails.	▪ The nail is shortened by cutting the nail at each side and then across the middle to give a straighter edge. ▪ Support the nail plate with one finger as you cut to avoid pulling the nail plate.	▪ Nail scissors have a light curve at the end to make it easier to cut nails. ▪ Avoid cutting the nail in one go as it is difficult to do and might tear the free edge rather than giving a neat cut.

Tool	Use	Technique	Additional information
Nail clippers	Used to shorten and remove nail length.	▪ Nail clippers have small pincers that are used to cut away small pieces of nail until the desired shape is achieved rather than cutting the nail in one go. ▪ Toenail clippers are designed to cut tougher nails and aim to cut off the length in three clips – one each side and one across the middle – to give a straight edge. They have a lever to help get a better grip and give stability. ▪ When you are clipping toenails, it is important to cut the toenail straight across. This helps to prevent the nails from curving at the sides and growing into the skin. File the nail very lightly to remove any rough edges and smooth the free edge. Do not shape the nail otherwise it might become ingrown. ▪ Support the nail plate with a finger when you are using clippers to prevent any movement in the nail bed and any discomfort.	▪ There are different designs of nail clippers depending on whether you are cutting fingernails or toenails and for different nail thicknesses (ie very thick toenails). ▪ Nail clippers are usually only used on the toenails. They can be used on fingernails if there is lots of free edge to remove and filing is not practical. ▪ The advantage of nail clippers is that they are less likely to cause shattering or splitting of the nail layers if the nail is very thick or brittle. **INDUSTRY TIP** The only time that toenails should be taken down at the sides is if they are actually ingrown. This should only be carried out by a foot specialist, such as a podiatrist or chiropodist who will have the tools to do this safely.
Foot files/rasps	Used to remove dead, hard skin from the heels and balls of the feet. A foot file usually has a pumice or rough surface to remove the dead skin. A rasp has a metal surface like a grater.	▪ Make firm contact with the skin and rub in one direction. ▪ The skin should be dry to prevent shredding of the skin. ▪ It is also easier to file the skin when it is dry.	▪ There are several different designs of foot rasp and files. They all have the same function of removing dead, hard skin but just have a different design to make them easier to grip or to make contact with the skin. ▪ When using a foot file, place a piece of tissue under the foot for hygiene reasons and to collect the dead skin (which can then be disposed of easily).

Tool	Use	Technique	Additional information
Nail buffers 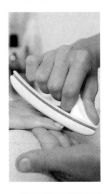	Nail buffers smooth the nail plate and remove any ridges or imperfections in the surface of the nail plate.	<ul><li>There are three different types of nail buffers:</li><li>Traditional buffers are made from chamois leather and are used with a tiny bit of buffing paste (the size of a grain of rice). The nail is buffed by stroking the buffer firmly in one direction – from the cuticle to the free edge – at an angle in several quick movements.</li><li>The second type of buffer has the same shape as an emery board but has a special coating. One side is slightly abrasive and the second side is smooth to give a shiny, natural-looking finish to the nail surface. They are not usually used with any product.</li><li>With a three-way buffer start by using the coarsest side and buff the nail plate in both directions taking the buffing across the nail plate in quick repetition. Move on to the next grade and finally use the smooth part to bring the nail plate to a shine.</li></ul>	<ul><li>Buffers can be quite abrasive and should not be used too frequently as excessive use can thin and weaken the nail plate.</li><li>The buffing action also stimulates the circulation which is good but too much buffing can cause friction (and heat) which is uncomfortable for the client.</li></ul>

HANDY HINTS

When carrying out manicure and pedicure treatments, you should be aware of the structure and function of the muscles, bones, arteries, veins and the lymphatic vessels of the lower arm, hand, leg and foot. You can find this information in the Anatomy and Physiology chapter on pages 49–85. It is recommended that you work through the relevant 'Test your knowledge' questions at the end of the Anatomy and Physiology chapter to make sure you have a good understanding as this will help you to apply more effective manicure and pedicure treatment techniques.

MANICURE AND PEDICURE TREATMENTS AND TECHNIQUES

Most salons offer a range of manicure and pedicure treatments ranging from standard treatments to luxury treatments (such as a paraffin wax). In this section you will learn about the range of treatments that are available, the techniques for carrying out the treatments and the sequence in which you should carry out the treatments.

MASSAGE

As part of a standard manicure and pedicure the client will receive a massage. This is usually carried out towards the end of the treatment before painting the nails. Most clients really enjoy this part of the treatment and find it very relaxing. Remember when working on the feet that you need to be confident with your techniques as light pressure on the feet can be ticklish and it might also cause the client's foot to twitch.

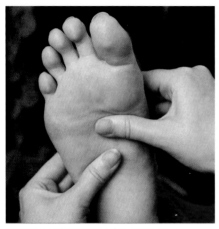

Massage will improve the circulation

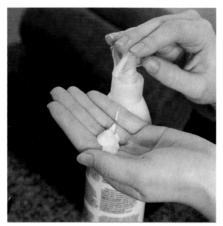

Pump dispensers make it easier to apply products

The physiological benefits of massage

Massage can be beneficial to the client in many ways as it:

- improves the texture of the skin by **desquamation** – the application of a suitable massage medium will have a smoothing, nourishing and softening effect on the skin and the massage itself also helps to keep the skin supple
- increases the circulation to the tissues where the massage is being carried out – the improved circulation gives the skin a healthy glow
- increases the oxygen and nutrients to the tissues and stimulates the removal of waste products from the intercellular tissues
- stimulates the activity of the glands in the skin, increasing secretions and making the skin more supple
- increases cellular activity (metabolism)
- relaxes the muscle fibres and relieves tension
- promotes relaxation – releases **endorphins** and gives the client an increased sense of wellbeing.

Desquamation
To remove dead skin cells.

Endorphins
Chemicals released by the brain that reduce feelings of pain.

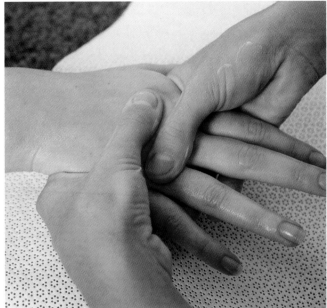
Frictions to the metacarpals

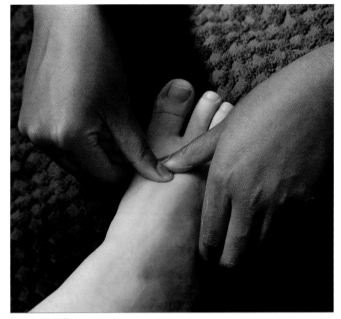
Massage relieves tension

Hydrate
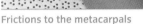
To add water.

Repetitive
Doing the same thing over and over again.

Massage mediums

The massage medium for manicures and pedicures is usually a massage cream. However, it can also be a rich lotion or an oil-based product. The product needs to provide lubrication for the hands so that they glide easily over the surface. The product needs to nourish the skin and not be absorbed too quickly by the skin otherwise the treatment routine has to be interrupted to reapply more product. The medium should also leave the skin feeling soft, **hydrated** and supple.

Massage techniques

Massage techniques will often follow a set routine for a manicure or pedicure. Your routine should be flowing, continuous, not too **repetitive** and use a variety of massage movements and techniques. The different massage techniques that you should include in your routine are:

- effleurage
- petrissage
- frictions
- tapotement/percussion
- vibrations
- joint manipulation.

Effleurage

A massage routine always starts with effleurage. It is the movement used to apply the massage medium. Effleurage is light, stroking movements that are applied with the palms of the hands, fingertips or thumbs. During effleurage, the movements should be linked together by moving the hands from one area to another to keep the massage flowing and continuous.

The effects of effleurage are:

- an increase in the circulation, bringing oxygen and nutrients to the skin tissues and removing waste products from the skin tissues
- the relaxation of the muscles and skin tissues
- the removal of dead skin cells (desquamation).

Petrissage

Petrissage is kneading movements that involve applying pressure and rolling or lifting the tissues in some way. Petrissage movements can use the whole of the palm of the hand, the pads of the thumb, the fingers or the knuckles. These movements are deeper and more stimulating.

The effects of petrissage are:

- an increase in the circulation, bringing oxygen and nutrients to the skin and removing waste products from the skin – a visible erythema will be seen on the skin's surface
- the relaxation of the skin tissues
- desquamation
- the stimulation of cell renewal
- the relaxation of muscles and the removal of lactic acid from the muscles, thereby reducing muscular aches
- assistance to the lymphatic system in carrying out its job.

Frictions

Frictions are a type of petrissage movement but they have a very different purpose. They are quick movements applied using the fingers or thumbs in either a rubbing or circular motion to stimulate the skin and create friction. They are good to use on the feet as they help to increase circulation.

The effects of friction are:

- vasodilation and a rapid increase in circulation (seen as erythema on the skin's surface)
- the loosening of the tissues in the skin (such as scar tissue) by stretching the collagen in the skin tissue
- the loosening of **adhesions** in the muscles to relieve muscular tension
- desquamation.

Tapotement/percussion

Tapotement is also known as percussion movements. Tapotement is stimulating movements that are light and brisk. Tapotement is rarely used on the hands but can be very effective for increasing circulation in the legs and feet. For example, in a pedicure, tapotement can be used as cupping on the calf area and toe plucking.

The effects of tapotement are:

- a rapid increase in the circulation, bringing oxygen and nutrients to the skin tissues and removing waste products from the skin tissues – a visible erythema will be seen on the skin's surface
- the stimulation of cellular renewal
- the relaxation of the muscles and the removal of lactic acid from the muscles, thereby reducing muscular aches
- assistance to the lymphatic system in carrying out its job.

Vibrations

Vibrations are mild trembling movements that are transferred from the therapist's lower arm through their fingers to the client's nerve path. These movements are applied sparingly.

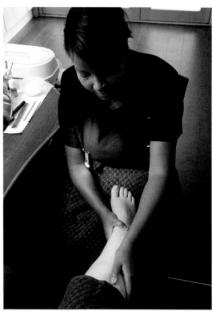

Support the client's leg during massage

Adhesions
Fibrous bands.

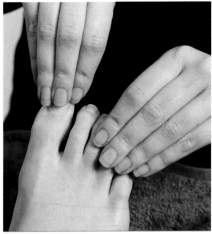

Tapotement using a finger plucking action is great for improving circulation in the toes

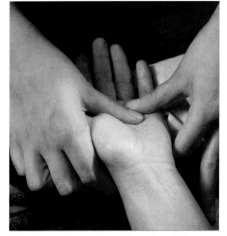

Thumbs can be used on the palm of the hand to apply deep circular kneading or frictions by sliding the thumbs back and forwards across the palm

The effects of vibrations are:

- the gentle stimulation of the deeper skin layers
- stimulation of the nervous system
- assistance in the removal of static lymph from the tissues.

Joint manipulation

This is used to help improve and maintain joint **mobility**. It is a **passive** movement meaning that the therapist moves the hand or foot while the client is relaxed. The hand or foot is supported with one hand and rotated, flexed or extended with the other. Care must be taken not to force a movement and to only move the joint within a comfortable range of movements.

Adapting massage techniques

Massage movements can be adapted to suit the clients' treatment objectives. Below are some examples of where you might need to adapt your technique.

- If a client has varicose veins in their lower leg then massage should not be applied to the calf area.
- If a client has poor circulation you could increase tapotement and deeper petrissage to stimulate the circulation.
- Poor nail growth and dry cuticles would benefit from concentrated movements along the fingers and toes, particularly around the nail plate and cuticles.

ACTIVITY

From memory, see how many names you can remember for the:

- bones of the hand and lower arm
- the main muscles of the lower arm
- the main blood vessels of the lower arm.

Suggested massage routine for a manicure treatment

Make sure you are familiar with the bones and muscles of the arm and hand before carrying out a massage. You can review these in the Anatomy and Physiology chapter on pages 57–58 (bones) and pages 69–72 (muscles).

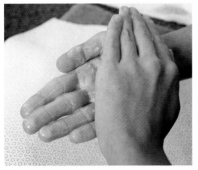

STEP 1 – Warm your chosen massage medium in your hands and apply to your client's left hand. Using effleurage movements, massage up the arm to the elbow.

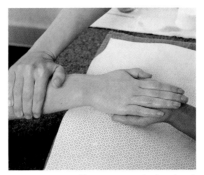

STEP 2 – Use effleurage over the hand and forearm in sweeping movements.

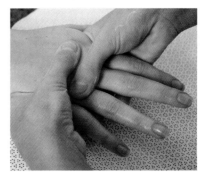

STEP 3 – Using effleurage movements, massage the back of the hands using your thumbs.

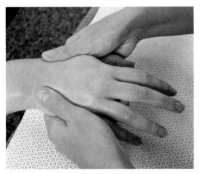

STEP 4 – Stretch the hand by sweeping your thumbs across the back of the hand and pushing up with your fingers into the palm.

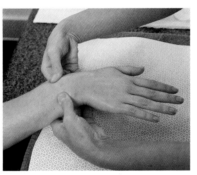

STEP 5 – Using effleurage movements, massage around the wrist using your thumbs.

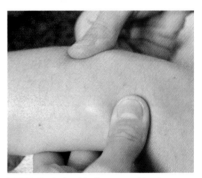

STEP 6 – Take this deeper and begin to knead around the wrist.

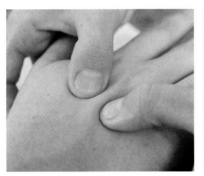

STEP 7 – Slide your thumbs down and knead in between the metacarpals and from the phalanges up to the carpals.

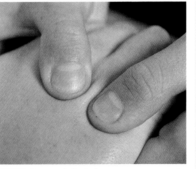

STEP 8 – Apply little friction movements in between the metacarpals using your thumbs.

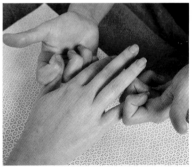

STEP 9 – Knead down each finger including the nail plate. Start with the little finger and finish with the thumb.

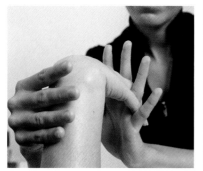

STEP 10 – Hook your hand into the client's hand and rotate their hand at the wrist. Flex and extend their wrist – remembering not to force any movement.

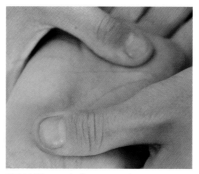

STEP 11 – Apply frictions to the inner wrist using your thumbs.

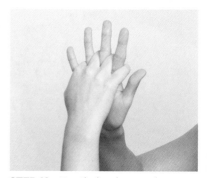

STEP 12 – Turn the hand over and massage the palm of the hand.

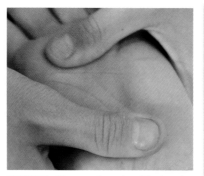

STEP 13 – Massage the palm of the hand and lower inside arm using your thumbs, then rotate the arm back to its original position.

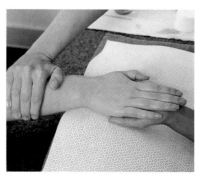

STEP 14 – Repeat step 1 using effleurage movements to massage up the arm to the elbow to finish. Now repeat the routine on the right hand.

WHY DON'T YOU...
look back at the Anatomy and Physiology chapter to remind yourself where the carpals, metacarpals and the phalanges are.

207/208 PROVIDE MANICURE/PEDICURE TREATMENTS

ACTIVITY

From memory, see how many names you can remember for the:

- bones of the foot and lower leg
- the main muscles of the lower leg
- the main blood vessels of the lower leg.

Suggested massage routine for a pedicure

Make sure you are familiar with the bones and muscles of the lower leg and feet. You can review these in the Anatomy and Physiology chapter on pages 58–59 (bones) and page 73 (muscles).

Gastrocnemius
Muscle forming the calf.

Tibialis anterior
Muscle on the front of the leg.

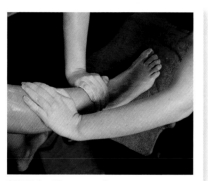

STEP 1 – Warm your chosen massage medium in your hands away from your client's feet and apply to their foot. Using effleurage movements, massage up the lower leg to the knee, taking the hand up the front and the back of the leg.

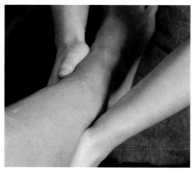

STEP 2 – Knead the **gastrocnemius** (calf) using your palms.

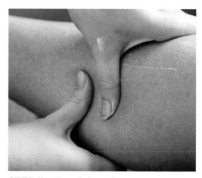

STEP 3 – Knead along the groove next to the **tibialis anterior** (side of the calf) using your thumb.

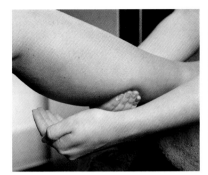

STEP 4 – Apply tapotement to the gastrocnemius – either cupping or finger slapping.

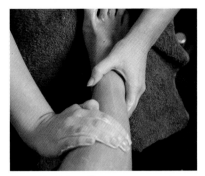

STEP 5 – Using effleurage movements, massage the lower leg down to the foot.

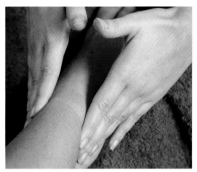

STEP 6 – Using effleurage movements, massage the top of the foot starting at the toes and moving up the foot. Divide your hands and circle around the ankle back to the toes.

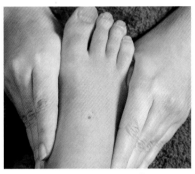

STEP 7 – Stretch the foot by pulling your fingers across the top of the foot and pushing your thumbs up under the sole of the foot.

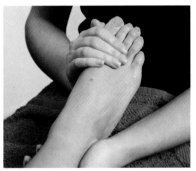

STEP 8 – Using effleurage movements, massage around the inside of the foot, starting at the big toe and moving along the side of the foot and around the ankle joint before finishing back at the big toe.

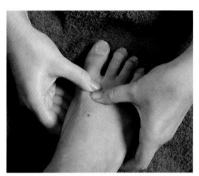

STEP 9 – Using your thumbs, knead in between the metatarsals from the phalanges up to the tarsals.

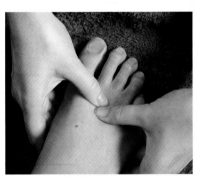

STEP 10 – Apply little friction movements in between the metatarsals using your thumbs.

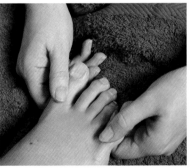

STEP 11 – Starting with the little toe, knead down each phalange, massaging the toenail well and finishing with the big toe.

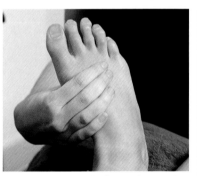

STEP 12 – Support the foot and rotate the foot at the ankle. Flex and extend the ankle – remembering not to force any movement.

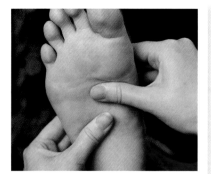

STEP 13 – Using your thumbs, with deep circles massage the sole of the foot working up to the pad of the foot.

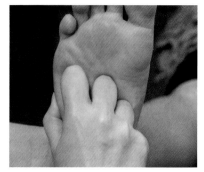

STEP 14 – Knead the sole of the foot with the palm of your hand.

INDUSTRY TIP

If a client has varicose veins, do not massage over their lower leg as this will put pressure on the varicose veins and might be very uncomfortable.

WHY DON'T YOU...
work with a colleague and carry out a foot massage. Make the first massage really light and then complete a second massage using firm and deep (but not rough) techniques. How did each pressure feel to receive and how did your feet feel after each massage?

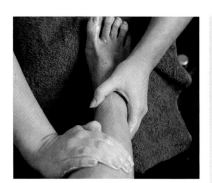

STEP 15 – Repeat step 1 using effleurage movements to massage up the lower leg to the knee.

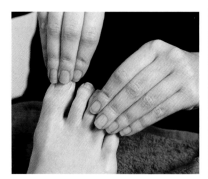

STEP 16 – Finish with tapotement – plucking of the toes. Repeat the routine on the right foot.

SPECIALIST HAND AND FOOT TREATMENTS
Hand and foot masks
In a manicure or pedicure, masks are used as part of a deluxe treatment to hydrate and nourish the skin.

The use and benefits of a mask

Mask type	Use and benefit
Cleansing	These have a clay base that absorbs surface impurities and excess oils. They also cause the skin to desquamate, absorbing and holding the dead skin.
Stimulating (thermal masks)	Thermal ingredients cause the mask to warm up when applied to the skin. The heat stimulates the blood's circulation and increases sweat and sebaceous activity.
Stimulating (cryo-masks)	Cryo-masks contain a cooling ingredient, such as camphor or mint, and cause a vasodilating effect. The cooling reduces the blood's circulation and decreases sweat and sebaceous activity. They are very refreshing on the feet in the summer.
Hydrating	Hydrating masks leave a film of moisture or oil on the skin's surface to nourish and rehydrate. Some of these masks can be left on and massaged into the skin

ACTIVITY

With a colleague, apply two different types of mask – one to each leg. How did the skin feel afterwards? Did you feel and see a difference?

Applying a mask

Masks are usually applied after the cuticle work and before the massage. Apply the mask to clean skin using a large brush or with the hands. It is important to make sure the mask is applied evenly and that the area is fully covered. Do not forget to apply in between the fingers and toes.

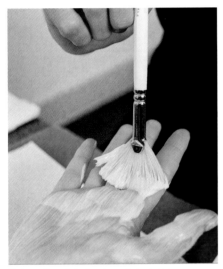

Using a brush helps to get an even application

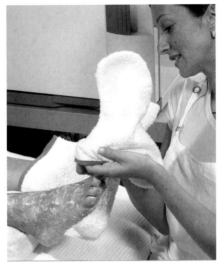

Towelling booties will help keep the feet warm while the mask is on

Clay-based cleansing foot masks should be left to dry naturally in the air. Moisturising masks can be covered with cling film and placed into thermal booties/mittens to enhance the effects.

Removing a mask

When the mask has been left on for the desired time (anything from 5–15 minutes) you can remove it. Unwrap the hands or feet if they are in plastic film or remove them from the thermal booties/mittens and remove the mask from the skin with warm water and a cloth or mittens. If you are using a clay mask, make sure you have removed all the residue from the mask before continuing with the treatment.

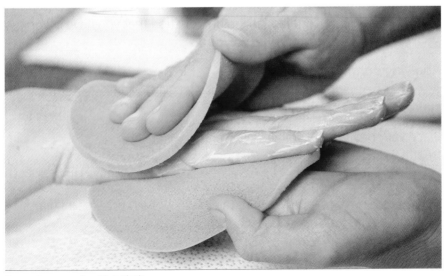

Removing a mask with a cloth

INDUSTRY TIP

Some moisturising masks are actually left on the skin and the residue is used as the massage medium.

INDUSTRY TIP

To maintain good standards of hygiene during nail treatments:

- use a spatula to remove products from containers
- keep tools in a container of disinfectant when not in use
- wipe debris from cuticle nippers onto a cotton pad or tissue, not onto towels
- use clean towels for each client
- place rubbish in a bin as you work
- use disposable files/orange sticks.

Distillation

The heating of a substance until it evaporates and then it condenses as it cools. The liquid that is left after this process is collected and used.

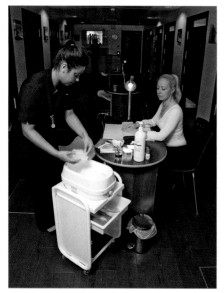

Therapist preparing paraffin wax

Paraffin wax treatments

Paraffin wax is used as a mask treatment during manicures and pedicures. Paraffin wax is obtained from the **distillation** of petroleum, producing a white colourless waxy substance. It comes as pellets or blocks of wax that are placed in a special heater. When heated it becomes clear and completely fluid. It has a working temperature of 40–48°C. At this temperature it can be applied easily and spread evenly.

The benefits of paraffin wax

Paraffin wax:

- softens the skin
- hydrates the skin
- promotes desquamation – the dead skin is then trapped in the wax as it sets
- increases the circulation as a result of the heat – this can be seen as erythema following treatment
- increases sweat and sebaceous activity
- soothes and relaxes the sensory nerves
- improves the skin's texture.

Preparing for a paraffin wax treatment

If a paraffin wax treatment is being included as part of a deluxe treatment, you must make sure you are prepared for it before you start the treatment.

- Make sure that the wax is fully melted.
- Make sure it is at the correct working temperature.
- Wear an apron.
- Protect the client with a towel to avoid any possibility of the product getting onto their clothes.
- Make sure your working area is protected as the wax can be messy.
- Never apply paraffin wax directly over towels as any spillage will mark them.

ACTIVITY

Write down a list of different skin types and conditions. Next to each skin type and condition write down which mask would be the most beneficial for that skin type or condition from the selection that you have in your salon. Check your answers with you tutor.

Applying paraffin wax

As with the other mask treatments, paraffin wax is applied after the cuticle work and before the massage.

Place your heater on a stable trolley and position it close to the treatment area.

It might be your salon's policy to place a small amount into a working bowl. If this is the case, make sure the bowl is covered with cling film so that you can lift the wax out easily.

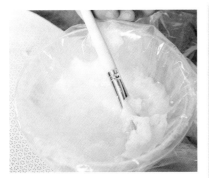

STEP 1 – Remove some paraffin wax and place it carefully into the bowl.

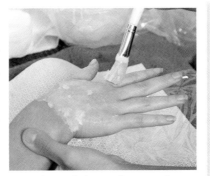

STEP 2 – Apply the paraffin wax to the treatment area using a large brush.

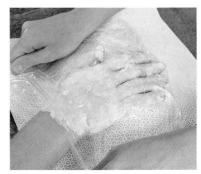

STEP 3 – Brush slowly and firmly building up the wax on the skin. Avoid flicking the brush as you must keep control of the wax.

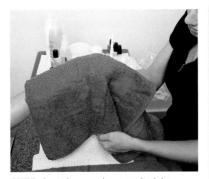

STEP 4 – When you have applied the paraffin wax, cover the hands or feet with cling film and wrap them in a towel to retain the warmth. Leave the paraffin wax on the skin for 10–20 minutes.

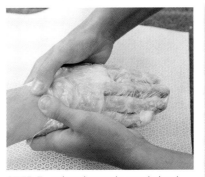

STEP 5 – When the wax has cooled and hardened it is ready to be removed. It should lift off the skin easily like removing a glove. Make sure you remove all the wax.

INDUSTRY TIP

It is advisable to offer paraffin wax as a separate conditioning treatment to avoid having to apply nail polish. The paraffin wax leaves a residue that needs to be removed thoroughly before applying polish as it can cause the nail polish to peel.

INDUSTRY TIP

Try to make the edges of the paraffin wax application slightly thicker as this will help with the removal and will prevent little bits of wax being left behind.

Dispose of the paraffin wax that has been removed from the skin in a bin. Any wax left in the bowl should be lifted out or wiped out with a piece of tissue.

Thermal mittens and booties

Thermal mittens and booties are often used in salons as part of a deluxe manicure or pedicure. They can be used with hydrating and cleansing masks and nourishing creams or oils. The heat from the mittens and booties warms the mask or cream and helps to increase the circulation, open the pores, soften the skin and aid penetration of the product into the skin. The gentle warmth is also a very relaxing experience for the client.

Benefits of thermal mittens/booties

Thermal mittens/booties:

- soothe painful or aching joints
- increase hydration of the moisturising product to soften the skin and cuticles
- improve circulation.

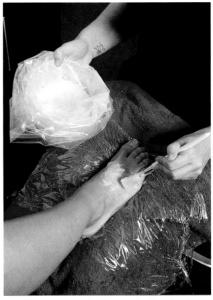

Paraffin wax can also be applied to the feet in the same way as the hands

INDUSTRY TIP

Never put paraffin wax down the sink as it will block the pipes when it sets.

427

Using thermal mittens/booties

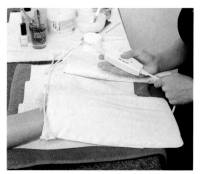

STEP 1 – Turn the mittens or booties on before use so that they warm up.

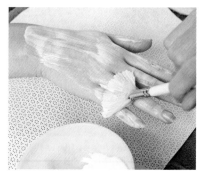

STEP 2 – For the maximum moisturising effect, apply hand or foot cream or a mask to the skin before placing the hands or feet into the thermal equipment. You can also use a moisturising, hydrating mask.

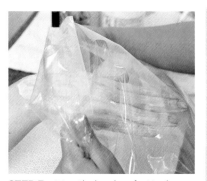

STEP 3 – Wrap the hands or feet in cling film to protect the insides of the thermal equipment and for hygiene reasons.

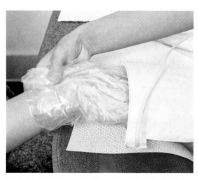

STEP 4 – Place the hands or feet inside the mittens or booties.

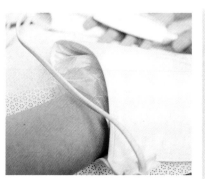

STEP 5 – Leave for the desired length of time to allow the heat to penetrate and heat the area. This is usually for 5–10 minutes.

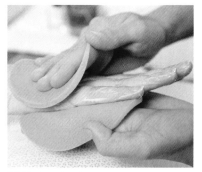

STEP 6 – After the correct time, remove any product (hand or foot cream or treatment mask) using warm water and a cloth or hot mittens.

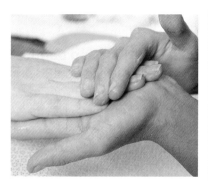

STEP 7 – Alternatively, if you have used a hydrating or moisturising mask you can massage it into the skin until it is fully absorbed.

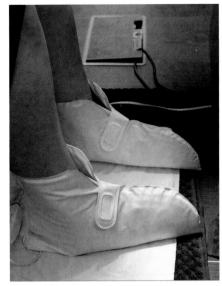

Thermal booties

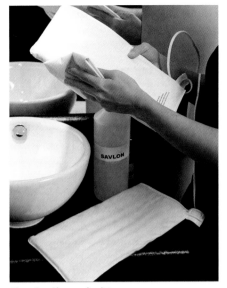

Cleaning thermal mittens

Storing thermal mittens/booties safely and hygienically

Always disconnect the mittens or booties from the mains electricity supply before cleaning.

To clean the surface, wipe over with a warm soapy cloth.

Spray the insides with a disinfectant spray when they have been wiped over.

Never place into water or soak them with water – this will damage the heating elements inside the gloves.

NAIL PAINTING

If the client has chosen to have their nails painted at the end of the treatment, you should make sure you leave plenty of time to apply the polish professionally. This is the part of the treatment where clients will have the greatest **expectations** so it is important to get it right. If nail polish has been applied well and allowed to dry, it should last between 10 and 14 days. It is suggested that you time your manicure and pedicure so that you give yourself enough time to apply a perfect finish.

It is important that when you apply nail polish that you follow a **sequence**. This is to avoid smudging or touching the nails that you have already polished. The same sequence applies to both the hands and the feet.

The finished polish application should come as close to the cuticle as possible but without any polish ending up on the skin. If the polish is too far from the cuticle, it will look like a growth line (ie the polish is old and has been applied a while ago). The whole nail plate should be covered so make sure you roll the finger or toe from side to side so that you can visually check the polish application. The finish should be a smooth, even, solid colour.

Expectation

A strong belief that something will happen.

Sequence

A particular order that you follow.

> **INDUSTRY TIP**
>
> Wearing nail polish without a break will cause discolouration of the nail plate making it look yellow. This can be limited by using a base coat. The discolouration is the result of the nail plate drying out and the keratin proteins on the surface of the nail plate becoming slightly rough. Using an abrasive buffer can help to smooth this and lift the colour. Encourage clients to apply products to condition the nail plate, even if they are wearing nail polish, as they will feed the new nail being formed.

> **INDUSTRY TIP**
>
> Clients often say they are leaving their nails to 'breathe' and are having a break from nail polish. The nail plate is dead and does not breathe. Using a product to continue to condition the nail can be beneficial.

Nail painting techniques
1 Solid colour

207/208 PROVIDE MANICURE/PEDICURE TREATMENTS

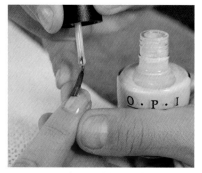

STEP 1 – Apply a single layer of base coat to each nail plate using three strokes.

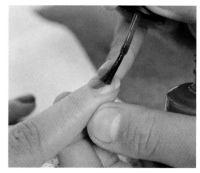

STEP 2 – Apply the first stoke down the centre of the nail from the cuticle to the tip.

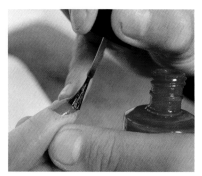

STEP 3 – Apply the second stroke. Curve around the cuticle and down the side of the nail plate.

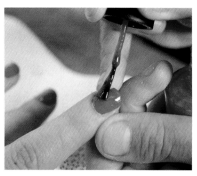

STEP 4 – Apply the third stroke down the other side of the nail plate and apply the second coat of nail polish and the top coat in the same way.

2 French polish

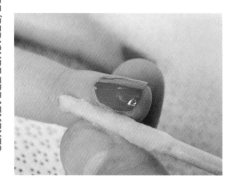

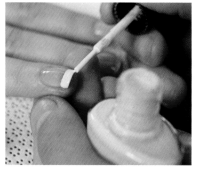

STEP 1 – Using a sweeping action, apply the colour across the top of the nail following the hyponychium line.

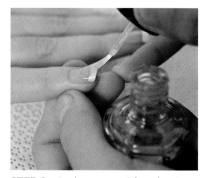

STEP 2 – Apply a cream, pink or clear top coat to create a French polish look, and complete with a top coat.

ACTIVITY

Apply ten different colours to ten different hands. Make sure you use a range of different colours and finishes from pale to dark and from cream finishes to frosted finishes. Record each colour you have used. Which colours and finishes did you find easier to apply? Write down three reasons why. Which colours and finishes did you find hardest to apply? Again, write down three reasons why.

French manicure

There are different ways of applying polish for a French manicure. The different techniques give a slightly different finish. The base colour can be applied first and then the white tip. This creates a more defined white free edge.

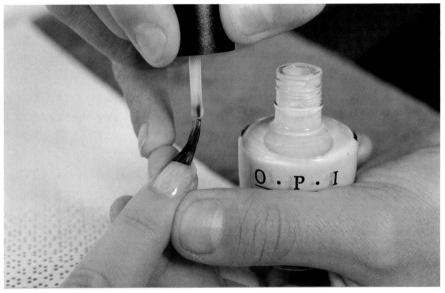

Applying French colour

Alternatively the white tip can be applied first. Some nail technicians like this as they can use a small brush to smooth along the smile line to get a crisp finish. The main colour is then applied over the whole nail plate. This gives a softer finish to the free edge.

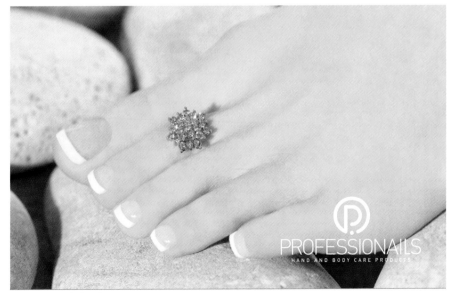

Classic French finish

COMPLETING THE MANICURE AND PEDICURE TREATMENT

When you have applied your final products, make sure you ask the client to check that they are happy with your work. If they are not satisfied, it gives you the opportunity to make any corrections before they leave. Now is a good time to give your client their personalised aftercare advice. Advise the client that they should wait about 10 minutes for their nails to dry for before they leave. It is a good idea to offer the client a drink while they are waiting. If the client has had a pedicure, you should help them put their shoes on (hopefully open-toed sandals or flip flops) when they are ready to leave.

COMPLETING THE CLIENT'S RECORDS

Now that you have finished the treatment, make a note of what you have done during the manicure or pedicure. Record details of any products you have used, especially the nail polish you have applied. Make a note of any products you have recommended and note any reactions the client had during treatment, particularly if they were adverse. When the information on the card is complete, file the card away. Always maintain confidentiality and privacy – never leave record cards lying around in the salon for other clients to see.

TIDYING YOUR WORK AREA – GOOD PRACTICE

Tidy your work area and leave the area ready for the next treatment. Make sure you place lids back on any pots securely. Dispose of rubbish carefully into the bin. Wipe any tools over with surgical spirit or a disinfectant spray to remove any debris and grease. Wash up your manicure bowl or pedicure bowl and put towels into the laundry area ready to be washed. If you are working in a larger salon, it is important to help the colleagues in your team and not expect others to clear up after you.

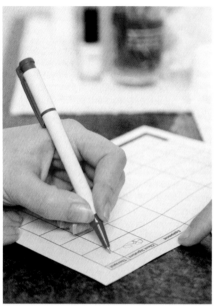

Completing a record card

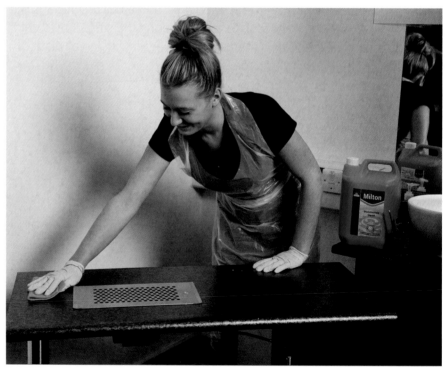

Therapist cleaning the work area

AFTERCARE AND HOME CARE ADVICE

AFTERCARE ADVICE

Following a manicure and pedicure you should give the client suitable aftercare advice to continue the treatment at home. This will help to maximise the benefits the client will get from the treatment.

Advice	Benefit
Drying time	<ul><li>Nail varnish might be touch dry in 20 minutes but will take about 2 hours to dry completely.</li><li>Clients should be advised to treat their nails carefully during this time to avoid any damage to the nail polish.</li></ul>
Regular treatments	<ul><li>Advise your client to have regular manicures or pedicures to maximise the results. Regular treatments will:<ul><li>help to maintain nail growth and keep the nails' free edges evenly shaped</li><li>keep the cuticles softened and in place</li><li>keep the nail polish immaculate</li><li>soften and condition the skin.</li></ul></li></ul>
When to book their next treatment	<ul><li>Manicure: it is that recommended clients have a manicure once every 2 weeks to maintain their nail shape and nail polish.</li><li>Pedicure: it is recommended that clients have a pedicure every 3–4 weeks to keep their nails tidy, keep the polish looking good and avoid any visible regrowth. It will also help to manage the build-up of hard skin.</li><li>It might be appropriate for the client to have a course of manicures or pedicures to help improve a particular problem, such as hard skin on their feet or overgrown dry cuticles. These courses can be offered at a special price as an **incentive** to encourage the client to come back.</li></ul>
Lifestyle changes	<ul><li>Where appropriate, discuss any lifestyle changes that the client could make to improve their hands and feet.</li><li>Be tactful and discuss only issues that have been raised to avoid offending the client.</li><li>You will need to explain the benefits of any suggestions you make so that the client understands why you are recommending the changes.</li></ul>

Incentive
A reason that encourages you to do something.

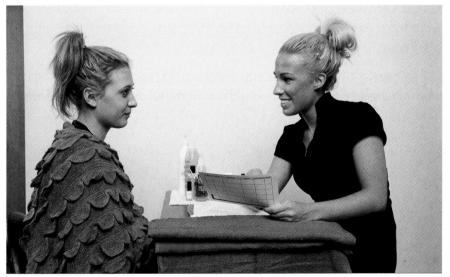

Therapist giving a client aftercare advice

Advice	Benefit
Following a home care routine	■ Suggest that your client follows a maintenance routine at home, ideally using products that you have recommended, such as cuticle oil, hand cream or foot spray, to maintain the treatment results.
Removing nail polish	■ Recommend that the client avoids acetone-based nail polish removers as these are very dehydrating. ■ When removing polish, advise the client to put a little nail polish remover onto a cotton pad and hold it on the nail for a few seconds until the polish dissolves and can be easily wiped from the nail plate.
Treating nails with care	■ Remind clients not to treat their fingernails as tools, for example using their nails to open a can of fizzy drink, as this will damage them.
Protecting the hands	■ Remind clients to wear suitable gloves when working with chemicals, cleaning products or gardening. ■ Rubber gloves can be quite drying as they make the hands sweat. Over long periods of time or if the hands are also in hot water, rubber gloves can be quite dehydrating. Make sure the client is aware of this and encourage them to moisturise regularly. ■ Protective cotton gloves might be more appropriate for some tasks, such as dusting.
Filing the nails	■ When filing the nails, advise your clients to file in one direction only and not to use a sawing action. ■ Advise them to use emery boards and avoid metal files as these can create friction and heat causing the nail to flake.
Cutting toenails	■ Advise your clients to cut toenails straight across to avoid ingrown nails.

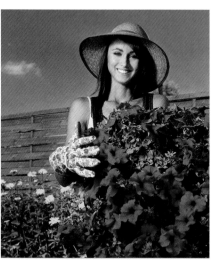

Gloves will protect hands

ACTIVITY

Write a list of all the times you have used yours nails as a tools. What could you have used instead to have prevented damaging your nails?

CONTRA-ACTIONS

A contra-action is an adverse reaction that can happen during or after treatments.

The following table lists the contra-actions that might occur during or after a manicure or pedicure and the action that should be taken if they do.

Contra-action	Cause	Action to take or recommend
Severe erythema	▪ This might be due to overstimulation of the skin (eg as a result of an overstimulating massage) or excessive use of an exfoliant. ▪ It could also be a sign that the skin is reacting to a product.	▪ Review what you are doing. If you are carrying out a massage, are you using appropriate techniques? ▪ If the skin feels warm, the client might be having an adverse reaction so you need to remove the product you are using with lukewarm water and apply a cold compress to the skin to reduce the circulation.
Allergic reaction to a product	▪ The client might suffer an allergic reaction to a product that has been applied to the skin.	▪ The skin will feel hot and the client will feel irritation, tingling or itching so you need to stop the treatment, remove the product completely with lukewarm water and apply a cold compress. Refer the client to a medical practitioner if the irritation does not subside. ▪ Sometimes this reaction can be delayed and it might occur when the client has returned home. In this case advise the client to bathe the skin with lukewarm water and apply a cool compress. They should seek advice from a medical practitioner or a pharmacist.
Tissue damage resulting in blood loss	▪ This can only happen as a result of poor practice. ▪ It can be the result of scratching the client with long or poorly manicured nails. ▪ It can also be the result of using products or tools in an inappropriate way that cause damage to the skin (eg nipping too much cuticle away with cuticles nippers or using sharp (poor quality) emery boards that catch the underside of the nail creating a cut similar to a paper cut).	▪ The area should be cleaned with an antiseptic solution. Advise the client that the skin has been broken and that they should take care.

TEST YOUR KNOWLEDGE

Use the questions below to test your knowledge of Chapter 207/208 to see how much information you have remembered. These questions will help you to revise what you have learnt in this chapter.

Turn to page 601 for the answers.

1. Which **one** of the following is the best method for cleaning the surface of thermal booties?
   a) Wipe them with surgical spirit
   b) Wipe them with a warm, soapy cloth
   c) Wipe them with bleach
   d) Spray them with antibacterial foot spray

2. What is the best method for sterilising a cuticle knife?
   a) In an autoclave
   b) Using chemical sterilising solutions
   c) In a UV cabinet
   d) Using surgical spirit

3. When filing a nail, at what angle should the emery board be to the free edge?
   a) 25°
   b) 35°
   c) 45°
   d) 55°

4. In what position should you hold a cuticle knife when removing cuticle from the nail plate?
   a) Flat to the nail plate
   b) Vertical to the nail plate
   c) At a 45°angle to the nail plate
   d) At a 35° angle to the nail plate

5. Which **one** of the following is the main benefit of using a base coat?
   a) It provides a protective layer
   b) It provides a smooth surface
   c) It gives a sheen to the nail polish
   d) It seals and protects the nail polish

6. Which **one** of the following is the main benefit of using a top coat?
   a) It provides a smooth surface
   b) It prevents discolouration
   c) It seals and protects the nail polish
   d) It acts as an adhesive agent

7. Overgrown thickened skin on the heels of the feet is referred to as:
   a) a callus
   b) a corn
   c) hyper-keratosis
   d) onychorrexis.

8. Which **one** of the following contra-indications would restrict a pedicure?
   a) Onychocryptosis
   b) Leuconychia
   c) Onychophagy
   d) Pterygium

9. Which **one** of the following is a benefit of using a paraffin wax treatment?
   a) It stimulates nail growth
   b) It stimulates the skin
   c) It cleanses deeply
   d) It softens the cuticles and the skin

10. What does cuticle remover do?
    a) It lifts and dissolves dead cuticle
    b) It softens and nourishes the cuticle
    c) It hydrates the nail plate
    d) It conditions the nail plate and nail wall

11. What is the name of the common active ingredient in cuticle remover?
    a) Potassium hydroxide
    b) Ethyl acetate
    c) Sodium hydroxide
    d) Butyl acetate

12. What should cuticle nippers be used for?
    a) Removing loose dead skin
    b) Shaping the cuticle
    c) Cutting untidy cuticle
    d) Neatening the cuticle area

13. Which **one** of the following is the main cause of yellowing of the nail plate?
    a) Continuous use of nail polish without a break
    b) Wearing nail polish without a base coat
    c) Wearing nail polish without a top coat
    d) Dryness and dehydration

14. Which **one** of the following is the main cause of white spots on the nail plate?
    a) Trauma
    b) Stress
    c) Diet
    d) Illness

15. Which **one** of the following reasons is the most important reason for checking the hands and feet prior to treatment?
    a) To check for contra-indications
    b) To check the condition of the skin
    c) To check the condition of the nail
    d) To formulate a treatment plan

Having enjoyed a successful career as a fitness instructor, I made the decision to incorporate beauty therapy into the fitness centre I owned and I caught the 'beauty bug'. Consequently, my next business venture was a hair, nail and beauty salon and all things nails became my passion. I quickly progressed into teaching at a local college and after 6 years of combining salon life and teaching I decided to sell up and become a full-time educator.

I thoroughly enjoy sharing the vast knowledge and expertise I continue to gain from working in this amazing industry. I have sat on an expert working panel at Habia to review and develop the new occupational standards for nail services. I work as a freelance Internal Quality Assurer and a Moderator for City & Guilds. I have written material for candidate logbooks. I have recently written a column in *Scratch* magazine.

My working life is varied, great fun and challenging. Nothing has given me more pleasure than teaching and performing manicures, pedicures and nail enhancements. Would you like to catch the 'beauty bug' and work with amazing people every single day?

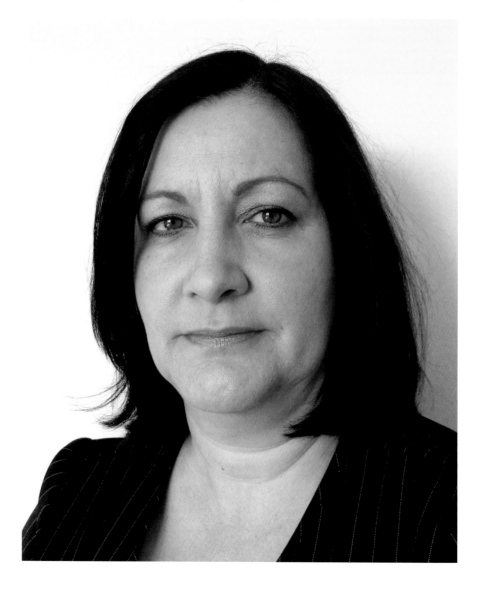

PROVIDE AND MAINTAIN NAIL ENHANCEMENT

This chapter is all about working with different nail systems to provide nail enhancement. Nail enhancement is a very competitive industry which is continually growing. You will learn about each of the different nail systems – UV gels, wraps and liquid and powder. You will gain understanding of the reasons why someone might want nail enhancements – for example, for a special occasion (a wedding or a party), a holiday or just to improve their own natural nails.

This chapter also covers how to maintain and repair nail enhancements professionally and how to remove them safely. Health and safety regulations are very important in the nail enhancement industry and it is important that you follow them. You will also acquire an understanding of how to behave in a professional manner throughout the service.

In this chapter you will learn how to:
- prepare for nail enhancement services
- provide nail enhancement services.

PREPARE FOR NAIL ENHANCEMENT SERVICES

Before you can apply nail enhancements, it is important to be prepared. You must follow health and safety requirements for every service. Knowing how to set up your service area, which products and tools you should use and how to carry out an effective consultation are essential for nail enhancements.

In this part of the chapter you will learn about:

- health and safety
- consultation for nail enhancement services
- the products required to carry out a nail enhancement service
- the tools and equipment required to carry out a nail enhancement service
- preparing your work area for a nail enhancement service.

HEALTH AND SAFETY

It is very important to **adhere to** all health and safety regulations when you are performing a nail enhancement service.

The main legislation affecting nail enhancement services is:

- Personal Protective Equipment (PPE) at Work Regulations
- Health and Safety at Work Act (HASAWA)
- Control of Substances Hazardous to Health (COSHH)
- Data Protection Act.

METHODS OF STERILISATION AND SANITISATION

You must sterilise tools and equipment prior to carrying out the service to ensure maximum health and safety and to stop **cross-contamination**. Use disposable tools where possible.

Prior to your client arriving for their service, sterilise the work surface. Isopropyl alcohol is a good sanitising agent. To kill off all micro-organisms, the metal tools you are using should have been sterilised in an **autoclave** and then placed in **Barbicide.**

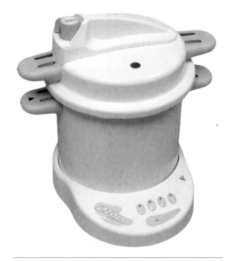

An autoclave

Adhere to

To have to follow.

HANDY HINTS

Look back at the Legislation chapter (pages 91–113) to refresh your memory on the relevant legislation.

 SmartScreen 201 Worksheet 3

 SmartScreen 202 Worksheet 6

Cross-contamination

Transfer of micro-organisms from one place to another, or from one person to another.

Autoclave

A machine that uses high-pressured steam to kill all micro-organisms. It is used to sterilise small metal tools.

Barbicide

A blue translucent liquid that is used to sanitise tools used for treatments.

HANDY HINTS

Look at Chapter 202 (pages 141–164) for more information on sterilisation and sanitisation.

INDUSTRY TIP

Throughout the service, make sure that you keep the lids on all products to prevent contamination.

Sterilisation is the process of destroying all micro-organisms and their spores. Sanitisation prevents bacteria from growing but does not destroy all micro-organisms.

When your client has arrived and prior to consultation, make sure they see you washing your hands. This will give the client confidence that you take health and safety very seriously.

THE NAIL SERVICE ENVIRONMENT

The salon environment is very important in making the client feel relaxed and comfortable throughout the service. You will need to think about the following factors.

Privacy

Although nail enhancements can be performed within the reception area, where clients are waiting or walking in to book an appointment, it can also be performed in a treatment room where your clients have more privacy.

Lighting

It is very important to have good lighting when you are applying nail enhancements. In addition to making sure that the room is well lit, it is a good idea to put a lamp on your workstation to give you a little bit of extra light for carrying out detailed filing work or during the application of enhancement products (which need precision). Make sure the wattage of the bulb is not too high – anything over 40 watts could interfere with the consistency of the products.

Heating

It is important to make sure that the room is warm for the client so they feel comfortable throughout their service. Make sure it is not too hot, as this could affect the consistency of the products you are using.

Ventilation

In the room in which you are carrying out nail enhancement services, you will need a ventilation system – an extractor fan or an open window – to remove dust, vapours and fumes that could lead to respiratory problems. Mobile nail technicians carrying out nail enhancement services will need to have a filter on their mobile workstation.

Music

Clients come into the salon to relax so some relaxing music playing in the background will help to create a calm and relaxing environment. However, always be aware of the volume of the music being played; it should be a background noise that allows your client to relax.

Health and safety

Hazards and risks could cause injuries. Make a quick check of your working area for hazards and either remove these, or reduce any risks that might cause hazards. Health and safety should be monitored constantly.

Refer to Chapter 202 (pages 141–164) for information on how to dispose of contaminated waste.

INDUSTRY TIP

If you have any highly flammable products that you have finished with, make sure you place them back in the locked COSHH cupboard.

INDUSTRY TIP

It is a good idea to contact the local authority and Habia (who write the National Occupational Standards) to see what their recommendations are for good ventilation.

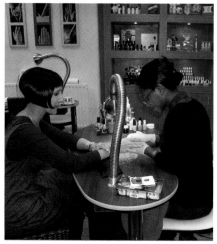
Good posture

POSITIONING THE CLIENT AND THE NAIL TECHNICIAN

It is very important to position yourself and your client correctly throughout the service. You are sat down for some time which could cause back pain to yourself and your client. Make sure when you are sat on a chair that you have both feet on the ground and that you are facing your client – this will eliminate any stress on your back. Tell your client that they can get up and move around if they need to.

CONSULTATION FOR NAIL ENHANCEMENT SERVICES

Before you carry out a nail enhancement service, you will need to have a consultation with your client as it is very important the client understands the service they are having and that they are sure it is the right service for them. There are three different systems used in nail enhancement and they suit different clients so it is essential when a client is booking their service to make sure they are aware of the different systems that are available.

Communication techniques are very important in ensuring an effective consultation. For more in-depth information, refer back to Chapter 203. The most important communication techniques used are:

- speaking
- listening
- body language
- reading
- recording information/writing
- following instructions
- using a range of related terminology.

 SmartScreen 203 Worksheet 1

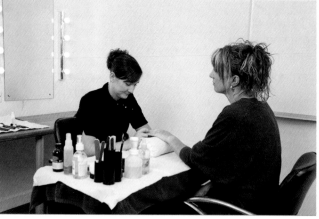
Nail technician/therapist looking at the client's skin and nails checking for contra-indications

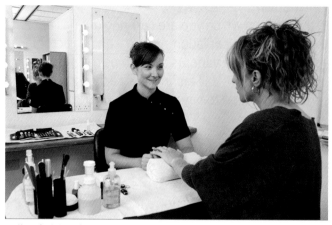
Nail technician/therapist asking the client questions to gain all the relevant information to carry out the treatment

CARRYING OUT THE CONSULTATION

The consultation stage is very important; this is where you gain all the information from your client to be able to give them the best service you have to offer. To carry out a professional consultation using the correct techniques, refer back to Chapter 203 where consultation is covered in more detail.

The most common consultation techniques used for gathering information include:

Verbal techniques – questioning and the use of language and tone of voice. Make sure that your questioning techniques are clear and understandable and talk in a calm, soft voice that is not too loud. Be aware that your clients will not always understand the technical terms, so always explain the service in terms they will understand and allow them to ask questions.

Non-verbal techniques – listening, **interpretation** of body language and facial expressions and the use of eye contact. These are all very important as you will be expressing yourself without words. Body language can be interpreted in many ways, such as the way you present yourself through your posture. Make sure you are sat upright and do not slouch. Make sure you are always smiling and keep good eye contact with your client.

Visual aids – the use of visual aids so that clients can see the finished results.

Reference to client records – it is important to record all of your client's details onto a record card. You need to record their telephone number in case you have to contact them and their address details so you can send them any special offers. In addition, you need to document the services they have had and the products used so that for future treatments you can make sure your workstation is prepared prior to the client arriving.

Below is a checklist of questions that you will need to ask your client during the consultation in order to gain all the information you need to advise them on the right nail enhancement system.

Interpretation
Your understanding.

INDUSTRY TIP
Information about clients should be kept in a locked cabinet where only the receptionist or therapist/nail technician can have access to it.

Questions	Tick
What are your main objectives from today's service?	
Have you previously had nail enhancements? If so which system did you have?	
What is your occupation?	
(This will help you determine which system to use – for example, if your client is a hairdresser who has their hands in water a lot, you would recommend the UV gel system as it is water resistant.)	
How long do you want nail enhancements for?	
Will you require regular infills and maintenance? (If the client wants to keep their nail enhancements on for some time, they can return to you to have them maintained.)	

INDUSTRY TIP
Do not forget to ask your client if they have any leisure interests or past-times that might affect the system you are going to apply.

Now you have determined the system that is best suited to your client, you will need to continue with the consultation to:

- gather further information on their nail shape
- find out if there are any possible contra-indications to treatment.

WHY DON'T YOU...
design your own consultation form as part of your evidence for your portfolio.

INDUSTRY TIP

Always make sure your client signs the consultation form before you carry out the service to safeguard yourself and the salon.

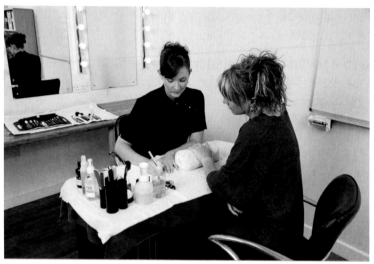

Checking and documenting any contra-indications present

INDUSTRY TIP

You will find that your clients shape their nails themselves at home to complement their own hand shape and will ask for longer artificial nails to enhance this shape further. It might be that the shape they have chosen is not the best shape and so, as a nail technician, you need to advise the client about which shape would be more beneficial and complementary.

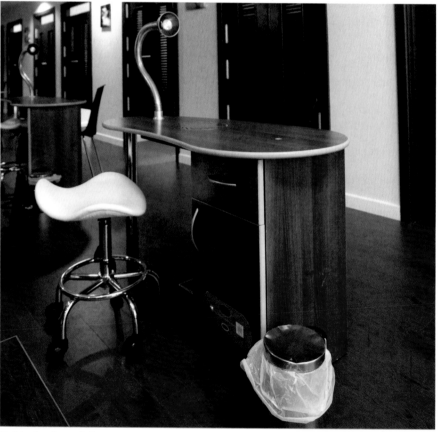

Nail technology station

Nail shapes

You need to determine your client's nail shape so that you can use the correct tip application. The main shapes you will come across are:

HANDY HINTS

Look at the Anatomy and Physiology chapter to remind yourself about the structure and function of the nails and surrounding skin.

Nail shape	Nail shape correction needed before tip can be applied
Oval	No correction needed.
Tapered	File the nails at the sides to create an oval/squoval shape for better tip application.
Square	File the corners so that they are slightly rounded.
Squoval	No correction needed.
Claw	File the nails down until they are level with the fingertip to give the nail plate a more suitable structure that allows the artificial tip to fit snugly.
Fan	File the nails at the sides to create an oval/squoval shape for better tip application.
Pointed	File the nails at the top to create an oval/squoval shape for better tip application.

Selecting the right nail enhancement system based on the client's needs

When deciding which nail enhancement system to use on your client, you need to think about what would be best for them by asking them all the relevant questions. You need to consider their:

Lifestyle – What do they do in their free time? Do they like gardening? Do they go swimming a lot? If so, suggest the UV gel system.

Occupation – What kind of job do they do? This could affect the nail enhancement system you decide to apply. If they have a manual job then acrylic would be best as it is the strongest system. Are they are allowed to wear nail polish at work?

The reason for having enhancements – Are the enhancements for a specific occasion? If so, then suggest the wrap system as it is easier to remove and causes less stress on the natural nail.

Contra-indications

During the consultation, you must ask your client if they suffer from any contra-indications that could **prevent** you from continuing with the service or **restrict** the service. You will need to look back to Chapter 207/208 Provide manicure/pedicure treatments to make sure you are familiar with the following contra-indications to nail treatments:

Prevent treatment: onychia, onychatrophia (atrophy), onychoptosis, fungal infections, bacterial infections, viral infections, infestations, severe nail separation, severe eczema, severe psoriasis and severe skin conditions.

Restrict treatment: onychogryphosis, onychauxis (hypertrophy), onychomalacia (eggshell nails), broken bones in the area being treated, recent fractures and sprains, recent scar tissue, hyper-keratosis, skin allergies, cuts and abrasions, varicose veins, epilepsy, **diabetes**, skin disorders, undiagnosed lumps and swellings, product allergies and phlebitis.

Nail conditions

Nail conditions can *prevent* and *restrict* you from performing a nail enhancement service, depending on the severity of the condition. During the consultation, you should look out for different types of nail conditions. Please refer to Chapter 207/208 Provide manicure/pedicure treatments for more details.

There will be a section on your consultation form that asks about the condition of the hands and nails. Make sure you fill this in with as much information as you can.

PRODUCTS REQUIRED TO CARRY OUT A NAIL ENHANCEMENT SERVICE

When you have completed the consultation with your client, you will need to select the best system to use and, therefore, the right products, tools and equipment. There are a lot of product ranges within the industry and it is best to try a few and find one that suits you and your clientele. Try to avoid mixing products from different manufacturers as some products can react chemically with others.

HANDY HINTS

Refer to the Anatomy and Physiology chapter for more information on contra-indications.

Prevent

To stop you from doing something (ie carrying out the service).

Restrict

To limit what you can do (ie working around the affected area and adapting the service if necessary).

Diabetes

A disease that prevents sufferers from breaking down glucose in their blood cells.

INDUSTRY TIP

An infection that to most people is small could be very serious to a person who is diabetic.

INDUSTRY TIP

If your client does suffer an allergic reaction during the service, apply a cold compress and stop the service. If the symptoms persist, seek medical attention.

HANDY HINTS

Refer back to the Anatomy and Physiology chapter for full descriptions of these skin conditions.

- **Pterygium**
- **Onychopaghy**
- weak nails
- dry nails
- brittle nails
- split nails
- hangnails
- longitudinal or horizontal ridges.

Pterygium

A nail condition where the cuticle is thick and overgrown.

Onychopaghy

Bitten nails.

Listed below are the products you will need for all three of the systems we will be looking at in this chapter.

Product	Description
	Sanitisers: these are used to **sanitise** your hands and your client's hands throughout the service.
	Polish remover: when you are using a polish remover, be sure that it is an **acetone-free** product as this will be kinder on the nail enhancement.
	Nail cleansers/sanitisers: these are used to sanitise the natural nail plate prior to the application of enhancements.
	Nail dehydrators: these will **dehydrate** the nail plate and remove any oils or moisture. The overlay will not adhere to the nail plate if there is any oil or moisture present.
	Primer: the primer allows the product to adhere to the natural nail plate.
	Adhesives: these are used to glue the tips to the natural nail plate.

Sanitise

To prevent the growth of micro-organisms.

Acetone free

A product that does not contain the harsh chemical acetone.

Dehydrate

The removal of moisture and oil from the natural nail plate.

INDUSTRY TIP

If the cuticles are overgrown, suggest to your client that they have a mini-manicure – ie their nails are filed and their cuticles are pushed back – prior to their nail enhancement service, as this condition can cause premature lifting of nail enhancements.

INDUSTRY TIP

You cannot perform a full manicure on the same day as the nail enhancement service since the products you will be using within the manicure will act as a barrier and stop the tips from adhering to the nail plate. Adapt the manicure for the client.

Monomer

A product that creates a chemical reaction when mixed with the powder to create an acrylic nail enhancement.

Product	Description
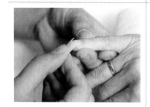	**Tips:** these are the structures you apply to the nail plate to achieve artificial length. There is a variety of tips designed to suit different natural nail shapes.
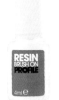	**Resin:** this is used when applying fibreglass or silk nail wraps. An activator is applied over the resin to set the product.
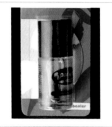	**Setting agents:** these are used to set the final look. Activators are used with resin and a sealant/gloss is used with UV gel and acrylic.
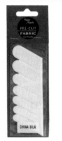	**Fibreglass/silk:** this is a mesh fabric embedded within the resin to add strength to wrap nail enhancements.
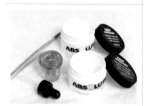	**Powders:** these are used when you are applying acrylic nail enhancements and come in a variety of different colours to complement the client's skin tone. Liquid **monomer** and powder are mixed together to create the nail enhancement.
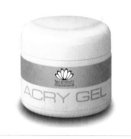	**UV gels:** these are used when applying UV gel enhancements. They come in a variety of different colours to suit your client's desired look. UV gel has to be cured and set under a UV (ultraviolet) lamp.
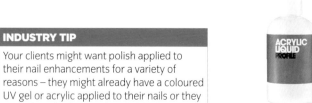	**Monomer liquid:** this is mixed with the powder used in the acrylic system to create the nail enhancement.

Product	Description
	Nail polish: polish adds colour to natural nails or enhancements. It must be removed with acetone-free polish remover.

TOOLS AND EQUIPMENT REQUIRED TO CARRY OUT A NAIL ENHANCEMENT SERVICE

Listed below are the tools and equipment you will need for the three systems we will be looking at in this chapter.

Product	Description
	Brushes: there is a variety of brushes available for the application of UV gel and acrylic. They come as either sable or synthetic brushes. Sable brushes are more commonly used for **sculpting** techniques as they keep their shape better.
	Tip cutters: these are used for cutting the artificial nail tips.
	Cuticle tools: these include cuticle nippers and a cuticle knife and are used to prepare the cuticle prior to a nail enhancement service. If your client has overgrown cuticles, suggest they have a manicure a couple of days before.
	Buffer: a buffer brings shine to the nail surface and smoothes out any ridges.
	Dappen dish: the dish used in the acrylic system to hold the monomer.
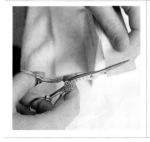	**Scissors (stalk scissors):** these scissors are used to cut fibreglass or silk to the desired size and length.

Sculpting

The use of UV gel or acrylic to build the nail without applying a nail tip.

Grit
The coarseness of the file.

Product	Description
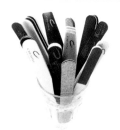	**Files:** there is a variety of files you can use when you apply nail enhancements. They all have a different **grit**. The higher the number of the grit, the finer the file. The lower the number of the grit, the coarser the file. The following files are available: ■ 400–900 grit – normally used in block buffers that are designed to smooth the surface ■ 360 grit – used as a natural nail file ■ 240 grit – this is the lowest grit that you should use on a natural nail ■ 180 grit – used for removing length, shaping artificial nails, removing overlays and blending tips ■ 100 grit – a course file used for removing overlays and overlay bulk. Use them with care.
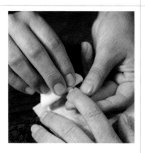	Consumables: ■ nail wipes – a square piece of lint used to remove nail polish and apply nail products (used instead of cotton wool so no fibres get caught in the artificial system) ■ nylon brush – used to remove dust from the natural nail and enhancements ■ couch roll – used to protect your workstation ■ dustbin bag – used to collect your waste ■ apron – used to protect your clothes ■ safety mask – prevents the inhalation of dust ■ tissues – used to dab excess products.
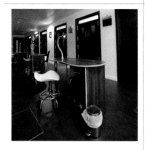	**Workstation:** most workstations for nail technicians come fitted with a filter to get rid of dust, vapour and fumes. If not, you can buy a portable filter. Always make sure you have adequate ventilation within your salon to deal with the fumes and dust from a nail enhancement service. Refer to the **manufacturer's instructions** for advice on ventilation.
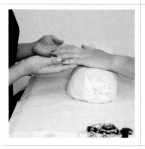	**Hand support:** this supports your client's hand and makes the service more comfortable.

Manufacturer's instructions
These should be supplied with every product. They must be adhered to for the correct application of products.

Product	Description
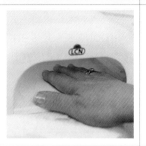	**UV lamp:** you need a UV lamp for applying UV gel nails as this cures the product. The wattage used in UV (ultraviolet) lamps varies between 36 and 45 watts – any higher and it would cause a heat reaction on the nail bed.
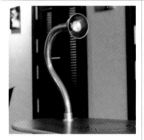	**Light:** if the lighting in your room is not sufficient then you can use a lamp to give you extra light.

INDUSTRY TIP

Your tools are your best friends so make sure you look after them with care. Clean and sterilise them after every use. If you do not look after your brushes then it will affect the end result.

WHY DON'T YOU...
create some laminated cue cards of how to set up your workstation. They will help you to remember.

PREPARING YOUR WORK AREA FOR A NAIL ENHANCEMENT SERVICE

Before you carry out the nail enhancement service, you must make sure that you have all the correct tools and equipment ready. The spider diagram below will act as a checklist to help you prepare your work area.

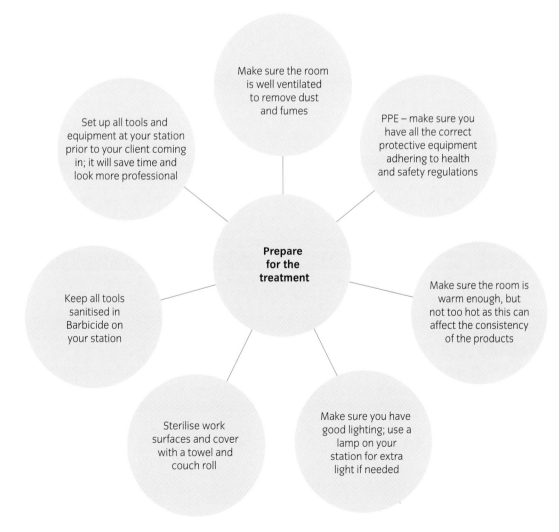

Set up all tools and equipment at your station prior to your client coming in; it will save time and look more professional

Make sure the room is well ventilated to remove dust and fumes

PPE – make sure you have all the correct protective equipment adhering to health and safety regulations

Prepare for the treatment

Keep all tools sanitised in Barbicide on your station

Make sure the room is warm enough, but not too hot as this can affect the consistency of the products

Sterilise work surfaces and cover with a towel and couch roll

Make sure you have good lighting; use a lamp on your station for extra light if needed

Now that you know about health and safety and the products, tools and equipment you will need, you are ready to carry out nail enhancement services.

In this part of the chapter you will learn about:

- applying and removing tips
- fibreglass/silk nail enhancement
- UV gel nail enhancement
- acrylic nail enhancement
- aftercare and home care advice
- contra-actions.

APPLYING AND REMOVING TIPS

SIZING NAIL TIPS

It is important to size the tips correctly. The box of tips will be numbered from 0 to 10, with 0 being the largest and 10 being the smallest. Always check though as each company might be different. The number is usually found on the lid of the box and also on the tip itself. Try to estimate the correct size to match the client's natural nail. Hold the tip at a 45° angle and press it down along the free edge to see if it fits snugly from side wall to side wall. If it does, then it is the correct size to use. If it is too big, go for the next number up and if it is too small, go for the next number down. Repeat this for each nail until you have the correct size of tip for all ten nails.

Clients' nails will not necessarily fit the artificial tips perfectly. If this is the case, go with a larger sized tip and file down the edges on each side of the tip to create the perfect size. Make a note of all the tip sizes on the client's record card for future reference.

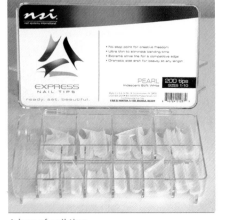

A box of nail tips

INDUSTRY TIP

The more tips you apply, the more accurate your eye will become and you will automatically know which size tip to use.

INDUSTRY TIP

If you get an air bubble, your only option is to remove the nail tip with acetone and start again.

INDUSTRY TIP

Always make sure you remove any existing products with lint-free pads rather than cotton pads so that you do not leave any loose fibres on the nail plate.

INDUSTRY TIP

A chemical tip blender can be used to dissolve the plastic tip at the seam. This helps to speed up the application and aid the blending of the tip. Brush the product along the seam of the tip and wait for it to soften. Use a 180–240 grit file to blend the tip and remove the seam.

INDUSTRY TIP

The procedures in this book show one way of applying enhancements but these might differ from the way you have been taught. Always refer to the manufacturer's instructions before carrying out nail enhancements.

APPLYING TIPS

The application of tips will be the same whichever system you are using, unless you are applying a natural nail overlay or sculpting. It is important to apply the perfect tip otherwise your final look will be ruined.

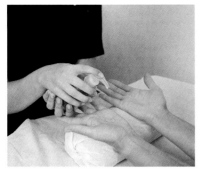

STEP 1 – Sanitise your hands and your client's hands.

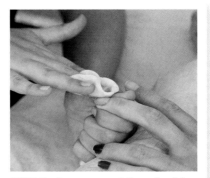

STEP 2 – Remove any existing nail polish.

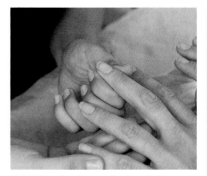

STEP 3 – Check your client's nails for contra-indications.

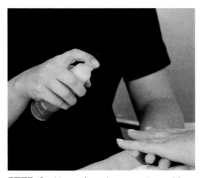

STEP 4 – Use a cleansing spray to sanitise the nail plate and to remove any **bacteria**.

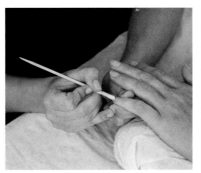

STEP 5 – Push the cuticles back using a covered orange stick.

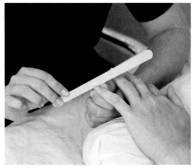

STEP 6 – File the natural nails on both hands (remembering to file in one direction only).

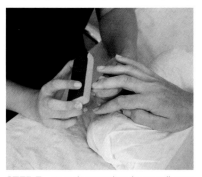

STEP 7 – To make sure that the tip adheres to the natural nail, buff away the shine using your block buffer.

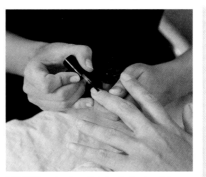

STEP 8 – Apply nail dehydrator to all ten nails.

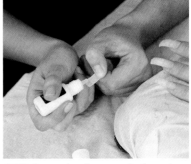

STEP 9 – Apply adhesive to the free edge of the natural nail and the contact area of the tip.

Steps 1–5 will be needed in each application technique throughout this chapter.

214 PROVIDE AND MAINTAIN NAIL ENHANCEMENT

INDUSTRY TIP

If you make a mistake and accidentally bond together any skin with glue during the procedure, get an orange stick with cotton wool on the tip and soak it in acetone before applying to the affected area. This will dissolve the glue quickly. However, you must do your best to make sure that you are applying the products correctly so that this does not happen.

Bacteria

Single-celled organisms that live on the skin's surface. Most are not harmful but others (pathogenic bacteria) are harmful and can cause skin diseases.

INDUSTRY TIP

Always check the manufacturer's guidelines before using enhancement products.

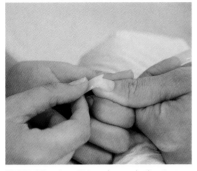

STEP 10 – At a 45° angle, apply the tip to the natural nail plate holding the edges of the tip firmly for about 10 seconds to make sure there are no air bubbles.

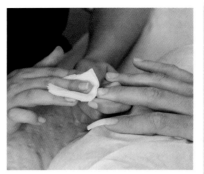

STEP 11 – Remove any excess adhesive from around the edges with a lint-free pad.

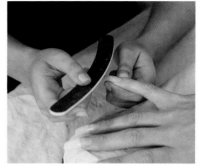

STEP 12 – With a 180–240 grit file, blend across the seam line, taking care not to damage the natural nail.

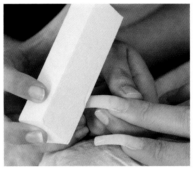

STEP 13 – When you have blended the seam, use a block buffer to remove the surface shine of the tip. This will prepare the nail so that the UV gel, fibreglass or acrylic will adhere to it better. Repeat this for all ten nails.

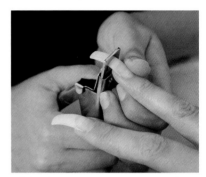

STEP 14 – Using your tip cutters, cut the tips to the desired length.

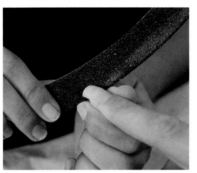

STEP 15 – Shape the tips according to your client's requirements.

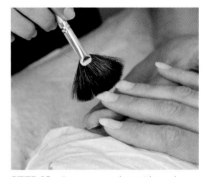

STEP 16 – Remove any dust with a nylon brush.

INDUSTRY TIP

Always advise the client to come to the salon to have nail enhancements removed professionally.

After applying the tips, you are now ready to move on to the application of your chosen nail enhancement system.

TIP REMOVAL

To remove the tips, soak each finger in acetone and buff each one with a four-way buffer to remove all the excess plastic.

FIBREGLASS/SILK NAIL ENHANCEMENT

This system is probably the oldest system on the market but it gives a very natural result. It gives a transparent finish, allowing the natural colour of the nail to show through. This system does not damage the natural nail plate as you do not have to apply a primer so it is a very good system for someone who wants to grow their natural nails. The table below outlines the advantages and disadvantages of the fibreglass system.

Advantages	Disadvantages
Quick and easy to remove	Expensive to apply
Strong	More time consuming
Flexible	
Natural looking	

PRODUCTS AND TOOLS REQUIRED

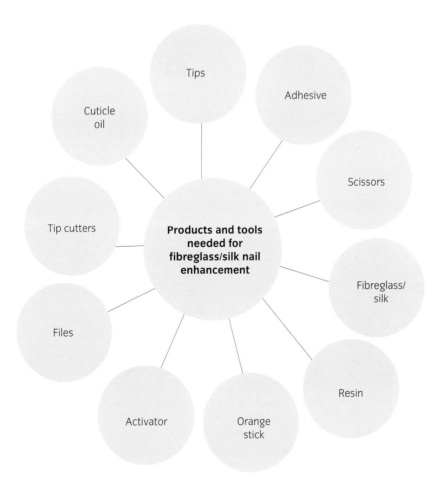

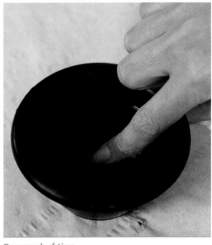

Removal of tips

APPLICATION

Approximate treatment time: 1½ hours.

First, follow steps 1–16 of the tip application routine (pages 453–454).

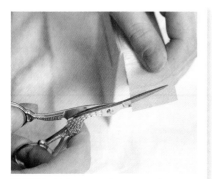

STEP 1 – Using your scissors, cut the fibreglass/silk to the width to be overlaid. Try to avoid touching the fibreglass too much. Remove the fibreglass/silk from its backing paper.

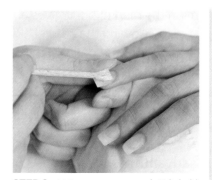

STEP 2 – Using an orange wood stick, hold the fibreglass/silk in place, place the fibreglass/silk onto the nail, making sure you do not touch the cuticle area.

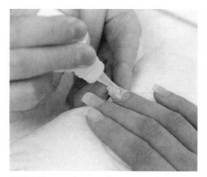

STEP 3 – Apply a small amount of resin to cover the fibreglass, making sure not to flood the nail plate.

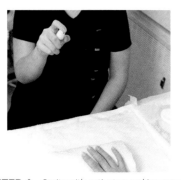

STEP 4 – Spritz with activator, making sure you do not hold it too close to the nail plate.

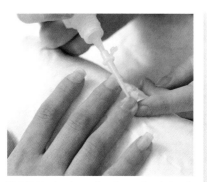

STEP 5 – Apply another layer of resin to all the fingers using the same method as before.

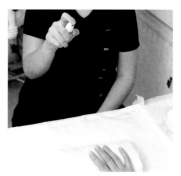

STEP 6 – Apply another layer of activator to all fingers using the same method as before.

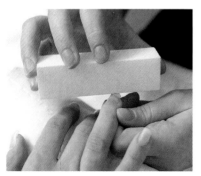

STEP 7 – Buff the surface of each finger until it is perfectly smooth.

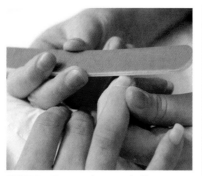

STEP 8 – Use your four-way buffer to create a flawless shine.

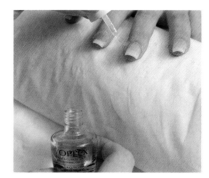

STEP 9 – Apply cuticle oil to finish.

INDUSTRY TIP

If you spray the activator too close to the hand or apply too much, the client might feel a sensation of heat. When you are spraying activator, allow a distance of 30 cm between the product and the natural nail.

OVERLAYS

In the fibreglass/silk system, an overlay is sometimes applied over the natural nail to add strength.

The process of applying an overlay is the same as the process for applying fibreglass/silk nail enhancements; you just do not apply the tips (step 1).

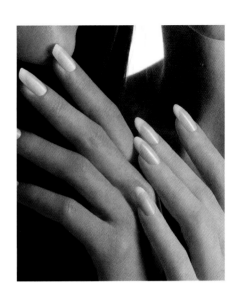

MAINTENANCE (INFILLS)

Maintenance of nail enhancements should be carried out every 2–3 weeks to keep the nails looking attractive and to prevent them from breaking or chipping.

1. Sanitise your hands and the client's hands with a spray or gel.
2. Remove any existing nail polish.
3. Check the client's nails for any contra-indications.
4. Use a cleansing spray to sanitise the nail plate to remove any bacteria.
5. Push back the cuticles using a covered orange stick.
6. Blend away any lifting with your file (be careful not to be too rough) and thin out the enhancement until there is no ridge between the product and the natural nail. There should be no visible lines left on the nail plate.
7. Buff the surface of the natural nail plate to remove the shine and use nail dehydrator to dehydrate the nail.
8. Apply a small amount of resin to the regrowth area and use the nozzle to spread it.
9. Apply a layer of activator (remembering to be 30 cm away).
10. With a fine grit file, buff the nail to create a smooth surface.
11. Using a four-way buffer, buff the nails to a shine.
12. Apply cuticle oil to finish.

REMOVING FIBREGLASS/SILK NAIL ENHANCEMENTS

1. Wash your hands and get the client to wash their hands too.
2. Remove any existing nail polish.
3. Using your tip cutters remove the free edge of the artificial nail, taking care not to cut the client's natural nail underneath.
4. With a medium grit file, file the whole surface of the nail to allow absorption of the acetone and aid removal of the artificial nail.
5. Place each hand into separate bowls filled with acetone and allow them to soak for 15–20 minutes. Make sure you do not overfill the bowl; you need enough acetone just to cover the fingertips.
6. Check the nails after 10 minutes and remove any dissolved artificial nail product with an orange stick.
7. After 20 minutes, the artificial nail should be completely dissolved. Use a white block buffer to remove any remaining product.
8. When you have removed the artificial nail product from all 10 nails, conduct a mini-manicure – remembering to apply cuticle oil to rehydrate the natural nail and cuticle area.

INDUSTRY TIP

A full set of nails should be removed at least every 3 months and a new set applied to allow the natural nail to breathe and rehydrate. During maintenance, always look out for possible bacterial or fungal nail infections.

UV GEL NAIL ENHANCEMENT

This system is widely used within the nail industry. UV gel can be used as a natural nail overlay, applied over tips and sculpted. It gives a natural-looking finish with a high-gloss shine. A variety of different colours are available to suit clients' requirements. This system is considered to be one of the easiest systems for beginners to master. The gel is set by a UV (ultraviolet) lamp. The table below outlines the advantages and disadvantages of the UV gel system.

Advantages	Disadvantages
Easy to apply	Not as strong as acrylic
Self-levelling	Outlay can be expensive because of the UV lamp
Natural looking	Best used with shorter nails as it is not as strong
Water resistant	Hard gels need to be buffed off to remove them which can be time consuming
A variety of colours is available	

Self-levelling
The product levels itself when applied to the nail plate.

INDUSTRY TIP

Most UV gels are self-levelling. Apply the gel down the centre of the nail and leave it for 30 seconds to level itself.

INDUSTRY TIP

If the client wants a polish on top of their enhancements, apply the polish, then apply a layer of sealant over the top and cure for the recommended time. This helps to prolong the polish and avoid chipping.

INDUSTRY TIP

Cure four fingers on one hand under the lamp, then the four fingers of the other hand. Cure the thumbs together.

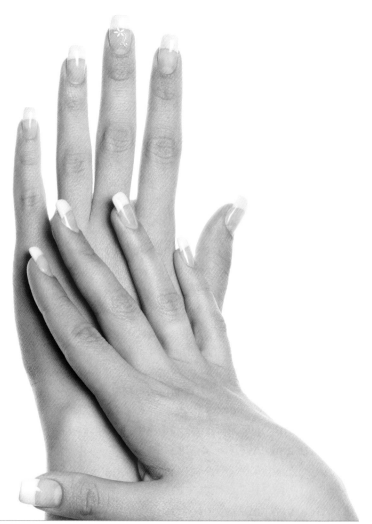

A set of nail extensions

PRODUCTS AND TOOLS REQUIRED

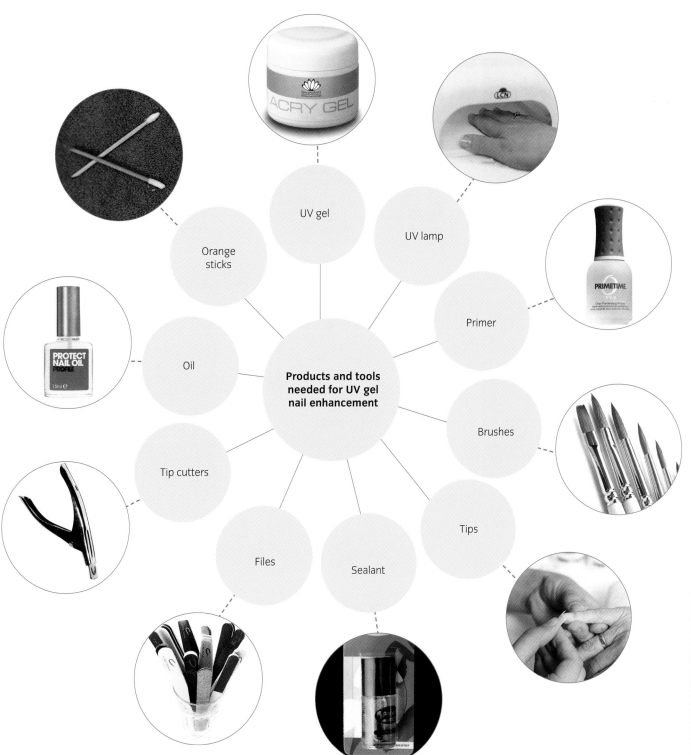

UV gel

UV lamp

Orange sticks

Primer

Oil

Products and tools needed for UV gel nail enhancement

Brushes

Tip cutters

Tips

Files

Sealant

APPLICATION

Approximate treatment time: 1½ hours.

First, follow steps 1–16 of the tip application routine (pages 453–454).

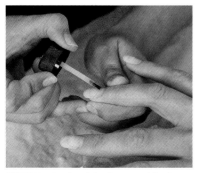

STEP 1 – Apply a dehydrator to dehydrate the nail plates on all 8 fingers.

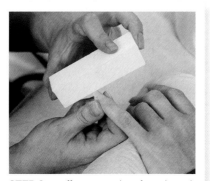

STEP 2 – Buff away any shine from the nail plate using a buffer.

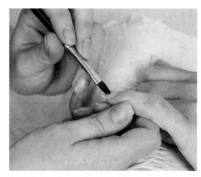

STEP 3 – Apply the UV gel primer to the natural nail plate on the fingers.

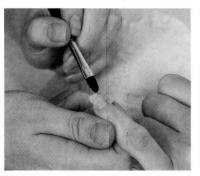

STEP 4 – Apply a layer of UV gel with the brush in accordance with the manufacturer's instructions. When you have applied the UV gel, make sure you have not flooded the cuticle and side walls.

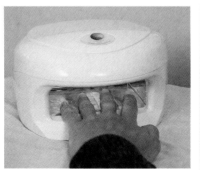

STEP 5 – Cure the UV gel by placing all fingers under the UV lamp for the recommended time stated in the manufacturer's instructions. (Gels from different manufacturers might cure for different times so always check.)

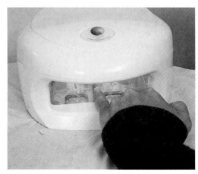

STEP 6 – Apply the gel to all the fingers but leave the thumbs for now. In between applying the gel you can **flash cure** individual fingers for 10 seconds to prevent the gel from moving.

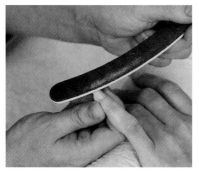

STEP 7 – When you have applied the UV gel to all 10 nails, file the enhancements with a 180-grit file to create a smooth surface. Look down the length of the fingers to make sure that you have achieved a perfect **'C' curve**.

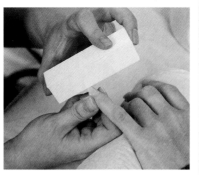

STEP 8 – Remove any dust and buff the nails to remove any scratches to the surface.

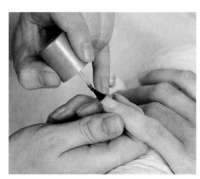

STEP 9 – Apply the sealant.

'C' curve

The natural curve of the nail from side wall to side wall. You need to look down the finger from the end to see the 'C' curve.

Flash cure

This stops the gel from moving while you apply it to the other nails. When the gel has been applied to the nail plate, flash cure it for 10 seconds to hold the gel in place.

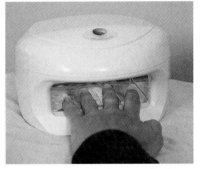

STEP 10 – Cure all the fingers under the UV lamp in line with the manufacturer's instructions.

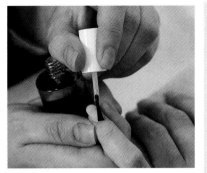

STEP 11 – Apply cuticle oil.

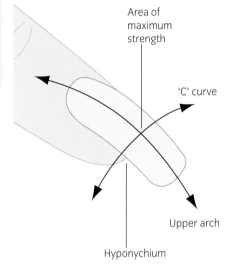

Area of maximum strength

'C' curve

Upper arch

Hyponychium

OVERLAYS

The process of applying a UV gel natural nail overlay is the same as the process for applying an enhancement but without the application of tips.

MAINTENANCE

Maintenance should be carried out every 2–3 weeks, depending on the rate of growth of the natural nail, to infill the growth area around the cuticle and to repair any damage. This will keep the nails looking attractive and prevent them from breaking or chipping.

1 Sanitise your client's hands with a spray or gel.
2 Remove any existing nail polish.
3 Check your client's nails for contra-indications.
4 Use a cleansing spray to sanitise the nail plate to remove any bacteria.
5 Push back the cuticles using a covered orange stick.
6 On each finger, file the edge of the overlay area with a medium grit file (180 grit) until the line between the product and the natural nail becomes invisible.
7 Buff the shine away from the natural nail plate and apply primer to the natural area only.
8 Apply a small ball of gel to the regrowth area and blend it out to the edges, making sure you do not get too close to the cuticle and nail wall.
9 Blend the gel into the existing gel and brush up over the existing UV get to the free edge.
10 Place the fingers under the UV lamp to cure.
11 Using a four-way buffer, buff the nails to give a smooth finish.
12 Apply sealant and cure the nails for a second time under the UV lamp.
13 Apply cuticle oil to finish.

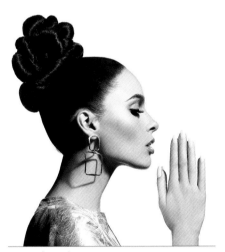

A set of overlays

INDUSTRY TIP

The client's nails might be dehydrated after the removal of nail enhancements so why not recommend a hot oil or paraffin wax manicure to replenish lost moisture. This should only be done if the enhancements are *not* being replaced.

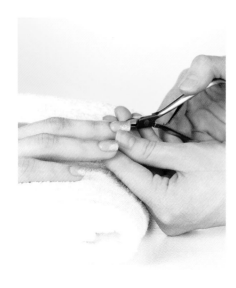

REMOVING UV GEL NAIL ENHANCEMENTS

1 Wash your hands and get the client to wash their hands too.

2 Remove any existing nail polish.

3 Using tip cutters, remove the free edge of the artificial nail, being careful not to cut the client's natural nail underneath.

4 With a medium grit file, file the whole surface of the nail gradually and carefully to remove the artificial structure. Work down the middle of the nail then out to the edges, being careful of the side walls and cuticle area.

5 When you have removed the product, use a block buffer to remove any residue still adhered to the natural nail.

6 Repeat with all 10 nails.

7 When you have removed the UV gel from all the nails, carry out a manicure.

ACRYLIC NAIL ENHANCEMENT

Acrylic nails are strong and durable. They are excellent for clients who have a manual job. This is probably the most used system. The table below outlines the advantages and disadvantages of the acrylic system.

Advantages	Disadvantages
Very durable	Produces a strong smell
Good for people who bite their nails	

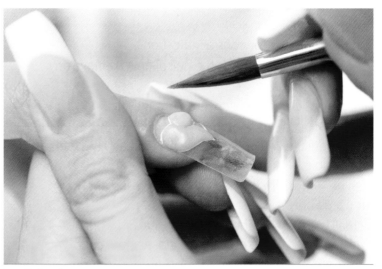

Acrylic bead

PRODUCTS AND TOOLS REQUIRED

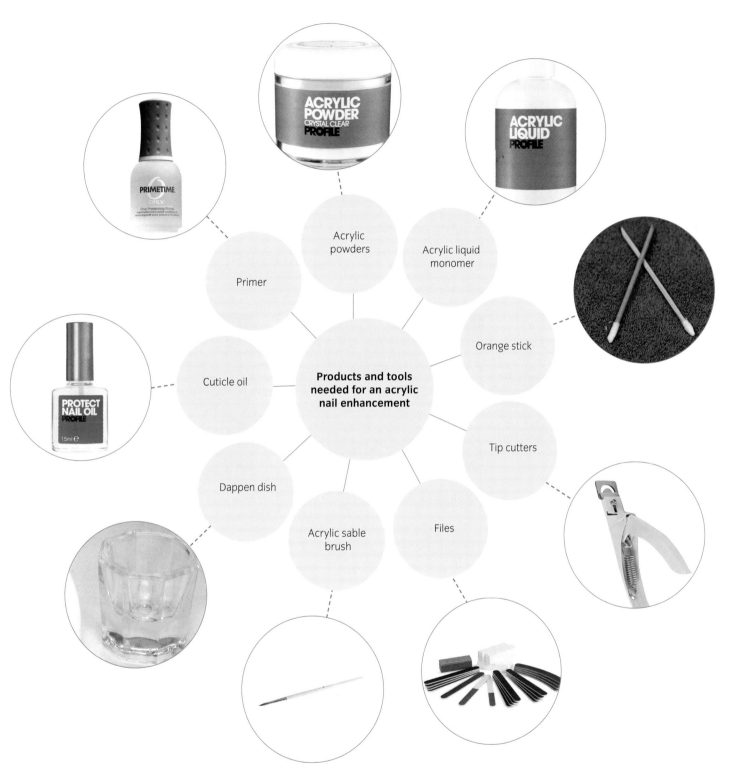

Products and tools needed for an acrylic nail enhancement

- Primer
- Acrylic powders
- Acrylic liquid monomer
- Orange stick
- Cuticle oil
- Tip cutters
- Dappen dish
- Files
- Acrylic sable brush

APPLICATION

Approximate treatment time: 1½ hours.

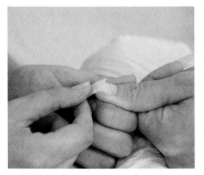

STEP 1 – Follow steps 1–15 of the tip application routine.

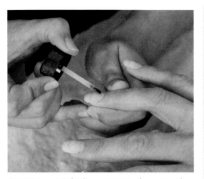

STEP 2 – Apply the primer to the natural nail plate area, being careful to follow the manufacturer's instructions.

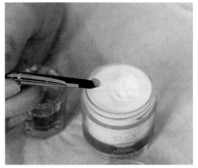

STEP 3 – Dip the brush in the liquid monomer, taking the excess off one side of the brush, and then dip it into the powder to pick up a small ball of acrylic (about the size of a pea).

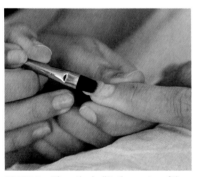

STEP 4 – Place the ball in the centre of the nail plate and with the flat of your brush, blend the acrylic out to the edges (remember you have to work quite quickly otherwise the acrylic will harden). Make sure the acrylic is thinner at the cuticle and nail walls.

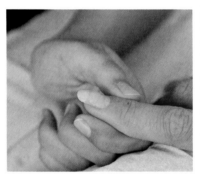

STEP 5 – Look down the finger to check that the nail is a natural shape.

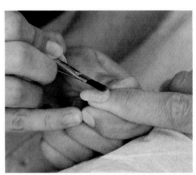

STEP 6 – You can always apply more acrylic if needed before it sets hard.

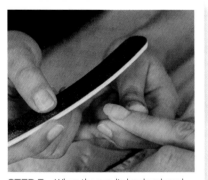

STEP 7 – When the acrylic has hardened, take a course grit file and file to the desired shape.

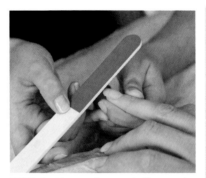

STEP 8 – Use your four-way buffer to make sure the product is well-blended and to create a high-gloss shine.

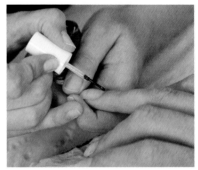

STEP 9 – Apply cuticle oil to finish.

INDUSTRY TIP

To make it easier, you can section the nail into three zones – the cuticle area, the middle and the tip. Apply small beads to each of these areas and, starting at the cuticle, work your way to the tip, overlapping slightly as you go.

INDUSTRY TIP

Acrylic that is applied too thickly will lift.

INDUSTRY TIP

When the powder and liquid monomer are mixed, a chemical reaction called polymerisation occurs.

OVERLAYS

The process of applying an acrylic overlay is the same as above – you just do not apply the tips (step 1).

MAINTENANCE

You should carry out maintenance every 2–3 weeks to keep the nails looking attractive and to prevent them from breaking or chipping.

1 Wash your hands and make sure the client washes their hands too.
2 Remove any existing nail polish.
3 Check your client's nails for contra-indications.
4 Use a cleansing spray to sanitise the nail plate to remove any bacteria.
5 Push back the cuticles using a covered orange stick.
6 Use your cuticle nippers to trim the cuticle area if necessary.
7 With a medium grit file, file down any uneven acrylic until the line between the acrylic and the nail plate is completely invisible.
8 Buff the surface of the natural nail plate to remove any shine.
9 Apply a small ball of acrylic to the regrowth area and blend it out to the edges, making sure you do not get too close to the cuticle and nail wall.
10 Blend the acrylic into the existing acrylic and brush up over the existing acrylic to the free edge.
11 Allow the acrylic to set hard and buff with a four-way buffer to achieve a high-gloss shine.
12 Apply cuticle oil to finish.

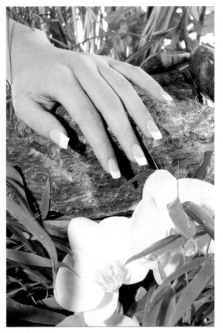

Overlays

REMOVING ACRYLIC NAIL ENHANCEMENTS

1 Wash your hands and get the client to wash their hands too.
2 Remove any existing nail polish.
3 Using your nail cutters, remove the free edge of the artificial nail, being careful not to cut the client's natural nail underneath.
4 With a medium grit file, file the whole surface of the nail to allow absorption of the acetone and aid removal of the artificial nail.
5 Place each hand into separate bowls filled with acetone and allow to soak for 15–20 minutes. Make sure you do not overfill the bowl – you need enough acetone just to cover the fingertips.
6 Check the nails after 10 minutes and remove any artificial nail that has melted with a nail wipe.
7 After 20 minutes the artificial nail should be completely dissolved. Wipe each nail to check that all of the artificial structure has dissolved and use your white block buffer to remove any remaining product.
8 When you have removed the artificial nail product from all the nails, carry out your full manicure, remembering to apply cuticle oil to rehydrate the nails.

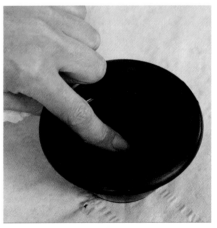

Removal of acrylic nails

WHY DON'T YOU...
make cue cards for each of the nail enhancement services and get them laminated. This will help when you are performing each of the services.

INDUSTRY TIP

All services need to be completed in a timely manner and to the satisfaction of the client. Make sure you get feedback from your client at the end of the service as this will allow you to improve. Also, write down your own feedback on how you feel the service went and if you would improve anything for next time.

INDUSTRY TIP

While you are waiting for the acetone to dissolve the artificial nail, give your client a mini-pedicure (file and polish). This will give your client that extra special treatment and care which in turn will promote business.

Aftercare advice

Advice that you need to give to your client immediately after their treatment.

Home care advice

Advice on what the client should do at home to maintain their nail enhancements.

AFTERCARE AND HOME CARE ADVICE

It is very important to give your client **aftercare** and **home care advice** before they leave so they:

- are aware of how to look after their nails at home
- know what they should avoid doing
- know when to come back for further services
- know what to do if they have an adverse reaction.

Always recommend other services and products to your clients when you are performing the treatment. Tell them about special offers, new services you are offering and products they can use to enhance their service at home – for example, a cuticle oil to help soften the cuticle area and a hand cream to protect the hands and keep them soft and supple.

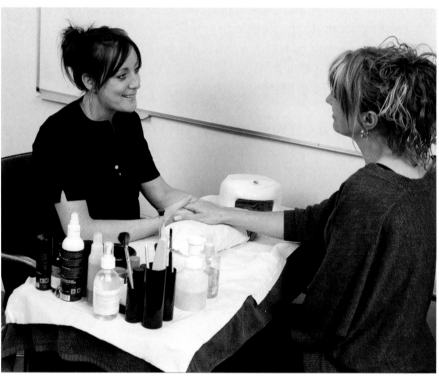

Therapist giving aftercare advice

AFTERCARE/HOME CARE ADVICE FOR NAIL ENHANCEMENT SERVICES

The following spider diagram shows the aftercare and home care advice you should provide your clients following a nail enhancement service.

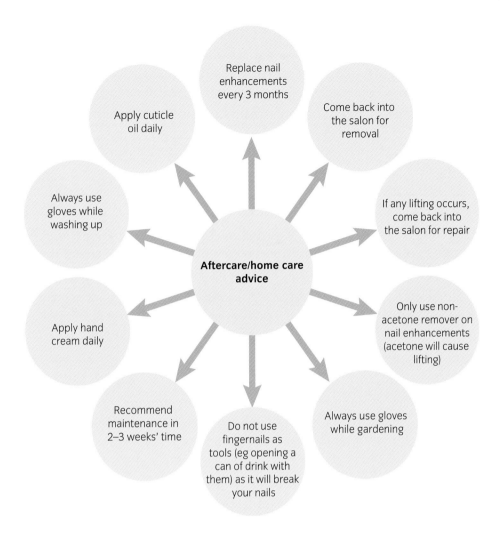

Aftercare/home care advice

- Replace nail enhancements every 3 months
- Come back into the salon for removal
- If any lifting occurs, come back into the salon for repair
- Only use non-acetone remover on nail enhancements (acetone will cause lifting)
- Always use gloves while gardening
- Do not use fingernails as tools (eg opening a can of drink with them) as it will break your nails
- Recommend maintenance in 2–3 weeks' time
- Apply hand cream daily
- Always use gloves while washing up
- Apply cuticle oil daily

CONTRA-ACTIONS

A contra-action is an adverse reaction to a treatment suffered by a client. It could happen during or after a nail enhancement service. If a contra-action occurs during the service, you need to stop the service straight away and remove the product causing it. If it occurs after the treatment, you should advise your client to seek medical attention by contacting their GP.

WHY DON'T YOU...
make a laminated card with all the contra-actions on and give one to each of your clients as they leave.

COMMON CONTRA-ACTIONS

It is important to be able to recognise the signs of the most common contra-actions.

Contra-action	Cause/treatment
Erythema	This is the dilation of blood capillaries that come to the surface of the skin. It is caused by friction or irritation of the skin. If this occurs, apply a cold compress to the affected area.
Allergic reaction	Your client might have an allergic reaction to a product you are using within your service. If this occurs, remove the product straight away and apply a cold compress. If the problem persists, suggest your client seeks medical advice.
Swelling	This could occur if your client is allergic to a product you are using. If swelling occurs, stop the service and apply a cold compress to the area.

CONTRA-ACTIONS CAUSED BY INCORRECT APPLICATION

As long as you are carrying out nail enhancement application correctly, the following contra-actions should not occur. You need to make sure you are taking care to prevent them from occurring and know how to treat them should they occur.

Contra-action	Cause/treatment
Lifting of the artificial nails	Make sure you apply the product evenly to the nail plate. If lifting occurs, the client should return to salon.
Incorrectly fitted tips	Make sure when you are applying the tip that you secure it correctly and that there are no air bubbles. Also, make sure it is the correct size for the natural nail.
Overexposure	When applying UV gel enhancements, make sure you do not **overexpose** the gel to the UV lamp as this can cause pitting. In addition, it is important not to overexpose your clients to chemicals, such as nail varnish remover, acetone and surgical spirit, as they might develop an allergy to these products.
Infection of the natural nail	Prior to application of enhancements, make sure the natural nail has not got any kind of infection. Make sure you work hygienically throughout the service to prevent any bacterial, viral or fungal infections.
Hygiene	Hygiene is one of the most important aspects of being a nail technician. Make sure you do not cross-contaminate and make sure you and your client sanitise hands regularly.
Incorrect application techniques	Make sure you apply products correctly, otherwise you could cause lifting, bubbling and pain to the client.
Accidental damage, such as a cut cuticle or broken nail	If you are too harsh with your file, you could accidentally cut your client's cuticle. If this happens, make sure you put on a pair of gloves (to prevent cross-contamination) and apply a cold compress to the area until the bleeding stops. Keep your gloves on for the remainder of the service if this occurs. At home, a client might accidentally break a nail.
Damage to the nail plate	You can sometimes file the nail plate too harshly and cause damage. Be very careful when you are filing and ask your client at all times if she is comfortable. If this occurs, apply a cold compress and keep the area protected. Do not file over the area.
Chemical damage	Be careful not to apply harmful products directly onto the client's skin. When you are applying UV gel enhancements, a chemical reaction occurs when the gel cures so be careful not to cure the gel for too long. Also, be aware that while under the UV lamp the nail plate can sometimes get rather hot. If this occurs, ask your client to remove their hands from under the UV lamp and press down on their fingers – the heat will quickly go away.
Contamination of products	Always put the lids back on products you are using otherwise they can become **contaminated**.
Mechanical damage	If you are using mechanical tools, such as an electronic file, be very careful you do not damage the nail plate. If this happens, avoid the area and apply a cold compress.

Overexpose
Expose something for too long a time.

Contamination
The presence of something unwanted that might be harmful.

TEST YOUR KNOWLEDGE

Use the questions below to test your knowledge of Chapter 214 to see how much information you have retained. These questions will help you revise what you have learnt in this chapter.

Turn to page 601 for the answers.

1. When you are applying a tip, what is the correct angle to hold the tip at?
   a) 30°
   b) 35°
   c) 40°
   d) 45°

2. Which product would you apply to the nail to remove grease and moisture?
   a) Dehydrator
   b) Enamel remover
   c) Soapy water
   d) Sanitising spray

3. Which grit file is best for blending the tip to the natural nail plate?
   a) 180–240 grit
   b) 260 grit
   c) 320 grit
   d) 400 grit

4. How often would you recommend clients come in for maintenance on their artificial nail system?
   a) Weekly
   b) Every 2–3 weeks
   c) Monthly
   d) As required

5. Polymerisation is a chemical reaction that occurs when you mix which of the following products?
   a) Acrylic powder with liquid monomer
   b) Acrylic liquid monomer and a primer
   c) Acrylic liquid
   d) Acrylic powder and a primer

6. 'Thick and overgrown cuticle' describes which **one** of the following conditions?
   a) Pterygium
   b) Lamella dystrophy
   c) Onychophagy
   d) Leuconychia

7. Which **one** of the following nail conditions would restrict nail enhancement?
   a) Diabetes
   b) Paronychia
   c) Tinea ungium
   d) Onycholysis

8. Which **one** of the following files is best for filing a nail enhancement?
   a) 80 grit file
   b) 180 grit file
   c) 240 grit file
   d) 320 grit file

9. Why should the surface of the nail plate be filed lightly before application of enhancements?
   a) To clean the nail plate
   b) To remove any loose bits of nail
   c) To remove surface shine
   d) To make it shine

10. Why is it important not to touch the nail plate during application?
    a) To maintain hygiene
    b) To avoid putting grease onto the nail plate
    c) To avoid contact with the product
    d) To avoid putting dust onto the working area

11. Which **one** of the following best describes the 'C' curve?

   a) The highest point of the nail

   b) The stress point of the nail plate

   c) The curved shape of the nail plate

   d) The area where the nail tip meets the nail plate

12. Prolonged exposure of the nail to the products used for creating nail enhancements can cause which **one** of the following adverse conditions?

   a) Allergies to products

   b) Lamella dystrophy

   c) Dehydrated nails

   d) Discoloured nail plates

13. In which **one** of the following pieces of equipment should acrylic and powder be mixed together?

   a) A plastic bowl

   b) The lid of the product

   c) A dappen dish

   d) A metal bowl

CASE STUDY: SAMANTHA WATKINSON

After studying beauty therapy it became clear that I had a talent for creative work on the hands and feet and that nails was the industry for me. I attended a number of nail courses and, over the years, my career has taken me all over the world, working in education management, competing nationally and internationally, gaining industry awards, judging competitions, working on photoshoots and at various high-profile events with celebrities. I am now back in the classroom as a tutor at Derby College and enjoy sharing my passion and knowledge with others.

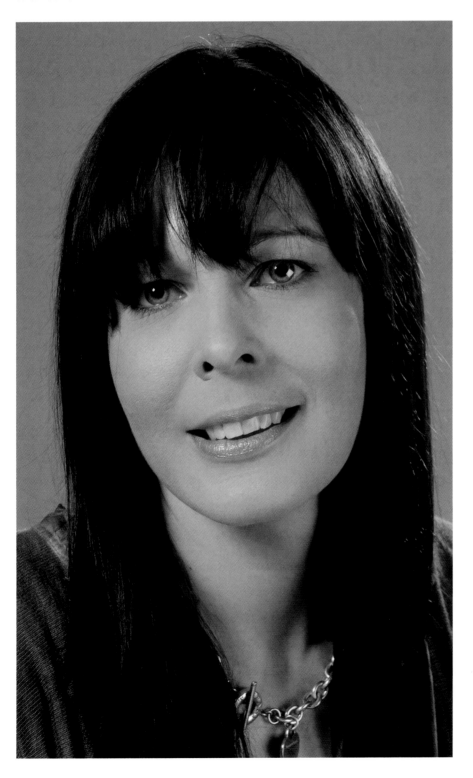

PROVIDE NAIL ART

This chapter is about using your imagination to create effective looks for your clients. Nail art is a creative additional treatment that can be carried out on both natural nails and nail enhancements, on the hands and the feet. Within this chapter you will learn how to create various designs using a variety of different techniques and tools, including polishing, application of gems, glitters and transfers, dotting tools and pens for creating inspiring freehand designs. Nail art is a growing industry and people are starting to become more adventurous with their looks. People will come to you to have nail art designs for a variety of reasons, such as special occasions including weddings, parties and holidays, or to wear as an everyday look.

In this chapter you will learn how to:

- prepare for nail art services
- provide nail art services.

Before you can perform nail art, it is important to be prepared. Health and safety requirements should be carried out for every service, but knowing how to set up your service area, which products and tools you should use and how to carry out an effective consultation are essentials for nail art.

In this part of the chapter you will learn about:

- health and safety
- products, tools and equipment required to carry out a nail art service.

HEALTH AND SAFETY

It is very important to adhere to all health and safety regulations when you are performing a nail art treatment. Please look back and refresh your memory on the legislation in Chapter 202 Follow health and safety practice in the salon and also Chapter 214 Provide and maintain nail enhancement.

ACTIVITY

Perform a risk assessment for your salon to check for any **risks** or **hazards**. Show it to your tutor when you have finished it.

The main legislation covered within nail art treatments are:

- **PPE**
- Health and Safety at Work Act
- **COSHH**
- Data Protection Act.

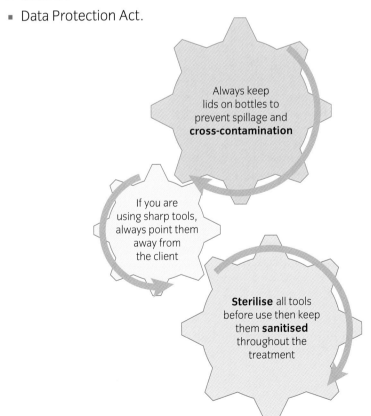

Always keep lids on bottles to prevent spillage and **cross-contamination**

If you are using sharp tools, always point them away from the client

Sterilise all tools before use then keep them **sanitised** throughout the treatment

You should always follow these basic rules

Risk
The danger that damage or injury will occur.

Hazard
Something with the potential to cause harm.

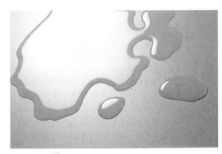
Water spillage

PPE (personal protective equipment)
Clothing and equipment to be used when carrying out services; might include the use of masks or aprons for nail services.

COSHH (Control of Substances Hazardous to Health)
Health and safety regulations require employers to identify hazardous substances used in the workplace and state how they should be stored and handled.

Cross-infection/cross-contamination
Transfer of micro-organisms from one place to another, or from one person to another.

Sterilise
Treat to kill all micro-organisms.

Sanitise
Treat to kill some micro-organisms.

PREPARING YOUR CLIENT

Make sure your client is sitting on a chair that is safe and secure, allowing them to touch the floor with their feet. Make sure the chair is stable.

PREPARING YOURSELF

To prepare yourself for the treatment, make sure:
- you are in the correct uniform
- your hair is tied back
- you have removed all jewellery
- your hands are washed
- all tools and equipment are laid out ready for use.

PRODUCTS, TOOLS AND EQUIPMENT REQUIRED TO CARRY OUT A NAIL ART SERVICE

Many different tools and products are available within the nail art industry. It is a large and growing industry and there are many companies out there to choose from. With nail art you can use just about anything to create fantastic designs and there is no right or wrong design. As long as you apply the products correctly, you can create anything you like. Let your imagination run wild!

It is very important to select your tools, products and equipment carefully to make sure that you have everything that suits your client's requirements; this will be done after the consultation has taken place and you are ready to set up your station.

PRODUCTS NEEDED TO PERFORM A NAIL ART TREATMENT

The following table lists all the products you will need to perform the nail art techniques we will be looking at in this chapter.

Product	Use
Coloured polishes	These can act as a base to your nail art design; you can use any colour.

Product	Use
Polish secure (sealer), top coat or sealer	This product secures your polish to protect the colour and prevent it from chipping. It is also used for securing glitters, flatstones, striping tape, foils and rhinestones in place.
Rhinestones	These are used to create a design and come in many different shapes, sizes and colours. They are usually made of glass which gives a very nice sparkle.
Flatstones	These come in many different shapes, sizes and colours. They are a cheaper version of rhinestones and sparkle well.
Pearls	Pearls add a more glamorous look to the nail. They come in a variety of shapes and sizes to enable a unique look.
Base coat	Apply this product before the coloured polish to prevent the nail from staining.
Glitters	These are a glitter dust and come in different colours. They are used to create a design on the nail. You do not have to use glitter all over the nail; it is just as effective in small areas like the **free edge**. **Free edge** The portion of the nail plate that extends beyond the fingertip. It protects the hyponychium, which lies at the edge of the nail bed.

Product	Use
Top coat	This is used to protect the coloured polish and prevent it from chipping.
Transfers	These come in a variety of different ready-made transfer designs – from flowers to birth signs. They are either stick-on with backing paper that peels off, or water release that you immerse in water and slide off the backing paper. They are very effective.
Foil	This comes on a roll in a variety of different designs and colours. You have to cut it to the necessary size and shape and then place it onto each nail. The end result is very effective.
Tape	This is used to create a striped effect over the nail and comes in a variety of different colours.
Striping pens	These can normally be used in two ways: you can use one side to give a dotting effect and the other to give a **freehand** effect. **Freehand** Using your imagination to create a design with your own artistic talents, eg using a striping pen or paints and brushes.
Paints	These come in pots and are thicker than enamel or polish. You would use paint pots for freehand work like dotting and marbling.

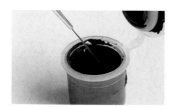

215 PROVIDE NAIL ART

TOOLS NEEDED TO PERFORM A NAIL ART TREATMENT

The table below lists all the tools you will need to perform all the nail art techniques we will be looking at in this chapter.

INDUSTRY TIP

Store your polishes/enamels in a cool dry place. This will prevent them from separating and becoming 'gloopy'.

Tool	Use
Tweezers	To help place and fix products to the nail surface.
Nail scissors	To cut nail art materials.
Orange sticks	To help apply nail art products.
Dotting tool	To create a dotting effect design on the nail.
Brushes, including fan brush, fine brush, liner brush, striping brush	To apply freehand designs: ■ Fan brush – to sweep away excess products from the nail; to create a fan effect. ■ Fine brush – for detailed work. ■ Liner brush – to create thick lines. ■ Striping brush – to create thin and long lines.
Glitter dust brush	To use when you are applying glitter to the nail.
Jewellery tool	To apply jewellery to the free edge of the natural or artificial **nail plate**. **Nail plate** Forms part of the nail structure and protects the nail bed.

EQUIPMENT NEEDED TO PERFORM A NAIL ART TREATMENT

The table below lists the equipment you will need to perform all of the nail art techniques we will be looking at in this chapter.

Equipment	Use/comment
Table/workstation 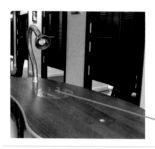 Extraction system	Make sure you have a big enough surface to lay out your products on and it is comfortable for yourself and your client to sit at. Alternatively, you can sit either side of a couch – you do not have to have a separate nail station. It is important that your workstation has a working extraction system. This will include a specialist filter that extracts the chemicals from the air. Filters might need changing regularly as they can become saturated quickly.
Hand support 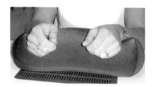	This supports your client's hand and makes the treatment more comfortable.
Light 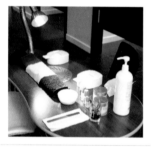	If the lighting in your room/reception is not sufficient, use a lamp to give you extra light.
Training hand 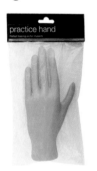	A training hand is a great piece of equipment for practising your nail art designs. It is suitable for sticking artificial nail tips onto.
Stool and client chair 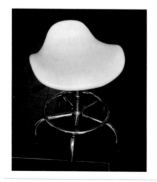	The client's chair must be static for health and safety regulations. Make sure your client's and your feet are flat on the floor for better comfort.

CONSULT, PLAN AND PREPARE FOR NAIL ART

There is a huge array of different designs in nail art that you could offer to your client – it usually comes down to the client's own style and personality.

Communication techniques are very important. For more in-depth information on communication, refer back to Chapter 203 Client care and communication in beauty-related industries.

The consultation stage is very important. This is where you gain all the information from your client to enable you to give them the best treatment you have to offer. In order to carry out a professional consultation, you must use the correct consultation techniques (refer back to Chapter 203 Client care and communication in beauty-related industries) for more in-depth knowledge.

Make sure that you carry out a detailed consultation with your client and find out if they suffer from any contra-indications. You will need to look back at Chapter 207/208 Provide manicure/pedicure treatments to make sure you are familiar with the contra-indications to nail treatments.

Prevent treatment: onychia, onychatrophia (atrophy), onychoptosis, fungal infections, bacterial infections, viral infections, infestations, severe nail separation, severe eczema, severe psoriasis and severe skin conditions.

Restrict treatment: onychogryphosis, onychauxis (hypertrophy), onychomalacia (eggshell nails), broken bones in the area being treated, recent fractures and sprains, recent scar tissue, hyper-keratosis, skin allergies, cuts and abrasions, varicose veins, epilepsy, diabetes, skin disorders, undiagnosed lumps and swellings, product allergies and phlebitis.

You might also need to adapt the treatment to suit the client's needs and nail conditions. For example, if the client is really set on having a specific design but their nail plates are too small, you might have to adapt the style to suit your client's natural nail size.

HANDY HINTS

Refer back to the Anatomy and Physiology chapter for more information on these contra-indications.

INDUSTRY TIP

Make sure you record all your client's details on a record card. This will be useful when the client returns to the salon, as you will have all their details to help you set up and provide an effective service.

HANDY HINTS

Refer back to Chapter 214 Provide and maintain nail enhancement for details on contra-indications that prevent and restrict a treatment, nail conditions and their descriptions.

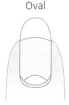
Oval

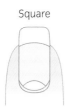
Square

ACTIVITY

Design your own record card for nail art.

You will need to make sure that you are working safely throughout the treatment process. Here are a few points to consider when you are performing your nail art treatment.

During the consultation you need to make sure that you find out why the client is having the treatment. You need to know what the client expects from the treatment. Sometimes you might have to carry out a mini-manicure prior to the nail art application to make the client's nails presentable.

HANDY HINTS

Refer back to Chapter 207/208 Provide manicure/pedicure treatments for more information on how to carry out a mini-manicure.

INDUSTRY TIP

When you are discussing treatment requirements with your client at the consultation stage, make sure they are not allergic to anything that you could be using within your nail art treatment.

Nail and skin analysis

It is very important to carry out a full skin and nail analysis of your client's hands prior to treatment. This will enable you to determine whether your client is suffering from any contra-indications that might prevent or restrict the treatment.

Make sure you look at the hands and nails and question your client about their condition. When you have carefully inspected these areas, make sure you document your findings on the consultation form.

Refer back to Chapter 207/208 Provide manicure/pedicure treatments for a more detailed look into skin and hand analysis.

Make sure you explain to the client the designs and colours that are available. Listen to your client's comments and give verbal advice on what you have to offer. It is a good idea to show your client photos of designs and colours to give them ideas of what they can have and help them to decide.

ACTIVITY

Research on the Internet or look through magazines for pictures and descriptions of contra-indications and skin conditions. Cut out the pictures and cut out the definitions without the names. Place them muddled up on a table and try to match the descriptions with the pictures.

ACTIVITY

Design a display board of your own nail art designs on artificial nail tips to show to your clients when they come in for a nail art treatment.

ACTIVITY

Design your own nail art consultation form.

Skin allergy

HANDY HINTS

Look back at Chapter 203 Client care and communication in beauty-related industries for more advice on consultation skills and communication techniques.

INDUSTRY TIP

Remember, you are not qualified to diagnose a contra-indication; you can only advise. Refer your client to their GP for a professional diagnosis.

INDUSTRY TIP

It is very important at the consultation stage to discuss with your clients the different nail shapes and what shape they prefer. (Refer back to Chapter 207/208 for in-depth information and pictures on nail shapes.)

Preparing for the treatment

When you are preparing for the treatment, make sure that you have all the correct tools and equipment ready. The spider diagram will help you to prepare your area.

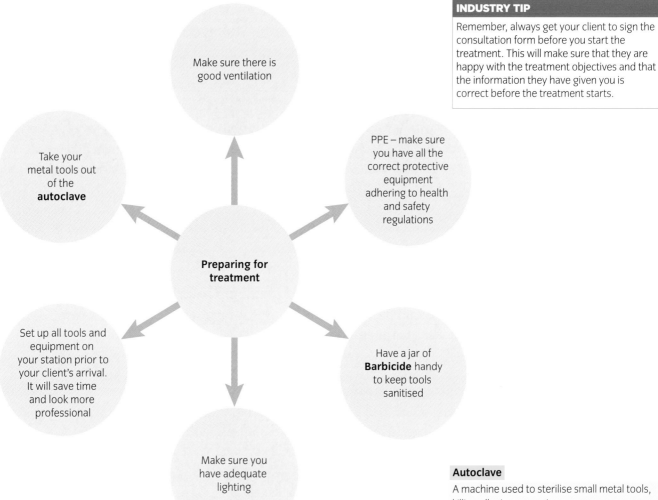

Preparing for treatment

- Make sure there is good ventilation
- PPE – make sure you have all the correct protective equipment adhering to health and safety regulations
- Have a jar of **Barbicide** handy to keep tools sanitised
- Make sure you have adequate lighting
- Set up all tools and equipment on your station prior to your client's arrival. It will save time and look more professional
- Take your metal tools out of the **autoclave**

Autoclave

A machine used to sterilise small metal tools, killing all micro-organisms.

Barbicide

A product used to keep tools sanitised, ready for the treatment.

PROVIDE NAIL ART SERVICES

When deciding what design to apply to your client's nails, you need to consider what would be best for her. Make sure you ask them all the relevant questions, including questions about their **lifestyle** and occupation, as this could affect the design you decide to apply. (Refer back to Chapter 214 Provide and maintain nail enhancement for more in-depth knowledge on environmental conditions.)

In this part of the chapter you will learn about:

- techniques
- aftercare and home care advice.

Lifestyle

How you live your life. Is it stressful? Do you have a good diet? Do you exersice? Do you have hobbies? Do you smoke?

It is very important that you explain to your client why you are asking them about their lifestyle and how it will affect the treatment outcome. Factors to consider when you are talking about your client's lifestyle are:

- Job – if your client has a manual job, the nail art might not last.
- Housework – if your client's hands are constantly in water or if they use detergents a lot then the nail art might not last.
- Hobbies – if your client rides horses or spends a lot of time gardening then the nail art will not last.

TECHNIQUES

You can use a variety of different techniques when you are applying nail art. Use your imagination and do not be afraid of trying a different design or technique; you will only ever learn by experimenting. Here are the techniques you will learn about in this chapter:

- polishing
- enamelling
- marbling
- blending
- application of glitter
- dotting
- application of striping tape

- application of foils
- application of transfers
- application of rhinestones
- application of flatstones
- application of pearls
- application of jewellery.

APPLICATION OF NAIL ENAMEL AND NAIL POLISH

These techniques are both very similar. They are applied in the same way but give slightly different effects as seen in the photo below.

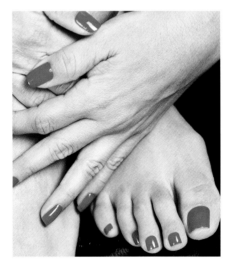
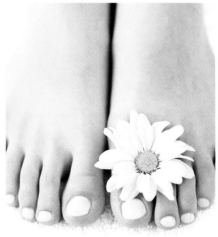

There are a variety of different polishes on the market that come in a variety of different consistencies:

- cream
- glitter
- matte

- shimmer effect
- crackle effect.

Enamel is slightly thicker than polish. It will set on the nail with a thicker consistency and tends to give a matte appearance. Polish has a thinner consistency than enamel and gives more of a shine to the nail.

Step-by-step application of enamel or polish

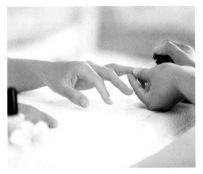

STEP 1 – Apply a base coat to the nails.

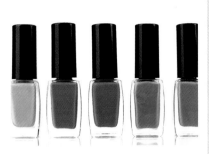

STEP 2 – Choose the desired colour in either enamel or polish.

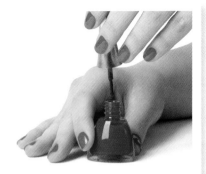

STEP 3 – Do not overload the brush – remove the brush from the bottle and wipe the polish off one side of the brush.

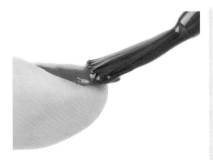

STEP 4 – Apply the polish to the nail using the side of the brush with polish. Starting at the cuticle, fan your brush out, making sure you do not flood the cuticle area.

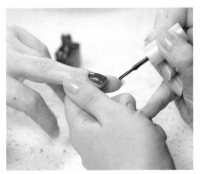

STEP 5 – With one stroke come up the centre of the nail plate, then do the same either side to cover the whole nail.

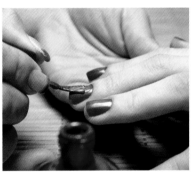

STEP 6 – Repeat this with every nail. When you have completed all 10, the first nail should be dry enough for you to apply the second coat.

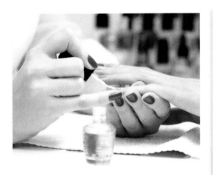

STEP 7 – When the polish is dry, apply the desired nail art or top coat.

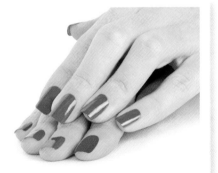

STEP 8 – Finish with cuticle oil to help set the nail polish and soften the cuticles.

ACTIVITY

Together with your friends, look at each other's painting techniques and score each other out of 10 for the end result. Always remember to give each other constructive feedback on ways to improve for next time.

MARBLING EFFECT

This effect is created by a marbling tool using two or more coloured paints.

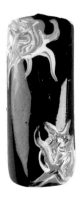 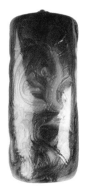 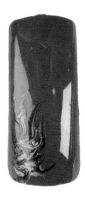 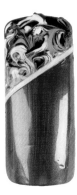

Step-by-step guide to creating a marbled effect

Apply a base coat to the nails and select two or three coloured paints.

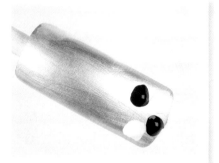

STEP 1 – Using your marbling (dotting) tool, apply two to three drops of each colour to the nail.

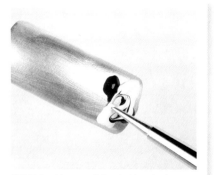

STEP 2 – Very carefully, start to mix the colours together in a swirling motion to create a marbling effect. Remember that you can add more colour if needed. When you have created the desired effect, allow to dry.

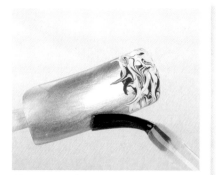

STEP 3 – Apply top coat or sealer.

BLENDING EFFECT

It is a lot easier and more effective to blend with opalescent paint. This will create an iridescent effect.

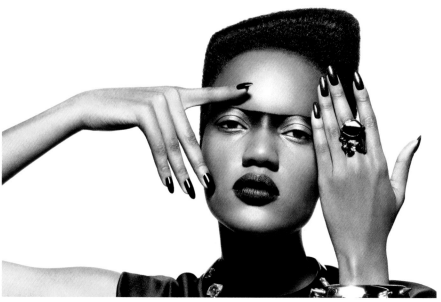

Step-by-step guide to creating a blending effect

Apply a base coat to the nails followed by your desired colour of polish/enamel.

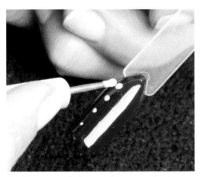

STEP 1 – Apply the opalescent paint in dots down either side of the nail using your dotting tool.

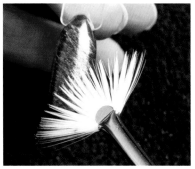

STEP 2 – Using your fan brush, sweep the colours from side to side. This will create the blended look.

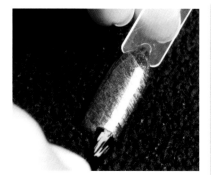

STEP 3 – Apply top coat or sealer when dry.

GLITTER EFFECT

This gives a very effective result and is great for the party season. Glitter is a fine powder and comes in many colours.

INDUSTRY TIP

You can apply glitter to a top coat to give the effect of a shimmer polish.

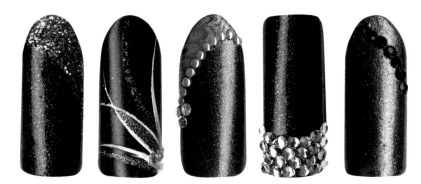

Step-by-step guide to creating a glitter effect

Before you begin, apply a base coat to the nails followed by your desired colour of polish/enamel.

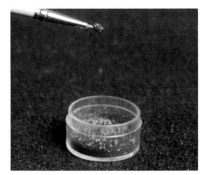

STEP 1 – Dip the end of your glitter brush into the glitter mixture to create a ball.

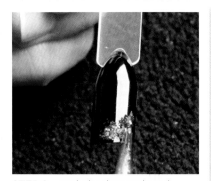

STEP 2 – Apply the glitter to the nail, spreading it evenly across the desired area. You can use as many different colours as you desire, but remember to clean the brush in between each colour.

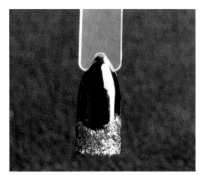

STEP 3 – Wait for the glitter to set before applying top coat or sealer.

DOTTING EFFECT

This creates small dots over the nail and can be used for floral designs, paw prints and other dotting effects.

Step-by-step guide to creating a dotting effect

Apply a basecoat to the nails followed by your desired colour of polish/enamel.

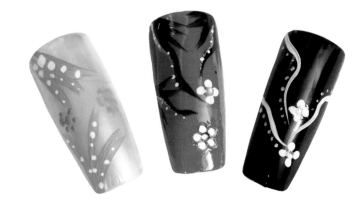

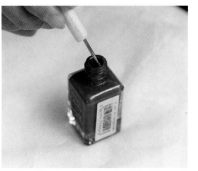

STEP 1 – Dip the end of your dotting tool into the desired colour of paint.

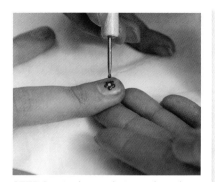

STEP 2 – Apply your design to the nail. When dry, apply top coat or sealer.

STRIPING TAPE

This is a self-adhesive product that comes on a roll. It can be used to create stripes or diagonal patterns and will enhance and add class to your design.

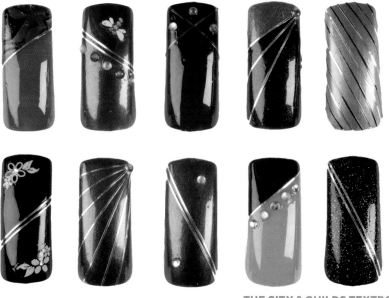

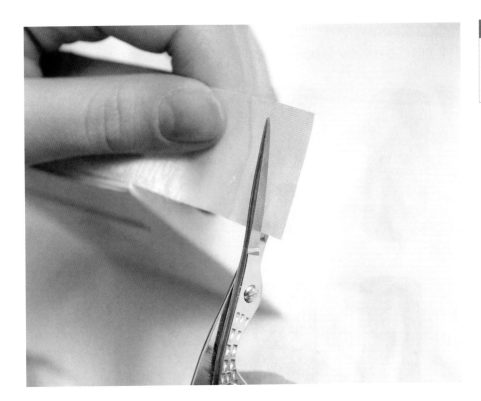

INDUSTRY TIP

Always use stalk scissors when you are applying striping tape as they are made for precise work and allow you to get into smaller areas.

Step-by-step guide to applying striping tape

Before you begin, apply a basecoat to the nails followed by your desired colour of polish/enamel.

INDUSTRY TIP

You can apply a rhinestone in between the tape to enhance the effect.

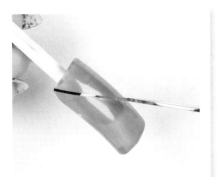

STEP 1 – Apply the striping tape across the chosen part of the nail and press down to secure it to the nail surface.

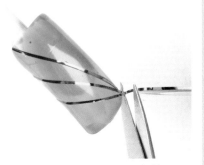

STEP 2 – Trim away any unwanted tape with your nail scissors.

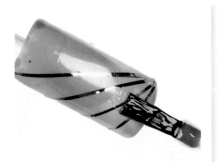

STEP 3 – Apply sealer or top coat to seal the design.

FOIL EFFECT

This effect gives you a fantastic result on the nails.

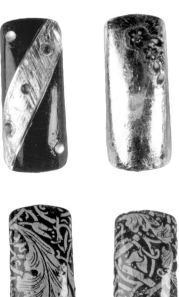
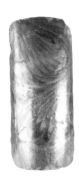
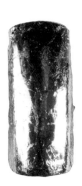
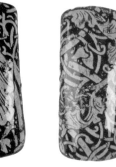
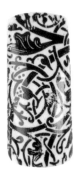
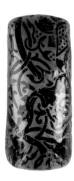

Step-by-step guide to applying foil

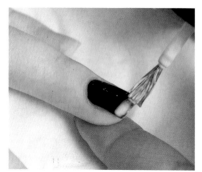

STEP 1 – Apply foil adhesive to the part of the nail where you want to apply the foil (you do not have to coat the whole nail). Leave it to dry and become clear.

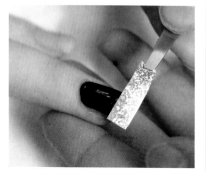

STEP 2 – When it is clear, apply the foil securely to the adhesive with the pattern facing upwards. Firmly roll a covered orange stick or cotton bud over the foil.

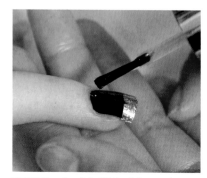

STEP 3 – Carefully lift the foil away, leaving the desired pattern on the nail. Apply top coat or sealer.

TRANSFERS

These can be used to create a fantastic design on the nails without too much artistic talent being required. There are many different designs available.

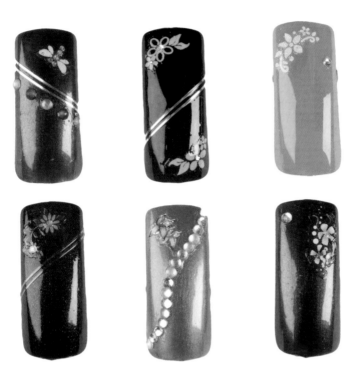

Step-by-step guide to applying transfers

Before you begin, apply a base coat to the nails followed by your desired colour of polish/enamel.

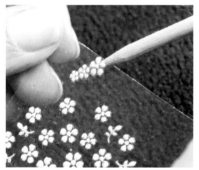

STEP 1 – Choose your transfer. Using the end of an orange stick, remove the transfer from its backing.

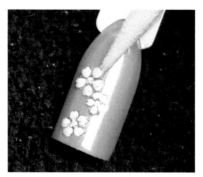

STEP 2 – Apply to the nail plate where required.

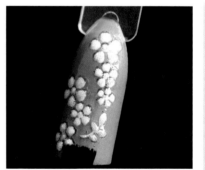

STEP 3 – Apply top coat or sealer.

RHINESTONES, FLATSTONES AND PEARLS

These give a really glamorous effect to the nail art. They come in many different colours, sizes and shapes.

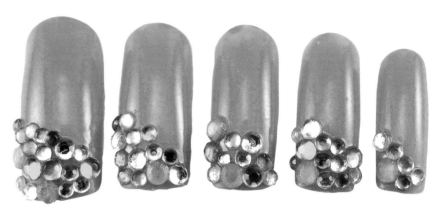

Step-by-step guide to applying rhinestones, flatstones or pearls

Before starting, apply a base coat and your desired colour/design to the nail.

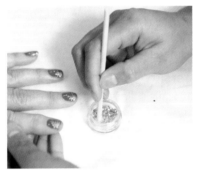

STEP 1 – Before the polish dries, select a rhinestone, flatstone or pearl and apply it to the nail using the end of an orange stick that has been dipped in water.

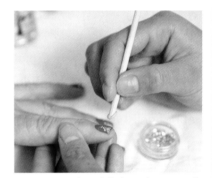

STEP 2 – As the polish dries, the stone will set into place.

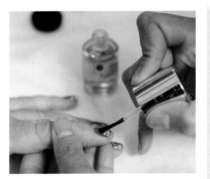

STEP 3 – Apply top coat or sealer.

Jewellery

You can apply a variety of different jewellery items to the nail. It is better to attach these to artificial nail structures to avoid damage to the natural nail.

Guide to applying jewellery

Before starting, apply a base coat and your desired colour/design to the nail, including top coat/sealer.

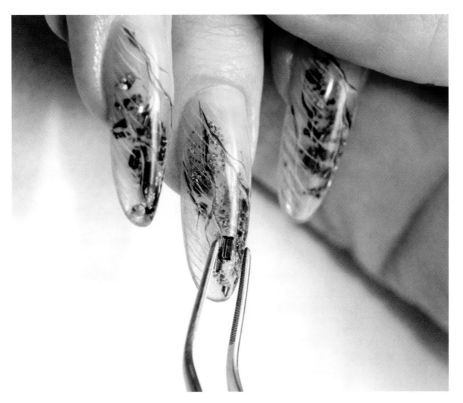

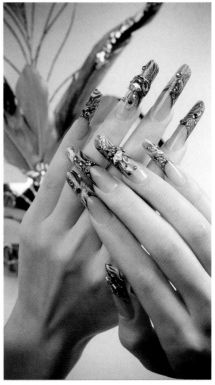

The finished result

Using a jewellery tool, carefully make a small hole on the free edge of the nail. Attach your jewellery.

AFTERCARE AND HOME CARE ADVICE

It is very important to give your client **aftercare** and **home care** advice before they leave so they are aware of how to treat and look after their nails at home. They need to know what to avoid and when to come back for further treatments. Also, if they have an adverse reaction you can advise your client what to do.

Aftercare
Advice to give to your client straight after their treatment.

Home care
What the client should do at home to maintain their nail art.

ACTIVITY

Create your own aftercare/home care advice leaflet to give to your clients at the end of the treatment so they can refer back to it at home.

INDUSTRY TIP
Always recommend other services and products to your clients when you are performing the treatment. Tell them about special offers, new treatments you are offering and products they can use to enhance their treatment at home, such as cuticle oil and hand cream.

INDUSTRY TIP
Always make sure you ask your client at the consultation stage if they have any known allergies to the products you will be using.

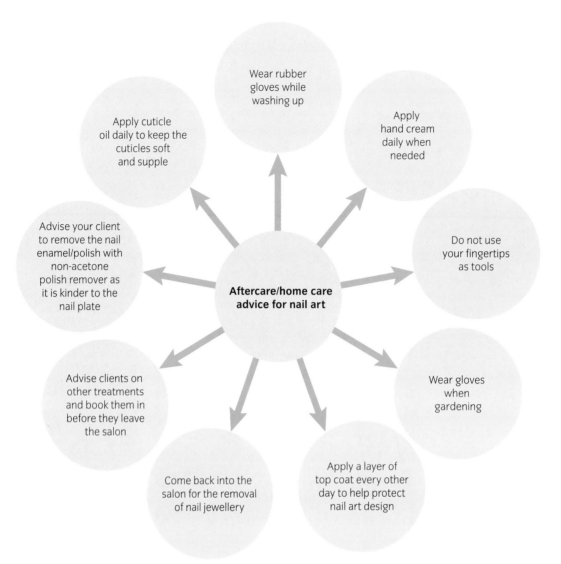

Wear rubber gloves while washing up

Apply hand cream daily when needed

Apply cuticle oil daily to keep the cuticles soft and supple

Do not use your fingertips as tools

Advise your client to remove the nail enamel/polish with non-acetone polish remover as it is kinder to the nail plate

Aftercare/home care advice for nail art

Wear gloves when gardening

Advise clients on other treatments and book them in before they leave the salon

Come back into the salon for the removal of nail jewellery

Apply a layer of top coat every other day to help protect nail art design

WHY DON'T YOU...
include the price of a nail varnish into your treatment price, then you can give the client their chosen polish/enamel colour to take home at the end of the treatment. It is a small gesture that will please clients.

Contra-actions

This is something linked to the treatment that causes a problem. It could happen during or after a nail art treatment.

If your client suffers from a contra-action, advise them to remove the products and seek medical attention by contacting their GP. Some common contra-actions are described in the table.

Contra-action	Cause/prevention
Severe erythema	A dilation of blood capillaries just beneath the surface of the skin. This can be caused by friction or if the skin is irritated. If this occurs, apply a cold compress to the affected area. If the erythema persists, advise your client to speak to their GP.
Allergic reaction	An allergic reaction is when your client has reacted adversely to a product you are using within your treatment. If this occurs, remove the product straight away and apply a cold compress. If the problem persists, suggest your client seeks medical advice.
Tissue damage resulting in blood loss	If you accidentally damage your client's skin and it results in blood loss, make sure the first thing you do is put on a pair of gloves to prevent cross-infection. Depending on the severity of the damage, apply pressure with a cold compress until the bleeding has stopped, then apply a plaster to the affected area if needed, making sure you ask the client if they are allergic to plasters beforehand. If the bleeding persists and it is a deep wound, suggest your client seeks medical advice.

TEST YOUR KNOWLEDGE

Use the questions below to test your knowledge of Chapter 215 to see how much information you have retained. These questions will help you to revise what you have learnt in this chapter.

Turn to page 601 for the answers.

1. How often should a client be advised to apply top coat to protect nail art?
   a) Only when re-varnished
   b) Every other day
   c) Every 3–4 days
   d) Once a week

2. Which **one** of the following is not a technique used for applying glitter dust?
   a) Dip a brush into sealer then into glitter and apply to the nail
   b) Apply sealer to the free edge and then dip into the glitter
   c) Shake the glitter onto wet nail enamel
   d) Apply straight from the bottle with the brush supplied

3. Which **one** of the following is the correct method to use to pick up rhinestones?
   a) Tweezers with pointed ends
   b) The end of an orange stick dipped in water
   c) An orange stick placed onto the tongue to moisten
   d) An orange stick dipped into sealer

4. Which **one** of the following nail conditions would restrict nail art designs?
   a) Splinter haemorrhage
   b) Dry nails
   c) Brittle nails
   d) Ridged nails

5. Which **one** of the following is a contra-action that might occur during, or after, a nail art service?
   a) Stained nails
   b) Dehydrated nails
   c) Ripples in the nail enamel
   d) An allergic reaction

6. Which **one** of the following would contra-indicate a nail art service?
   a) Paronychia
   b) Lamellar dystrophy
   c) Koilonychia
   d) Leukonychia

7. Which **one** of the following contra-indications would restrict nail art?
   a) Hangnail
   b) Onychophagy
   c) Blue nail
   d) Paronychia

8. How should nail enamel be stored to stop it separating and becoming 'gloopy'?
   a) In a cupboard
   b) In a warm room
   c) In a fridge
   d) In a cool dry place

9. Which **one** of the following enamel removers should be avoided when removing nail enamel before nail art?
   a) Oily
   b) Acetone-free
   c) Non-oily
   d) Ethyl acetate

10. When you are applying polish secures, they must be applied onto:
    a) a top coat
    b) a clear base coat
    c) a sealer
    d) nail polish.

11. Which **one** of the following is the nail plate made up of?
    a) Melanocytes
    b) Keratinised cells
    c) Collagen
    d) Fibroblast cells

12. Which **one** of the following is not nail art?
    a) Blending
    b) Transfers
    c) Marbling
    d) Shading

13. Which **one** of the following contra-indications should be referred to a GP?
    a) Onycholysis
    b) Pterygium
    c) Onychophagy
    d) Onychorrhexis

14. Which **one** of the following is the best surface on which to mix or blend acrylic paints for nail art deigns?
    a) Plastic palette
    b) Glass bowl
    c) Lid of the paint pot
    d) Dappen dish

15. Which **one** of the following tools would you use to create a flower design?
    a) Orange stick
    b) Striping brush
    c) Fine brush
    d) Dotting tool

CASE STUDY: JACKIE O'SULLIVAN

I first got into nails when I watched a mobile technician apply a set of acrylics to my mum. I am now a busy nail technician, college lecturer and judge at international nail competitions. I am very passionate about education, and want to share my experiences and ideas with everyone.

Nail art is my passion. I love the creativity I get to use with nails as I do not get that from other beauty disciplines.

I love seeing my students gain confidence and progress, then go on to become great nail technicians. One of the best things about teaching is when you see the information click in the student's mind. All of a sudden they understand it, and there's no stopping them!

My job has a huge amount of variety to it, which is so much fun! Along with teaching, doing clients' nails and competing, I also work on photoshoots with make-up and nails and advise other nail technicians on competitions. Every day holds something different. It keeps me interested and motivated, I'm literally never bored!

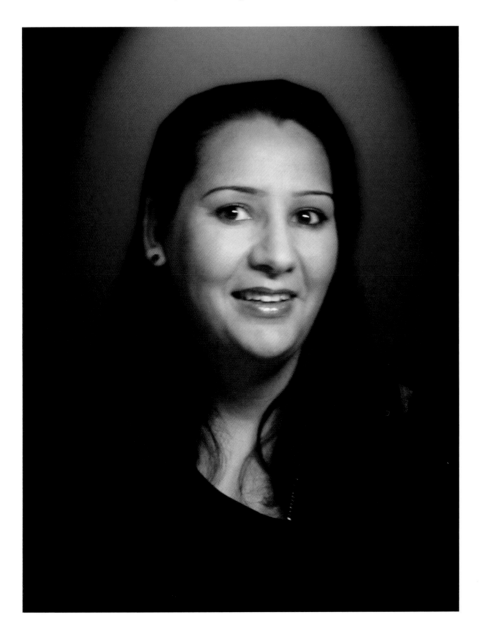

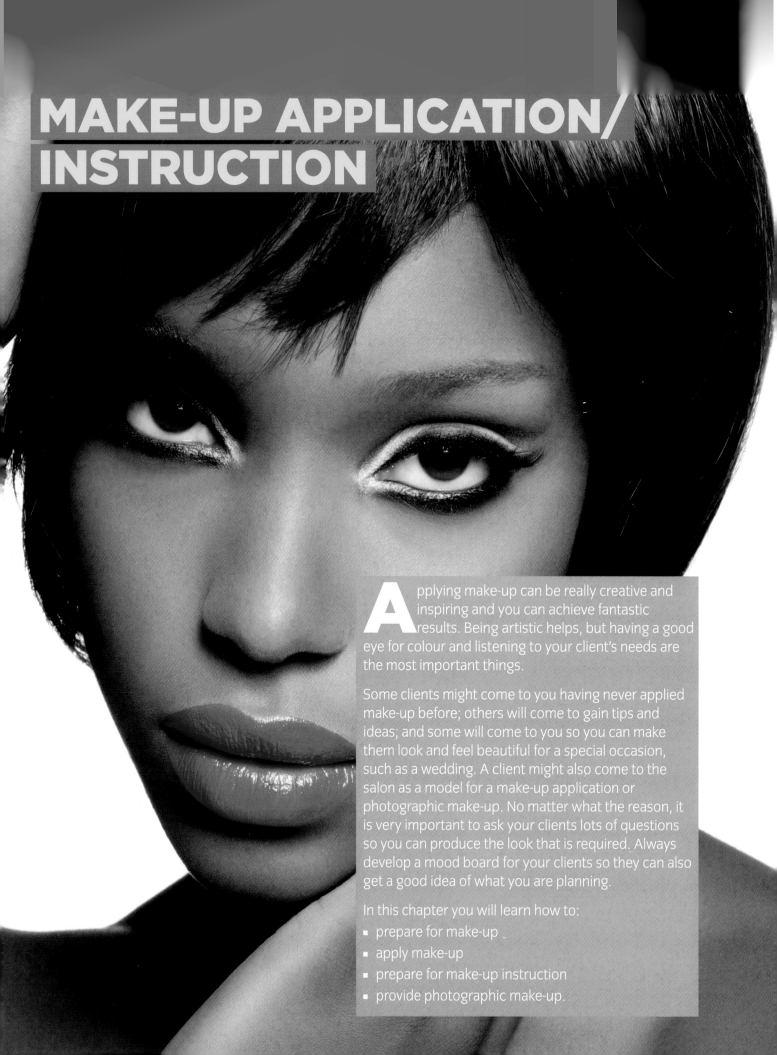

MAKE-UP APPLICATION/ INSTRUCTION

Applying make-up can be really creative and inspiring and you can achieve fantastic results. Being artistic helps, but having a good eye for colour and listening to your client's needs are the most important things.

Some clients might come to you having never applied make-up before; others will come to gain tips and ideas; and some will come to you so you can make them look and feel beautiful for a special occasion, such as a wedding. A client might also come to the salon as a model for a make-up application or photographic make-up. No matter what the reason, it is very important to ask your clients lots of questions so you can produce the look that is required. Always develop a mood board for your clients so they can also get a good idea of what you are planning.

In this chapter you will learn how to:

- prepare for make-up
- apply make-up
- prepare for make-up instruction
- provide photographic make-up.

You must prepare for make-up application before you can create your looks. It is important to pay attention to health and safety regulations, tools and equipment and consultation techniques.

In this part of the chapter you will learn about:

- health and safety
- preparing yourself and your client
- preparing the work area
- consulting, planning and preparing for make-up treatments
- contra-indications.

HEALTH AND SAFETY

It is very important to follow all health and safety regulations when you are performing a make-up treatment. Look back and refresh your memory on the legislation in Chapter 201 Follow health and safety practice in the salon.

The main legislation covered within make-up treatments are:

- **PPE**
- Health and Safety at Work Act
- **COSHH**
- Data Protection Act
- Workplace Regulations.

METHODS OF STERILISATION

It is very important to sterilise tools and equipment prior to carrying out a make-up treatment for maximum health and safety and to stop **cross-contamination**. Use disposable tools where possible and sterilise your brushes after every client, as **micro-organisms** will start to develop and cross-contamination might result. As you cannot use the **autoclave** to sterilise your brushes, make sure you get a sterilisation spray, such as isopropyl alcohol.

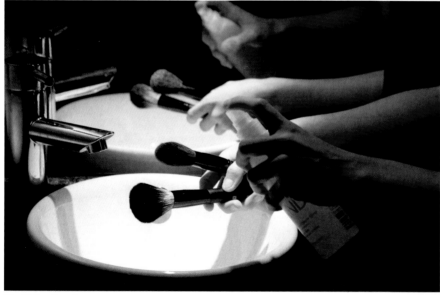

Sterilising brushes

PPE
Personal protective equipment.

COSHH
Control of Substances Hazardous to Health.

 SmartScreen 206 Worksheet 4

Cross-contamination
When micro-organisms are transferred from one place to another, eg through unhygienic practices.

Micro-organisms
Tiny microscopic organisms that live in colonies, eg bacteria and fungi.

Autoclave
A machine that produces steam at up to 121–134°C; used to sterilise all small metal tools, killing all micro-organisms.

HANDY HINTS
Refer to Chapter 202 to find out more about sterilisation.

INDUSTRY TIP
Throughout the treatment, make sure that you keep lids on all products to stop contamination from harmful airborne micro-organisms. Also, make sure you remove the products with a spatula and not your fingers, and do not put brushes directly into products.

PREPARING YOURSELF AND YOUR CLIENT

It is very important to position yourself and your client correctly throughout the treatment. Make sure your client is comfortable at all times. Depending on what kind of environment you are in, some salons apply their make-up using a couch for the client. If that is the case, make sure it is at the correct height so you do not strain your back; and make sure the client is sitting with their back against the back of the couch as this will prevent their back from aching. Other salons have a make-up station with a mirror that has light around it and a chair in front of it; this will allow you to stand to the side of the client to apply the make-up. Make sure that the chair is at the correct height for you and that you are not straining your back. Also, remember to make sure that when you are instructing a make-up lesson that your client or clients, depending on the size of the group, all have comfortable chairs to sit on with a mirror in front of them to allow them to clearly apply the make-up themselves while you are instructing them.

PREPARING THE WORK AREA

When preparing for the treatment, make sure that you have all the correct tools and equipment ready. The spider diagram below will help you prepare your work area.

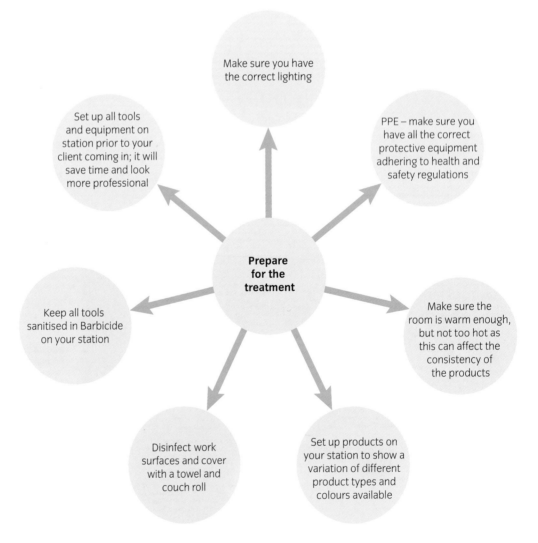

Make sure you have the correct lighting

PPE – make sure you have all the correct protective equipment adhering to health and safety regulations

Set up all tools and equipment on station prior to your client coming in; it will save time and look more professional

Prepare for the treatment

Make sure the room is warm enough, but not too hot as this can affect the consistency of the products

Keep all tools sanitised in Barbicide on your station

Disinfect work surfaces and cover with a towel and couch roll

Set up products on your station to show a variation of different product types and colours available

WORK LOCATIONS

There are many different environments that you might be asked to work in when applying make-up as a therapist or a make-up artist. You might need to go out on location if you are doing photographic make-up. Or it might be in a studio, salon or a film set, so make sure you are prepared and that you have all the correct tools and equipment available to you. It might be worth taking a stool of your own and a mirror, just in case they are not provided for you.

ENVIRONMENTAL CONDITIONS

The salon environment is very important. The working area should be clean and tidy. A pleasant atmosphere and ambience in the salon will make your working environment and the client's treatment more pleasurable.

Lighting

Lighting is the most important environmental condition you need to think about for make-up treatments – it is essential to have good lighting when you are applying and instructing make-up. Daylight is the best light to work in, but if there is not enough daylight entering the room you are working in, the next best thing is to use natural daylight bulbs to give the illusion of daylight. If you are working in a room that does not give you enough natural light, it will affect the end result. When your client steps outside into the natural daylight, the make-up will appear completely different to what it looked like under the dull or fluorescent lighting inside.

The different types of lighting and their effects on make-up are:

- **Fluorescent lighting:** this type of lighting contains the colours blue and green that take away the depth of colour and make the complexion look dull. Try to avoid very dark colours as fluorescent lighting intensifies the tones.
- **Natural daylight:** this type of lighting contains all the colours of the rainbow and intensifies every colour. This is the best lighting to apply make-up in as it always gives a perfect finish and you can see every shade and tone you apply.

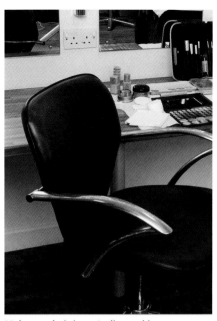

Make-up chair in a studio working area

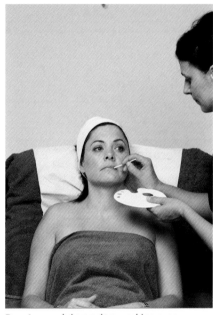

Beauty couch in a salon working area

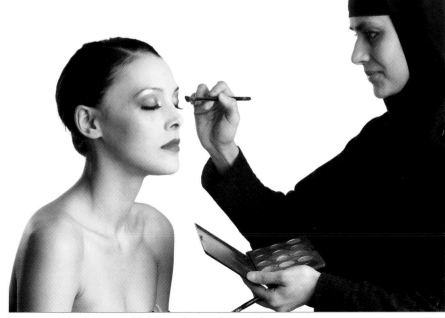

it is essential to have good lighting when applying make-up

- **Filament lighting:** this type of lighting contains the colours red and yellow that create a very warm look. You can use almost every colour under this lighting apart from browns, which will appear a lot darker.

INDUSTRY TIP

Make sure the room is warm enough for the client so they feel comfortable throughout their treatment, but make sure it is not too hot as this could affect the consistency of the make-up products. For more advice on environmental conditions, see Chapter 201 Working in beauty-related industries.

PRODUCTS, TOOLS AND EQUIPMENT

It is important that you use the correct products, tools and equipment for make-up treatments. There are several different product ranges within the industry and it is best to try a few and find one that suits you and your clientele.

INDUSTRY TIP

To make sure you are using the best products for you and your clientele, have a wide variety of products available with lots of different colours to choose from.

When instructing a make-up lesson, always make sure you explain to your client what everything is, what equipment you are using and how they could use it at home. Talk clearly through what all the products do and how they should be stored and used at home to gain the maximum effects.

There is more information on products later in the chapter, next to the make-up techniques.

The tools needed to perform a make-up treatment are described in the tables below.

Tool/equipment	Use
Sponges 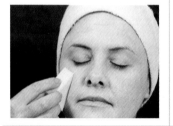	You need sponges or brushes to apply and **blend** the foundation – these come in all different shapes and sizes. It does not matter which ones you use as long as you are comfortable using them. **Blend** Merge two or more colours together to provide a seamless transition from one colour to the next.
Palette 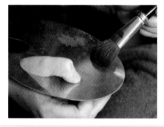	This is used for **dispensing** all products onto and to prevent cross-contamination occurring. **Dispense** Remove the product from its container with a spatula for use on the client.
Headband 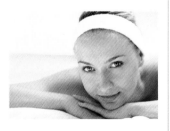	A headband protects the client's hair and keeps it off their face. A headband must be worn to make sure you meet health and safety regulations.

Tool/equipment	Use
Gown/apron 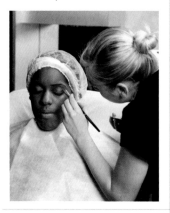	Always use a gown or an apron on the client as this will protect their clothes.
Disposable applicators 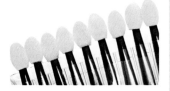	These are used to stop cross-contamination. They can be thrown away after every client and prevent transfer of micro-organisms from one eye to the other, or one client to another. They are plastic tools with the appearance of a real sponge applicator or mascara brush.
Spatulas 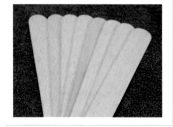	Always make sure you dispense your products with a spatula as this will prevent cross-contamination. You can get plastic and metal spatulas. The plastic ones are disposed of after use, while the metal ones can be placed in an autoclave to sterilise them between clients.

Brushes

You can get a wide range of different brushes with different fibres and textures, including ox, pony, sable, camel and **synthetics**. When you are giving a make-up lesson, explain to your client what all the brushes do, what techniques they create and how they could use them at home. Here are the most common brush types and their uses.

Synthetic

Made artificially by chemical synthesis to resemble a natural product.

Brush type	Use
Foundation brush 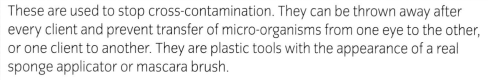	Used to apply foundation to the skin; using a foundation brush can cause fine lines, you might need to blend afterwards with a sponge.
Concealer brush	Used to apply concealer to the correct place.
Powder brush	Used to apply powder or remove excess powder dust.

Brush type	Use
Contouring brush 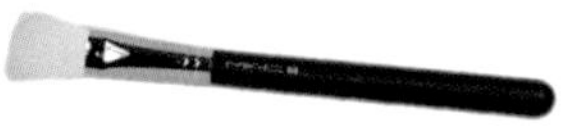	Used to apply highlighter and shading products to the skin to create contouring.
Small rounded eyeshadow brush 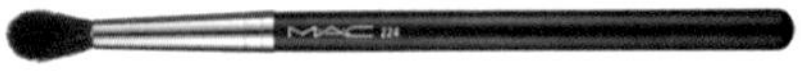	Used to apply eyeshadow and to blend colours.
Flat angle brush 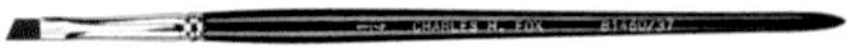	Used to apply eyeshadow to the socket area and to blend colours.
Coarse eyeshadow brush 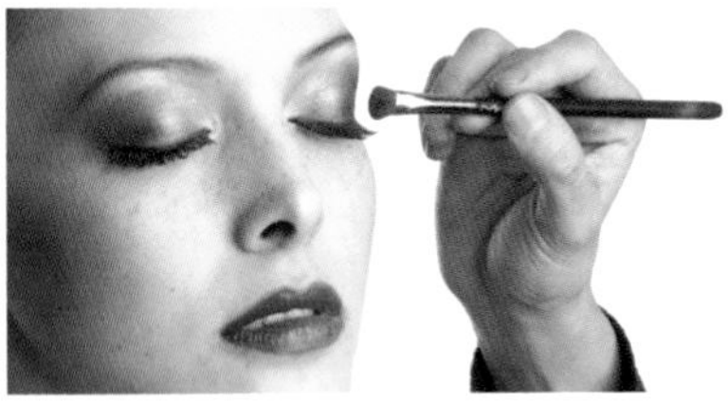	Used to soften harsh lines.
Blusher brush 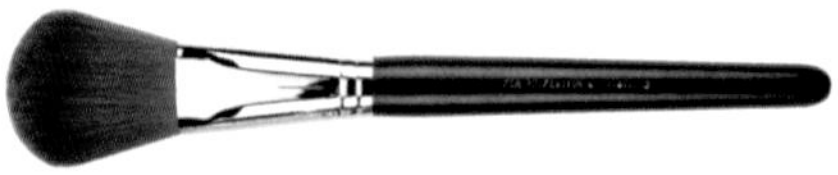	Used to apply powder blush.
Angle-ended brush 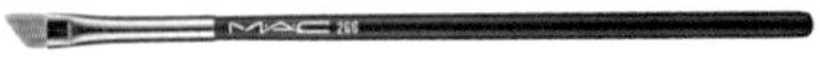	Used to apply eyeshadow or liquid liner to small areas.
Eyeliner brush 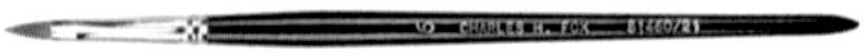	Used to blend pencil eyeliner and to apply eyeshadow directly above and below the lashes.
Mascara brush/comb 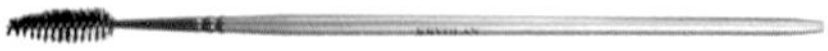	Used to apply mascara and to remove clumps in the mascara.
Lip brush 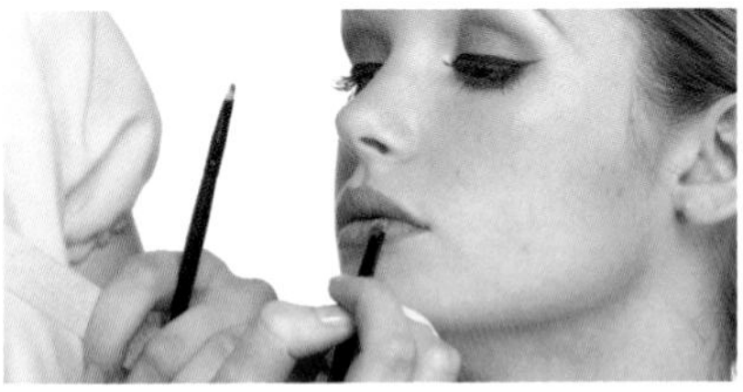	Used to apply lipstick, lip gloss and tint.

INDUSTRY TIP

The best way to start collecting brushes is to purchase one a month and build your collection gradually, in addition to the brushes you will receive from your college kit. Trade shows and wholesalers are good places to buy brushes.

INDUSTRY TIP

Using a brush pouch is a great way of keeping all your brushes together. They come in different sizes and you can even get ones that attach around your waist like a belt.

ACTIVITY

Research the different types of synthetic brushes and write down their advantages over natural fibre brushes.

INDUSTRY TIP

There are a variety of different brushes to use for applying make-up. They all give different effects and have their own uses. It is a good idea to have lots of brushes handy as you need to sterilise them between each use and they can take up to 24 hours to dry.

The equipment needed to perform a make-up treatment is described in the table below.

Equipment	How to use
Make-up chair/couch 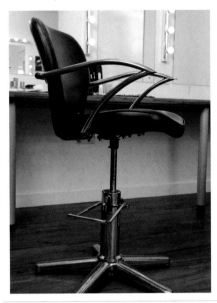	You can apply make-up on either a couch or a chair. Make sure both you and your client are comfortable throughout the service. Refer to earlier text on positioning of the client.
Trolley 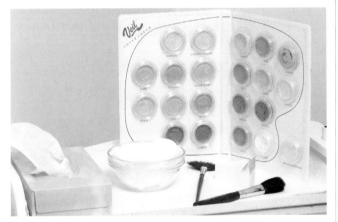	Make sure you have a big enough surface to place all your products and brushes on. You need to make sure your station is clean and tidy at all times. You can use a trolley table or any flat surface.
Lights and mirror 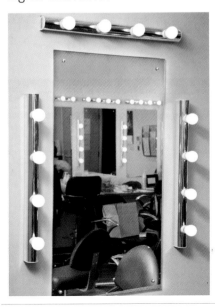	Make sure you have enough lighting in your room – try to apply the make-up in natural daylight if possible. If you do not have a mirror on the wall, make sure you have a hand-held mirror available so you can show your client what you are applying step-by-step and make sure they are happy with the colour selection. Make-up always looks different on the skin from what it does in the pallette. If you are instructing the client on how to apply make-up, make sure they have their own mirror for when they apply the make-up themselves.

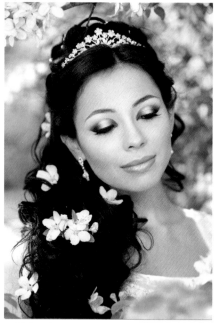

Bridal make-up

CONSULTING, PLANING AND PREPARING FOR MAKE-UP TREATMENTS

The consultation stage is very important. This is where you gain all the information from your client to make sure you give them the best treatment you have to offer. It is very important that the client is comfortable with the treatment they are having and that the treatment is right for them.

Your client will normally have an idea of what type of make-up they would like before their appointment, unless they are coming in for a make-up lesson. Most clients will book in to have their make-up applied for a special occasion, but that could mean a day or an evening look. If your client is coming in for wedding make-up, you would normally offer them a trial run first. You will need to try out a few different looks and to make sure that the client is happy with the end result as this will be their special day and they will want to look their best.

ACTIVITY

Look through a magazine and find a make-up look that really catches your eye. Practise it on yourself in front of a mirror.

CONSULTATION TECHNIQUES – QUESTIONING

Here is a checklist of questions to ask while you are carrying out a thorough consultation. These will enable you to gain all the information you need to be able to advise your client on the correct make-up look.

- What are the main objectives of today's treatment?
- How long do you want your make-up to last for?
- Is there a certain look you want to achieve?
- Do you wear make-up on a daily basis?
- What are the colours of the bride's flowers, bridesmaids' dresses and accessories? (If the make-up is for a wedding.)
- What type of lighting will you be under?
- Why do you need a lesson? (If the client is coming in for a make-up lesson.)
- Have you got any ideas of what you do not like?
- Is there any make-up that you never use? Why not?
- Is your skin/are your eyes sensitive?

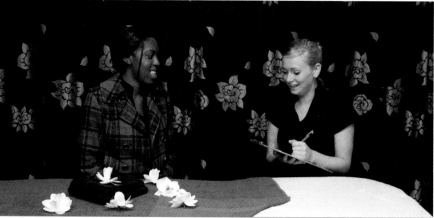

A consultation being carried out

SKIN TYPES AND CONDITIONS

Everyone has a certain skin type (see below). Adverse skin conditions can happen for various reasons, eg if someone does not drink enough water their skin might be dehydrated, or if a person has reached the age of 25, they can be **deemed** to have mature skin.

If your client is coming in for a make-up lesson, you should also instruct them on how to cleanse, tone and moisturise their skin correctly. Advise them of their skin type and make them aware of the effects that different products have on the skin. You should also do this as part of the aftercare/home care advice you give your client.

It is very important to cleanse, tone and moisturise the skin prior to the application of make-up. This removes any existing make-up the client/model might be wearing. It also removes any dirt and bacteria on the skin's surface.

Explain to your client/model what you are doing and why you are doing it throughout the cleansing process; explain the products and their benefits as you apply them, and give your client/model advice on how to continue this process at home. Recommend that they should be cleansing, toning and moisturising twice daily.

The four main skin types you will come across are:

- oily
- dry
- combination
- normal.

HANDY HINTS

Look back at the Anatomy and Physiology chapter for information on the structure and function of the skin.

Deem

If you think something.

HANDY HINTS

Refer back to Chapter 204/224 Provide facial skin care/facial care for men for step-by-step guides on cleansing, toning and moisturising the skin.

 SmartScreen 209 Worksheet 2

HANDY HINTS

Refer back to Chapter 204/224 Provide facial skin care/facial care for men for in-depth details on each of the skin types and skin conditions below.

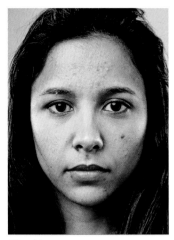

Oily skin

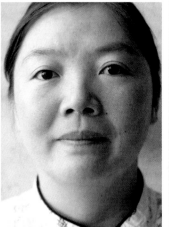

Dry skin

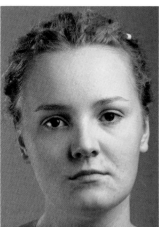

Combination skin

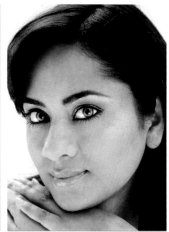

Normal skin

The three main skin conditions are:

- dehydration
- sensitivity
- maturity.

INDUSTRY TIP

Use a **dehydration pen** to correctly detect your client's moisture balance in the skin. Record it on their consultation form and record card. Advise them to drink plenty of water to rehydrate their skin and test them again when they next come into the salon to see if it has improved. You can purchase a dehydration pen from a beauty supplier. It is an electronic device and calculates the moisture in your skin when pressed against it.

Dehydration pen

Detects the percentage of water in the skin.

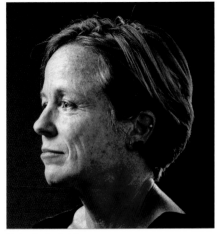

Dehydrated skin

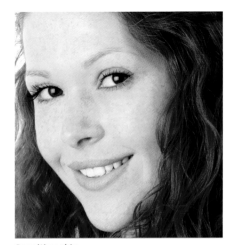

Sensitive skin

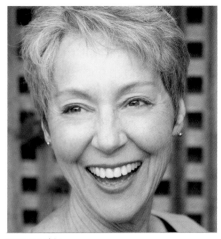

Mature skin

SKIN COLOUR

It is very important that you have a good idea of what colours suit what skin tone so you are able to apply make-up to all skin colours.

Fair, redhead skin

This skin will flush easily and tends to have freckles. To help reduce the redness in the skin, you can apply a green tint by adding a small amount of green concealer to your foundation, making sure you do not apply too much. Apply a peach or warm, rose-coloured blush. The use of green, peach, rust and brown eyeshadows, lipsticks and blush colours tend to suit this skin tone the best. Apply a light peach, gold or pink-coloured lipstick.

Oriental skin

This skin tone can appear quite sallow. Apply warm colours to add warmth to the skin tone. Use a brown or warm, peach blusher and highlight the eyes as they can appear quite dark. Use pastel colours to really lift the eye area, while a deep pink or reddish orange lipstick will complement this tone.

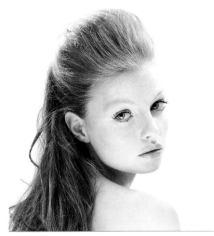

Fair, redhead skin

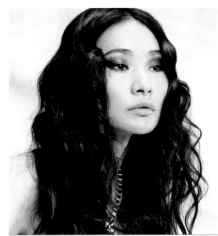

Oriental skin

Black skin

Black skin tones can appear very shiny, so apply a foundation with a yellow tone and avoid pink tones as this could make the skin appear chalky. Do not forget that you might have to mix your foundation colours together to create the perfect match. You can use most colours on black skin as long as it has a high pigmentation. Choose bright colours for the lips, such as reds and deep pinks.

Olive skin

Olive skin can sometimes appear quite sallow. Make sure you choose the correct foundation shade. Avoid pinks and orange tones around the eyes as this can cause a reddening effect and make the eyes look sore. Browns and greens are a very good colour to use around the eyes. Choose warm reds for the lips.

Asian skin

This type of skin can have warm, yellow undertones. Dark circles under the eye area are common in Asians, so use an orange corrective colour to lighten the dark patches. Make sure you mix the foundations to get the required colour. Almond and warm, coffee tones are good for blushers, but make sure you do not make the blusher too dark. Warm colours will be most effective around the eye area – gold, browns and bronzes. For a more dramatic look, choose silver, deep blue and burgundy colours. Use deep berry or brown colours on the lips.

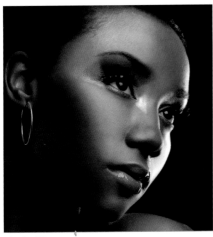

Black skin

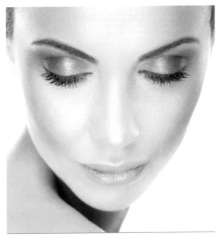

Olive skin

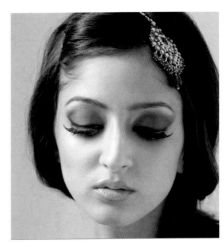

Asian skin

CORRECTIVE MAKE-UP TECHNIQUES

You will need to determine your client's face shape, eye shape and lip shape at the consultation stage. This will enable you to use make-up techniques to alter the shape of the features, giving an illusion of perfection. This is achieved by using **shading** and **highlighting** techniques. You will need to use a colour two shades darker to **diminish** a feature and a colour two shades lighter to **accentuate** a feature. You can highlight or shade using either a powder- or a cream-based product.

Shading
A make-up product/technique that draws attention away from and minimises a facial feature.

Highlighting
A make-up product that draws attention to and emphasises a facial feature.

Diminish
To reduce the appearance, eg to shade down either side of a wide nose to make it appear narrower.

Accentuate
To highlight an area to make it stand out, eg to highlight under the cheekbone to make them stand out.

> **INDUSTRY TIP**
> Use shading to hide any facial features that the client does not like or wants to reduce, eg a hooked nose. Use highlighting to bring out what the client wants to show off, eg high cheekbones.

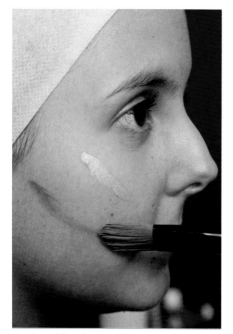

Testing of foundation colour

INDUSTRY TIP

If your client is having their make-up applied for a special occasion and they have already had their hair done, apply a hairgrip instead of a headband so you do not spoil the hairstyle.

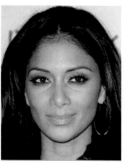

Oval face

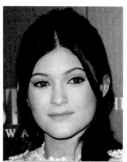

Round face

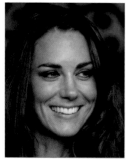

Oblong face

INDUSTRY TIP

Recording your client's eye colour on your consultation form in addition to the eye shape will give you an idea of what colour eyeshadows to use. However, eyeshadow does not have to match the eye colour. It can actually make the eyes look more effective if you contrast the colours.

To determine your client's face shape, eye shape and lip shape, first make sure their hair is away from their face. Clients will often have a hairstyle that disguises their natural face shape. Clients should wear a headband for health and safety regulations in the salon, to protect the hair and to stop any product getting into the hairline.

It is very important that as a make-up artist you have a good eye and a clear understanding of the facial structure, colourings, contouring and highlighting required, particularly when you are applying make-up for a photoshoot.

Place yourself in front of your client and look closely at their face structure to determine the shape. Make sure you tell your client why you need to determine their face shape, and the reason why you will be applying the shading and highlighting techniques. You need to explain this because you can highlight or shade areas of the face you might want to either make more noticeable or hide.

If you are performing a make-up lesson, you will need to instruct your client on how they can achieve the following techniques at home.

ACTIVITY

Practise shading and highlighting on yourself in front of the mirror to learn the techniques required.

Not everyone has the same face shape, or their face might be a mixture of different face shapes. It is generally thought that the perfect face shape is oval because it is symmetrical. Below are the techniques to use for different face shapes.

Oval

This is said to be the perfect face shape. When you are correcting a face shape, this is the shape you should aim to achieve. All you need to do with this face shape is apply blusher to the cheekbones to add definition.

Round

Apply a highlighter to the centre of the face in a narrow strip. This will give the illusion of length. Add shading to the sides of the jaw and temple area, and create a triangle shape under the cheekbone with the point facing towards the nose. Apply blusher to the inner jawbone.

Oblong

Apply shader to the point of the chin and the top hairline to reduce the length. Highlight the temple and lower the jaw to create width. Apply blusher to the outer jawbone.

Square

Apply shader to the angles of the jawbone and create a triangle shape under the cheekbone with the point facing towards the nose. Apply blusher in a circular pattern to the inner cheekbone.

Heart

Apply highlighter to the angles of the jawbone and shader to the point of the chin and the sides of the forehead. Apply blusher under the cheekbone.

Pear

Highlight the forehead, shade the sides of the chin and jawbone. Apply blusher to the whole cheekbone.

ACTIVITY

Practise on your friends and family at home to gain confidence in instructing make-up. If you want a trial run before practising on real people, practise on a mannequin's head first.

ACTIVITY

Look at your friends' and families' faces and try to determine their face shapes.

Techniques to use for eye shapes

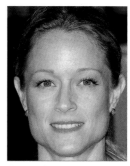

Square face

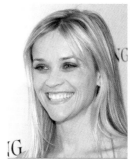

Heart face

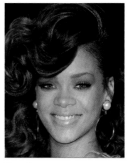

Pear face

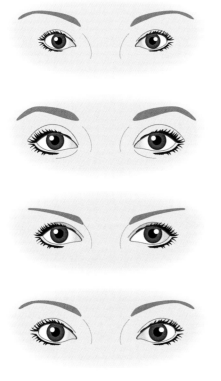

Small eyes – apply a light-coloured shadow all over the eyelid, do not use dark colours as this will make the eyes look smaller. Apply a medium-coloured tone to the outer corners of the eyes and blend upwards and outwards just above the socket line. Apply liner to the outer corners of the eyes, highlight the browbone and apply mascara.

Prominent eyes – apply a dark-coloured shadow to the prominent upper eyelids. Apply a darker shade to the outer section of the eyelids and blend it upwards and outwards. Make sure you highlight the browbone as you want to draw attention to this area. Apply mascara.

Deep set eyes – apply a light-coloured eyeshadow all over the eyelid, then apply a slightly darker tone to just above the socketline and blend lightly upwards. Apply eyeliner or fine shadow underneath the lower lashes and blend. Apply mascara.

Round eyes – apply a light-coloured shadow all over the eyelid, then with a darker shade apply to the outer socketline blending outwards. Apply an eyeliner or shadow to the outer corners of the upper and lower lids. Apply mascara.

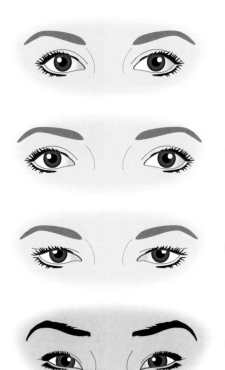

Close set eyes – apply a light-coloured shadow to the inner corners of the eyes, then use a darker shade on the outer corners of the eyes to give a lengthening effect. Apply eyeliner to the outer corners of the upper lid.

Wide set eyes – apply a dark-coloured shadow to the inner section of the eyelids then use a lighter shade on the outer corners of the eyes to give the illusion of bringing the eyes closer together. Apply a dark eyeliner to the inner section of the eyes and apply mascara.

Overhanging eyelids – apply a light-coloured shadow to the middle of the eyelids and apply a darker shade to the socket area and blend it upwards creating a higher crease. Apply mascara.

Oriental eye shape – apply a light-coloured shadow all over the eyelids. With a medium-coloured shadow create a half-moon effect from the top of the lashline up to the socketline. Apply a darker shadow to the outer corners of the lower lashes and blend around the lashline. Apply mascara.

Techniques to use for lip shapes

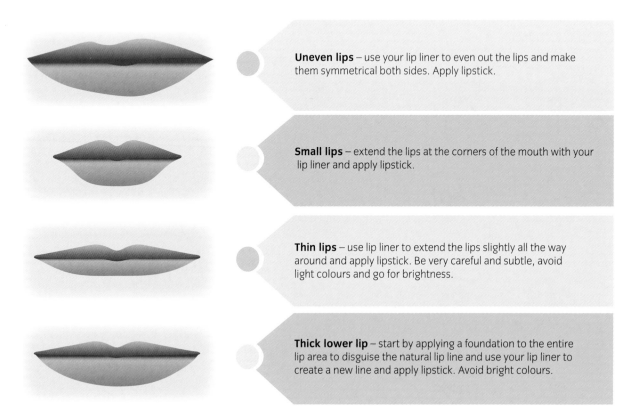

Uneven lips – use your lip liner to even out the lips and make them symmetrical both sides. Apply lipstick.

Small lips – extend the lips at the corners of the mouth with your lip liner and apply lipstick.

Thin lips – use lip liner to extend the lips slightly all the way around and apply lipstick. Be very careful and subtle, avoid light colours and go for brightness.

Thick lower lip – start by applying a foundation to the entire lip area to disguise the natural lip line and use your lip liner to create a new line and apply lipstick. Avoid bright colours.

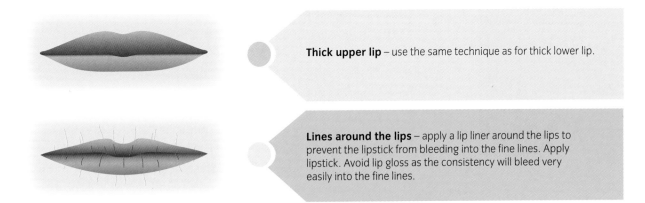

Thick upper lip – use the same technique as for thick lower lip.

Lines around the lips – apply a lip liner around the lips to prevent the lipstick from bleeding into the fine lines. Apply lipstick. Avoid lip gloss as the consistency will bleed very easily into the fine lines.

INDUSTRY TIP

When correcting a lip shape, make sure you do not go too far away from the natural lipline, only enough to gain the correction required.

Techniques to use for nose shapes

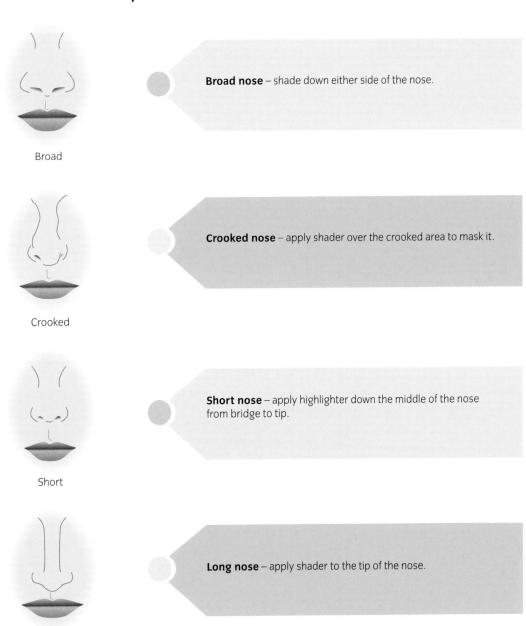

Broad nose – shade down either side of the nose.

Broad

Crooked nose – apply shader over the crooked area to mask it.

Crooked

Short nose – apply highlighter down the middle of the nose from bridge to tip.

Short

Long nose – apply shader to the tip of the nose.

Long

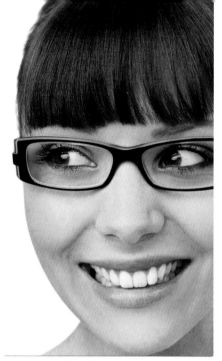

A client wearing glasses

Elasticity

Stretchiness – the skin is made up of elastin fibres, which give it elasticity.

Wrinkles

These form as you age and as your skin loses its elasticity.

Capillaries

Tiny blood vessels with walls, that are one cell thick, can be seen on the surface of the skin.

Glasses and contact lenses

Your client might be wearing glasses or contact lenses. As part of a make-up lesson you can advise the client on how this can affect the make-up routine and different techniques they could use at home.

- If clients wear contact lenses they should avoid mascaras that have a high filament content and loose-particle eyeshadows, as these could both cause irritation to the eye if they come into contact with the eyeball. Small particles could drop into the eye during application.
- When purchasing glasses, clients tend to select a shape and size that complements both their face and eye shape. However, it is important to avoid applying too much mascara and lengthening the lashes as this can cause the lashes to rest on the lens, resulting in irritation.
- If the lenses in the glasses are strong they will give the illusion of magnifying the eyes, making the make-up appear bolder.
- When applying eyeshadow, clients should make the strength of the colour darker so it is seen through the glasses.

Age correction techniques

As well as the factors described above, you also need to consider the client's age. This can have a big impact on the application of make-up and choosing the right products to use on your client's skin. As you get older your skin loses its **elasticity** and fine lines and **wrinkles** start to appear. The appearance of your skin and face shape changes. The colour of the skin becomes more sallow and small, broken **capillaries** might start to form on the cheek and sides of the nose.

You can use corrective make-up, such as a concealer, to hide skin pigmentations, dark circles under the eye area and small broken capillaries. You can also use techniques to lift the appearance of the face, eg by applying a highlighter under the browbone to give the illusion of lifting the eye area and under the cheekbones to define them and give an instant lifting effect. What you do not want to do is use products that will bring out the fine lines or wrinkles. Be very careful when you are applying powder as this will sit in the wrinkles, and try to avoid cream eyeshadows as this will crease into the wrinkles. The graph on the next page illustrates what happens to your skin as you age.

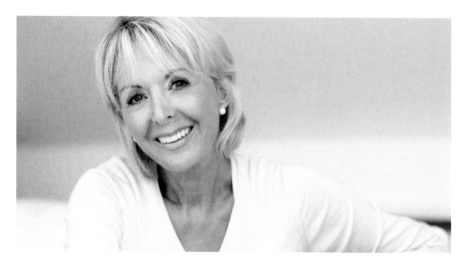

How we age and when it occurs

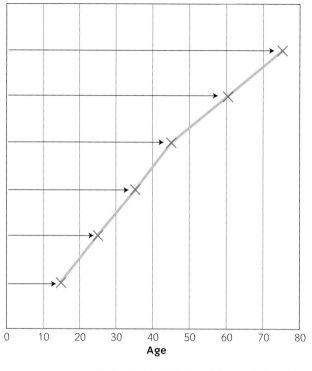

The skin has the appearance of being soft. Deeper lines appear from the corner of the nose towards the lips and from the outer mouth down to the chin. The throat, neck and chest appear are lined, like tissue paper

Wrinkles and fine lines are very visual, pigmentation starts to appear. And sagging worsens around the eye

Wrinkles start to form, skin tends to be more dehydrated, sagging starts around the eye area

Fine lines appear more defined under the eye area with small amounts of loss in elasticity

Fine lines start to appear and pores slightly enlarge

Skin feels soft and smooth. There are no fine lines and pores are small

Aging characteristics (y-axis)

Age (x-axis): 0 10 20 30 40 50 60 70 80

CONTRA-INDICATIONS

Ask your client if they suffer from any contra-indications as these could prevent or restrict you from carrying out the treatment. Remember though, you are not qualified, as a therapist/make-up artist, to diagnose a condition; you can only advise them and ask them to visit their GP for a professional opinion.

You must remember that not all contra-indications are visible. Make sure that you use your communication skills to gain all the information required. If your client is suffering with a contra-indication that might prevent you from performing the treatment but it is not contagious, a letter from the client's doctor giving permission for you to carry out the treatment will be sufficient for you to go ahead. Make sure you attach it to your client's record card.

CONTRA-INDICATIONS THAT PREVENT MAKE-UP TREATMENT

The contra-indications listed in the following table will prevent you from carrying out make-up treatments.

Contra-indication	Why it prevents treatment
Fungal infection	It might make the condition worse or it might be contagious.
Bacterial infection	It might make the condition worse or it might be contagious.
Viral infection	It might make the condition worse or it might be contagious.
Severe eczema	It might make the condition worse.
Severe psoriasis	It might make the condition worse.
Severe skin conditions	Risk of cross-infection.
Eye infections	Risk of cross-infection.

INDUSTRY TIP

Everyone's skin ages slightly differently depending on health, environment, product use and genetics. Our skin is also classed as mature at the age of 25.

INDUSTRY TIP

'Prevent' means you cannot continue with the treatment. 'Restrict' means you can work around the affected area and amend your usual way of working.

HANDY HINTS

Refer to the Anatomy and Physiology chapter for more in-depth understanding of these contra-indications.

CONTRA-INDICATIONS THAT RESTRICT MAKE-UP TREATMENT

The following contra-indications will restrict you from carrying out the treatment. If the contra-indication is visible, you can work around the affected area, using very light pressure.

- broken bones, for example a broken nose would affect the make-up treatment
- recent scar tissue
- hyper-keratosis
- skin allergies
- cuts and abrasions
- skin disorders
- recent fractures and sprains
- undiagnosed lumps and swellings
- product allergies.

 SmartScreen 209 Worksheet 1

APPLY MAKE-UP

Now you know how to set up for the make-up treatment and what tools and equipment you need, you are ready to learn how to apply make-up products.

In this part of the chapter you will learn about:

- products needed and application
- daytime, evening and special occasion make-up
- aftercare advice
- home care advice
- contra-actions.

SmartScreen 209 Worksheet 3

PRODUCTS NEEDED AND APPLICATION

CLEANSERS, TONERS AND MOISTURISERS

Always cleanse, tone and moisturise your client's skin before you apply any make-up. This should not be as in-depth as a facial, but you do need to remove surface dirt. This process **enables** you to clean the skin and remove any existing dirt from the surface. You might ask your client to remove their existing make-up before they come in for a make-up treatment as it will allow you more time on the application. However, some clients/models might feel uncomfortable with this, so be aware of their feelings. Unless they are having a make-up lesson, it is best to ask them to come in with what they normally wear so you can get an idea of their look and their make-up capability. You can also advise them on how to correctly remove their make-up at home. Make sure you analyse your client's skin type so you can perform a quick cleanse and tone with the correct products. Cleansing will remove dirt and existing make-up and a toner will remove any trace of cleanser and close the **pores**.

Enables

Allows you to.

HANDY HINTS

Refer back to Chapter 204/224 Provide facial skin care/facial care for men for more in-depth knowledge and understanding of cleansing, toning and moisturising products.

Pores

Openings in the skin that allow absorption of cosmetics; also secrete oils onto the surface.

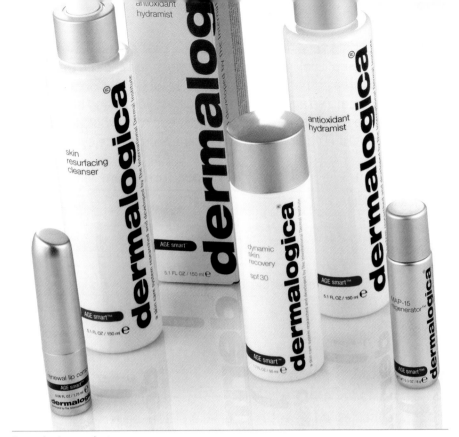

Dermalogica products

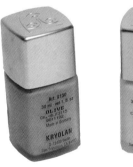
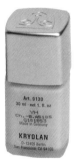

INDUSTRY TIP

Make sure you fill out an in-depth skin analysis chart at the consultation stage to determine the client's skin type and condition. As well as keeping a copy for your records, give your client a copy with detailed product recommendations so they can purchase products in the future without the need for another skin analysis. But remember, skin can change over time so recommend that your client has regular facials.

When you have cleansed and toned, apply a moisturiser to add moisture to the skin and protect it from the environment. It is advisable that your client uses a moisturiser with an SPF as this will protect the skin from pollution and the sun's rays.

When you are performing a make-up lesson, you will need to explain all of the products and techniques listed below as part of the lesson. You are providing a service to enhance the client's image; you are also giving them knowledge and understanding of the different products and techniques available for them to take away and use at home. When you have learned about all the products and techniques below, practise teaching your classmates how to apply them.

BASES

This is applied either before or after the moisturiser but before the foundation. Check the manufacturer's instructions prior to application to see when to apply. It acts as a base for the foundation to adhere to, which will allow it to last a lot longer. It comes either matte or with an iridescent shimmer, which will give your skin a natural glow. Some product ranges have a variety of base primer products that are applied before or after a moisturiser.

CONCEALERS

One of the first products you apply after you have cleansed, toned, moisturised and primed is a concealer. This product hides any imperfections, for example blemishes, dark circles under the eyes and thread veins.

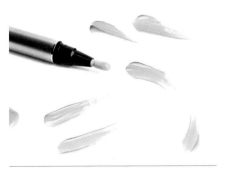

Concealer

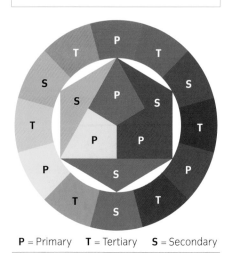

INDUSTRY TIP

A colour wheel can be used to work out how different colours hide blemishes and dark circles.

P = Primary   T = Tertiary   S = Secondary

Primary and secondary colours

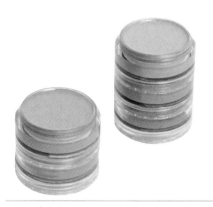

Concealer

INDUSTRY TIP

Use these products with caution – a little goes a long way. Using too much can have the reverse effect and can make your client look ill! You can use these colours mixed in with your foundation to give a subtle effect.

INDUSTRY TIP

Write down the product reference numbers in case your client wants to come back and have the treatment done again, or if the client wants to buy the product at a later date. This will remind you what colours you used last time.

Colour correction is very important to achieve the flawless coverage you desire in a make-up. Looking at the colour wheel, you can see that it gives you the three primary colours and the secondary colours produced by them: red and yellow make orange; yellow and blue make green; and blue and red make purple. With this in mind you can colour-correct redness, dull complexions and darkness under the eyes.

Imperfection	Colour correction
Dull/sallow skin	Violet
Redness	Green
Dark circles	Orange

Concealer products are available in three types:

- stick
- fluid
- compact

Application

1 Use a small soft brush.
2 Apply to the desired areas to create your picture-perfect base.
3 Apply small amounts gradually (you can always apply more if needed).
4 Blend in at the edges.
5 Apply foundation (as stated below), making sure you go carefully over the concealed areas.

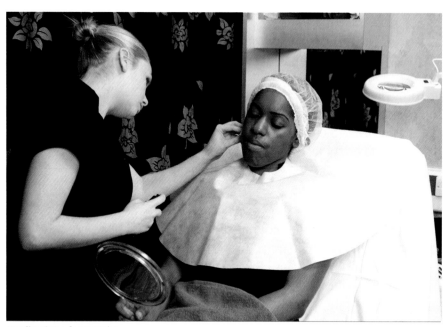

Application of concealer

HIGHLIGHTERS/SHADERS

As explained in the corrective methods section above, highlighters and shaders are used to improve, mask or enhance the shape of the face, nose, eyes and lips. The products are available in three different types:

- cream
- powder
- liquid.

You can use either shaders or highlighters to learn the techniques – it is just a case of what you prefer to use. Both come in a variety of different colours so try them both and find your preference.

Application

Apply the shader or highlighter with a sponge or brush to the areas you need to mask or highlight. Remember to **decant** all of your products with a spatula. The effect will look uneven at this stage as the colours will not match the client's natural skin tone.

FOUNDATIONS

There are many types and colours of foundations within the beauty industry. This is the most important part of your make-up. It is the base (foundation) from which to create an even, smooth and healthy looking skin, adding coverage to hide any imperfections and give a flawless complexion. The different types of foundations on the market are:

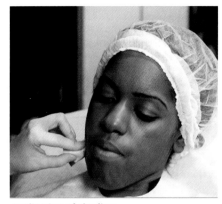

Application of shading

Decant

To pour from one container into another.

Foundation	Reason for use	Skin type
Liquid	This gives a light-to-medium coverage and is either oil or water based depending on the supplier.	Normal/combination.
Cream	This gives you quite a heavy coverage and is oil based.	Normal/dry.
Mousse	This gives a light-to-medium coverage and is oil based.	All skin types light coverage.
Tinted moisturiser	This gives a very light coverage and is kind to the skin, with a high moisture content.	Young men; all skin types.
Mineral	This gives a medium-to-heavy coverage and contains micro-minerals.	All skin types; not great for mature skin.
Two-in-one/ powder	This gives a heavy coverage; applied as a cream then sets as a powder.	Oily.
Stick	This is great for camouflage make-up to cover skin disorders, scars and birthmarks.	Most skin types; not great for mature or very dry skin.
Camouflage	This gives you a thick coverage and is used to hide birth marks, tattoos and skin imperfections, such as hypo- or hyper-pigmentation. Apply with a brush and set with powder.	Problem skin; heavy coverage.
Airbrush	This gives a flawless complexion using the airbrush machine and is great for photographic make-up. Apply by using the airbrush machine and gun; there is no need to apply powder over the top.	All skin types.

INDUSTRY TIP

Remember – two shades lighter than your client's skin tone to *highlight* and two shades darker to *shade*.

Velous hair

Very fine hair that grows on the face and the body.

SmartScreen 209 Worksheet 5

Application

Foundation is professionally applied using a sponge or brush. Both are effective methods of application. Make-up artists tend to use a brush for a thicker application and a more flawless complexion. When you are using a sponge, make sure it is disposable as germs and micro-organisms can bread freely in sponges and could cause cross-contamination.

1 Apply the foundation all over the face and neck to include the eyelids and lips, so you can work from a blank canvas.
2 Make sure you blend the foundation down the neck if it is darker than the natural skin tone for photographic work, and blend into the jawline for day/evening make-up.
3 There is nothing worse than a tidemark where you can see where the foundation stops.
4 Take care when you are blending the foundation around the eyebrows and hairline – try to avoid getting it on the hair as it can add a coloured tinge.

Make sure you have a variety of different-coloured foundations for fair skin, black skin and Asian skin. Everyone has a different skin colour – no skin colour is the same. You might not find a perfect foundation match, in which case mix the foundations together to get the colour required.

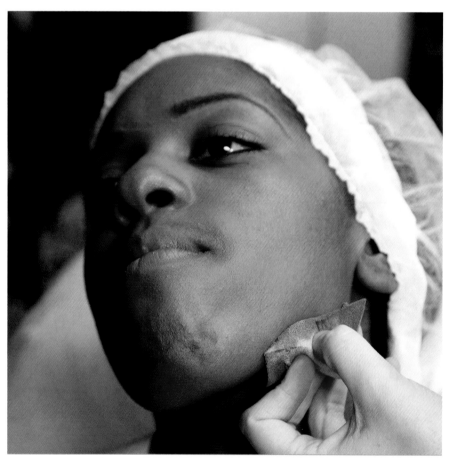

Application of foundation

POWDERS

A powder is an important part of the make-up and comes in different shades for a variety of skin colours. You use a powder to set the foundation and to remove shine from the skin. It also protects the skin from the environment as it acts as a barrier.

There are two main types of powder:

- loose
- compact/pressed.

These come in different varieties as listed in the table.

Powder	Reason for use
Transparent	Allows the colour of the foundation to come through.
Tinted powder	Should match the colour of the foundation exactly.
Bronzing powder	Used to give a sun-kissed look to the skin.
Iridescent powder	Creates a shimmer to the skin; good as a highlighter.

Application

1 Apply a small amount onto your make-up palette and with a powder puff or firm brush.

2 Apply to the skin in a downwards motion in the direction of hair growth to avoid unevenness.

3 Use a matte powder for a daytime look and an iridescent shimmer powder for an evening look.

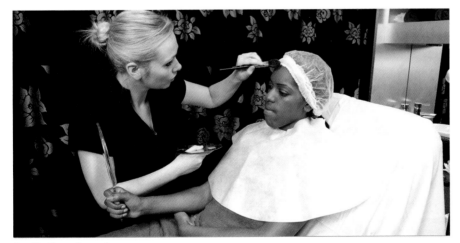

Application of powder

INDUSTRY TIP

You could also use translucent powder under the eye area when you are applying eyeshadow. The powder will collect the unused eyeshadow and this can then be swept away with a fan brush after the eyeshadow is complete. Translucent powder will also set the finished make-up.

BLUSHERS

Blushers come in a range of different colours to emphasise and add contour to the cheekbones and to add colour to the cheeks. You can apply the blusher either after the powder or at the end of the make-up. Choose which method is best suited to you or what you have been taught by your tutor as routines can vary. Blusher comes in three main types:

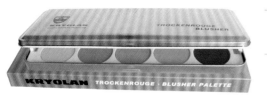

Blusher

Blusher	Reason for use
Powder	This is a mineral-based product used to achieve a lighter tone.
Cream	A wax-based product that smoothes onto the skin; can be applied quite strongly to give a vivid colour; apply prior to powder to prevent unevenness.
Liquid	Comes as a tint and gives a lasting finish; must be applied prior to powder application so it does not create an unevenness on the skin.

Application

Powder blusher

1 Apply powder blusher with a medium sized brush, remembering to **dispense** from container to palette.
2 Place the end of the brush into the product and with the other end of the brush, tap the product down into the bristles to prevent loss of product.
3 Apply to the skin in a light, outward movement from the apple of the cheekbone to the hairline.

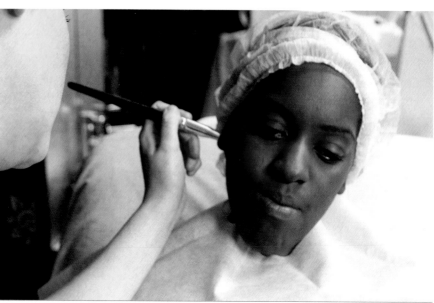

Application of blusher

Cream blusher

1 Apply cream blusher using your fingertips, making sure you dispense first.
2 Dot the cream blusher from the apple of the cheekbone, moving up to the hairline and blend with your fingertips.
3 Always remember to set the cream blush with powder.

Liquid blusher

1 Apply liquid blusher with a small brush.
2 As with the cream blusher, dot the liquid from the apple of the cheekbone, working up to the hairline.
3 Blend with the fingertips then set with powder.

Dispense

Remove the product from its container with a spatula for use on the client.

INDUSTRY TIP

Make sure that you blend the blusher well to prevent harshness.

INDUSTRY TIP

Remember, liquid blush dries very quickly, so apply it and blend straight away to prevent staining.

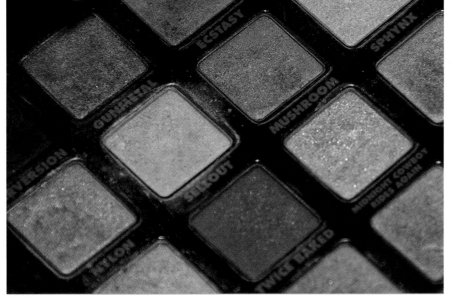

Different-coloured eyeshadows

EYESHADOWS

The reason for using an eyeshadow is to add colour and definition to the eyes. The eyeshadow need not match the eye colour; it can actually make the eyes look more effective if you contrast the colours. For example, you can enhance brown eyes by using green shades and use gold colours around blue eyes to make them look bluer. There are a variety of different eyeshadows and they come in matt, pearlised, metallic or pastel finishes. They also come in different types as described in the table.

Eyeshadow	Description
Compact powders	These can be used on all skin types and come in a vast array of different colours. They are talc based and mixed with oils to give smooth application.
Loose powders	Same as above but the powder is loose rather than compact and has no oil content.
Creams	These can be used on all skin types but are not advisable for use on mature skin as they will collect in the wrinkles and create creasing. Very smooth application; gives a very strong colour.
Crayons	These are very similar to eyeliner but are bigger and can be applied all over the eyelid; again, best avoided with mature skin.

Application

Powder eyeshadow

1 Choose the coloured eyeshadows required and transfer a small amount of each eyeshadow onto the palette.

2 Keep the skin taut using your fingers covered with a tissue to prevent the natural oils in your fingers from dislodging the make-up. Apply the eyeshadows with your chosen brush.

3 Make sure you blend the colours together to create a professional look. Using a blending brush, lightly feather the shadow to prevent the colour from appearing too bold.

4 When you have completed the application of shadow, you can use your fan brush to remove the excess translucent powder from under the eye in a sweeping movement. Do this very gently – you do not want the brush to ingrain the flecks of shadow onto the skin.

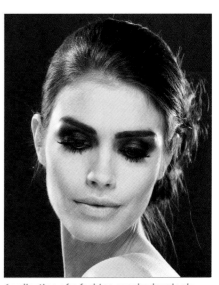

Application of a fashion eyeshadow look

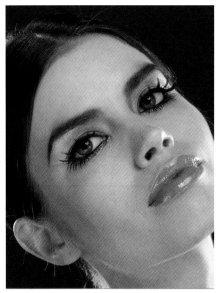

Photographic fashion make-up

Cream eyeshadow

1 You do not need to protect underneath the eye with cream eyeshadow as you will not get small particles falling onto the skin.

2 Select your desired colours and dispense them onto your palette.

3 Keeping the skin taut, apply the eyeshadow with a brush or sponge applicator.

Crayon eyeshadow

1 You do not need to protect underneath the eye with cream eyeshadow.

2 Select your desired colours and either apply them straight from the crayon, making sure you sharpen before and after use and when you change eyes to prevent cross-contamination, or dispense onto a palette using the side of a spatula, then apply with a brush or sponge applicator.

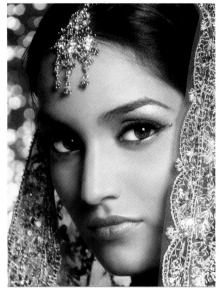

Bollywood fashion make-up

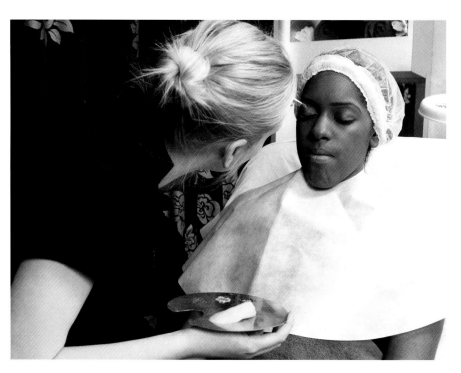

EYE PENCILS/EYELINERS

Eye pencils and eyeliners define and emphasise the eye area. They come in a variety of different colours and types.

Eye pencil/ eyeliner	Description
Liquid liner	Comes in a small container and either has a brush applicator or a nib.
Pencil liner	Made of wax and comes as a pencil.
Gel	An eyeliner that gives you the look of a liquid liner with the ease and feel of a gel formula.
Kohl	A soft powder available in a variety of matte shades. It is most often used in black to outline the eyes. It comes in pencil, pressed powder or loose powder form.
Cake	Comes dry; you need to mix it with a small amount of water to apply.

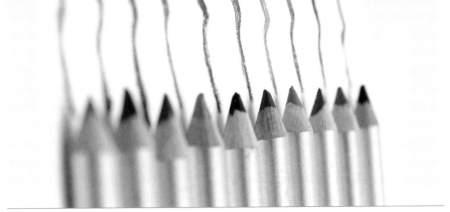

Eyeliners

Application

1 Keeping the skin taut and supported, draw a fine continuous line along the base of the eyelashes either on top or underneath (if you find that your hand is not that steady use small fine strokes).

2 If you are using a pencil, you can smudge the eyeliner to give a softer appearance.

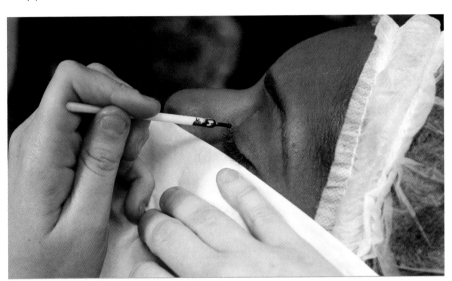

Application of eyeliner

INDUSTRY TIP

Make sure you sharpen the pencil between eyes to prevent any cross-contamination.

EYEBROW PENCILS

These are used to define the eyebrows and add colour and shape. They can create the illusion of thicker eyebrows and can also fill in gaps. Eyebrow pencils are available in three types.

Eyebrow pencil	Description
Pencil	This is made of wax and is firmer than an eyeliner.
Liquid	This is a liquid that is quick-drying on the eyebrows.
Powder	This is a matte powder used with a brush and a stencil to create a perfect brow shape and define the colour.

Application

1 Keeping the skin taut and supported, brush the eyebrows with a clean eyebrow brush to set the brow into place.

2 Choose your desired product and with light strokes apply the liner, liquid or powder to the brow, creating the appearance of a natural browline.

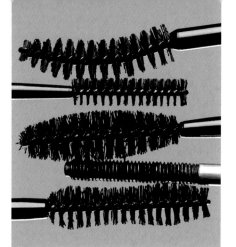
Mascara brushes

MASCARA

Mascara is used to lengthen, enhance, volumise and thicken the natural lashes. There is a wide variety of mascaras that come with different shaped brushes to create different looks. They can be found in a variety of different colours and some are waterproof. There are two types of mascara available:

Mascara	Description
Liquid	This is the most common and most used mascara. It comes in a variety of different colours and is made from a mixture of gum and alcohol.
Cake	This comes in a block form. You need to add water to it before application. It is made from waxes and mineral oils.

Application

1 Using a disposable mascara wand, hold the brush horizontally to the top lashes and coat from the base to the tip. Depending on how thick you want the lashes to be, apply more coats as necessary to gain your desired look. Remember that you can only dip a brush once into the applicator as you do not want to cross-contaminate from one eye to the other, so have three or four disposable brushes to hand.
2 Coat the lower lashes with the mascara wand, using the tip of the wand to get up tight to the base of the lashes.
3 Brush through the lashes with a comb to make sure there are no clumps.

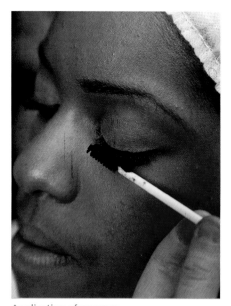
Application of mascara

LIP LINERS

These are used to create a perfect shape and define the lips. They are also used to prevent the lipstick from bleeding into the lines around the mouth.

When you are selecting a lip liner, be sure to find the nearest colour match to your lipstick. If you cannot find a perfect match then choose one that is slightly darker.

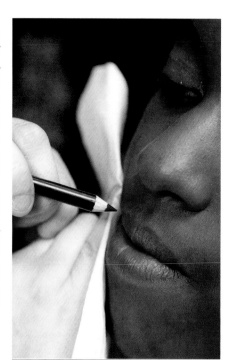
Application of lip liner

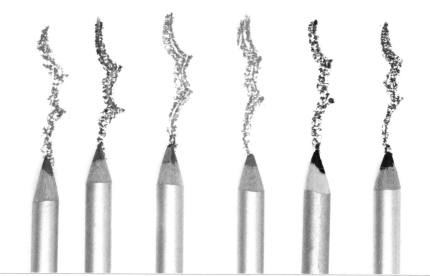
Lip liners

Application

1 Make sure you have sharpened the pencil before use.

2 Apply to the lips to create a **symmetrical** finish.

3 Using small light strokes, work from the tip of the lips down to the sides and underneath.

LIPSTICKS/GLOSSES

These give a **brightening effect** to the lips and can make a real difference to the finished make-up look. A variety of different products are available to create a colour on the lips.

Lipstick/gloss	Description
Lipstick	Made of wax and oils with pigment added to create the desired colour. They often also contain moisturiser to keep the lips soft and smooth. You can get matte or high-shine lipsticks.
Lip gloss	Provides a high shine to the lips and comes in a variety of different colours. You can apply gloss on its own or over lipstick. Lip gloss does not tend to last for long.
Lip balm	Contains beeswax and vitamin C to protect and soften the lips. This can be applied on its own or under lipstick.
Lip tint	This will stain the lips and last for a long time. It comes in a wide range of colours and is made of glycerine and water.

Application

1 Using a disposable lip brush, apply the lipstick/glos/tint within the lines of the lip liner.

2 Blot with a tissue.

3 For more density, apply another coat to get your desired colour.

The flow chart on the right summarises the procedure you should follow when applying make-up for any occasion – daytime, evening, special occasion or photographic.

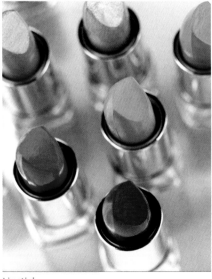
Lipstick

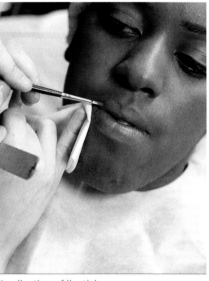
Application of lipstick

INDUSTRY TIP

You will come across different ways of applying make-up. Some might involve applying a highlighter before the foundation and some might involve applying it after. Try both ways and see which you prefer.

Symmetrical

A look that is identical on both sides.

Brightening effect

Adds colour and gloss to create a brighter look.

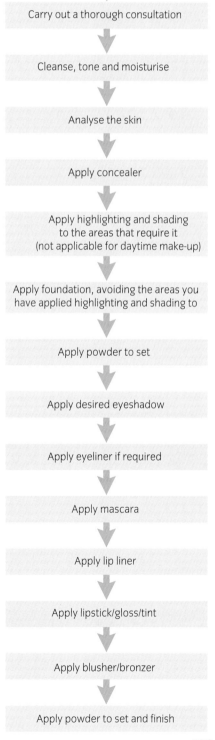

Sanitise your hands

↓

Carry out a thorough consultation

↓

Cleanse, tone and moisturise

↓

Analyse the skin

↓

Apply concealer

↓

Apply highlighting and shading to the areas that require it (not applicable for daytime make-up)

↓

Apply foundation, avoiding the areas you have applied highlighting and shading to

↓

Apply powder to set

↓

Apply desired eyeshadow

↓

Apply eyeliner if required

↓

Apply mascara

↓

Apply lip liner

↓

Apply lipstick/gloss/tint

↓

Apply blusher/bronzer

↓

Apply powder to set and finish

DAYTIME, EVENING AND SPECIAL OCCASION MAKE-UP

You now have all the underpinning knowledge of how to use your equipment and products and how to apply basic make-up. Within this section you will learn how to apply daytime, evening and special occasion make-up and the differences between them.

DAY MAKE-UP

This is a very subtle make-up and should be kept to a minimum. The key things to remember are:

- The foundation should be the same colour as the skin and blend into the neckline perfectly.
- Use light, neutral colours that flatter the natural hair and eye colour. Avoid strong colours as natural daylight really emphasises colour and can make dark tones appear darker.
- The mascara should be the same colour as the client's lashes, but this also depends on your client's preferences.
- Eyeliner can be used but make sure it is blended and not too strong.
- Apply lip liner and lipstick in a natural colour unless your client is used to darker, brighter colours.

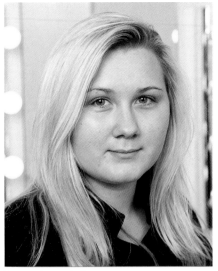

Day make-up: before

EVENING MAKE-UP

Ask your client what kind of lighting they are going to be in as this will have different effects on the colours you are applying (look back at the information on different lighting to recap). Artificial lighting dulls colour, so if your client is going to be under artificial lighting, choose brighter colours. The key things to remember for evening make-up are:

- Highlight and shade the contours of the face and highlight around the eye area as this will diminish shadows caused by artificial lighting.
- Add darker blush and emphasise the cheekbones with an iridescent highlighter.
- Apply darker/brighter tones around the eyes.
- You can also use a shimmer frosted shadow as this looks beautiful under artificial lighting.
- Apply darker mascara and also apply extra coats to make the lashes appear longer and thicker.
- There are also several high-fashion-coloured mascaras that can be used in an evening make-up – purples, blues and greens – these will really electrify the look.
- Apply thicker, darker eyeliner to frame the eyes and open them up.
- You can apply any lip colour as long as it matches the rest of the make-up. Apply a high gloss over the top.

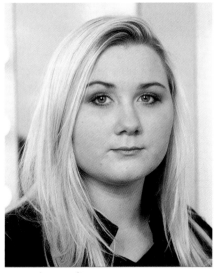

Day make-up: after

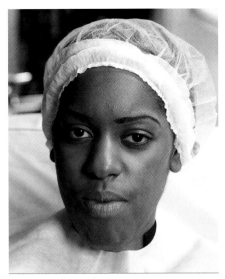

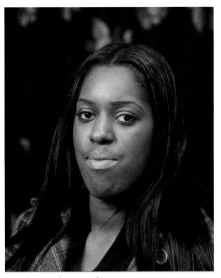

Evening make-up: before

Evening make-up: after

SPECIAL OCCASION MAKE-UP

A special occasion, such as a wedding or prom, is an important event for your client, so they want to look dazzling. You need to sit down initially with your client and find out exactly what their needs are. As it is a special occasion, it is a really good idea to have your client in for a trial run. It gives your client piece of mind and assurance that they are going to be happy with the end result. It gives you a chance to see the colours your client is wearing and to have more of an idea of what event it is, what type of lighting it will be in and how long it will be worn for. When you have all of this information from your client, you can choose the make-up that you think will best suit them.

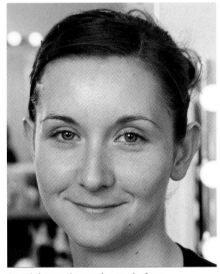

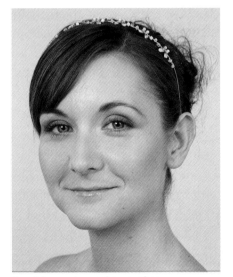

Special occasion make-up: before

Special occasion make-up: after

INDUSTRY TIP

Remember, if you are applying the make-up for a bride, be sure to talk through with her exactly what she wants, as she will still want to look at herself in the photos. Going over the top will not please your client, even if you think it looks great! When she is having her make-up applied, make sure she is not wearing something she needs to take off over her head as this could spoil the make-up.

AFTERCARE ADVICE

Upon completion of the treatment, it is important you give the appropriate aftercare advice to make sure the client is able to maintain the results. Giving aftercare advice is very important as it gives your client the confidence in themselves to go away and maintain the results. These are the main aftercare advice points you should give to your client at the end of their make-up treatment. Make sure you sit them down and advise them face-to-face, letting them ask questions at any time.

- Do not touch the face.
- Come back in for a make-up lesson.
- Book in for an eyelash tint or eyebrow shape.

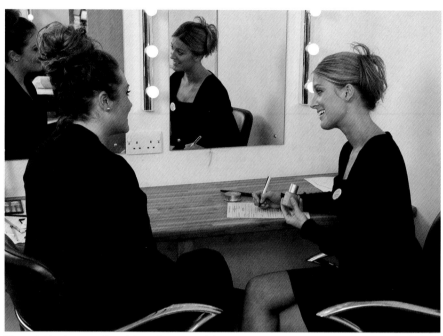

Therapist/make-up artist giving aftercare advice

HOME CARE ADVICE

Homecare advice is also given to every client but is more specific to their individual needs and will include product recommendations and advice on removal and reapplication techniques. It is the advice you offer your clients so they can use the techniques at home to complement the treatment. Here is a list of the home care advice you should give your client for make-up treatments:

- Cleanse, tone and moisturise twice a day.
- Apply eye cream/gel morning and night.
- Use a brush/sponge to apply foundation and sterilise it after each use.
- Do not pump the wand in the mascara container as this will introduce air and dry the product out.
- Look at the 'use by' dates on products. They usually only have a 12-month period for use once opened.
- Use a base (primer) under foundation for lasting effect.
- Use a moisturiser and/or foundation with an SPF of at least 15 to protect your skin from the environment.
- Use colours that complement you and meet your objectives.
- Use a lip pencil prior to lipstick to stop the colour bleeding.
- Use a lip balm daily.
- When removing make-up, make sure you are careful around the eye area. Do not stretch the skin.

ACTIVITY

Design an advice leaflet for your clients to take away with them, listing all the aftercare and home care advice.

CONTRA-ACTIONS

A contra-action is something that could happen to cause a problem during or after a make-up treatment. If your client suffers from a contra-action, advise them to seek medical attention by contacting their GP if it is severe. You must also inform the salon. If a client experiences a contra-action during a make-up treatment, you should:

- stop the treatment
- remove the product.

The table describes some of the most common contra-actions that follow make-up treatments.

Contra-action	Cause/prevention
Severe erythema	A dilation of blood capillaries at the surface of the skin, making them visible. This is caused by friction or if the skin is irritated. If this occurs apply a cold compress to the affected area.
Allergic reaction – rash; swelling; irritation	Your client might react adversely to a product you are using within your treatment. If this occurs, remove the product straight away and apply a cold compress. If the problem persists, suggest your client seeks medical advice.
Perspiration	If your client is perspiring during the make-up application, dab the area gently with a dry tissue, trying to avoid the removal of products that are already on the skin. Advise your client to keep a pack of tissues with them and not to rub or wipe too harshly over the areas that are perspiring. Application of powder will take away any shine on the skin surface but there are no products that will prevent you from perspiring.
Watery eyes	Some clients might have very sensitive eyes that will water very easily. Make sure you work around the eye very carefully; try not to spend to much time on the eye area if they are prone to watery eyes. Avoid direct light shining into your client's eyes. Make sure your client is not allergic to any of the products you will be using around the eye area. If the eyes do water, take a dry tissue and dab the tear away, being careful not to take away the make-up you have already applied. Avoid cotton wool pads as these contain filaments that could irritate the eye more.

ACTIVITY

Create a glossary of words or terms you are unsure about and keep it at the front of your portfolio so you can refer to it when you are unsure about something. Pictures would help in this.

 SmartScreen 209 Worksheet 7

PREPARE FOR MAKE-UP INSTRUCTION

Your clients will come into the salon to get advice from you on how to apply their own make-up at home. This is different to your client just coming into the salon for a special occasion as you will not be applying the make-up, just instructing them in how to apply it themselves at home.

When you are giving instruction on make-up application, it is not necessarily just about the application. Some people might want to find out what colours best suit them or how to use certain products to get the maximum results. You will usually get the client to apply the make-up themselves in front of a mirror, with your help step-by-step. Alternatively you can apply make-up to one side of the client's face and then instruct the client in doing the same the other side. There is little point in you applying it for them as they are unlikely to be able to achieve the same look when they get home.

In this part of the chapter you will learn about:

- reasons for a make-up lesson
- make-up lesson procedure.

REASONS FOR A MAKE-UP LESSON

Your client might want:

- advice on application – they might not have worn make-up before
- to change their appearance
- to be able to follow the trends
- to find out what colours suit them most
- to find out how to create a look they have seen on TV or in a magazine
- to increase their confidence.

When you have gained all the information you require from your client at the consultation stage, explain to your client what you will be doing throughout their make-up lesson. Do not forget that your client might be quite nervous, so put them at ease.

MAKE-UP LESSON PROCEDURE

This is only a guide to help you; your tutor might teach you a different routine. There is no right or wrong, as long as your instructions are clear and the client is happy.

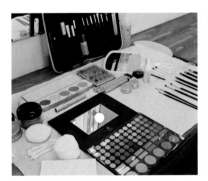

STEP 1 – Prepare for the treatment – lay out all of the tools, equipment and products you will be using and explain to your client what they all are and how you would use them.

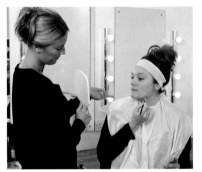

STEP 2 – Give your client a mirror and talk through their needs with them. What are their expectations of their make-up lesson? Explain the importance of looking after their skin and applying a cleanser, toner and moisturiser before make-up.

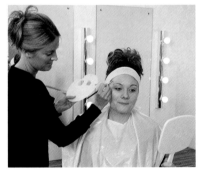

STEP 3 – Explain to your client the application of a concealer and why this is applied to the skin prior to foundation.

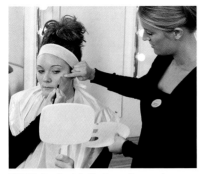

STEP 4 – Explain the importance of shading and highlighting – how to give the illusion of a perfect face shape; how to hide unattractive features and enhance attractive features.

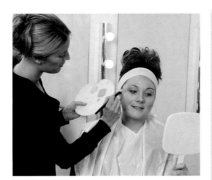

STEP 5 – Apply shader and highlighter to one side of your client's face, then allow your client to do the same on the other side, with your instruction. (Depending on preference you can do step 6 before step 5.)

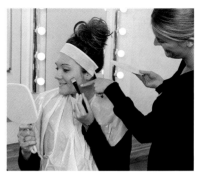

STEP 6 – Explain to your client the best way to choose the correct foundation colour by applying it to the jawline and blending it to match the natural colour of their own skin tone.

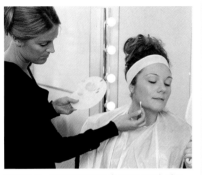

STEP 7 – Instruct your client to apply the foundation to their skin and blend into the neckline.

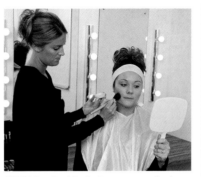

STEP 8 – Explain the importance of using powder and instruct your client to apply it in a downwards motion.

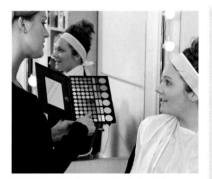

STEP 9 – Talk to your client about the colours they would normally choose and what they would usually apply at home. Give them advice on colours that would enhance their eye colour and skin tone. Ask them about the type of eye make-up they want instruction in. Is it for daytime, evening or a special occasion?

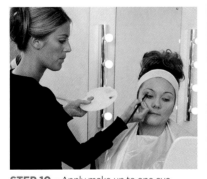

STEP 10 – Apply make-up to one eye, talking through your techniques and your colour choices. Instruct the client in applying the same techniques and colours to the other eye themselves.

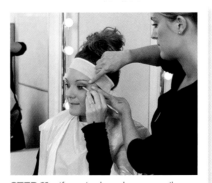

STEP 11 – If required, apply eye pencil or liquid liner to one eye, explaining to the client the different looks it can give and how it can enhance features. Allow your client to apply the same to the other eye.

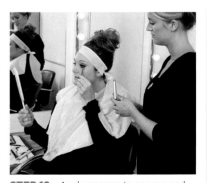

STEP 12 – Apply mascara to one eye and explain to your client the different types of mascaras available and how they produce different looks. Allow your client to apply mascara to the other eye.

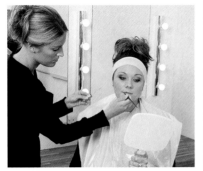

STEP 13 – Explain to your client the different types of lip products available and the different looks they can achieve. Also advise your client that you can correct lip shapes using different techniques.

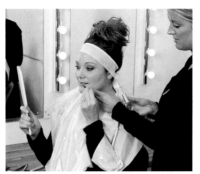

STEP 14 – Apply lip pencil and lipstick/gloss to one side of the lips, then get your client to apply the same techniques to the other side.

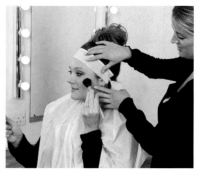

STEP 15 – Explain the different types of blushers available and what looks they achieve. Apply blusher to one side of the face and allow your client to do the same on the other side, instructing them all the time.

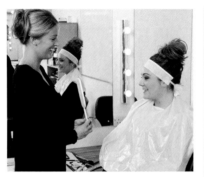

STEP 16 – Allow your client to look in the mirror for a couple of minutes to digest the make-up and to think of any questions they want to ask.

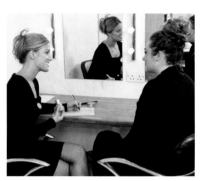

STEP 17 – Allow your client to ask you as many questions as they want. Make sure you clarify the procedure with your client step-by-step. In addition to verbally telling your client, write the procedure down for them, together with the colours and techniques used.

INDUSTRY TIP

If your client would like ideas on different looks, a good idea would be to start off with a day look and then turn it into an evening look, always allowing them to apply it themselves on one side.

INDUSTRY TIP

Make sure that you write down every product you have used and instructions on how you have applied it so that your client can refer to it when they get home.

INDUSTRY TIP

Talking through the make-up look with your client gives you a great opportunity to sell the products you have used on your client.

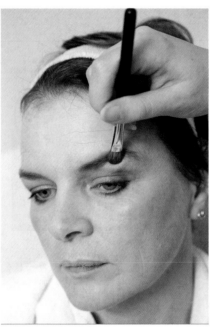

Instructing the client

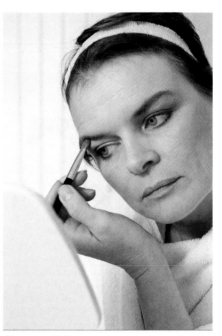

Client practising

ACTIVITY

Make your own techniques guide with hints on how to create different looks, for example smokey eyes, evening eyes and day eyes.

PROVIDE PHOTOGRAPHIC MAKE-UP

For make-up artists, the opportunity to create a photographic look is very exciting. It might be a high-fashion shoot for a catwalk show or a family photograph – either way you will have to make sure you listen to the photographer and get along with them.

Here are some situations when you might need to create photographic make-up:

- A professional magazine shoot or catwalk show, where your client/ model wants to look completely flawless.
- A personal shoot, at a professional photographer's studio, where you will create the perfect look for your models/clients with family, friends or just on their own.
- A catalogue shoot, where your client/model is advertising clothes or accessories.
- A showcase, where the pictures will be mounted and displayed to advertise a company brand, or could also be used for a billboard or advertisement on the sides of buses.
- Competition work, where you would be competing with others within the make-up industry.
- A total look, where the make-up should always match the clothes and accessories of the model. Refer to Chapter 212 Create an image based on a theme within the hair and beauty sector for more information on total looks.

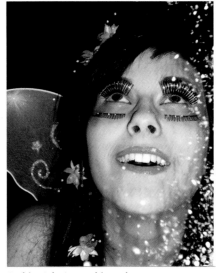

Fashion/photographic make-up

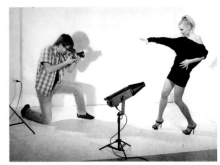

A photoshoot

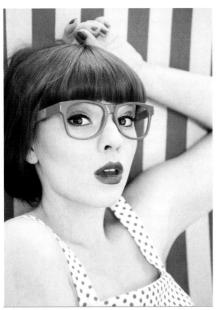

Fashion photogaphic make-up

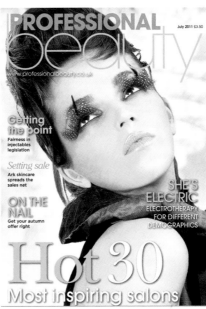

High fashion photogaphic make-up

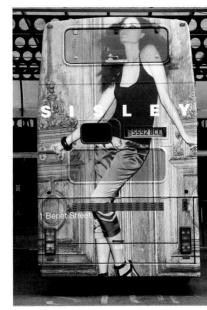

Advertising make-up

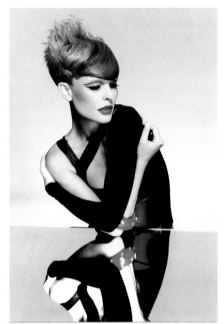

Professional photoshoot

In this part of the chapter you will learn about:

- the purpose of the shoot
- mood boards
- getting ready for a shoot
- black-and-white photography
- lighting for photographic make-up
- backdrops
- evaluating the make-up treatment.

PURPOSE OF THE SHOOT

You will need to get the full brief from the client prior to the shoot (the client is the company the model is modelling for) and you will need to know exactly what they require for the model. The make-up is a very important part of the image. If the model looks good it will sell the product. For example, if the photoshoot is advertising a fun, colourful object, the model's make-up should also be fun and colourful, or if it is advertising a horror book, the make-up should be very dark and gothic.

ACTIVITY

Cut out pictures from magazines and build up a scrapbook of different looks and ideas to show your clients.

Applying make-up for a photoshoot is very personal. Your client has to be happy and confident with their make-up and the way they look, as they might be purchasing their pictures at the end of the day for their own personal use. If it is a model they will be sending the photos to an agency or an advertising company. You do not want them to look like a completely different person, which they might not feel comfortable with. Gain as much information as you can from your client prior to the application and keep them updated throughout so they can see what you are doing.

Your client will have a clear picture in their mind of what they would like. As a make-up artist you are there to provide advice and guidance.

MOOD BOARD

You will need to plan and develop a mood board for your photographic make-up look. The main purpose for creating a mood board is to present the collective ideas from the research you have undertaken; showing the journey from where you obtained your inspiration to creating your image. You will then be able to sit down with your client/model to discuss the required look. A mood board is not set in stone; it is a board full of inspirational ideas, pictures and write-ups that you discuss with your model/client to get an overall picture for the look. You would normally create two boards – one 'before' board with all your ideas and another 'after' board that you can compile when you have discussed all the ideas and have come up with the look. You can then take the second board with you to the photoshoot.

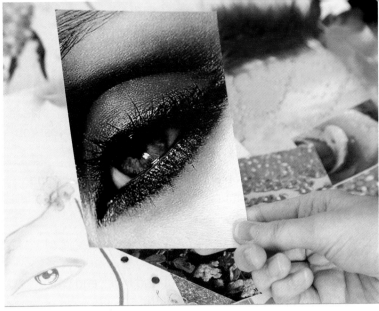
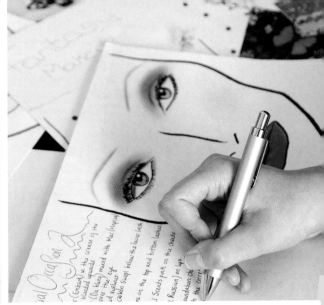

Creating a mood board

GETTING READY FOR A SHOOT

There is a lot to think about and prepare when you are applying make-up for a photoshoot:

- Make sure you are fully prepared the night before the shoot, and that you have all necessary products, tools and equipment. If you are working on location there is no going back as you might be in the middle of a field or on top of a mountain. You need to have a clear idea of the photoshoot before you arrive on location so you can pack everything you need.
- What will your model be wearing? Will you need to do their make-up before or after they get changed? How will their hair will be fashioned? For example, are they having a headpiece applied?
- Health and safety is very important, so make sure you follow the health and safety regulations at all times.
- What will you have as a workstation? Will you have one? Or will you need to bring your own?
- Is it an outdoor shoot? Will you need to be undercover?
- Is it an indoor shoot? Will they have electricity?
- What is the theme (so you can design your mood board)?
- What clothing will be worn? Will you need to match the make-up?
- What accessories will be used? Is the model wearing accessories that will affect your application of make-up?
- Will the weather impact upon the choice of make-up? What time of year is it? The photoshoot might be outside. If it is raining you might need to apply a waterproof mascara or set the make-up with a waterproof spray. You also need to be aware of the lighting outside.
- How many models are there (so you can allow enough time for each one)?

BLACK-AND-WHITE PHOTOGRAPHY

As you become more skilled at applying make-up you will start to focus more on shades and tones. These are particularly important in black-and-white photography. If the photoshoot is to be in black and white, it is a good idea to use neutral colours on the eyes, such as browns,

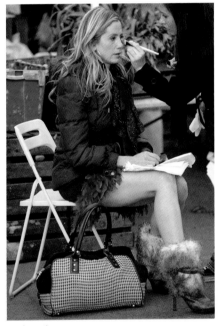

On location

INDUSTRY TIP

Make a list of everything you need to remember to pack in your box if you are going out on location.

INDUSTRY TIP

Be aware of the weather outside if you are on location. Always wrap up warm and take an umbrella with you as a precautionary measure.

INDUSTRY TIP

You need to make sure your model's make-up is flawless. The lens will pick up every speck of dust, so make sure you check with the photographer before they start snapping.

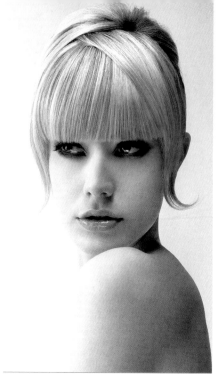

Black-and-white make-up

209/211/220 MAKE-UP APPLICATION/INSTRUCTION

INDUSTRY TIP

When you are working with colour images, ask the photographer to also take the photo as a black-and-white image so you can get used to the different tones the colours achieved.

Accentuate

To highlight an area to make it stand out, eg to highlight under the cheekbone to make them stand out.

INDUSTRY TIP

Always have your products with you so you can top up your make-up throughout the photoshoot. Your model might be there for some time.

INDUSTRY TIP

Powder application should be kept to a minimum over wrinkled skin as well as hairier areas, such as the sides of the face and upper lips, as this will show through a camera lens.

blacks, creams and greys, as it is a lot easier to judge their tone level. Reds and browns are the best colours to use on the lips as they are vibrant and will show up in black and white.

Make sure you contour the face; it is usually advisable to go four shades darker than your model's skin tone so it will show up in the photos. You can also go up to four shades lighter when highlighting.

Always use matte colours when you are creating a look for black-and-white photography; shimmery colours will look very dull and lifeless in the photo.

ACTIVITY

Take a photo of your make-up palette in colour and black and white so you can see the differences in tones of each of the colours.

LIGHTING FOR PHOTOGRAPHIC MAKE-UP

Outdoor light varies according to the time of day and this will change the colour of your make-up when photographed. Here are a few hints to help you gain an understanding of the effects of morning, afternoon, evening and studio lighting.

MORNING LIGHTING

Apply soft tones to enhance your surroundings. At this time of the day make-up will photograph darker than it will appear to the natural eye because the light is soft. Choose a fluid foundation to get that dewy look. Choose soft, warm tones for the eyes, remembering not to apply them too strongly as the lighting will **accentuate** the colours. Lips should be kept light, soft and natural looking.

AFTERNOON LIGHTING

This is the best light to be photographed in as afternoon light is at its most golden. It will give a softer, warmer look to your make-up so you can go slightly more dramatic. You can apply more colours at this time of day and use darker shades on the eyes and cheek. Lip colour can also be stronger.

EVENING LIGHTING

This time of day allows you to go very dramatic as evening light will give way to darkness. Most photographers will use a flashlight at this time of day, which has a tendency to wash away colour, so make sure that you apply the products quite liberally.

STUDIO LIGHTING

When you are filming in a studio, the lighting tends to make the area get very hot. Make sure you are there at all times so you can apply powder to any shiny areas. The photographer will tell you when they look through their lens if they can see any shadows or shine.

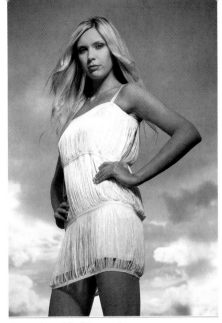
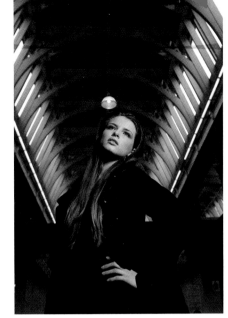

Examples of fashion make-up

BACKDROPS

When working in a photographic studio, you need to be aware of the different backdrops and what colour backdrop your model will be photographed in front of. The most common backdrops used within photography are:

- Black – with a black background make sure your model's make-up is strong as the black will fade the colours that you apply.
- White – this will show every imperfection that your model has; make sure that the contouring and foundation application is flawless.

The photographer is very important. You must always listen to them as they are the professional looking through the camera lens and they can see every imperfection. They will also be able to shoot the model in the best lighting and position. Always ask to see the pictures after the first couple of takes so you are both happy with the results.

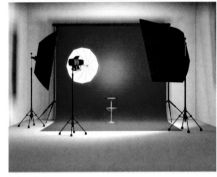

A backdrop

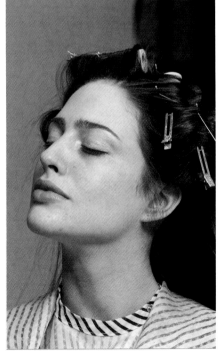

High fashion: before

High fashion: after

Constructive

To be able to give feedback to enable people to improve.

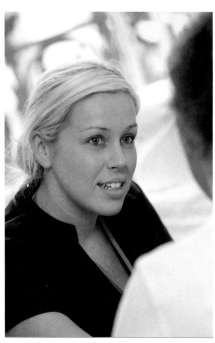

Evaluating the make-up service

The procedure for the application of photographic make-up is the same as when applying make-up for a day, evening or special occasion. The only differences are that the make-up has to be completely flawless and contouring of the face can be made darker by two shades. You might also need to apply the make-up for the eyes and lips slightly thicker, depending on what lighting your model/client is being photographed in. Try to avoid shimmer/glitter as this will just look like a sheen on the face.

EVALUATING THE MAKE-UP TREATMENT

During your preparation you will need to evaluate how well your photographic look is progressing. After the event you will need to evaluate the service provided and whether it met with the expectations of the client. You will also need to evaluate the effectiveness of your make-up instruction.

You will have the opportunity to both offer and receive **constructive** verbal feedback from meetings with the model/client during the planning process. Always listen to this feedback as it will help you to develop and improve your skills.

You will receive feedback from your tutors and, occasionally, from your peers too. When you have worked hard on a task and someone criticises you, constructively or otherwise, it can hurt. Do not take it to heart – consider how you can benefit from the feedback. If the overall results improve because of the comments/feedback you receive, then you have learnt something and progressed with your skills; this can only be a positive outcome.

SELF-EVALUATION

Throughout the whole of the process – the planning, constructing and developing your mood board and creating your look to be photographed – you should be evaluating yourself. You will be using a combination of technical skills, some of which you might not have used together before. You will be learning new skills along the way and you should evaluate your progress. Often in life, we are our own worst critics, so keep a diary/journal of how you felt as you planned and created a photographic look or completed your instruction on make-up application.

TEST YOUR KNOWLEDGE

Use the questions below to test your knowledge of Chapter 209/211/220 to see how much information you have retained. These questions will help you to revise what you have learnt in this chapter.

Turn to page 601 for the answers.

1. Which **one** of the following skin tones would benefit from a green concealer and beige foundation?
   a) Red
   b) Peach
   c) Beige
   d) Sallow

2. Which **one** of the following is the main reason why lipstick should be applied with a brush?
   a) To maintain hygiene
   b) To be able to apply more than one coat
   c) It gives even application
   d) To be able to blend colours

3. Which **one** of the following skin types/conditions is a cream blusher most suitable for?
   a) Sensitive skin
   b) Dry skin
   c) Oily skin
   d) Normal skin

4. A natural make-up is usually created under the category of:
   a) an evening make-up
   b) a special occasion make-up
   c) a day make-up
   d) an avant-garde make-up.

5. Which type of lighting contains the colours blue and green and gives a cool effect on make-up?
   a) Incandescent
   b) White
   c) Natural
   d) Fluorescent

6. Shading can be used to achieve which **one** of the following?
   a) Draw attention away from and minimise a feature
   b) Draw attention to and enhance a feature
   c) Cover a prominent feature
   d) Change the colour of a product

7. For which **one** of the following face shapes would this corrective make-up be applied? Apply a highlighter to the centre of the face and shade at the sides of the jawline and hairline.
   a) Round
   b) Oval
   c) Heart
   d) Oblong

8. A light colour used over the entire lid would benefit which **one** of the following eye shapes?
   a) Small
   b) Wide set
   c) Prominent
   d) Deep set

9. Which **one** of the following lip shapes would benefit most from the use of a dark lip colour?
   a) Full lips
   b) Uneven lips
   c) Thin lips
   d) Small lips

10. Which **one** of the following nose shapes would benefit from the application of shader to the tip?
    a) Wide
    b) Short
    c) Long
    d) Broken

11. Which **one** of the following is the main purpose of a face powder?
    a) To give a flawless finish
    b) To give a matte finish
    c) To set the make-up
    d) To apply an SPF protector

12. A foundation brush can be used to:
    a) mix foundation colours
    b) apply loose powder over the foundation
    c) blend and remove streaking in foundation
    d) apply foundation to the skin.

13. Which **one** of the following SPFs is recommended for daily use to protect the skin?
    a) SPF 6
    b) SPF 10
    c) SPF 15
    d) SPF 30

14. Which **one** of the following describes the main reason why a lip balm should be recommended to the client?
    a) To prevent chapped lips
    b) To help lipstick last longer
    c) To keep their lips soft and rehydrated
    d) To give a smooth surface for lipstick to be applied to

15. Where is the most effective place to test the colour of a foundation on your client's skin?
    a) Wrist
    b) Temple
    c) Jawline
    d) Cheekbone

16. Which **one** of the following contra-indications will prevent a make-up treatment?
    a) Blushing
    b) Acne vulgaris
    c) Recent piercing
    d) Scar tissue

17. Which **one** of the following should be avoided when applying make-up to an elderly client?
    a) Iridescent colours
    b) Cream blusher
    c) Cool colours
    d) Lip liner

18. When applying photographic make-up for morning light conditions, which **one** of the following should you do?
    a) Apply products liberally
    b) Apply extra powder
    c) Use darker eye colours
    d) Use soft, warm eye colours

19. Which **one** of the following is the main reason why shimmer should be avoided when applying photographic make-up?
    a) It will make the skin look oily
    b) It will give a sheen to the finish
    c) It will have a lightening effect
    d) It will highlight the look

20. What type of make-up should be used to get the best effect from a black-and-white photo?
    a) Shimmery
    b) Frosted
    c) Matte
    d) Dark

21. What effect will a black backdrop have on the appearance of make-up?
    a) It will fade the colours
    b) It will highlight imperfections
    c) It will enhance (brighten) the colours
    d) It will hide imperfections

22. What effect will the flash on a camera have on an evening make-up?
    a) It will reflect any shine
    b) It will wash out the colours
    c) It will exaggerate the colours
    d) It will highlight flaws

CASE STUDY: JENNIFER LENARD

I started out as a competitive ice skater, going on to become an ice-skating teacher and then a performer in various ice shows. I toured the world performing in skating roles and took every opportunity offered to learn new skills. Alongside performing I helped out with making and fixing the costumes and props and with dressing the performers and setting their wigs. I also took some make-up training and loved it so much I decided to change my career.

Following unpaid work experience on film sets and in the theatre, I landed my first paid job for the BBC and have since worked on period dramas, soap operas and films. Once I was even part of a BAFTA-winning team for make-up and hair! I went on to teach make-up application and hair styling, and really enjoyed passing my knowledge onto keen students. It makes me feel very proud to see them working as successful make-up artists in their own right. I also became a member of the Habia Skills team and was involved in writing the standards for Habia.

I now run my own make-up academy (The Biz Media Make-Up and Hair Academy, in Derbyshire) and The Biz Wigs Ltd. We make and supply wigs for film and television, as well as providing NHS approved wigs to cancer and alopecia patients.

As a make-up artist you get to do so many different things, including meeting lots of interesting people and working in some amazing places. Although it might seem very glamorous, be prepared for unsociable hours, split shifts and all kinds of weather conditions! Despite all that, working as a make-up artist is a very rewarding job and I feel very lucky to be doing something I love.

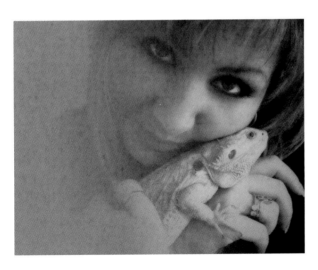

212

CREATE AN IMAGE BASED ON A THEME WITHIN THE HAIR AND BEAUTY SECTOR

Creating an image based on a theme is a chance to show off your creativity and really have some fun. Let your imagination run wild. Go out and take inspiration from all around you – the countryside, the buildings in the town centre, art and media, or just people-watch at a train station. Ideas will come to you in a flash. However, to create the overall image, you will need to work hard, plan effectively and have a vision in your head that you can transform onto a mood board; eventually creating the image for real. Do not forget to enjoy yourself and photograph your work as you progress with your theme.

In this chapter you will learn how to:

- plan an image
- create an image.

PLAN AN IMAGE

You must plan an image before you can create it. This means doing your research and creating a **mood board**, but it is still important to pay attention to health and safety regulations and consultation techniques.

In this part of the chapter you will learn about:

- health and safety
- planning for the event
- professional consultation.

HEALTH AND SAFETY

The main legislation covered within this chapter are:

- **PPE**
- Health and Safety at Work Act
- COSHH.

As with all previous chapters, the health and safety of you, your client (or model in some instances) and those around you is vital! Preparing for a fashion show, a themed event or planning a special occasion naturally puts you under pressure as there are deadlines and time scales that need to be met. However, you must always follow health and safety legislation.

PREPARING YOUR WORK AREA

Wherever your event is taking place, some of the work is likely to take place in the salon. Of course this is not always the case – it could also be a competition setting or out on location.

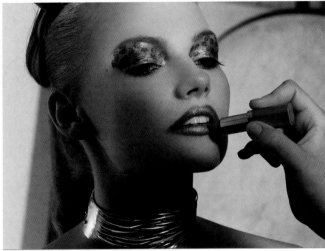

Creating an image

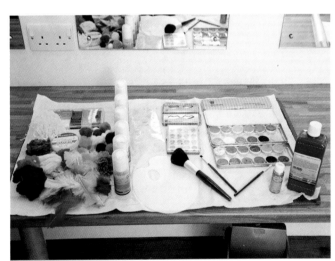

A set up of your station ready to create your image

When you are preparing the salon for your client's or model's arrival, the usual standards of safety and hygiene need to be **adhered** to. Make sure that your work area is clean, hair free and sterilised before starting. Wipe the chairs and work surfaces down with hot soapy water and spray with disinfectant. Prepare your tools and equipment, making sure they have been cleaned and sterilised prior to use or packing them in your **day-box**.

Mood board

This is where you apply all of your ideas onto a board, using pictures and written explanations of what you are going to achieve with your look. We will look at creating your mood board later on in the chapter.

PPE

Personal protective equipment.

SmartScreen 212 Worksheet 2

HANDY HINTS

Refer back to Chapter 202 Follow health and safety practice in the salon for more in-depth knowledge and understanding on legislation, sterilisation and disposal of waste.

Adhered

Followed or stuck to.

Day-box

A small container where you pack all your small tools and equipment that are needed on a day-to-day basis, for example a moulding tool, spatula, brushes, spirit gum, acetone, etc.

If you are working off-site (ie not in a salon), take spray sterilisers with you; make sure your tools and equipment are always cleaned and ready for each model/situation. When you are using electrical equipment in the salon or off-site, make sure that they are in good working order. Check the wires and plugs for damage and follow the Electricity at Work Regulations. Before you plug your equipment in, untangle the wires and check the equipment again prior to use. To be extra prepared, take a spare spay gun, pair of tongs and hairdryer. Hopefully you will not be travelling by bus as you will have lots to carry!

ACTIVITY

Try to list from memory all the things you need to put together for preparation of your image.

PREPARING YOURSELF

On the day you create your masterpiece, follow the plan in the diagram below.

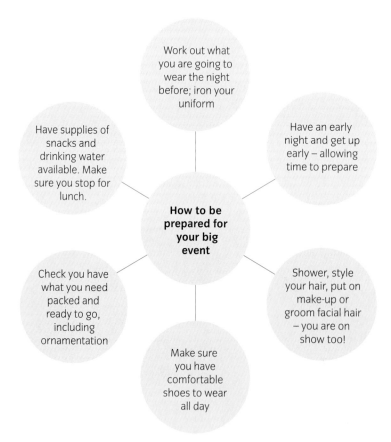

PLANNING FOR THE EVENT

Preparation for events is very important. You must make sure you are organised and work in a logical manner; good planning is the key to your success! Planning and creating your mood board will be calm and leisurely compared to creating your finished image on the actual day. To help the event run smoothly, plan in advance, think about what could go wrong and plan for that too.

RESEARCH

You need to decide individually or as a group what your theme is going to be. When this has been decided you will need to research ideas for your image. You can use the following resources to find ideas for creating your theme:

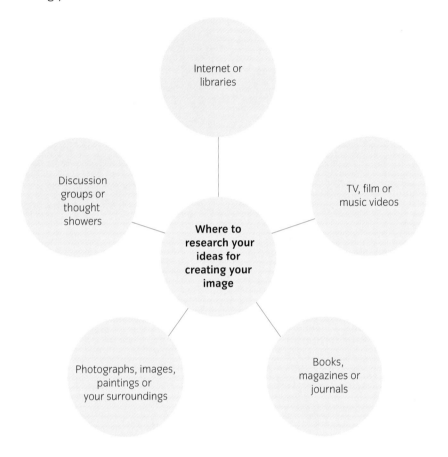

Internet or libraries

Discussion groups or thought showers

TV, film or music videos

Where to research your ideas for creating your image

Photographs, images, paintings or your surroundings

Books, magazines or journals

212 CREATE AN IMAGE BASED ON A THEME WITHIN THE HAIR AND BEAUTY SECTOR

INDUSTRY TIP

You can achieve the objectives of this chapter by working independently – creating the total look yourself with your own theme. Alternatively you could work as part of a group and create a total theme together by recreating a specific look, for example recreating the characters from *The Lion King* or a **fantasy** film like *Pirates of the Caribbean*. If you are working as part of a team it is very important that you support each other on the overall image and organisation.

Fantasy
Something that is not real, for example a fairy or a unicorn; Peter Pan is a fantasy film as it could never happen in the real world.

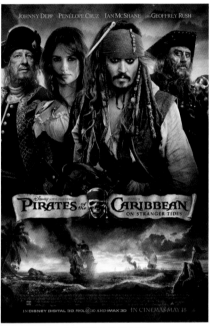

An example of fantasy make-up

ACTIVITY

With your colleagues, discuss ideas for resources and places you could visit to research for ideas.

These resources should give you ideas and inspiration to develop your own theme. For example, you might use a character from a Disney film to develop a more grown-up look based on that.

TECHNICAL SKILLS USED TO CREATE AN IMAGE

You need to think about the skills you need to help you create the total look. The technical skills that could be considered to complete your look are:

- hairstyling
- make-up
- nail art.

All of these elements must be covered to complete your total look; they must all fit into the theme you are aiming to create.

Although you are beauty therapists, make-up artists or nail technicians, it is important that you include the hairstyling to give you a better overall look. You will not be assessed on your ability to create a hairstyle; it will just come into the end result, so enjoy and have fun with it. You will be surprised at how enjoyable creating the look from head to toe will be.

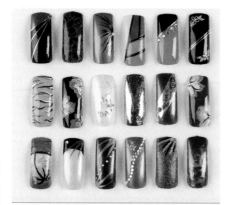

Samples of nail art designs you can create as part of your image

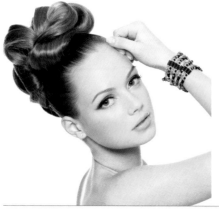
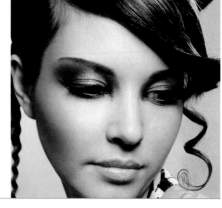

Create the perfect hairstyle for your image

CHOOSING CLOTHES AND ACCESSORIES

Depending on the topic of your event, you could have accessories that range from a bridal gown for a special occasion, or tree branches to add to your competition entry or a pair of Disney Mickey Mouse ears to create your fantasy image.

To help you decide on where to get your clothing and accessories from, consider the following ideas:

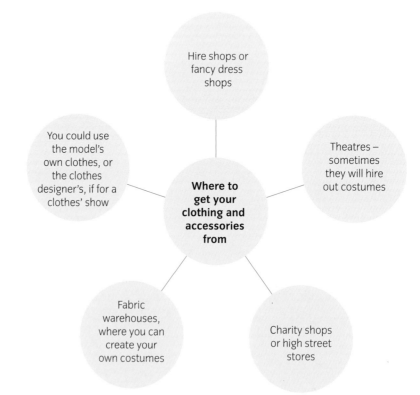

Hire shops or fancy dress shops

You could use the model's own clothes, or the clothes designer's, if for a clothes' show

Theatres – sometimes they will hire out costumes

Where to get your clothing and accessories from

Fabric warehouses, where you can create your own costumes

Charity shops or high street stores

INDUSTRY TIP

Ask one of the hairdressing tutors to give you some ideas to help you on your way.

INDUSTRY TIP

When you are choosing your theme, remember this is a total look you are creating – you will need to blend in the hairstyle with the facial make-up and the clothing. You will need to think about the detail of your image, so it all comes together to create the overall look you are trying to achieve. Check the balance of the style regularly – you will need a keen eye for detail. Stand back from your model and look at the image you have created. Use fresh eyes and try to imagine what other people are seeing.

ACTIVITY

With your peers, discuss other places you could visit to obtain your clothes and accessories.

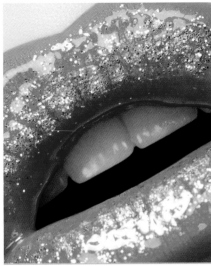

A high-fashion look

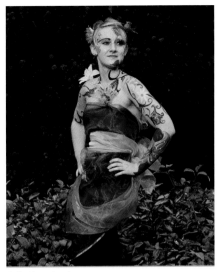

A fantasy look

ACTIVITY

If you were planning a fantasy theme, what resources could help you? List all the tools, materials, clothes, accessories, products and tools/ equipment you would need for this event.

PLANNING FOR A SPECIAL OCCASION – A WEDDING

A bride's special day! In this case your client is definitely someone who needs to be treated with extra care and attention. It is your job to make the occasion fun, relaxing and special.

Before the big day you should have a trial run, experimenting with ideas that will suit your client's hair and skin type, and also match the dress. When a style has been agreed upon, discuss the need for any hair accessories. Arrange a final practice a week or two before the big day so you are confident with the look on the day. During the trial practices discuss with your client other services that might be beneficial, such as eyelash and eyebrow tinting, eyebrow shaping, manicure, nail extensions, facials or a tanning treatment.

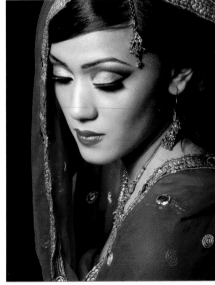

A complete look

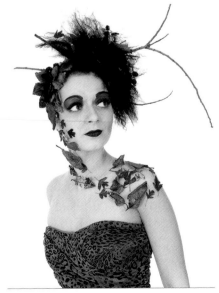

A high-fashion look

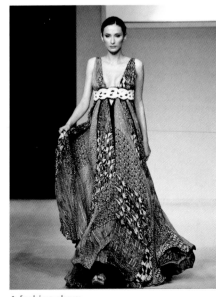

A fashion show

PLANNING FOR A COMPETITION

If your event is a competition, this could be a college in-house competition or a national event. The competition could have a set theme or have a variety of options, such as a fantasy look. Whichever event you have decided to enter into, plan, practise and prepare.

PLANNING FOR A THEMED EVENT – FASHION SHOW

Again this could be a salon fashion show to show off the talents of the salon staff, or an in-house college fashion show for students in hair and beauty. Get into the spirit of what the show is all about and take this opportunity to experiment and 'think outside the box'. Let your imagination and creativity go wild.

Semi-professional fashion show

Your themed event might be for a clothes' designer who has asked your college to style the look for the show. If this is the case, it is likely that the clothes' designer will want some input into the ideas behind the looks. Listen to their ideas and, of course, make some suggestions of your own. You will need to know about the clothes that the models will be wearing to make sure the look suits the style of clothing. If the clothes designed are wacky and way out, then the hair and make-up must be too. If the clothes are more traditional daytime wear, this should also be reflected in the overall look.

PURPOSE OF A MOOD BOARD

Not only do you need to plan your event, you will need to plan and develop your mood board. The main purpose for creating a mood board is to present the linking ideas from the research you have undertaken, showing the journey you took to obtain your inspiration for creating your image.

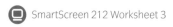
SmartScreen 212 Worksheet 3

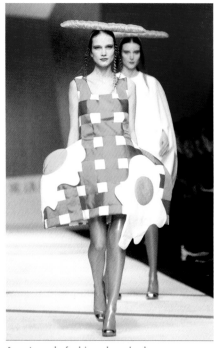
Avant-garde fashion show look

ACTIVITY

Research different mood boards and how they can be used to help you with your planning.

The resources you use for your research could include:

- media images – newspaper or magazine articles, music videos, Internet sites or TV programmes relating to the industry or the theme of your event
- photographs of where your inspiration came from
- sketches of ideas you have had along the way
- materials – textures, fabrics or materials that have given you a brainwave or a motivating idea.

How to present a mood board

Your mood board needs to be large enough to show everything from your first ideas through to your end results. Make it colourful and exciting, but make sure it tells your story.

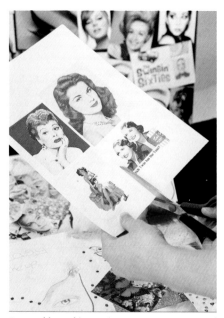
A mood board in progress

Your mood board should outline how your **concepts** and ideas were developed to create your image. It should show links from the **inspiring** ideas to your creative thoughts and the end result – your model. Describe what technical skills you expect to be using to create your **vision** and how you would advertise/present your idea to others.

Your mood board will need a heading. Remember that it needs to give the viewer a first impression of what your image is all about, so make sure the theme is mentioned.

Around the heading, attach your photos, sketches and magazine/newspaper clippings, showing the hair, clothes, make-up, etc. Add brief text descriptions about your ideas and how the images link to your theme.

Use combinations of images, such as the fabrics and materials used that **enthralled** you. These can be anything, from drinks cans – as used to set hair in Lady Gaga's music video – to candy floss or chopsticks. Add anything and everything you used that inspired you.

Often for a college fashion show you will be asked to present your mood board to your client/assessor, explaining what **motivated** you and where you obtained this inspiration from, so be prepared to talk about your journey too.

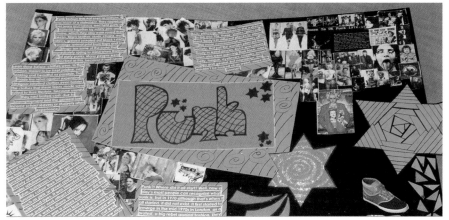

An example of a mood board

SmartScreen 212 Worksheet 4

ACTIVITY

Search for images of avant-garde make-up on the Internet. You will be amazed at what materials make-up artists use on the skin or in the hair to create their images.

ADVERTISING TO YOUR TARGET AUDIENCE

When planning the event, you will also need to consider who your targeted audience is. It might be your family or friends that have been invited in for your end-of-year show or it might be a photographer who will be taking pictures at a competition.

If you are putting on a show, you will need to advertise the event to make sure that you have an audience on the day. If the show has a fantasy theme and is a loud, high-colour, funky event, your target audience is more likely to be younger. If the show is about 'hair through the ages', for example, it will appeal to a wider audience.

Concept
An idea that you form in your mind.

Inspiring
Something that motivates you.

Vision
How you see something as an end result.

Enthralled
To be interested and excited about something.

Motivated
Driven to complete the task.

INDUSTRY TIP
Your attention to detail and planning who to invite is as crucial as planning your model's appearance.

If your salon is putting on an event to show off your skills, you will want to capture new trade and custom, so make sure that the invite list and advertisements are distributed further afield, not just to the regular client base.

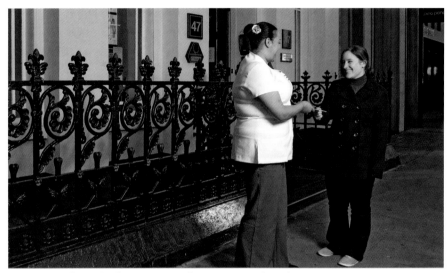

A therapist offering leaflets to passers-by to promote the salon

PROFESSIONAL CONSULTATION

To be able to carry out a professional consultation using your mood board, you must use the correct techniques. Refer back to Chapter 203 for more in-depth knowledge.

COMMUNICATION TECHNIQUES

Communication techniques are very important when you are creating an image. The planning of these types of event requires a whole-team approach to make sure that it runs smoothly and the day itself goes to plan. The lead-up will require frequent team meetings to establish everyone's responsibilities. A plan of who is doing what, where and when should be drawn up and issues that arise from the meetings should be discussed tactfully with others. Always treat your peers with respect. Address any issues politely, clearly and calmly. Make sure that you follow any instructions that you have been given and be a team player, assisting others where you can.

INDUSTRY TIP

There's no 'I' in TEAM! Work harmoniously together and create a great team effort that your salon/college can be proud of.

HANDY HINTS

Look back at Chapter 203 Client care and communication in beauty-related industries for more information on communication techniques.

 SmartScreen 203 Worksheet 1

CREATE AN IMAGE

When planning a themed event, you might think you have a very good memory, but it is always sensible to write checklists to make sure that nothing gets forgotten on the day. Sometimes fashion shows or similar events involve the make-up artist/therapist starting early in the morning and when you start it is go, go, go! By the time you are ready for the event itself, you will have a completed mood board to help remind you of what you need, but it is always best to have a written list to hand as an **aide-mémoire**.

Aide-mémoire

Something to help the memory.

In this part of the chapter you will learn about:

- preparing your model
- creating your theme-based image
- avoiding disasters and dramas
- evaluating the effectiveness of the theme-based image.

PREPARING YOUR MODEL

By the time the big event arrives, you would have practised creating your image many times, probably starting on your peers in the classroom. By now you should know whether you prefer your model's hair to be freshly washed, or washed the night before. Whichever you prefer, make sure you agree these arrangements with your model (or client).

You will probably want to start creating your vision using a blank canvas, so make sure the hair is free of products and the face is clean and make-up free (unless you have requested otherwise). Depending on the style of clothing you have chosen for the image, you might even need to discuss what type of underwear your model should wear – your image will not look so good if you have visual bra straps or strap marks.

ACTIVITY

Make sure that you practise your look on several occasions. 'Practice makes perfect'! Take photos and recap on the total look.

ON THE DAY

On the day you are likely to be running on adrenaline, but you are bound to get a little stressed and nervous. This is normal – even celebrity make-up artists and hairdressers get nervous. To help you deal with the pressure on the day, make sure you:

- plan the event
- follow the plan.

INDUSTRY TIP

As you prepare for the day ahead, pack your day-box – your accessories, model's clothing, make-up, spare false nails or polish, pins, grips, styling products, etc and make sure you have plenty of hairspray. Tick these off your checklist as you pack and prepare them. If you are working in a salon environment, it is always handy to have a needle and thread and some tape – you never know when these might come in handy.

INDUSTRY TIP

When you are packing your day-box do not forget your gown and towels – your model will need her clothing protected.

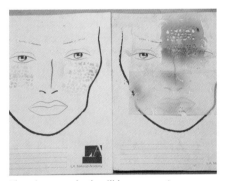

Planning your look will keep you stay focused

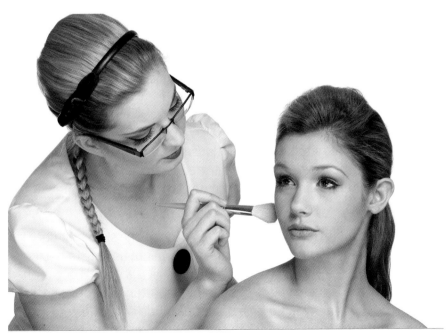

A make-up artist/therapist working on their model

On the day of the event, demonstrate positive body language and be confident. Believe in yourself – you know you can do it; you have practised and you have prepared – you are ready! If you are running ahead of schedule, you can help others by responding to their needs. Make sure you look after your model and make sure they are comfortable and have had some refreshments. If your model is nervous, speak to them in a reassuring manner to put them at ease.

CREATING YOUR THEME-BASED IMAGE

For your assessment you will need to create one mood board and a theme-based image from the following options:

- a competition
- a themed event
- a special occasion.

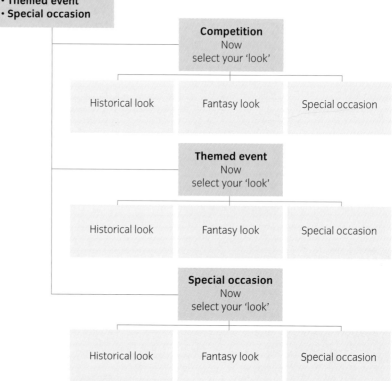

COMPETITION

Depending on whether this is held in-house at your college, or at a regional event, the theme might be decided for you. If your college is holding a competition for your assessment, a theme needs to be decided.

If the theme is **historical**, you will need to choose one style that fits with the chosen theme. If the theme is fantasy, you might be able to decide on the look or a look might be chosen for you. If it is a special occasion theme for a competition, you might get the opportunity to practise your bridal styles. Whether you go for a traditional bride or create your own masterpiece – this is for you to decide.

Historical

An event in the past.

ACTIVITY

Research the 'IMATS' or UK Skills shows for help or ideas on entering competitions and creating your own avant-garde image.

THEMED EVENT

You will need to include one of the theme-based options:

- a historical look
- a fantasy theme
- a special occasion.

All of these options have lots of room for flexibility and creativity. You can pretty much create any look you want.

A historical look

Creating a themed event based on a historical look could include:

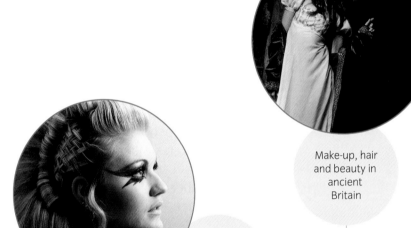

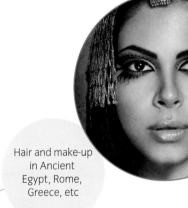

Make-up, hair and beauty in ancient Britain

Hair and make-up in Ancient Egypt, Rome, Greece, etc

Make-up and hair trends from times past, such as punk, rock, goth, etc

Historical look

Fashion from a chosen decade

Fashion through the ages – 20s, 40s, 60s, 80s, etc

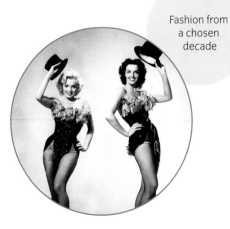

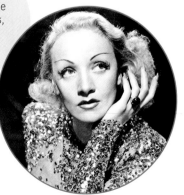

 SmartScreen 212 Worksheet 1

A fantasy theme

Open your mind and go wild; you have the chance to create a fantasy image so basically anything goes.

This could include:

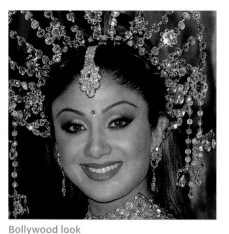

Bollywood look

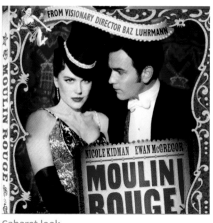

Cabaret look

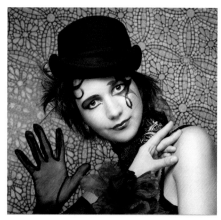

Clown look

ACTIVITY

Search on the Internet for 'themed venues', as they might give you inspirational ideas for a theme, or ideas for props that you could use to create your image.

A special occasion

If you choose a special occasion as your theme, this could be a prom-night style or a traditional bridal look. However, people are becoming more creative with their weddings these days, so a themed wedding might be your choice. A winter wonderland, or Las Vegas style or even Charlie and the Chocolate Factory are not unheard of for wedding themes.

Going back in history is also quite popular for special occasions. The 1940s' style is making a comeback, so you might choose a historical look for your style.

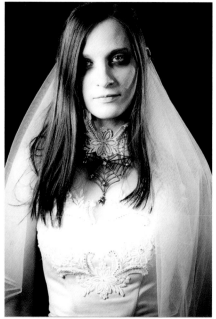

A creative look

MEDIA

Whichever theme you undertake, you will need to consider the following:

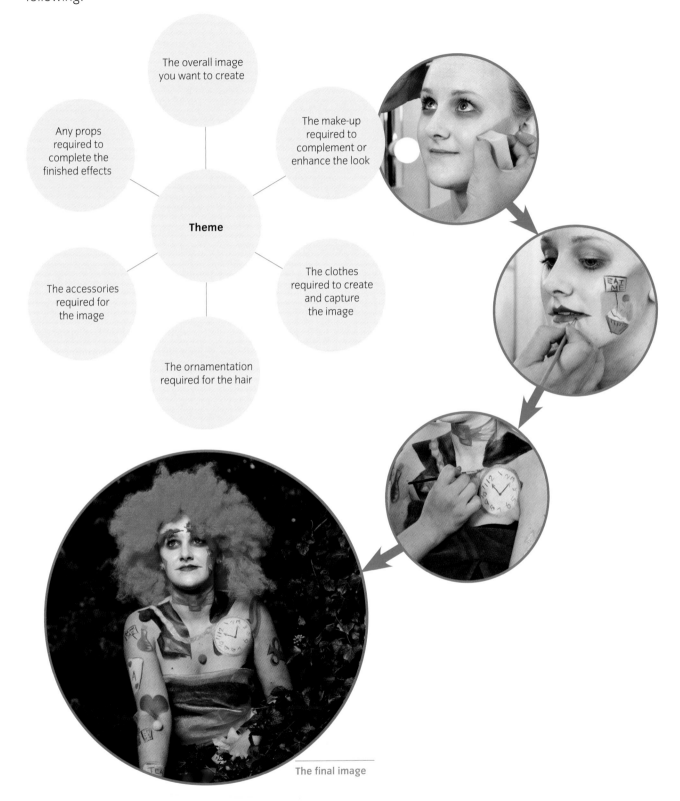

The overall image you want to create

The make-up required to complement or enhance the look

Any props required to complete the finished effects

Theme

The clothes required to create and capture the image

The accessories required for the image

The ornamentation required for the hair

The final image

AVOIDING DISASTERS AND DRAMAS

After all your careful preparation and planning, what could possibly go wrong on the day? Well, hopefully nothing, but always plan for the worst case scenario, then you will know you are covered for all eventualities. See the table below for ideas.

Disaster/drama	What to do next!
Missing or broken accessories	A needle and thread can always come in handy, and do not forget that sticky tape! If accessories break or snap, which makes them difficult to secure, you can help hold them in place with a needle and thread or some tape.
Wardrobe malfunction, eg if the clothing is ripped or has a hole	Where's that sticky tape and needle and thread? Again, do not panic. Think outside the box and improvise. Add a sash or a piece of material to hide any rips or gaps in clothing, but make sure it matches the rest of the clothing.
Power failure	If you are using a spray machine to create your look and the power fails, always make sure you have back-up make-up and brushes, so you can still create the look you desire but with a different product. Make sure you always bring a spare hairdryer or styling tongs.
Your model's taken ill	This cannot be helped and is totally out of your control. Hopefully, when you planned your event you had a reserve in mind in case of illness. Remember, you have practised this look many times on peers. All you need to do is rope in a friend and recreate the look on them! As long as the clothing will fit you can adjust the style a little to suit.
You are taken ill	If this is a wedding day, who will fill in for you? When you are completing your bridal practices, always make sure another work colleague is familiar with the bride and the look chosen. Make sure your mood board is available for the make-up artist/therapist covering for you, so they can follow your plan. If you are absent for a competition, sadly you will just have to miss out and enter again next year, putting this year's entry down to good experience but bad luck. If you are supposed to be creating the look for a fashion show, someone should be able to fill in for you. It will make their day extra busy and put them under more pressure, but that is what teamwork is all about. They will have to follow your mood board and the plan for the day.

INDUSTRY TIP

Always take plenty of pins and grips with you; they always come in handy and you can never have too many.

INDUSTRY TIP

If you did not have a 'plan B' in place allowing for the absence of a model, you should record this and evaluate what you have learnt from this valuable experience in readiness for next time.

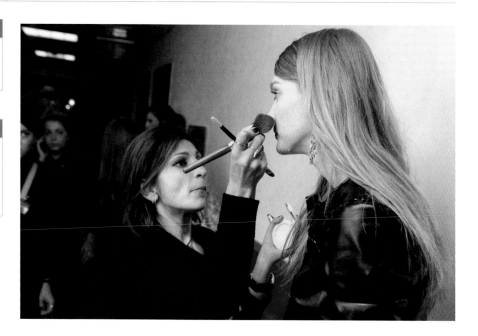

EVALUATING THE EFFECTIVENESS OF THE THEMED-BASED IMAGE

During your preparation you will need to record how well your theme-based image is progressing. After the event you will need to evaluate it and decide whether the service provided met with expectations.

You will receive feedback from team meetings throughout the planning process, and will have the opportunity to offer and receive constructive verbal feedback. This will be particularly useful when you are planning the event and you should always listen to this feedback, as it might help you to develop and improve your themed image.

You will receive feedback from your tutors and, occasionally, from your peers too. When you have worked hard on a task and someone criticises you, constructively or otherwise, it can hurt. Be positive; consider how you can benefit from the feedback. If the overall results improve because of the comments/feedback you receive, then you have learnt something and progressed with your skills. This can only be a positive outcome.

SELF-EVALUATION

Throughout the whole of the event – the planning, constructing and developing your mood board and creating the image – you should be evaluating yourself. You will be using a combination of technical skills, some of which you might not have used together before. You will be learning new skills along the way and you should evaluate your progress. Often in life we are our own worst critics, so keep a diary/journal of how you felt on your journey to create an image based on a theme.

INDUSTRY TIP

On a record card or in a journal, record the comments that you received that were valuable and those you learnt from.

INDUSTRY TIP

If you identify any requirements for your model's/client's future treatments, write these on the client record card. This will enable you to have something in readiness for her next appointment, or if you have the opportunity to use her as a model again.

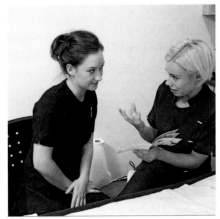
Evaluating the final image

INDUSTRY TIP

Keep photographs of your work each time you practise your image, so you can see your progress and evaluate it too.

 SmartScreen 212 Revision guidance, Revision crossword and Sample questions

A fantasy image

Use the questions below to test your knowledge of Chapter 212 to see how much information you have retained. These questions will help you to revise what you have learnt in this chapter.

Turn to page 601 for the answers.

1. Which **one** of the following is the best method of sterilising make-up brushes?
   a) Barbicide
   b) UV cabinet
   c) Autoclave
   d) Isopropyl alcohol

2. Which **one** of the following is the best resource to access ideas when creating a theme-based image?
   a) Journals
   b) Textbooks
   c) Magazines
   d) Internet

3. Which **one** of the following products would you use to create the wide-eyed look of the 60s?
   a) Eye shadow
   b) Liquid eyeliner
   c) Eye pencil
   d) Mascara

4. Which **one** of the following best states the purpose of a mood board?
   a) To link themes and demonstrate creativity
   b) To provide a visual aid
   c) To plan for the activity
   d) A place for all the material samples

5. Which **one** of the following best describes the reason for self-evaluation?
   a) To critique work and see where changes could be made
   b) To gain feedback and make improvements
   c) To alter work that you are unhappy with next time
   d) To write a review of what went well

6. Photographic evidence of an image can be used for all of the following except:
   a) keeping a record
   b) evaluating work
   c) advertising
   d) portfolio.

7. Which **one** of the following is the most important consideration when selecting a model for a make-up competition?
   a) Availability
   b) Height
   c) Skin type
   d) Posture

8. Which **one** of the following is a non-technical skill that can be used to enhance your image?
   a) Hair styling
   b) Nail art
   c) Nail enhancements
   d) Clothing

9. Written feedback is a form of:
   a) evaluation
   b) demonstration
   c) technical skills
   d) behaviour.

10. Which **one** of the following is the main benefit of a mood board?
    a) Allows the artist to show creativity
    b) Gives a colourful visual
    c) Demonstrates thought processes
    d) Shows technical skills

CASE STUDY: SITA GILL

After studying Media Studies, it was clear to me that the media and make-up world was where I wanted to be. Now I am a professional, specialist make-up artist and teacher, specialising in make-up artistry, hair artistry and styling. I love teaching make-up skills to those who share my passions. I also believe that knowledge is an extremely powerful tool which is why I attend further training; this helps me to excel within my area of expertise. My work has been featured in a number of respected publications and I have worked with highly esteemed professionals within the industry.

I love my career as a make-up artist as every day is different and you never know who you might be working with and I love the fact I can be creative and diverse in creating an amazing look with the brief I am given.

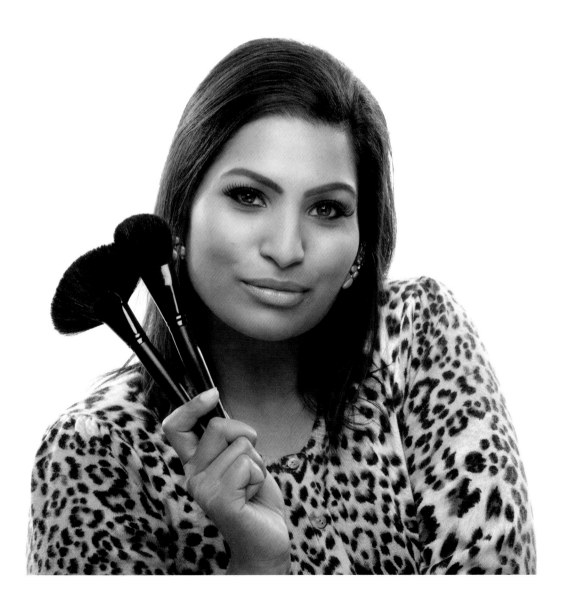

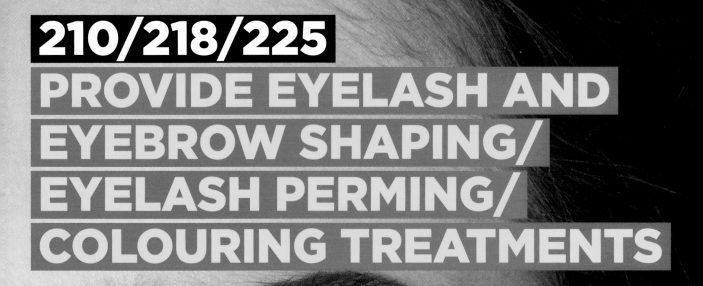

210/218/225
PROVIDE EYELASH AND EYEBROW SHAPING/ EYELASH PERMING/ COLOURING TREATMENTS

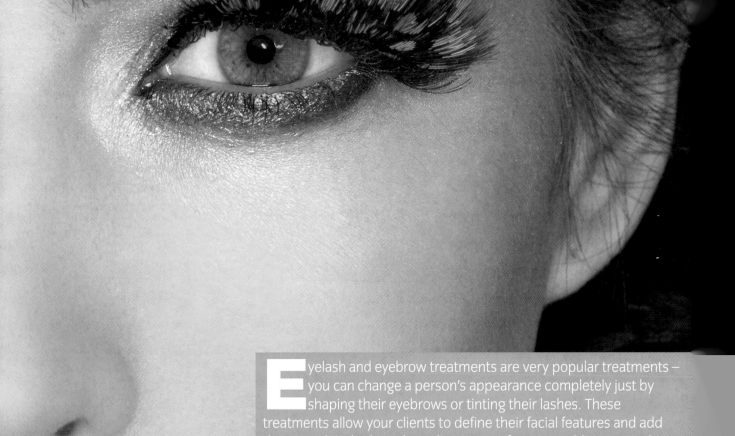

Eyelash and eyebrow treatments are very popular treatments – you can change a person's appearance completely just by shaping their eyebrows or tinting their lashes. These treatments allow your clients to define their facial features and add drama to their look. Lash application is a fantastic addition to make-up and it is this attention to detail that can enhance an appearance.

Within this chapter we will be looking at eyebrow shaping, lash and brow tinting, lash perming and the application of individual and strip lashes.

In this chapter you will learn how to:

- prepare for eye treatments
- provide eye treatments.

PREPARE FOR EYE TREATMENTS

Before you carry out eye treatments it is important to be prepared. Health and safety requirements should be followed for every treatment, but knowing how to set up your treatment area, which products and tools you should use and how to carry out an effective consultation are essential for eye treatments.

In this part of the chapter you will learn about:

- health and safety
- eye treatment products
- consultation.

HEALTH AND SAFETY

It is very important to follow all health and safety regulations when you are preparing for and performing eye treatments. Look back and refresh your memory on legislation in Chapter 201 Follow health and safety practice in the salon.

The main legislation covered within eye treatments are:

- **PPE**
- Health and Safety at Work Act
- **COSHH**
- Data Protection Act
- Work Place Regulations.

METHODS OF STERILISATION

It is very important to sterilise tools and equipment prior to carrying out any type of eye treatment to maximise health and safety and prevent cross-contamination. Use disposable tools where possible and always follow these instructions when you are preparing for eye treatments:

- Sterilise tweezers before use.
- Make sure you wash your hands prior to the treatment.
- Use disposable applicators where possible (eg disposable mascara wands, brushes, eye shields).
- Do not risk cross-contamination – make sure you use different applicators on each eye.

ENVIRONMENTAL CONDITIONS

You must make sure that both you and the client are comfortable. Make sure the working area is clean and tidy; the atmosphere and ambience of the salon will make your working environment and the client's treatment more desirable. Refer to Chapter 203 Client care and communication in beauty-related industries for in-depth information on environmental conditions. Here are a few that are specific to eye treatments:

PPE

Personal protective equipment.

COSHH

Control of Substances Hazardous to Health.

HANDY HINTS

Look back at Chapter 202 to remind yourself about PPE, COSHH and other health and safety practices.

 SmartScreen 202 Worksheet 6 and SmartScreen 210 Handout 2

INDUSTRY TIP

Throughout the treatment, make sure that you keep the lids on all products to stop contamination. Remove any product with a spatula and not your fingers.

Intricate

Fine detail.

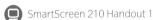

SmartScreen 210 Handout 1

- **Lighting** – when you are carrying out an eye treatment, the lighting within the treatment room needs to be clear, as it is very **intricate** work. This is especially important when you are performing an eyebrow shape – you need to see those fine hairs under the brow. If the lighting in the salon is not sufficient, you can use a magnifying lamp with a light to show fine detail.
- **Smell** – you work very close to your client when you are tweezing, tinting or perming lashes, so make sure you apply deodorant on a regular basis and suck a mint prior to your client coming in to give yourself fresh breath.

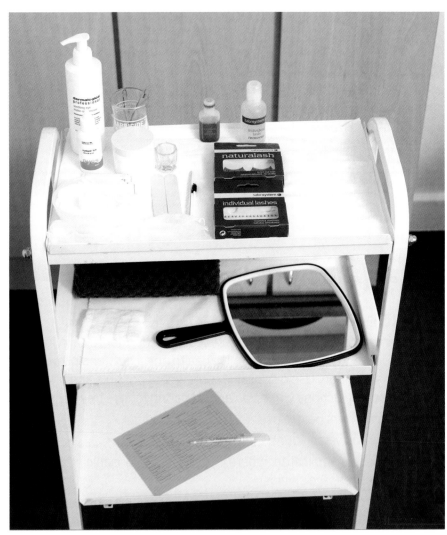

Set-up trolley for eyelash application

INDUSTRY TIP

It is very important to position both yourself and your client correctly to avoid causing harm to yourself or your client. Make sure that the stool you are sitting on is at the correct height, so that you can place both of your feet flat on the floor. Always ask your client if the back of the couch is at the correct height for them and do not lie them flat.

INDUSTRY TIP

Remember, you cannot treat any persons under the age of 16 without parental consent and a signed letter. The parent or guardian must also accompany the minor while they are having the treatment.

EYE TREATMENT PRODUCTS

Listed in the tables below are all of the products, tools and equipment needed to perform various eye treatments.

EYELASH/BROW TINTING

Product	What does it do?	How to use
Oil-free eye make-up remover	This product removes eye make-up, including waterproof mascara, by breaking down the product and gently removing it.	Dampen down and fold a cotton wool pad into a half-moon shape; apply under the bottom lashes. Apply the make-up remover to a cotton bud and gently remove any make-up on the eye area. When you are sure it has been removed, apply another dampened cotton wool pad over the eye and sweep over the lashes from the inner eye to the outer, also removing the pad under the lashes. Repeat if needed.
Tint	This product applies a semi-permanent tint to the lashes and comes in different colours: blue, black, grey, blue-black and brown. The tint lasts for 4–6 weeks.	Apply protecting shields under the bottom lashes with petroleum jelly. Using a small brush, apply the tint to the lashes, making sure you get right to the root. Coat them well but not so much that it becomes messy. Leave for the stated time and remove with cotton buds and warm water.
Hydrogen **peroxide**	This is a chemical that is mixed with the tint to activate it.	Check the manufacturer's instructions before use.

Manufactuer's instructions

A leaflet that comes with the product that explains how to use the product correctly.

Peroxide

A chemical that is mixed with the tint to activate the oxidisation of the colour molecules.

Product	What does it do?	How to use
Stain remover	Removes any excess tint that is on the skin.	Apply to the affected area of skin with damp cotton wool or a cotton bud to remove the stain.
Petroleum jelly	Acts as a barrier to the tint by preventing it from staining the skin. Apply to the skin surrounding the treatment area.	Apply with a cotton bud to the required areas; make sure you use a spatula to remove it from the pot to prevent cross-infection.
Sanitising agent	This acts as a sanitiser for metal and plastic tools, eg Barbicide.	Check the manufacturer's instructions before use.

Tool	What is it for?
Disposable brushes (applicators)	Use these to brush through the lashes and eyebrows.
Orange wood sticks	Use these to separate the eyebrows, allowing the tint to penetrate to the root of the lashes.

Tool	What is it for?
Glass mixing dish	Use this to mix your tint and peroxide to form a paste.
Mirror	This allows your client to view the results during and after the treatment process.

Equipment	What does it do?	How to use
Paper eye shields	These are used to protect the delicate skin under the eyes from tinting when you are performing the treatment.	Remove from the packet and apply petroleum jelly to one side. They are all one size but you can cut them to the correct shape with a small pair of scissors if required. Apply beneath the bottom lashes, petroleum jelly-side down. Make sure your client is comfortable with them.
Cotton wool pads	This is used to remove products.	Try to split your cotton wool pads into two – this will be more **cost-effective**. Always try to use damp cotton wool to seal in the fibres and prevent irritation to the eye. **Cost-effective** More value for money.
Tissue	You can use tissues to rest your products on to keep your station tidy.	Split your tissues into two to make it more cost-effective.

Product	What does it do?	How to use
Oil-free eye make-up remover	This product removes eye make-up, including waterproof mascara, by breaking down the product and gently removing it.	Dampen down and fold a cotton wool pad into a half-moon shape; apply under the bottom lashes. Apply the make-up remover to a cotton bud and gently remove any make-up on the eye area. When you are sure it has been removed, apply another dampened cotton wool pad over the eye and sweep over the lashes from the inner eye to the outer, also removing the pad under the lashes. Repeat if needed.
Sanitising agent	This acts as a sanitiser disinfectanct for metal and plastic tools, eg Barbicide.	Check the manufacturer's instructions before use.
Witch hazel	This is a soothing product and comes in liquid or gel form. Use the gel form around the eye area to prevent it from running into the eye and causing irritation.	Apply to the skin with a piece of damp cotton wool to soothe the area.
Eyebrow powder	This looks like an eye shadow and adds colour and definition to the eyebrows. You can also use it with a stencil and it will give you a perfect shape.	Using a small brush, apply the product to the eyebrow, following the natural shape. Alternatively, you can use a stencil: position the stencil correctly over the eyebrow and apply the eyeshadow to create a perfect shape.
Eyebrow pencil	This product allows you to fill in any gaps within the eyebrow.	Make sure you sharpen your eyebrow pencil before and after use to prevent any cross-infection. Apply the liner to the eyebrow with light, stroking movements to create your desired look.

Tool	What is it for?
Manual and automatic tweezers 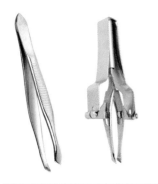	Tweezers are used to remove the unwanted hair from the eyebrows. Manual tweezers are designed to remove stray hairs and for more accurate work when creating a shape. Automatic tweezers are designed to remove bulk hair and are set on a spring. Both manual and automatic tweezers come with different shaped ends – slanted, pointed and flat. It is your own personal preference as to which type you use.
Orange wood sticks 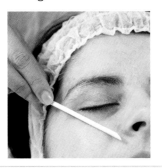	These are used to measure the eyebrows for the perfect shape to suit each individual client.
Mirror 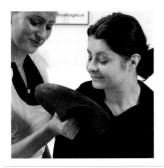	A mirror allows your client to view the results during and after the treatment process.

INDUSTRY TIP

Make sure you check your tweezers when you are buying them to make sure the ends meet and there is no gap.

INDUSTRY TIP

Never lend your tweezers to anyone else; they are a personal piece of equipment and need to be kept sterile at all times.

Equipment	What does it do?	How to use
Cotton wool pads 	This is used to remove products.	Try to split your cotton wool pads into two – this will be more cost-effective. Always try to use damp cotton wool to seal in the fibres and prevent irritation to the eye.
Ice pack 	You can use an ice pack to relieve discomfort when you are performing an eyebrow shape.	Keep the ice pack in the freezer until needed. Remove, wrap in a flannel or a towel and apply to the area required.
Tissue 	You can use tissues to rest your products on to keep your station tidy.	Split your tissues into two to make it more cost-effective.
Warming device (hot towels) 	These can be applied before an eyebrow shape to open up the pores and to make the treatment more comfortable for your client.	When you are using hot towels, remove them from the cabinet just before you need them. Test the heat on yourself first, then tell your client you will be testing it on the side of their face. If the temperature is OK, apply the towel over the eyebrow area. The heat is not retained for long, so as soon as the towel cools down, remove it and start your treatment.

INDUSTRY TIP

Make sure the warming device (hot towel unit) is switched on prior to your client coming in.

EYELASH PERMING

Product	What does it do?	How to use
Oil-free eye make-up remover	This product removes eye make-up, including waterproof mascara, by breaking down the product and gently removing it.	Dampen down and fold a cotton wool pad into a half-moon shape; apply under the bottom lashes. Apply the make-up remover to a cotton bud and gently remove any make-up on the eye area. When you are sure it has been removed, apply another dampened cotton wool pad over the eye and sweep over the lashes from the inner eye to the outer, also removing the pad under the lashes. Repeat if needed.
Lash conditioner	This product adds nourishment to the lashes.	Apply the product at the end of the eyelash perming treatment to replace the **nutrients** that were removed by the perming process. Apply with a disposable mascara wand like you would a mascara. **Nutrients** Substances that help us grow.
Perm lotion	This product is used to create the curl as part of an eyelash perming treatment.	Apply to the lashes with a small brush or cotton bud when you have applied the perming rods. Apply it directly onto the lashes where you want to create the curl. Cover with cling film to speed up the perming process (check the manufacturer's instructions for timings).
Neutraliser	This product is applied after the perming lotion and sets the curl.	Apply in the same way as the perming lotion. Cover with cling film and check the manufacturer's instructions for timings.
Sanitising agent	This acts as a sanitiser for metal and plastic tools, eg Barbicide.	Check the manufacturer's instructions before use.

Tool	What is it for?
Disposable brushes (applicators)	These are used to brush through the lashes and eyebrows.
Perm rod	These are used to create the curl during an eyelash perm. They come in different sizes (small, medium or large) depending on the type of curl your client requires and also the length of your client's lashes.
Mirror	A mirror allows your client to view the results during and after the treatment process.

Equipment	What does it do?	How to use
Cotton wool pads	This is used to remove products.	Try to split your cotton wool pads into two – this will be more cost-effective. Always try to use damp cotton wool to seal in the fibres and prevent irritation to the eye.
Tissue	You can use tissues to rest your products on to keep your station tidy.	Split your tissues into two to make it more cost-effective.
Cling film	Cling film is used to quicken up the perming process as it creates heat.	Remove from the container and apply to the lashes, making sure you do not cover the nostrils.

APPLICATION OF STRIP/INDIVIDUAL LASHES

Product	What does it do?	How to use
Oil-free eye make-up remover	This product removes eye make-up, including waterproof mascara, by breaking down the product and gently removing it.	Dampen down and fold a cotton wool pad into a half-moon shape; apply under the bottom lashes. Apply the make-up remover to a cotton bud and gently remove any make-up on the eye area. When you are sure it has been removed, apply another dampened cotton wool pad over the eye and sweep over the lashes from the inner eye to the outer, also removing the pad under the lashes. Repeat if needed.
Strip lashes	These come in many colours; they add thickness and length to the natural lashes.	Remove the lashes from the packet with a pair of tweezers. Apply lash glue to the base of the lashes, making sure you coat **sufficiently** but do not overload. Ask your client to close their eyes and apply the strip lashes to the base of your client's natural lashes, using your tweezers and fingers to secure the lashes in place. **Sufficiently** In enough detail.
Individual lashes	These are applied individually to the natural lashes. They come in black or brown colours, and different lengths and thicknesses.	Remove the individual lashes from the packet with a pair of tweezers. Dip the end into the glue and apply the lashes to the base of the client's natural lashes. Try to add the same number of lashes to each eye to make them even.
Lash glue	This product is used to attach the strip lashes and individual lashes to the client's natural lashes.	Squeeze a small amount of lash glue onto a palette. Make sure you seal the glue straight away with its lid as it will dry out very quickly.
Sanitising agent	This acts as a sanitiser for metal and plastic tools, eg Barbicide.	Check the manufacturer's instructions before use.

Tool	What is it for?
Tweezers (slant, claw, pointed and automatic)	Tweezers are used to help in the application of individual and strip lashes. **INDUSTRY TIP** Make sure you look after your tweezers. Do not drop them as this could lead to a loss of grip.
Disposable brushes (applicators)	These are used to brush through the lashes and eyebrows.
Mirror	A mirror allows your client to view the results during and after the treatment process.

Equipment	What does it do?	How to use
Cotton wool pads	This is used to remove products.	Try to split your cotton wool pads into two – this will be more cost-effective. Always try to use damp cotton wool to seal in the fibres and prevent irritation to the eye.
Tissue	You can use tissues to rest your products on to keep your station tidy.	Split your tissues into two to make it more cost-effective.

ACTIVITY

Design your own word search puzzle with all the tools, products and equipment described above. Time your friends on how long it takes to find all the words. It is also a good idea to leave a word out for them to figure out at the end.

CONSULTATION

The consultation stage is very important. This is where you gain all the information from your client to enable you to give them the best treatment you have to offer. Communication techniques are very important when you are carrying out a professional consultation (refer back to Chapter 203 Client care and communication in beauty-related industries for more in-depth knowledge on consultation and communication skills).

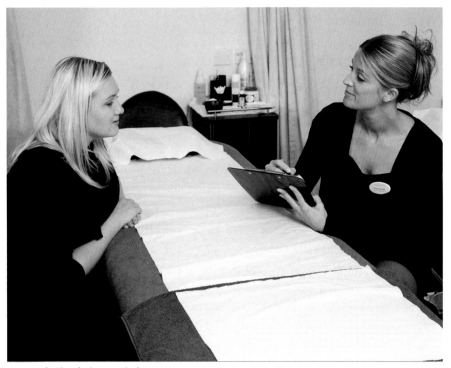

A consultation being carried out

INDUSTRY TIP

Remember to always keep good eye contact throughout the consultation process.

ACTIVITY

Test your knowledge and understanding on communication techniques by getting into pairs and practising a full eye treatment consultation on each other. Give each other constructive feedback on ways to improve the consultation process.

ACTIVITY

Design your own professional consultation form to use when you are performing eye treatments. Remember to include all the ranges stated in your assessment book.

FACTORS TO CONSIDER

There are certain things you need to think about when you are performing an eye treatment. These are called factors. They need to be fully explained to your client so they are aware of the treatment and how it will enhance their natural features. Listed below are the factors you need to explain to your client during the consultation. You also need to make sure that the client's objectives can be met and that there are no limitations. For example, you cannot perm lashes if they are too short to fit around the smallest rod size.

Eyelash/eyebrow tint

This treatment helps to enhance facial features and to change the natural colour of the client's eyelashes/eyebrows. The factors that you should consider when tinting someone's eyebrows or eyelashes are:

- Client's natural hair colour – lashes/eyebrows might already be dark and cannot be made any darker; client might have red hair; you will have to be careful not to go too dark.
- **Density** of eyebrow hair – there might not be enough hairs to dye, perhaps due to an illness or over-plucking.
- Client's eye colour – you want to enhance your client's natural eye colour.
- Strength of hair – the lashes/eyebrow hair might be too fragile to tint due to medication.

Eyebrow shape

Eyebrows are shaped to add **definition** and to **enhance** facial features. The factors that you should consider when shaping someone's eyebrows are:

- Age of client – as a client approaches her 50s, the hair becomes coarser, longer and thicker.
- Natural shape of the brow – always try to complement the client's natural browline. It can sometimes be impossible to create the look your client desires as their natural shape will not allow it. In this instance you can use a brow pencil to help achieve your client's look.
- Fashion – always keep an eye on the fashion trends as these tend to change with the seasons; there is always a different brow shape and make-up trend so keep these in mind, especially with your younger clientele.
- Client's expectations – ask them questions to determine exactly what they require.
- Eye shape/face shape – you want to enhance your client's own features, so look closely at your client's eye and face shape to maximise their good features.

Eyelash perming

Eyelashes are permed to curl them. The factors that you should consider before perming someone's eyelashes are:

- The client's natural lash length – they might be too short to wrap around the curling rods.
- Texture – the lashes might be too course to sit around the rod, making perming difficult.
- Tinting of lashes – make sure that your client has not had their lashes tinted in the past 24 hours.

Density
Thickness and colour depth of the hair.

Definition
Making the area stand out.

Enhance
To bring out.

- Type of curl – make sure you determine exactly what type and shape of curl the client wants.

Application of individual and strip lashes

False lashes add length and volume to the client's natural lashes. The factors that you should consider before applying false lashes are:

- Length of lashes required – make sure the client's required length is viable.
- Style of lashes – make sure the required style suits the client.
- Colour of lashes – make sure the false lash colour matches your client's natural colour.
- Occasion – determine why your client wants the lashes applied.
- Client's expectations – make sure the client is aware of the final look.
- Fashion – always make sure that you keep an eye on the fashion trends to make sure you have a full variety of different lashes available to suit all clientele.

CONTRA-INDICATIONS

You need to find out about any contra-indications the client has at the consultation. For a more in-depth description on all the contra-indications listed below, refer to the Anatomy and Physiology chapter. The following contra-indications will prevent you from carrying out eye treatments:

- fungal infection
- claustrophobia – your client's eyes will be closed for a substantial amount of time when tinting and perming, so it is very important that you ask if they are **claustrophobic**
- styes
- conjunctivitis
- bacterial infection
- viral infection
- severe eczema
- severe psoriasis
- severe skin condition
- infestations
- eye infections
- watery eyes
- client is undergoing chemotherapy
- client is undergoing radiotherapy.

The following contra-indications will restrict you from carrying out the treatment:

- recent scar tissue
- hyper-keratosis
- skin allergies
- cuts and abrasions
- high/low blood pressure
- skin disorders

INDUSTRY TIP

Always make sure you listen carefully to your client throughout their consultation to obtain knowledge of what your client's expectations are. Guide them to make a sensible choice; give advice on what shape would best suit their face shape and enhance their facial features.

Claustrophobia
The fear of being closed in.

INDUSTRY TIP

Remember, you are not qualified to diagnose a contra-indication; you can only advise and recommend your client seeks medical advice.

INDUSTRY TIP

'Prevent' means you cannot carry out the treatment. 'Restrict' means you can work around the affected area.

SmartScreen 210 Worksheet 1

- recent fractures and sprains
- undiagnosed lumps and swellings
- product allergies
- erythema
- hyper-sensitive skin.

SKIN TESTING

It is very important to perform a skin sensitivity test on every client at least 24 hours before their eye treatment. If these are not carried out there is the risk of the client suffering from an allergic reaction or, even worse, blindness. Some clients are very sensitive to the tinting product and will react almost immediately after contact; others might react a few hours later. You can test your client either behind the ear or inside the elbow. Make sure that you cleanse the area with a cleansing product before testing to remove any products that might be on the skin. Make sure that you always document the test results on your client's record card to protect yourself.

- Testing for eyelash/eyebrow tinting: mix a small amount of tint with peroxide and apply with either a cotton bud or a small brush.
- Testing for eyelash perming: apply each of the products (perming solution, neutraliser and cleanser) with a cotton bud.
- Testing the glue for individual or strip lashes: apply a small amount of glue with a cotton bud in accordance with the manufacturer's instructions.

Make sure you ask your client to avoid cleansing the area and to check for any changes in appearance. Ask them to let the salon know immediately if any reactions occur.

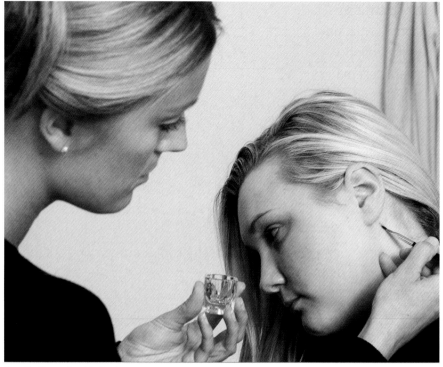
Application of a skin test

ACTIVITY

Design your own cue cards for each of the above skin tests with all the products required for each one.

There will be two outcomes to a skin sensitivity test:

- Positive – the skin will appear irritated, inflamed and might also look swollen. If any of these occur, advise your client to seek medical advice and do not continue with the treatment.
- Negative – the skin will appear normal with no visible reaction. If this is the case, you can continue with the treatment.

Make sure that you record the results of the skin tests onto the client's record card to safeguard yourself.

INDUSTRY TIP

Make sure the tint is fully dry before you allow your client to roll her sleeves down if you are testing on the inside of their elbow, to avoid staining their clothes. You can always blot excess tint until it is dry.

PROVIDE EYE TREATMENTS

In this part of the chapter you will learn about:

- eyebrow shaping and colouring
- eyelash and eyebrow tinting
- eyelash perming
- false lash application
- contra-actions
- evaluating the treatment.

INDUSTRY TIP

Subscribe to a professional beauty magazine. These usually come out monthly and are a great read as well as having a classified section in the back that lists available jobs in the industry.

ACTIVITY

Design your own posters, displaying the benefits of each of the eye treatment procedures. Make them colourful and eye-catching so the clients notice them.

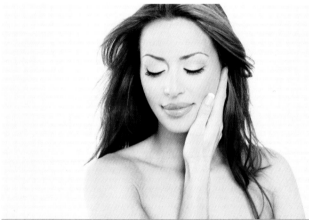

Example of perfect eyebrows

There are many different eyelash and eyebrow treatments available. Listed below are the most popular.

Treatment	Description
Depilatory waxing 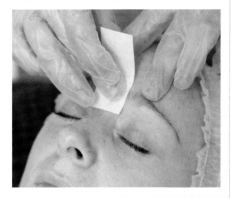	Removes the hair bulb and can last up to 4 weeks.
Electrolysis 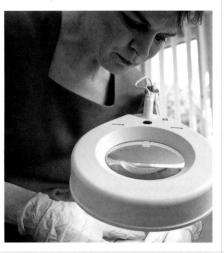	Permanently removes the hair over time by using a current to cauterise the hair bulb.
IPL (intense pulse light) 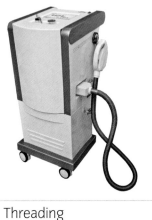	Permanently removes the hair using a laser.
Threading 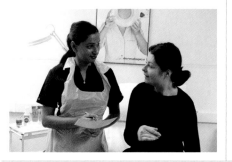	Removes the hair by using thread and can last up to 4 weeks.

Treatment	Description
Semi-permanent make-up 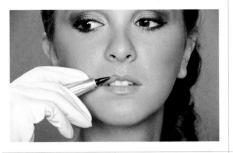	Make-up applied to the eyebrows that can last between 3 and 5 years.
Lash extensions 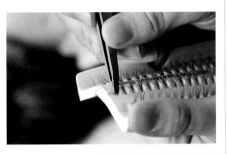	Individual lashes are applied to existing lashes to create length and fullness; can last up to 6 weeks.
Lash perming 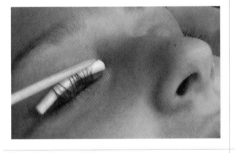	Creates a curl to the natural lash.
Eyebrow colouring (using eyebrow pencil and powder) 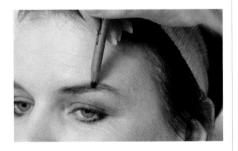	Gives the illusion of fuller eyebrows and enhances the colour.
Eyelash and eyebrow tinting 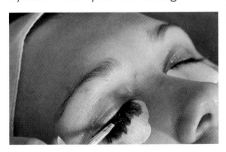	Gives the natural lashes and eyebrows definition and changes the colour, also giving the illusion of thicker, fuller lashes; can last up to 6 weeks.

The treatments you need to learn for Level 2 are covered below.

EYEBROW SHAPING AND COLOURING

Eyebrow shaping:

- adds definition to the face
- softens the facial features
- lifts the eye area
- helps change the shape of the eye
- adds colour to the brow.

Eyebrow shaping is a very popular treatment within a salon. Everyone's eyebrow shapes are different; some people have very bushy eyebrows with very coarse, curly hair and others have fine, thin eyebrows.

The purpose of shaping the eyebrows is to add definition to the face and enhance the facial features. It also acts as an instant face lift for more mature clients as it gives the illusion of lifting the browbone.

Always make sure you listen carefully to your client throughout the consultation to gain knowledge of your client's expectations. Give advice on what shape would best suit their face and enhance their facial features.

You can adapt the treatment at any time if necessary. The client might have a low pain threshold and you might have to amend the treatment by not taking as many hairs out, perhaps completing the treatment in two sessions so the client feels more comfortable.

ACTIVITY

Create a collage of 'before and after' photos of all your favourite celebrities. On one side stick pictures of before they were famous and the other side pictures of after they where famous. Note the difference in their eyebrow shapes.

EYEBROW SHAPES

These are the shapes that you can achieve to enhance your client's natural features, face shape and eye shape. Refer back to Chapter 209/211/220 Make-up application/instruction for more in-depth knowledge and understanding of face and eye shapes.

HANDY HINTS

See Chapter 209/211/220 Make-up application/instruction for detailed information on applying make-up to the eyes.

INDUSTRY TIP

The function of an eyebrow is to protect the eyes from dust and moisture and to act as a cushion to physical injury.

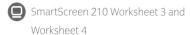 SmartScreen 210 Worksheet 3 and Worksheet 4

Eyebrow shape	Reason for use
Arched	An arched-shaped brow will enhance most features and face and eye shapes.
Straight	A straight-shaped brow will enhance an oblong face shape as it will give the illusion of a wider shape.
Angular	An angular-shaped brow will enhance a pear/triangular face shape as it will give the illusion of lifting.
Thin	A thin brow suits most face shapes and the majority of clients will opt for a thinner brow. This shape is great for more mature clients as it gives an instant lifting effect. It will not suit a client with a large nose as it will make their face look disproportionate.
Thin – thick	A thicker brow is good for younger clients but also suits most face shapes (long, square, heart, round and diamond).
Longer	Good for clients with close-set eyes. You need to create the illusion of width between the eyes, so extend the length of the eyebrows either side to help.
Shorter	Good for clients with wide-set eyes. You will need to create the illusion of the eyes being closer together, so bring the eyebrow length in at the bridge of the nose and keep the outer brows to the correct length.

Choosing a brow shape for your client

When you have determined your client's requirements and had a look at their natural features, you can advise your client on what you feel best suits them. Remember, the eyebrows should be balanced with the rest of the facial features. You are now ready to measure your client's eyebrows. Here are the three main guidelines to work from to determine the correct length of your client's eyebrows.

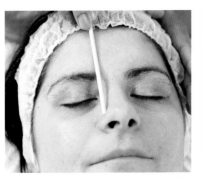

STEP 1 – Take an orange wood stick and place it to the right-hand side of your client's nose, keeping it straight as if you were pointing it towards their forehead. Remove the hair that grows to the left of the orange wood stick with tweezers. Repeat the same process on the left-hand side of the nose.

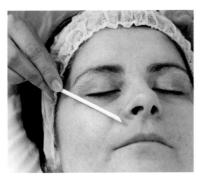

STEP 2 – Place the orange wood stick at the base of the nose, from the nostrils to the corner of the outer eye. Remove with tweezers any hairs to the left of the stick on the left eye and any to the right on the right eye.

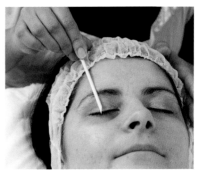

STEP 3 – Take your orange wood stick and place it in line with the centre of your client's pupil. This is where the highest part of the arch should be.

To make tweezing less painful for your client, follow these simple rules:

- Make sure your client is in a comfortable position.
- Make sure you are also in a comfortable position.
- Pre-heat the area with a hot towel or steamer to open up the pores.
- Apply pressure to the area.
- Stretch the skin while tweezing.
- Make sure you remove the hair in the direction of hair growth.
- Apply soothing lotion after tweezing.

ACTIVITY

Write down the advantages of having an eyebrow shape and how you would promote this treatment to your clients.

Step-by-step procedure for eyebrow shaping

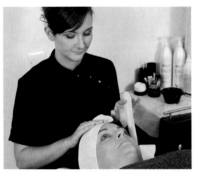

STEP 1 – Wash your hands and position yourself and your client comfortably. Apply a headband to your client.

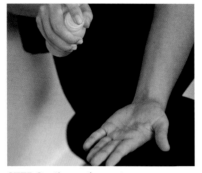

STEP 2 – Cleanse the area to remove make-up (refer to Chapter 204 Provide facial skin care/facial care for men for the correct techniques for cleansing the eye area).

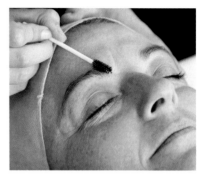

STEP 3 – Brush the brows with a disposable brush.

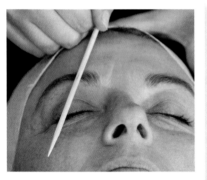

STEP 4 – Measure the brows with your orange wood stick.

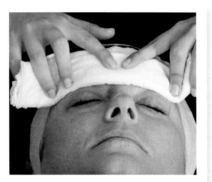

STEP 5 – Warm the area with hot towels. This will help to open the pores and will make the treatment more comfortable for your client. Place a cotton wool pad to the side of your client's head to put the tweezed hairs onto.

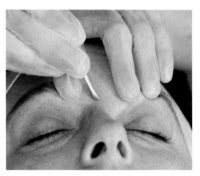

STEP 6 – Stretch the skin and start tweezing the unwanted hairs in the direction of hair growth. It is advisable to start in the middle the bridge of the nose as this area is said to be less sensitive.

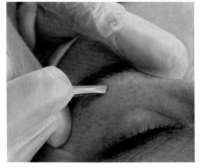

STEP 7 – Tweeze under each of the browbones, keeping the skin stretched; remove the unwanted hair in the direction of hair growth until you have achieved the desired shape.

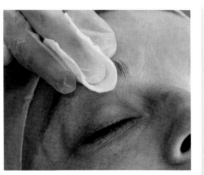

STEP 8 – Keep a cold compress to hand to soothe the area when it has been tweezed.

> **INDUSTRY TIP**
>
> You do not need to wear gloves when you are doing an eyebrow shape. If you do wear gloves, they will protect you against contact with body tissue fluid.

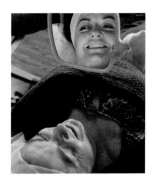

STEP 9 – Make sure you show your client the results in a mirror when you have completed one eyebrow.

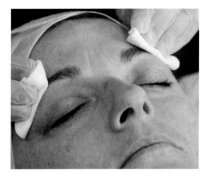

STEP 10 – When you have achieved your look and agreed the shape with your client, apply a soothing agent with cotton wool.

AFTERCARE ADVICE FOR EYEBROW SHAPING

It is very important to give your client aftercare advice after you have completed the treatment. This will enable the client to look after their eyebrows at home and you can also make sure they are not going to apply any products that will affect the result.

- Rebook your client for a maintenance eyebrow shape in 4–6 weeks' time.
- Advise your client to avoid the following for 24 hours:
  - heat treatments (sauna, steam room, sun bed)
  - sunbathing
  - application of make-up to the treated area
  - application of perfumed products to the treated area, including moisturisers
  - touching the area.
- Advise your client to apply a soothing product (witch hazel).
- Home grooming – your client can brush their eyebrows into place if they are a little unruly.
- Advise your client to tweeze any stray hairs between appointments.

ACTIVITY

Design your own aftercare advice leaflet to give to your clients at the end of their treatment.

ACTIVITY

With a group of three friends, test each others' knowledge by writing 10 questions each about eyebrow shaping and asking each other as part of a game to see which has the most knowledge.

EYELASH AND EYEBROW TINTING

Eyelash and eyebrow tinting are very popular treatments within the salon and give your clients an instant result. The benefits of tinting are:

- it gives the illusion of thicker/longer lashes
- it adds colour and definition
- it is good for clients who wear glasses or contact lenses
- it is great for holidays and special occasions.

INDUSTRY TIP

Your eyelashes protect your eyes from dust and moisture in the same way as your eyebrows do. Your eyelashes and eyebrows together add definition to your face.

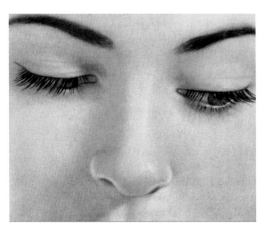

Example of eyelash and eyebrow tinting

The purpose of an eyebrow or eyelash tinting treatment is to add colour to the lashes and the eyebrows. You will find that most of your clients' lashes are lighter at the tips, so having a tint will give the illusion of longer lashes. There are a variety of different colours to use for tinting the eyebrows and lashes, and they also come in different types of product.

The colours available are blue, black, brown, blue/black and grey.

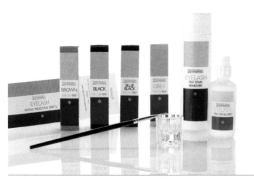

Eyelash and eyebrow tinting products

Consistency
Thickness of the product.

Tint product type	Advantages/disadvantages
Gel	Thick **consistency**
	Easy to apply and remove
Cream	Thick consistency
	Easy to apply and remove
Jelly	Easy to apply and remove
Liquid	Consistency is thin, which makes it harder to apply and could seep into the eye area

The most popular type of tint product is the cream as it is thicker in consistency and there is less risk of it running into the eye. It is also very easy to mix, apply and remove. The different colours are your client's preference, but it is best to use brown on the eyebrows and black only if your client already has dark brows. On the lashes you can use any of the colours to define your client's features.

Before the tint is applied to the client's lashes or brow, it has to be mixed with hydrogen peroxide. This causes a chemical reaction that activates the tint. Make sure you always check the manufacturer's instructions to see how much hydrogen peroxide to use. It should also be stated clearly on the bottle.

Molecule
A group of two or more atoms.

Cortex
The middle layer of the hair that forms the bulk; it contains melanin, which gives the hair its natural colour.

When the two products are mixed together the reaction occurs and the small **molecules** form large molecules. These then get trapped in the **cortex** of the hair and permanently add colour to the hair. Like any hair tint, the colour will start to fade and the hairs will grow and be replaced with new ones. The tint will last from 4–6 weeks before the brows or lashes will need re-tinting.

ACTIVITY

If you college has a hairdressing department, ask if you could cut a small amount of hair from their dolls' heads and test each of the tinting colours so you can get a true impression of the colours.

CHOOSING THE RIGHT COLOUR FOR YOUR CLIENT

INDUSTRY TIP
Make sure your client has a skin test 24 hours prior to application of a tint.

Make sure you sit down with your client before the treatment to determine their requirements so you can suggest the correct colour choice for them. Here is a list to help you:

- Skin colour – look at your client's skin tone and choose a tint colour that will complement it.
- Hair colour – look at your client's hair colour and try and match the tint colour (this will not work for a redhead).
- Eye colour – the colour of the tint should complement the eye colour.
- Mascara/eyebrow colour normally worn by the client – ask your client what colour mascara they usually wear and if they currently use an eyebrow pencil.
- Colour desired by the client – always ask your client what colour they would prefer; you can then advise them on the colour you think will suit them, taking into consideration the factors listed above.

- Occasion – your client might be coming in for an eyelash tint for a special occasion, for example a wedding. They might not want to wear mascara as they might get a little teary; tinting the lashes will add the definition they require without the risk of smudging.

STEP-BY-STEP PROCEDURE FOR EYELASH TINTING

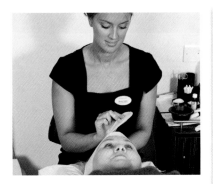

STEP 1 – Wash your hands and position yourself and your client comfortably. Apply a headband to your client.

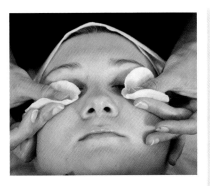

STEP 2 – Cleanse the area with a non-oily cleanser to remove make-up. Blot to remove any moisture.

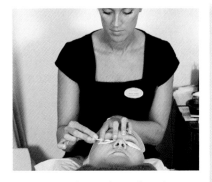

STEP 3 – Apply petroleum jelly to the eye shields and place these directly under each bottom lash, making sure there are no gaps for the tint to seep into.

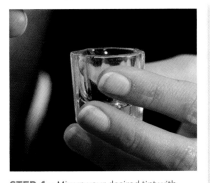

STEP 4 – Mix up your desired tint with hydrogen peroxide (checking the manufacturer's instructions for the correct amount of peroxide to use) using your mixing dish and brush.

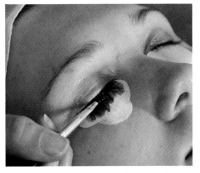

STEP 5 – Apply tint to the lashes with your disposable brush, making sure you cover all the lashes from root to tip and avoiding the skin. Repeat on the other lash, using a new disposable brush. Leave for 12–15 minutes to develop, checking the manufacturer's instructions for the correct time.

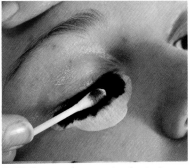

STEP 6 – Start by removing the tint from one eye with a cotton bud, brushing down the lashes and removing as much of the tint as you can. Repeat this until the cotton bud stays clear. Cover the lashes with a damp cotton wool pad. Repeat on the other eye.

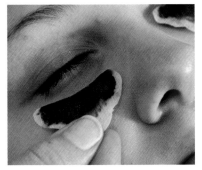

STEP 7 – Ask your client to keep their eyes closed and remove the cotton wool pads and eye shields from each eye.

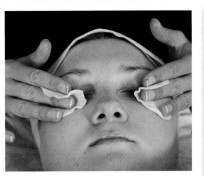

STEP 8 – Cover both eyes with damp cotton wool pads and wipe the lashes with a sweeping outwards motion.

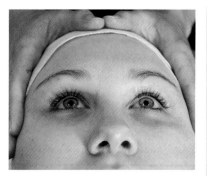

STEP 9 – Ask your client to open their eyes. If the removal has been correctly carried out there will be no tint left on the lashes (when you are training, you might leave a small amount on the lashes – just ask your client to close their eyes and remove the remaining tint with a cotton bud).

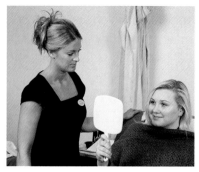

STEP 10 – Ask your client to sit up slowly and make sure they are comfortable. Give your client a mirror to show them the tinting results.

STEP-BY-STEP PROCEDURE FOR EYEBROW TINTING

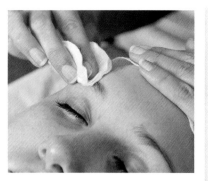

STEP 1 – Wash your hands and position yourself and your client comfortably before you begin. Apply a headband to your client. Cleanse the area to remove make-up and blot to remove any grease.

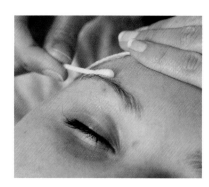

STEP 2 – Apply petroleum jelly above and below the eyebrows to protect the surrounding skin from staining.

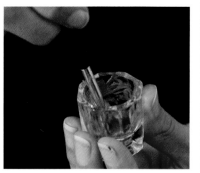

STEP 3 – Mix up your desired tint with hydrogen peroxide (checking the manufacturer's instructions for the correct amount of peroxide to use) using your mixing dish and brush.

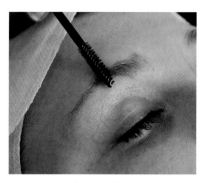

STEP 4 – Brush the eyebrows in the opposite direction to how they naturally lie.

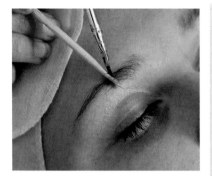

STEP 5 – Place an orange wood stick under the brow hairs. Paint the tint onto the hairs, starting from the inner brow and working your way outwards. Repeat on the other brow.

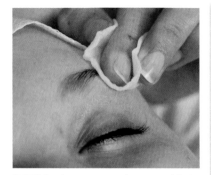

STEP 6 – As soon as you have completed both brows, remove the tint from the first brow with a damp cotton wool pad, sweeping it from inner brow to outer brow. Repeat on the other brow.

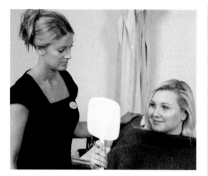

STEP 7 – Show your client the end result. If they would like them to be darker, repeat the same process again.

> **INDUSTRY TIP**
>
> It is always better, especially with eyebrows, to start off with a lighter colour. Then you can add more colour as required until the client is satisfied with the colour.

AFTERCARE ADVICE FOR EYELASH/EYEBROW TINTING

- Rebook your client for another eyelash or eyebrow tint in 4–6 weeks' time.
- Advise your client:
  - to avoid the application of mascara for 12 hours
  - not to wear contact lenses for 12 hours if you have performed an eyelash tint
  - to avoid touching the area
  - not to have an eyelash perm for at least 24–48 hours.
- Advise on suitable home care products, for example a clear mascara.

EYELASH PERMING

Eyelash perming is a popular treatment in the salon. It allows you to permanently curl the lashes, giving the appearance of longer lashes and giving the lashes an instant lift. The results are very effective and they will last as long as the hair growth cycle.

The benefits of an eyelash perm are:

- it creates a natural curl
- it adds definition to the lashes
- the lashes appear longer
- it is great for special occasions and holidays.

> **INDUSTRY TIP**
>
> If you accidentally stain your client's skin with tint, use the stain remover to lift the product off the skin.

> **INDUSTRY TIP**
>
> If you are inclined to be a little messy with the tint, wear gloves to prevent yourself from staining your skin and nails.

INDUSTRY TIP

Refer to the Anatomy and Physiology chapter to recap on the hair growth cycle.

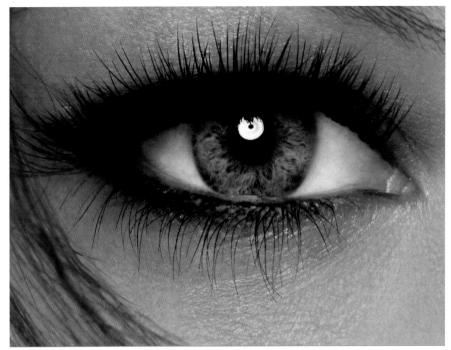

An example of eyelash perming

The process is the same as for curling the hair on the head. You will be setting the curl into place with rods, then neutralising to fix the curl into place.

When the perming solution is applied to the lashes, the bonds within the cortex of the lash hair are broken down by the hydrogen within the solution. This softens the hair and allows you to make a new shape with the perming rod. You then apply the neutraliser to fix the hair into place and stop the action of the perming solution. The bonds are reformed by the addition of oxygen and removal of hydrogen.

Different sized perming rods are available. The size will determine the type of curl – the smaller the rod the tighter the curl.

- Small – used for finer, shorter lashes.
- Medium – used for most lashes. This rod will create an uplifting, loose look for finer lashes and more of a definite curl for longer, thicker lashes.
- Large – used for thicker, longer lashes to create a natural uplifting curl.

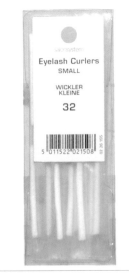

Small perming rods

ACTIVITY

When you are practising on your peers, take a picture of the eyelashes after using a small, medium and large rod size. This will give you photo evidence to show your clients the differences between each rod size and the effects they give.

STEP-BY-STEP PROCEDURE FOR EYELASH PERMING

Always make sure that you fully explain the treatment to your client before you start to put them at ease. Eyelash perming is a long process and your client will have their eyes closed for about an hour.

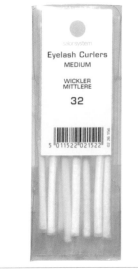

Medium perming rods

INDUSTRY TIP

Make sure you choose the correct sized rod for your client's lashes. Listen very carefully to their requirements.

Before you start the perming treatment, wash your hands, allow contact lens wearers to remove their lenses, position yourself and your client comfortably, apply a headband to your client, cleanse the area to remove make-up and blot to remove any grease.

INDUSTRY TIP

Before you apply the products, make sure that the bottom lashes are not attached to the rods.

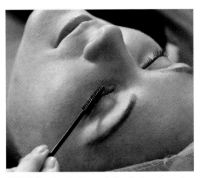

STEP 1 – Comb through the lashes to make sure they are evenly separated and dry.

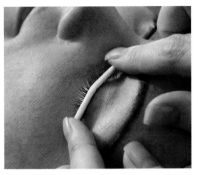

STEP 2 – Select the correct size rods for your client. Placing your fingers at either end of the rod, bend it so you get a curved contour in the middle. If you find that the curler is too long you can cut the rod to the correct size.

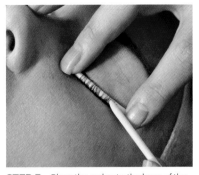

STEP 3 – Place the rod onto the base of the lashes and start to curl the lashes around using an orange stick. Make sure that the lashes are straight and do not overlap each other. If you have difficulty sticking the lashes to the rod, you can use a small amount of glue. Repeat with other eye.

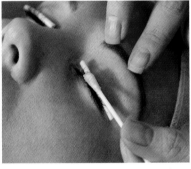

STEP 4 – Apply the perming lotion to the lashes using a cotton bud. Leave for 12 minutes (check the manufacturer's instructions for timing as some products might differ). Covering the eyes with a piece of cling film and a small towel will speed up the perming process.

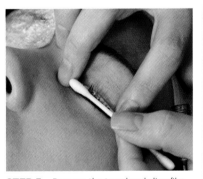

STEP 5 – Remove the towel and cling film, apply the neutralising lotion to the lashes over the perming lotion (there is no need to remove the perming lotion), re-cover the eyes with cling film and a small towel and leave for 12 minutes (check the manufacturer's instructions for timing as some products might differ).

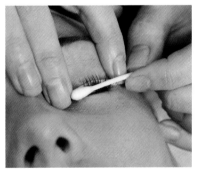

STEP 6 – Remove the cling film and, using a dry cotton pad, remove the neutralising product from both lashes.

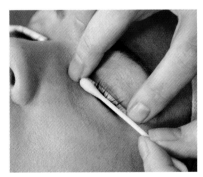

STEP 7 – Apply the collagen lotion to both lashes and leave for 3 minutes (this will add the nutrients back into the lashes)

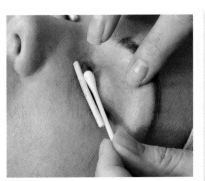

STEP 8 – Apply eyelash perming cleanser to a cotton bud and very gently use your cotton bud in a rolling motion to remove the rods from both eyes.

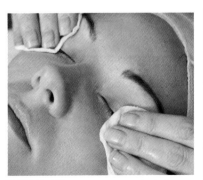

STEP 9 – Wipe any excess products from the eye area with a piece of damp cotton wool and slowly sit your client up, asking them to slowly open their eyes.

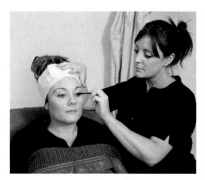

STEP 10 – Using a disposable mascara wand, gently stroke through the lashes.

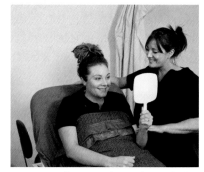

STEP 11 – Allow your client to have a look in the mirror.

Ineffective results (when things go wrong)

There are a few things that can go wrong when you are performing an eyelash perming treatment. See the table below for possible solutions.

Problem	Possible cause	Correction
Too curled	Wrong rod size, too small for the lashes.	Choose a larger rod.
Hairs pointing in different directions	Lashes not straight when placed onto the rods and have overlapped each other.	Make sure you place all the lashes correctly onto the rod and that they are secure.
Hooked ends	Tip of lashes not positioned correctly onto the rod.	Make sure that the lashes are flat when they are on the rod and the tips of the lashes are not hooked over each other. You can use a little glue to make sure they are flat.

AFTERCARE ADVICE FOR EYELASH PERMING

- Rebook your client for another eyelash perm in 4–6 weeks' time.
- Advise your client:
  - to avoid the application of mascara for 12 hours
  - to avoid touching the area
  - not to have an eyelash tint for at least 24 hours.
- Advise suitable home care products, for example a clear mascara.

FALSE LASH APPLICATION

Application of false lashes is a great way to enhance your client's eyes. They are made up of small threads of real hair or nylon and they come in either individual lashes or as strip lashes. They are great to add with evening or special occasion make-up, adding thickness and length to your client's natural lashes.

False lashes come in a variety of different thicknesses, lengths and colours. If you want to create an avant-garde catwalk look you can get some amazing designs. A selection of strip and individual lashes are illustrated.

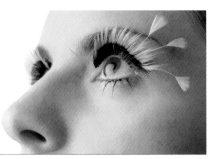

Funky strip lashes

The benefits of applying false lashes are:

- they enhance a make-up
- they add definition and give the illusion of thickness
- they add length to the natural lashes
- they are great for special occasions (photoshoots, weddings, holidays, fancy dress parties)
- they are a good alternative to someone who is allergic to mascara.

Strip lashes: these are designed only to be worn for a short period of time, like a special occasion or a photoshoot. They are attached to the base of the natural lashes and they come in many different lengths and colours.

Individual lashes: these come as individual hairs; they are a cluster of about three lashes attached to one small bulb. These are placed onto the natural lashes at the base and you can apply as many as you like to get your desired look. They can last for up to 3 weeks if looked after correctly. Due to the natural lashes' own hair cycle, you might find that some of the individual lashes will fall out naturally. They can be replaced very easily and quickly by the therapist.

ACTIVITY

Design a crossword with all the equipment and materials needed to perform a strip or individual lash application. Get your friends to complete it.

INDUSTRY TIP

To make sure the client is happy with the length of the lash you are going to apply, hold the lashes up to their eyes so they can see the effect or, if it is an individual lash application, apply one and ask your client to look in the mirror and check that it is what they want.

STEP-BY-STEP PROCEDURE FOR STRIP LASH APPLICATION

Preparation

Wash your hands, position yourself and your client comfortably and apply a headband to your client.

INDUSTRY TIP

There are many different varieties of strip and individual lashes. Make sure you keep a good stock to suit all types of client.

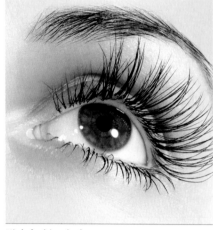

High-fashion lashes

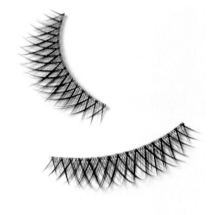

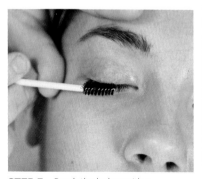

Individual lashes

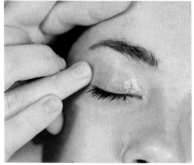

STEP 1 – Cleanse the area to remove make-up (however, you might be applying strip lashes over mascara if it is to be used with a fashion make-up).

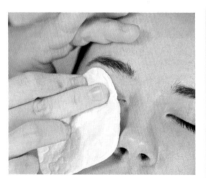

STEP 2 – Blot to remove any moisture.

STEP 3 – Brush the lashes with a disposable mascara brush, making sure they are all separated.

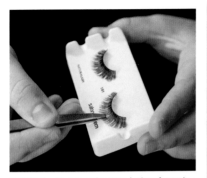

STEP 4 – Remove the strip lashes from the packaging with a pair of tweezers, being careful as they are very delicate.

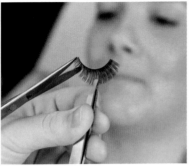

STEP 5 – Size up the strip lash with your client's natural lashes. If necessary, use a pair of small scissors to cut them to make them fit your client's natural lashline. Make sure you leave a 2 mm gap from the corner of the eye for comfort.

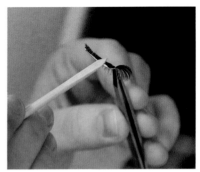

STEP 6 – Take an orange wood stick and apply a small amount of glue to the rim of the strip lash.

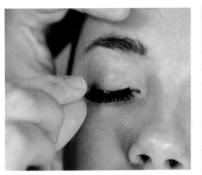

STEP 7 – Carefully take the strip lash, ask your client to close their eyes and place the lash at the base of the natural lashes. Use your fingers and place your strip lash firmly into place.

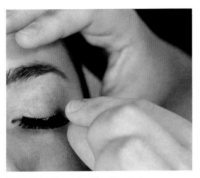

STEP 8 – Repeat with other eye.

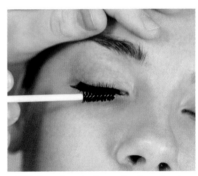

STEP 9 – Allow 3 minutes for the adhesive to dry, making sure that your client keeps their eyes closed.

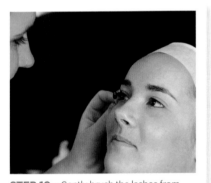

STEP 10 – Gently brush the lashes from underneath the natural lashes using a disposable mascara brush. This will allow the lashes to bond together.

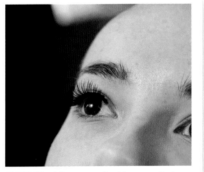

STEP 11 – Allow your client to open their eyes slowly and to look directly at you. Make sure they are in place and that they look balanced.

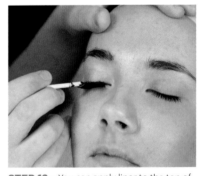

STEP 12 – You can apply liner to the top of the lashes to add extra definition.

INDUSTRY TIP

You apply all strip lashes in the same way, whether they are standard black ones or dramatic fashion lashes.

INDUSTRY TIP

Advise your client that strip lashes are re-usable and explain how to clean them when they are removed.

INDUSTRY TIP

Remember that the lashes come in a left and a right, so make sure you attach the correct lash to each eye.

INDUSTRY TIP

Make sure that the strip lashes are firmly stuck to the base of the natural lashes before you allow your client to open their eyes.

STEP-BY-STEP PROCEDURE FOR INDIVIDUAL LASH APPLICATION

Preparation

Wash your hands, position yourself and your client comfortably and apply a headband to your client.

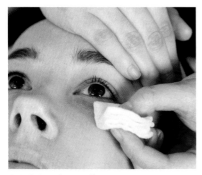

STEP 1 – Cleanse the area to remove make-up.

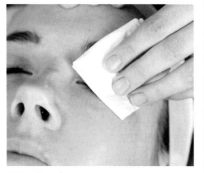

STEP 2 – Blot to remove any grease.

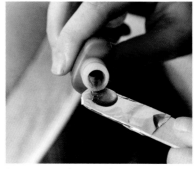

STEP 3 – Apply some glue to a wooden spatula.

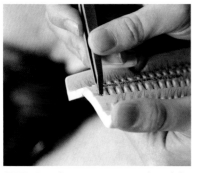

STEP 4 – Take your tweezers and carefully pick up an individual lash from the pack. Dip the bulb at the very top of the lashes into the glue, making sure there is just enough glue on the bulb but not too much.

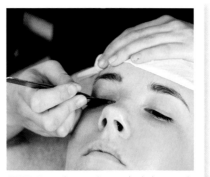

STEP 5 – Ask your client to look down and close their eyes and apply the individual lash to the base of the natural lash hair where you want it to be. It is best to start at the inner eye and work your way outwards.

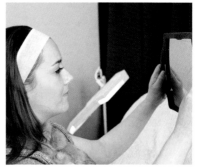

STEP 6 – When you have added the desired amount of individual lashes and checked that they are even on both sides, show your client in the mirror.

> **INDUSTRY TIP**
>
> The lash length chosen will depend on how many individual lashes you are going to apply. It is best to apply shorter ones from the inner eye to the middle, then longer ones to the outer lashes as this gives a better result.

AFTERCARE ADVICE FOR FALSE LASH APPLICATION

Show your client how to safely remove the strip lashes at home.

Advise your client:

- to avoid the application of mascara as this will break down the adhesive bond
- to avoid oil-based products as this will break down the adhesive bond
- to avoid touching or rubbing the area, or picking at the lashes
- to come back into the salon for an infill if required
- to come back into the salon for removal of individual lashes.

> **INDUSTRY TIP**
>
> Be very careful when removing the individual lashes from the packet; you do not want to break them or ruin their shape.

> **INDUSTRY TIP**
>
> Make sure both eyes are even and have the same number and length of lashes.

> **INDUSTRY TIP**
>
> Make sure you do not apply the lashes to the eyelids – they are a very sensitive area and can sometimes be irritated by the glue.

> **INDUSTRY TIP**
>
> You can switch from one eye to the other to make sure they are applied evenly on both sides. Remember to leave a 2 mm gap from the inner eye for comfort.

CONTRA-ACTIONS

This is something that could potentially happen during or after the treatment. Advise your clients of the contra-actions that are relevant to the treatment they have had and ask them to contact you if any occur. If the symptoms of the contra-actions are severe, suggest your client seeks medical advice from their GP. The table describes the normal contra-actions to eyelash/eyebrow treatments. Some more severe contra-actions are described at the end of the table.

Contra-action	Relevant treatment	Description and action
Erythema	All treatments	A dilation of blood capillaries that come to the surface of the skin. This is caused by friction or if the skin is irritated. If this occurs apply a cold compress to the affected area.
Swelling	All treatments	If swelling occurs, stop the treatment and apply a cold compress to the area.
Weeping eyes	All treatments	The eyes might be very sensitive and might weep slightly; the fumes from the adhesive, coloured tint or perming gel can be quite strong. Advise your client to keep their eyes closed for 3 minutes after application. If a small amount of glue/tint/perming gel enters the eye, immediately apply an eyebath. The eyes might also weep when you are tweezing. If this occurs, sit your client up and apply a cold compress to the eyebrow area to soothe it.
Stinging	All treatments	The eyes might sting a little after these eyelash/brow treatments as your client will have had their eyes closed for some time. If a small amount of glue, tint or perming gel has accidentally entered the eye and is causing real discomfort, apply an eyebath immediately. Your client's eyebrow area might sting slightly after you have tweezed. Apply a cold compress or witch hazel to ease the stinging. If the eyes continue to sting when the client reaches home, suggest they seek medical advice from their GP.
Bruising	Eyebrow shaping	This might occur during an eyebrow shaping treatment. If your client has sensitive skin be very careful not to add too much pressure.
Staining	Eyelash/ eyebrow tinting	Staining might still occur even though you have added petroleum jelly as a barrier. If this happens you can remove it with stain remover. Apply to a piece of cotton wool and lightly rub the affected area.
Severe erythema	All treatments	A dilation of blood capillaries that come to the surface of the skin. This is caused by friction or if the skin is severely irritated; the skin will become very red. If this occurs apply a cold compress to the affected area.
Tissue damage resulting in blood loss	Eyebrow shaping	If you accidentally damage your client's skin it can result in blood loss. Depending on the severity of the damage, apply pressure with a cold compress until the bleeding has stopped. If the bleeding continues and it is a deep wound, advise your client to seek medical attention.
Allergic reaction to product	All treatments	If your client suffers an allergic reaction, remove the product immediately and apply an eyebath. If the problem continues, advise your client to seek medical attention.

EVALUATING THE TREATMENT

It is very important to evaluate your work when you have completed your treatment. The different ways of evaluating are:

Verbal feedback: at the end of the treatment ask your client if there is anything they would change. Are they happy with the end result? Talk through the aftercare advice and ask your client if they have any questions. If your client feels they received a good service, they are more likely to keep coming back to the salon.

Written feedback: allow your client to give feedback on your consultation form. When you have completed the treatment, evaluate yourself and list what you think you did well, together with areas of improvement for next time. Remember, you are always learning and refining your skills.

Photographic evidence: always take pictures of your work to put into your portfolio. This will help you in the future with interviews, when yo are applying for higher education or for a job. You can also use your portfolio to advertise yourself to your clients. Always make sure that your clients are happy with you taking photos and tell them how you will be using them.

Repeat business: you can always evaluate yourself by seeing how much repeat business you get. If your client comes back after their first treatment, it means they are happy with the service they received.

ACTIVITY

Design your own feedback form to give to your client to fill out at the end of their treatment.

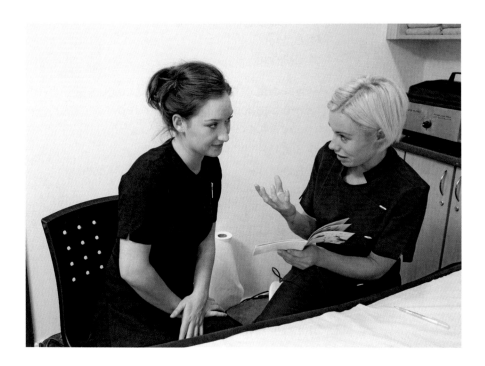

Use the questions below to test your knowledge of Chapter 210/218/225 to see how much information you have retained. These questions will help you to revise what you have learnt in this chapter.

Turn to page 601 for the answers.

1. Which **one** of the following is the best method of sterilisation for tweezers?
   a) Autoclave
   b) Chemical solution
   c) UV cabinet
   d) Surgical spirit

2. Which **one** of the following describes the best method for removing waste at the end of the day?
   a) Remove bin liner and tie up securely
   b) Put into a sealed bag and dispose of in an outside bin
   c) Put into a yellow bag and place in the bin
   d) Remove bin liner from the working bin and place into a black sack

3. Which **one** of the following best describes how to prevent client discomfort during a brow-shaping treatment?
   a) Pluck against the direction of hair growth
   b) Pluck in the direction of hair growth
   c) Apply soothing lotion on a cotton wool pad
   d) Wipe dry cotton wool over the skin between hair removal

4. The percentage of hydrogen peroxide that is safe for use in eyelash tinting is:
   a) 3 per cent
   b) 5 per cent
   c) 7 per cent
   d) 10 per cent.

5. Which **one** of the following would have a negative effect on the tinting process?
   a) Grease on the lashes
   b) Non-oily eye make-up remover
   c) Applying the tint with an orange wood stick
   d) Leaving the tint on for 10 minutes

6. Which **one** of the following best describes a positive reaction to the skin following a skin-sensitivity test?
   a) Swelling and itching sensation
   b) Pain and swelling
   c) Erythema and skin peeling
   d) Red raised papules

7. If a client has wide-set eyes, which **one** of the following should be recommended to the client during an eyebrow shape?
   a) Increasing the distance between the eyebrows
   b) Increasing the arch of the eyebrow
   c) Reducing the distance between the eyebrows
   d) Reducing the arch of the eyebrow

8. Which **one** of the following is the ideal eyebrow shape for a heart-shaped face?
   a) Arched
   b) Straight
   c) Angular
   d) Oblique

9. Which **one** of the following tint colours should be recommended to a client with red hair to achieve a natural look?
   a) Black
   b) Brown
   c) Blue/black
   d) Grey

10. Automatic tweezers are best for use in:
    a) removing stray hairs
    b) defining the eyebrow shape
    c) removing the bulk of excess hair
    d) increasing the speed of the technique.

11. Which **one** of the following treatments can open up the eyes and make short, straight lashes appear longer and curled?
    a) Eyebrow tint
    b) Eyelash perm
    c) Semi-permanent eye make-up
    d) Eyelash tint

12. What function does the neutraliser or fixing lotion have within an eyelash perming treatment?
    a) Opens the cuticle
    b) Breaks down the sulphur bonds
    c) Reforms the sulphur bonds
    d) Causes the cuticle to swell

13. During an eyelash perm, which **one** of the following would cause a 'hooked end' to the lash?
    a) Damp eyelashes prior to application of perming solution
    b) Chemical process too long
    c) Incorrect position of the point of eyelash on the curler
    d) Incorrect sized roller used

14. Which **one** of the following is the main benefit of placing cling film over the lashes while perming?
    a) Keeps the product on the lashes
    b) Creates warmth and speeds up the process
    c) Keeps the client's eyes closed
    d) Prevents the product from drying out

15. At what stage should tint be mixed to apply to the eyelashes/eyebrows?
    a) When the client arrives
    b) After the consultation
    c) When the client is on the couch
    d) Directly prior to application

While studying for my A levels, I worked part time in a salon and soon realised that the beauty industry had a lot to offer me as a career. This led to the decision to take my beauty therapy qualifications. Once qualified, I progressed to Head Therapist carrying out managerial duties and the day-to-day running of the salon. I also secured the role of Salon Trainer, which gave me the responsibility of training staff in new products and treatments. The experience I gained through this training inspired me to start teaching.

I am currently working in a college teaching beauty therapy and theatrical media make-up. I find it exciting and rewarding passing my knowledge onto others and seeing them progress.

Beauty therapy continues to grow and offers a diverse and exciting career in which there are lots of opportunities to specialise. I believe the role is to make a difference to people and provide a service that allows the client to feel good and confident about themselves. What I love about working in the industry are the prospects to develop new skills in the latest trends. As an example, I trained in lash perfect semi-permanent individual lash extensions, which remains one of the fastest growing salon services internationally. A demand in the market for more 'dramatic-looking' eyes is providing a renewed focus on eye treatments and industry experts are experimenting with the appearance of new and innovative products and treatments to meet this need.

A career in the beauty sector offers you the opportunity to provide a service to others using your own creative talents in an ever-expanding industry.

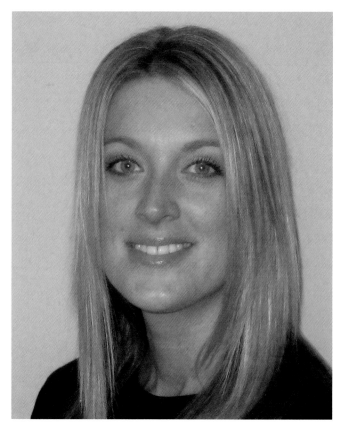

Anatomy and physiology

1 d, 2 a, 3 a, 4 d, 5 b, 6 c, 7 d, 8 a, 9 d, 10 b,
11 d, 12 b, 13 c, 14 c, 15 c, 16 c, 17 d, 18 a,
19 d, 20 b, 21 b, 22 c, 23 a, 24 c, 25 a

Legislation

1 b, 2 c, 3 a, 4 b, 5 b, 6 b, 7 b, 8 b, 9 d, 10 b

201 Working in beauty-related industries

1 b, 2 c, 3 c, 4 c, 5 d, 6 b, 7 b, 8 c, 9 b, 10 a

202 Follow health and safety practice in the salon

1 b, 2 c, 3 d, 4 c, 5 b, 6 c, 7 b, 8 d, 9 b, 10 a

203 Client care amd communication in beauty-related industries

1 b, 2 b, 3 a, 4 c, 5 d, 6 a, 7 a, 8 d, 9 b, 10 c

205/213 Promote products and services/display stock

1 b, 2 a, 3 b, 4 a, 5 c, 6 d, 7 a, 8 a, 9 d, 10 d,
11 a, 12 d, 13 b, 14 a, 15 d

216 Salon reception duties

1 d, 2 a, 3 a, 4 a, 5 b, 6 b, 7 b, 8 c, 9 b, 10 b

204/224 Provide facial skin care/facial care for men

1 a, 2 b, 3 a, 4 a, 5 d, 6 b, 7 b, 8 a, 9 b, 10 a,
11 d, 12 a, 13 d, 14 a, 15 b

206/219 Remove hair using waxing/threading techniques

1 a, 2 a, 3 c, 4 a, 5 c, 6 d, 7 d, 8 b, 9 c, 10 b,
11 a, 12 a, 13 d, 14 a, 15 c

207/208 Provide manicure/pedicure treatments

1 b, 2 a, 3 c, 4 a, 5 b, 6 c, 7 a, 8 a, 9 d, 10 a,
11 a, 12 a, 13 a, 14 a, 15 a

214 Provide and maintain nail enhancement

1 d, 2 a, 3 a, 4 b, 5 a, 6 a, 7 a, 8 b, 9 c, 10 b,
11 c, 12 a, 13 c

215 Provide nail art

1 c, 2 c, 3 b, 4 d, 5 d, 6 a, 7 a, 8 d, 9 a, 10 d,
11 b, 12 d, 13 a, 14 a, 15 d

209/211/220 Make-up application/instruction

1 a, 2 c, 3 b, 4 c, 5 d, 6 a, 7 a, 8 a, 9 a, 10 c,
11 c, 12 d, 13 c, 14 c, 15 c, 16 b, 17 a, 18 d,
19 b, 20 c, 21 a, 22 b

212 Create an image based on a theme within the hair and beauty sector

1 a, 2 d, 3 b, 4 a, 5 a, 6 c, 7 a, 8 d, 9 a, 10 c

210/218/225 Provide eyelash and eyebrow shaping/eyelash perming/colouring treatments

1 a, 2 b, 3 b, 4 d, 5 a, 6 a, 7 c, 8 a, 9 b, 10 c,
11 b, 12 c, 13 c, 14 b, 15 d

INDEX

A

abbreviations for services/treatments 249
abrasive mitts 380
accident books 103, 161
accidents, reporting and recording 102, 103, 160–161
acne 22, 23, 272
acrylic nail enhancements 462–465
advertising 216–217, 549–550
Afro-Caribbean skin 13, 15, 507
age correction make-up techniques 512
ageing, skin 13–14, 269, 271, 311, 513
agranulocytes 76–77
air conditioning 178
albinism 19
alcohol 13, 269, 284
allergens 21, 26
allergic reactions 17, 21, 317, 373, 402, 435, 467, 596
alopecia 37
alpha hydroxyl acids (AHAs) 287, 288, 330
ampoules 312
anaphylactic shock 21
androgenic alopecia 37
anonychia 42
appointments, booking 245, 248–252, 466
    dealing with client expectations and needs 246–247
aprons 147, 148
arms
    blood vessels in 79
    bone structure 57–58
    muscles 69–72
arrector pil muscle 8, 9, 32
arteries 77
Asian skin 15, 507
athlete's foot 29, 398
atrophy, nail 47, 398
Austin, Jayne 236
autoclaves 152
awarding organisations 129, 130

B

bacterial infections 28–29, 36, 150, 151, 398
balms 310
Barbicide 335, 405, 440
bases, make-up 515
beau lines 42
beta hydroxyl acids (BHAs) 287
bikini line waxing 353–355, 376
birthmarks 18, 21
blackheads 8, 22, 23, 289, 290, 293
blood 75–77
blood pressure 80–81
blood vessels 8, 74, 77–80

blue nail 44
blushers 519–520
body language 169–170, 183, 193, 265, 443
body lice 30, 399
boils 28, 398
bone shapes 50–51
    see also skeletal system
breaks, work 136
brittle nail syndrome 45, 396
broken and fractured bones 59, 400
Brown, Janice 383
bruising 46, 81, 373, 596
brushes, make-up 501–502
bunions 59, 394
by-laws 95, 96, 97

C

calluses 25, 394
cancer 25, 86, 87, 88
capillaries 20, 78
carbuncles 28, 398
cardiovascular system 74–81
    basic structure of 74
    blood composition 75–77
    blood functions 75
    blood vessels 8, 74, 77–80
    disorders 80–81
career
    case studies x, 140, 188, 236, 324, 383, 438, 471, 495, 541, 559, 600
    opportunities 118–124
cash payments 254–255, 258
Caucasian skin 15
cells 3
    of the dermis 6–9
    of epidermis 3–5
    keratinised 31, 32, 33, 34, 38
cellular growth skin disorders 26
chemotherapy 88
cheque payments 212, 256, 258
chin hair removal 361, 368
chloasma 19
circulation disorders 20–21
cleansers 199, 275–278
    for men 320
cleansing brush, manual 282–283
cleansing routine 279–283
cleansing wipes 277
client care, providing 177–186
    client comfort 177–179
    client feedback 183–184
    dealing with complaints and problems 184–186
    learning from mistakes 186
    professionalism 179–182
closed questions 168, 173, 192, 241, 246

codes of practice 142–143
cold sores 27
collagen 6, 7, 13, 14, 15, 16
colour charts 194
colour correction 516
combination skin 17, 268, 271, 291, 505
comedogenic 277
comedones (blackheads) 8, 22, 23, 289, 290, 293
commercial radio 218
communicating with clients 166–177, 442
    client care legislation 166
    consultation process 174–176
    methods of 166–174
    personal space 176–177
    at reception 241–247
communication skills 191–195, 238, 266, 442
    and teamwork 550
competitions 548, 552–553
complaints and problems, dealing with 184–186
complementary therapists 119
computer screens, working with 103–104
concealers 515–516
confidentiality 105, 106, 176, 251–252
conjunctivitis 29
consultation process 174–176
    for eye treatments 573–577
    for facial care 265–266
    make-up 504
    for manicures and pedicures 391–392
    for nail art 479, 481
    for nail enhancement treatments 442–446
    waxing and threading 328
consumables 129, 214, 264, 334, 450
Consumer Protection Act 1987 106–107
Consumer Protection (Distance Selling) Regulations 2002 107–108
contact lenses 266, 512, 588, 589
continuing professional development (CPD) 126, 195
contra-actions
    eye treatments 596
    facial skin care treatments 317
    make-up 529
    manicure treatments 434–435
    nail art services 492
    nail enhancement 467–468
    pedicure treatments 434–435
    waxing 371–375
contra-indications 12, 174–175
    eye treatments 575–576
    facial skin care treatments 272
    lymphatic system 85–88
    make-up 513–514
    manicure treatments 397–402
    nail art services 479

nail enhancement 446
   pedicure treatments 397–402
   threading 371, 372, 374, 375
   waxing 330–331
contract of employment 135–136
contract work 125
Control of Substances Hazardous to Health
   Regulations (COSHH) 2002 96–97, 144,
   157, 222
Copyright, Designs and Patent Act 1998
   112
corns 25, 394
cortex 33
cosmetic or beauty consultants 120
cosmetic science 273
covering letters xiv
credit and debit cards 212, 257, 258
curriculum vitae xii–xiv
cuticle diseases and disorders 48–49
cuticle knives 156, 414
cuticle nippers 156, 414
cysts 23

D

Data Protection Act (DPA) 1998 105–106,
   162, 171, 176, 252
debit and credit cards 212, 257, 258
dehydrated skin 17, 268, 271, 308
dehydration pens 505
delivery notes 231
depilatory creams 378
dermal papilla 9, 32, 377
dermatitis 26, 149
dermis 5–9
diabetes 87, 88, 330, 402, 446
diet 13, 40, 269, 316, 395, 396
dilated capillaries 20
direct marketing 218–219
discrimination, legislation to prevent
   111–112
disinfection 153–155
display area 221–230
   dismantling 233
   lighting 229, 230
   maintaining 230–233, 240
   organising 223–224
   purpose of 224–226
   safety considerations 221–223
   setting up 226–229
display screen equipment (DSE), working
   with 103–104
dress code 131
dry skin 16, 17, 268, 270, 291, 292, 298,
   342, 394, 505

E

eczema 26, 330, 399, 446, 479, 513, 575
editorials 217
effleurage 296, 418
eggshell nails 47, 400, 446, 479

elastin 6
electrical appliances and equipment 97–98,
   264, 388
electrical depilators 343, 380
Electricity at Work Regulations (EAWR)
   1990 97–98
electrolysis 20, 22, 24, 377, 578
emails 172, 218, 245
emergency procedures 158–163
emery boards 386, 413, 434, 435
Employers' Liability (Compulsory Insurance)
   Act 1969 112
employment legislation 135–137
Employment Rights Act 1996 135–136
employment, types of 124–125
emulsions 273–278
enquiries, dealing with client 241–247
ephilides (freckles) 18
epidermis 3–5, 9
epilepsy 87, 272, 330, 401, 476, 479
Equality Act 2010 111–112
erythema 17, 81, 317, 372, 377, 419, 435,
   467, 492, 529, 576, 596
erythrocytes/red bood cells 76
exfoliants 285–286, 406
exfoliation 288–289
extraction 293
eye creams and gels 310
eye make-up remover 277–278, 563
eye pencils/eyeliners 522–523
eye protection 148
eye shapes, make-up techniques for
   509–510
eye tests 104
eye treatments, preparing for 561–577
   consultation 573–577
   contra-indications 575–576
   eyebrow shaping 334, 566–568
   eyelash/brow tinting 563–565
   eyelash perming 569–570
   false eyelash application 571–572
   health and safety issues 561–562
   skin testing 576–577
eye treatments, providing 577–597
   contra-actions 596
   evaluation 597
   eyebrow shaping and colouring 579,
      580–584
   eyelash/brow tinting 579, 585–589
   eyelash perming 579, 589–592
   false eyelash application 592–595
   types of treatment available 578–579
eyebrow pencils 523
eyebrow shapes 580–581
eyebrow shaping
   and colouring treatment 579, 580–584
   consultation 574
   products, tools and equipment 334,
      566–568
   threading 367
   waxing 357–359, 578
eyelash/brow tinting
   consultation 574

products, tools and equipment 563–565
   treatment 579, 585–589
eyelash perming
   consultation 574–575
   products, tools and equipment 569–570
   treatment 579, 589–592
eyeshadows 508, 521–522

F

face
   blood vessels in 78
   bones of 56
   cleansing 279–283
   muscles of 61–67
   shape 508–509
face masks 302–307
face-to-face enquiries 244
facial expressions 193
facial scrubs 285, 286, 289
facial skin care treatments, preparing for
   262–272
   consultation 265–266
   contra-indications for 272
   health and safety 262
   preparing the client 266–267
   skin analysis 267–269
   skin care products 265
   skin types and conditions 269–271
   treatment environment 262–264
   trolley and equipment 264
facial skin care treatments, providing
   273–321
   aftercare and home care advice
      314–316
   cleansers 275–278
   cleansing 279–283
   clearing up 318
   completing 314
   contra-actions 317
   emulsions 273–278
   exfoliants and facial scrubs 285–286
   exfoliating 288–289
   extraction 293
   face masks 302–307
   facial massage 294–302
   features and benefits (FABS) 200
   male clients 264, 268, 281, 288, 289
   male grooming 318–321
   moisturisers 307–313
   and recommending lifestyle changes
      316
   record cards 318
   toners 283–284
   toning 285
   warming devices 289–293
facial threading 367–368
facial waxing 330, 349, 357–361
false eyelashes 526, 579
   application 592–595
   consultation 575
   products, tools and equipment 571–572
fantasy themes 545, 547, 554

fashion shows 548, 550
features and benefits (FABS) 198–201, 206
feedback, client 183–184, 465, 557, 597
feet
blood vessels in 80
bone structure of 58–59
masks 424–425
massage 417–420, 422–424
muscles of 73
waxing 350
fibreglass/silk nail enhancements 455–457
files 416, 434, 450, 459, 463
finance, principles of 213–214
fire and emergency procedures 162
Fire Precautions Act 1971 and Fire
Precautions (Workplace) Regulations
1997, Amended 1999 98–99
fire safety and fire-fighting equipment
158–159
first aid 102–103, 160
first impression, creating a good 130
fixed costs 213–214
flat-head wax applicators 346
flyers 194, 210, 219
folliculitis 36, 379
foot care 133
foot files/rasps 387, 415
foot scrubs 404
foot/spa bath 387
forged bank notes 255
foundations 517–518
fragilitis crinium (split ends) 37
franchises 123
freckles 18
French manicure 431
French polish 430
frictions, massage 297, 419
fungal infections 29–30, 150, 151, 272, 330,
398, 446, 479, 513, 575
furuncles (boils) 28, 398

G

gas safety 162
Gill, Sita 559
glass bead steriliser 152–153
glasses 498, 512
gloves, disposable 147–148, 149, 293, 317,
327, 334, 343, 362
removing 148
gross and net 214
guide dogs 247

H

Habia 129, 326, 332
habit tic 43
hair 31–37
diseases and disorders 36
follicles 9, 31–32, 36
growth cycle 34
shaft structure 32–33

texture 33
types and where found 35, 347
hair care 133
hair removal 376–380
see also threading, preparing for;
threading, providing services for;
waxing, preparing for; waxing,
providing treatments for
hammer toes 59
hand cream 410
hands
blood vessels 79
bone structure 58
dominant 40
exercises 298
hand and nail care for therapists
133–134
masks 424–425
massage 417–422
muscles 72
protecting 148–149, 410
sanitising 447, 453, 468
washing 148
hang nail 48, 396
hard selling 201, 202, 205
hazard labels 97
hazards and risks 144–146
head
blood vessels 78
bone structure 55–56
major lymph nodes 84
muscles 61–67
head lice 36, 151
health and safety
codes of practice 142–143
for creating images 543–544
for eye treatments 561–562
for facial skincare 262
hand protection 148–149
hazards and risks 144–146
hygiene and infection control 149–156
legislation 92–104, 142
for make-up treatments 497
for manicure and pedicure treatments
385–388, 425
for nail art services 473–474
for nail enhancements 440–442
personal protective equipment (PPE)
100, 147–148, 223, 327, 473
for threading and waxing 327
waste disposal 155, 156–157
workplace policies 143–144
Health and Safety at Work Act (HASAWA)
1974 92–93
Health and Safety (Display Screen
Equipment) Regulations 1992 103–104
Health and Safety (First Aid) Regulations
1981 102–103
heart 74
herpes simplex (cold sores) 27
herpes zoster (shingles) 28
highlighters/shaders 516–517
historical looks 552, 553–554

Hobbs, Nicola 600
holiday entitlement 136
hoof sticks 386, 414
hordeolum (stye) 29
hormones 12, 14, 16
hot towels 292–293
hot wax 338
hot wax technique 347–349, 359
hours of work 136
human papilloma virus (HPV) 27
humidity 177
hygiene and infection control 149–156
hyper-keratosis 24, 330, 401, 446, 479,
514, 575
hypertrophy, nail 46, 400
hypodermis (subcutaneous layer) 9

I

images based on a theme, creating
advertising to target audience 549–550
avoiding disasters and dramas 555–556
choosing clothes and accessories 546
competitions 548, 552–553
creation process 550–557
evaluation of work 557
fantasy themes 545, 547, 554
fashion shows 548, 550
health and safety 543–544
mood boards 548–549, 552
planning 543–550
preparing the model 551–552
professional consultation 550
research 545
technical skills needed 545–546
themed-events 553–554
weddings 547, 554
impetigo 28
infection control and hygiene 149–156
infestations 30, 151, 399
influenza 86
ingredients
cosmetic 273–275
massage 295
nail products 403–404
ingrown hairs 289, 321, 343, 371, 375, 380
ingrown nails 49, 133, 415
injuries, reporting 102, 103, 160–161
Intense Pulsed Light (ILP) 377, 578

J

jewellery
client 163, 266
nail art 491
therapist 134, 411
job applications xi–xvi
job interviews xiv–xvi
joints 51–54
manipulation 420
types of movement in 54

K

keloid scarring 15
keratinised cells 31, 32, 33, 34, 38
keratinocytes 3
koilonychia (spoon-shaped nails) 43

L

lamellar dystrophy (peeling nails) 45, 395
Langerhans cells 4
laser hair removal 377
late cancellations and no-shows 246
leaflets 194, 215, 216, 219, 550
legislation
    client care and 166
    consumer protection 105–111
    Copyright, Designs and Patent Act 1998
        112
    creating an image and 543
    Employers' Liability (Compulsory
        Insurance) Act 1969 112
    employment 135–137
    Equality Act 2010 111–112
    eye treatments and 561–562
    health and safety 92–104, 142
    make-up treatments and 497
    nail art services and 473
    nail enhancement services and 440
    reception duties and awareness of 252
legs
    blood vessels 80
    bone structure 58
    full and half leg wax 349–352
    muscles 73
Lenard, Jennifer 541
lentigines (age spots) 14, 18
leukocytes 76
leukonychia (white spots) 43
lifestyle factors 269, 316, 446, 482
lifting objects 100–101, 145, 223
ligaments 53–54
lighting 179
    display areas 229, 230
    for eye treatments 562
    for facial skincare 263
    for make-up treatments 499–500, 503
    for manicures and pedicures 388
    for nail services 441, 451
    for photographic make-up 536
    for waxing and threading 326
Linforth, Pamela 188
link-selling 206
lip cleansing 279
lip liners 524–525
lip products 312, 314, 524–525
lip shapes, make-up techniques for
    510–511
lipids 4
lipsticks/glosses 525
listening skills 166, 173, 193, 205
liver spots 14, 18
Local Government Miscellaneous

Provisions Act 1982 95–96
longitudinal furrows, nail 43
lymph nodes 83, 84, 85
lymphatic capillaries 83
lymphatic system 82–88
    basic structure of 82–84
    contra-indications 85–88
    diseases and disorders 84–85
    function of 84
lymphatic vessels 8, 83

M

magazines 194, 209, 239, 474, 577
magnifying lamps 331
mail shots 218–219
make-up, applying 514–527
    aftercare and home care advice
        527–528
    bases 515
    blushers 519–520
    bridal 518, 527
    cleansing, toning and moisturising
        514–515
    concealers 515–516
    contra-actions 529
    day make-up 526
    evening make-up 526–527
    eye pencils/eyeliners 522–523
    eyebrow pencils 523
    eyeshadows 508, 521–522
    foundations 517–518
    highlighters/shaders 516–517
    home care advice 528
    lip liners 524–525
    lipsticks/glosses 525
    mascara 524
    powders 519
    special occasion 527
make-up artists 118–119
make-up lessons 529–533
make-up, photographic 533–538
    application 538
    backdrops 537–538
    black-and-white photography 535–536
    evaluating 538
    getting ready for a shoot 535
    lighting for 536
    mood board 534
    purpose of shoot 534
make-up, preparing for 497–524
    brushes 501–502
    client and therapist preparation 498
    colour charts 194
    consultation 504
    contra-indications 513–514
    corrective techniques 507–512
    equipment 503
    eye shape 509–510
    face shape 508–509
    glasses and contact lenses 512
    health and safety 497
    lighting 499–500, 503

lip shape 510–511
nose shape 511
skin colour 506–507
skin types and conditions 505
testers 194
tools 500–501
work area preparation 498–503
male clients 264
    exfoliants 288, 289
    facials 264, 268, 281
    grooming 318–321
    manicures 392
    products for 278, 319–320
    skin 16
malignant tumours 25
manicure treatments, preparing for
    385–411
    consultation 391–392
    contra-indications 397–402
    health and safety 385–388, 425
    nail care products 402–410
    preparing client and technician for 411
    preparing treatment area 389
    skin and nail analysis 392–397
    tools 385–386, 389
    treatment environment 388
manicure treatments, providing 411–435
    aftercare and home care advice
        433–434
    completion of 432
    contra-actions 434–435
    hygiene standards 425
    masks 424–427
    massage 417–422
    nail painting 429–431
    sequence 412
    thermal mittens 427–429
    tools 413–416
manual handing 100–101, 145, 223
Manual Handling Operations Regulations
    1992 100–101
manufacturers 128
    advice 209
    promotional packages 228
marketing and publicity 171, 215–220
mascara 524
masks
    face 302–307
    hand and foot 424–425
masks, particle 148
massage
    facial 294–302
    hand exercises for 298
    of hands and feet 417–424
    media 294–295, 409–410, 418
    routine 299–302
    techniques 296–298, 418–420
mature skin 14, 271, 308, 310, 311, 315,
    342
medical advice, seeking 175
medications 269, 393
medulla 32
melanin 15, 18

melanocytes 4, 9, 15, 19
men's grooming 318–321
mentoring 116
messages, taking correct 247–248
micro-organisms 7, 150–151
milia (whiteheads) 22
minimum wage 137
mirrors 333
mobility needs, clients with 247
moisturisers 199, 307–313
    for men 319
moles 18, 330
mood boards 534, 548–549
muscular system 60–73
    head and face muscles 61–67
    of the lower leg and foot 73
    in shoulder, arm and hand 69–72
    structure and function of 60
    thorax muscles 68
    types of tissue 60–61
music in the salon 112, 263, 388, 389, 441

N

nail art services, preparing for 473–481
    consultation 479, 481
    contra-indications 479
    equipment 478
    health and safety 473–474
    nail and skin analysis 480
    preparing client and nail technician 474,
        481
    products 474–476
    tools 477
nail art services, providing 481–492, 546
    aftercare and home care advice
        491–492
    applying nail enamel and nail polish
        482–483
    blending effect 484–485
    contra-actions 492
    dotting effect 486
    foil effect 488
    glitter effect 485
    jewellery 491
    lifestyle questions 482
    marbling effect 484
    rhinestones, flatstones and pearls 490
    striping tape 486–487
    techniques 482–491
    timing 482
    transfers 489
nail-biting 44, 396
nail buffers 416
nail care products 402–410
    ingredients in 403–404
nail clippers 415
nail enhancement, preparing for 440–451
    consultation 442–446
    contra-indications 398, 446
    health and safety 440–442
    nail shapes 444, 445
    positioning client and nail technician 442

products required 446–449
    salon environment 441
    tools and equipment 449–451
    work area preparation 451
nail enhancement, providing 452–468
    acrylic 462–465
    aftercare and home care 466–467
    applying tips 452–454
    contra-actions 467–468
    fibreglass/silk 455–457
    maintenance (infills) 457, 461, 465
    products and tools required 455
    tip removal 455
    UV gel 458–462, 468
nail painting 429–431, 482–483
nail polish 408–409, 427, 429
    colour charts 194
    drying times 431, 433
nail ridges 397
nail scissors 414
nail shapes 41–42, 402, 444, 445
nail technicians 119
nails 37–48
    and cuticles types and conditions
        48–49, 395–397
    diseases and disorders 42–49, 393–394
    function of 38
    growth cycle 40
    shape of 41–42
    staining 398, 429
    structure of 38–40
National Minimum Wage Act 1998 137
neck
    blood vessels 78
    location of major lymph nodes 84
    whiplash injury 299
neck creams 311
net and gross 214
nevi (birthmarks) 18, 21
night creams 310
non-verbal communication 166, 169–172,
    193, 443
normal skin 16, 270, 292, 505
nose shapes, make-up techniques for 511

O

oily skin 8, 16, 23, 270, 291, 292, 295, 505
onychatrophia (atrophy) 47, 398
onychauxis (hypertrophy) 46, 400
onychia 49, 397
onychocryptosis (ingrown nail) 49, 133, 415
onychocyanosis (blue nail) 44
onychogryphosis 46, 400
onycholysis (severe nail separation) 48, 399
onychomalacia (eggshell nails) 47, 400,
    446, 479
onychomicosis (ringworm of nail) 47
onychopaghy (nail biting) 44, 396
onychoptosis 46, 398
onychorrexis (brittle nail syndrome) 45, 396
open questions 167, 183, 192, 204, 246
oral hygiene 132, 562

O'Sullivan, Jackie 495
overgrown cuticles 48, 396

P

packaging 194
papillary layer 5–6
parabens 209
paraffin wax 407
paraffin wax treatments 426–427, 461
parasites 30
parasitic infections of scalp 36
parental consent 562
paronychia 49
payments 252–257
    discrepancies and disputes 257–258
    end-of-day totals 258
    handling 253–257
    methods of 212
    security of 259
pediculosis capitis (head lice) 36, 151
pediculosis corporis (body lice) 30, 399
pediculosis pubis (pubic lice) 36
pedicure treatments, preparing for
    385–411
    consultation 391–392
    contra-indications 397–402
    health and safety 385–388, 425
    preparing client and technician for 411
    preparing treatment area 390–391
    products 402–410
    skin and nail analysis 392–397
    tools 387, 389
    treatment environment 388
pedicure treatments, providing 411–435
    aftercare and home care advice
        433–434
    completion of 432
    contra-actions 434–435
    hygiene standards 425
    masks 424–427
    massage 417–420, 422–424
    nail painting 429–431
    sequence for 412
    thermal booties 427–429
peeling nails 45, 395
Penford, Sally 324
personal development 126, 195
personal hygiene 132
personal presentation 130–134, 190
personal protective equipment (PPE)
    147–148, 223, 327, 473
Personal Protective Equipment (PPE) at
    Work Regulations 1992 100
personal space 176–177
petrissage 296–297, 418
petroleum jelly 335
pH levels 10, 275
phagocytic cells 7, 76
phlebitis 330, 402
photo-ageing 269
photographic make-up
    see make-up, photographic

pigmentation disorders 18–19
pitting 45
plasma 77
platelets 77
portfolios 597
posture when sitting 104
powders 519
press releases 217
price lists 197, 242
Prices Act 1974 111
privacy, client 263, 328, 441
product launches 224, 226, 228
products and services to clients, promoting
    communication skills 191–195
    features and benefits (FABS) 198–201,
        206
    increasing client awareness 225
    knowledge of products and services
        195–197
    marketing and publicity principles
        215–220
    product demonstrations 206
    product knowledge 195–197
    promotions 220–221, 226, 254
    sales process 202–211
    selling principles 201–202
professional organisations 126–129
professionalism 125–126, 179–182
promotional events 217–218
promotional materials 171, 215–220
promotions and special offers 220–221,
    226, 254
Provision and Use of Work Equipment
    Regulations (PUWER) 1998 95
psoriasis 24, 330, 399, 446, 479, 513, 575
pterygium (overgrown cuticles) 48, 396
pubic lice 36

Q

qualifications 115–117
    awarding organisations 129, 130
questioning skills 167–168
    closed questions 168, 173, 192, 241,
        246
    in discussing new services and
        treatments 192
    and gathering feedback 183
    and job interviews xv–xvi
    in make-up consultation 504
    open questions 167, 183, 192, 204, 246
    in sales process 203–204
questionnaires 175, 183

R

razors 318–319.379
reception duties
    attending to clients and enquiries
        241–246
    booking appointments 245, 246–247,
        248–252

busy periods 246
client confidentiality 251–252
communication skills and behaviour
    241–247
dealing with payments 252–257
legislation 252
list of duties 238
maintaining reception area 239–241
managing client needs and expectations
    246–247
taking messages 247–248
receptionist careers 120
record cards 171–172, 174–175, 182
client purchases 195
facial treatments 318
nail treatments 432, 443, 479
organisation of 251
skin tests 576
threading and waxing 376
recruitment consultants 123
red blood cells 76
Repetitive Strain Injury (RSI) 442
Reporting of Injuries, Diseases and
    Dangerous Occurrences Regulations
    (RIDDOR) 1995 102, 160
reticular layer 6
reward schemes 466
ringworm
    of beard 30
    of body 29
    detection 31
    of nail 47
    of scalp 30
risks and hazards 97, 144–146
roller application of wax 345–346
rosacea 20, 283, 297

S

safety glasses 148
Sale of Goods Act 1979 and Sale and
    Supply of Goods Act 1994 109–110
sales
    increasing 225
    link-selling 206
    selling principles 201–202
    stages in process 202–211
    targets 205, 225, 232
    up-selling 201, 392
sales representatives 122
salon or spa managers 122
salon owners 123
samples 209, 211
sanitisation 153–155
sanitisers 405, 447, 564
sarcoptes scabiei (scabies) 30
scalp infections and conditions 36
scanners 231
scar tissue 11–12, 15, 330, 394, 401, 446,
    479, 514, 575
scissors 333, 487

scrubs
    facial 285, 286, 289
    foot 404
search engines 220
sebaceous cysts 23
sebaceous glands 8, 9, 32
    disorders of 22–23
seborrhoea 23
seborrhoeic keratosis (senile warts) 24
security 162–163, 232, 254, 259
self-employment 125
selling, principles of 201–202
senile warts 24
sensation 10
sensitive skin 17, 271, 276, 286, 287, 297,
    330, 342, 506, 576, 596
sensitivity tests 19, 251, 329, 576–577
serums 312, 319
shaving 288, 318–321, 379
shaving rash 319, 321
shelf life of products 233
shelf talkers 205, 228
shingles 28
shoes 264, 342
shoulder girdle 57
shoulder muscles 69
skeletal system 49–59
    conditions that restrict treatment 59
    feet 58–59
    function 50
    head structure 55–56
    joints 51–54
    lower limbs 58
    structure 50–51
    torso 57
    upper limbs 57–58
    vertebral column 56–57
skin 2–30
    ageing 13–14, 269, 271, 311, 513
    around eyes 279
    characteristics 12–13
    colour 506–507
    diseases and disorders 17–30
    functions of 9–12
    normal structure 2–8
    tones 15–16
    types and conditions 16–17, 269–271,
        505
skin analysis 267–269, 515
    nail and 392–397
    waxing 341–342
skin cancer 25
skin tags 24, 335
skin tests 19, 251, 329, 576–577
sleep 11, 12, 269, 310
smoking 13, 269, 393
social networking sites 215, 220
spas 118, 122, 127, 128
spatulas 332, 358, 501
special offers and promotions 220–221,
    226, 254
specialist roles in beauty industry 120–121
SPF 18, 313

splinter haemorrhage 44
split ends 37
spoon-shaped nails 43
sprains 59, 400
stationery stock 240
steamers 289, 290–292, 582
sterilisation 152–153
    of eye treatment tools 561
    of make-up tools 497
    of manicure and pedicure tools
        385–388, 391
    for nail enhancement tools 440–441
sterilising fluid 405
steroids 331
stock
    inventory 231, 232
    maintaining 240–241
    missing and damaged deliveries 231
    rotation 233
    security 232
    software to monitor 230–231
stress 12, 13, 269
styes 29
sugar paste and wax 337
sugar paste application 347
sun protection products 18, 19, 313
suppliers 129
Supply of Goods and Services Act 1982
    108–109
sweat glands 8, 9
swollen glands 85
synovial joints 52–53

takings' sheet 256
tapotement/percussion 297, 419
teachers, lecturers or assessors 124
telangiectasias (dilated capillaries) 20
telephone enquiries 243
temperature regulation, body 10
temperature, salon 177, 328, 388, 441, 500
testers 194, 229, 230
text messages 172, 245
thermal mittens and booties 427–429
thorax 57, 68
thread veins 394
threading, preparing for 326–342
    consultation 328
    equipment and tools 331–338
    health and safety 327
    products for 335–336
    service environment 327–328
    treatment timing 338, 339
    work area preparation 339, 341
threading, providing services for 363–370
    advantages and disadvantages 363
    aftercare and home care advice
        369–371
    chin 368
    completing a service 368–369
    contra-indications 371, 372, 374, 375

eyebrow shaping 367
home care advice 371
record card 376
threading techniques 363–366
tidying work area after 376
upper lip 367
thrombocytes/platelets 77
times for services/treatments 250, 294, 482
    threading 338, 339
    waxing 338–339
tinea barbae 30
tinea capitis 30
tinea corporis 29
tinea pedis (athlete's foot) 29, 398
tinea unguium 47
toe separators 387, 388
toners 199, 283–284
toning the face 285
tonsils 84
torso, bone structure 57
Trade Descriptions Act 1968 and 1972 110
Trading Standards 92
traffic stoppers 215, 219
trainers 123
treatment couches 263, 340, 342
treatment plan 175
tricology 37
tweezers 156, 333, 477, 567, 572
    automatic 567, 584

ultrasonic treatment 378
underarm waxing 355–356
up-selling 201, 392
upper lip
    threading 367
    waxing 360
urticaria 21
UV Cabinet 153, 156
UV gel nail enhancement 458–462, 468
UV lamps 315, 451, 460, 461, 468
UV rays
    overexposure to 13, 25
    protection from 11, 18
    and skin damage 14, 15, 269

value added tax (VAT) 214, 253
variable costs 214
varicose veins 81, 330, 331, 401
vascular nevi 21
veins 78
ventilation 177–178, 328, 388, 441, 450
verbal communication 167–168, 192–193,
    443
verrucae 27, 398
vertebral column 56–57
vibrations, massage 298, 419–420
viral infections 27–28, 151, 398

visual aids 173, 194, 443
vitamins 11, 13
vitiligo 19
vouchers 212, 221, 225, 254, 255, 256

W

Ward, Hellen 140
warm wax 337
warm wax techniques 343–344, 358,
    360–361
warming devices, facial 289–293
warts 24, 27, 134
waste disposal 155, 156–157, 327, 388
Watkinson, Samantha 471
wax heaters 331, 334, 335, 338
wax strips 332, 335
wax, types of 337–338
waxing, preparing for 326–342
    The Code of Practice for Waxing 326
    consultation 328
    contra-indications 330–331
    equipment and tools 331–338
    health and safety 327
    preparing the client for 341–342
    products for 335–338
    sensitivity tests 329
    treatment environment 327–328
    treatment timing 338–339
    work area preparation 339–340
waxing, providing treatments for 342–362
    advantages and disadvantages 343
    aftercare and home care advice
        369–371
    bikini line wax 353–355, 376
    completing treatment 361–362
    contra-actions 371–375
    eyebrow shaping 357–359, 578
    facial waxing 349, 357–361
    feet 350
    full and half leg wax 349–352
    record card 376
    tidying work area after 376
    underarm waxing 355–356
    wax application techniques 343–349,
        350
websites 220, 245
weddings 547, 554
    bridal make-up 518, 527
whiplash injury 299
white corpuscles 76
white spots 43
Whitehead, Carole 438
whiteheads 22
Wilce, Sara x
Working Time Regulations 1998 136
Workplace (Health, Safety and Welfare)
    Regulations 1992 93–94
workplace policies 143–144
wrinkles 14, 512, 513
written communication 170–172

THE CITY & GUILDS

LEVEL 2 VRQ DIPLOMA IN

BEAUTY THERAPY

INCLUDES NAIL TECHNOLOGY

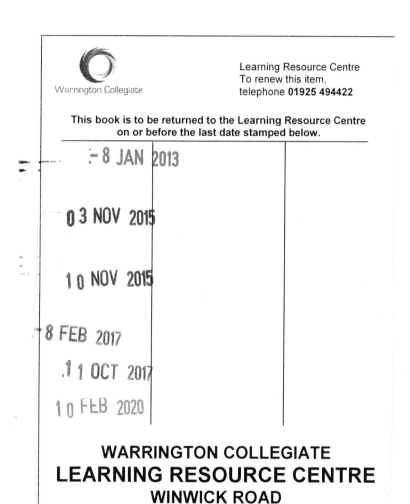

About City & Guilds

City & Guilds is the UK's leading provider of vocational qualifications, offering over 500 awards across a wide range of industries, and progressing from entry level to the highest levels of professional achievement. With over 8500 centres in 100 countries, City & Guilds is recognised by employers worldwide for providing qualifications that offer proof of the skills they need to get the job done.

Equal opportunities

City & Guilds fully supports the principle of equal opportunities and we are committed to satisfying this principle in all our activities and published material. A copy of our equal opportunities policy statement is available on the City & Guilds website.

First edition 2012
Reprinted 2012

ISBN 978 0 85193 204 0

Text design by Purpose
Cover design by Select
Page layout by GreenGate Publishing Services
Edited by Rachel Howells

Printed in the UK by Sterling

Publications

For information about or to order City & Guilds support materials, contact 0844 534 0000 or centresupport@cityandguilds.com. You can find more information about the materials we have available at www.cityandguilds.com/publications.

Every effort has been made to ensure that the information contained in this publication is true and correct at the time of going to press. However, City & Guilds' products and services are subject to continuous development and improvement and the right is reserved to change products and services from time to time. City & Guilds cannot accept liability for loss or damage arising from the use of information in this publication.

City & Guilds
1 Giltspur Street
London EC1A 9DD

T 0844 543 0033
www.cityandguilds.com
publishingfeedback@cityandguilds.com